Autoimmunization and the Autoimmune Hemolytic Anemias

Autoimmunization and the Autoimmune Hemolytic Anemias

BERNARD ⌊PIROFSKY, M.D.

Professor of Medicine
Head, Division of Immunology, Allergy and Infectious Disease
University of Oregon Medical School
Portland, Oregon

The Williams & Wilkins Company
Baltimore · 1969

Acknowledgments

Grateful acknowledgment is made to the University of Oregon Medical School and to the Commonwealth Fund of New York who provided the means to approach this task. The Instituto Nacional de la Nutrición, Mexico City, Mexico, and most particularly Drs. L. Sanchez-Medal and Ma. de la Soledad Cordova, supplied the stimulating environment for development of this book. Research studies cited throughout this volume as being performed in the author's laboratory were supported by the John A. Hartford Foundation, New York, the United States Public Health Service Cancer Institute, Grant CA-07941, and the Atomic Energy Commission, Grant AT-(45-1)-581. Their generous support permitted the development of many of the concepts presented here.

Particular thanks are due to my colleagues, Dr. Robert H. Bigley, Dr. Robert D. Goldman, Dr. Richard Jones, Dr. Robert D. Koler, Dr. Edwin E. Osgood, Dr. Demetrios J. Rigas, Dr. Marvin B. Rittenberg and Dr. Arthur J. Seaman. These associates contributed their extensive knowledge of patient care and technical procedures. The autoimmune hemolytic anemias frequently comprise aspects of great interest to other subspecialized areas of hematology, immunology and internal medicine. The opportunity to discuss these problems and to utilize the research skills and facilities of these scholars has proven invaluable. The benefits obtained from working closely with this group of well qualified hematologists and investigators cannot be overemphasized. Accordingly, many of the concepts presented in this volume reflect detailed discussions among fellow workers. Autoimmunization is constantly changing as a theoretical and experimental field. Even among our own colleagues differences were common in the interpretation of the clinical data and the resulting theoretical implications. For this reason the author must assume personal responsibility for the errors which will surely appear with further study. The concepts presented are personal ones and do not necessarily reflect the views of my associates who have been of such great aid.

Most of the laboratory studies reported in this volume were performed by research assistants in the Divisions of Immunology, Allergy, and Infectious Disease and Experimental Medicine. Mrs. Zelma Stocklen, M.T. (ASCP), directed the general hematologic laboratory. The serologic and immunohematologic investigations were carried out by Anne August, M.T. (ASCP), Katherine Pratt, M.T. (ASCP) and Marna Vaughn, M.T. (ASCP). These workers applied their considerable talents to the performance of accurate and precise laboratory procedures. Rather than approaching the many problems in a routine cookbook manner they frequently initiated new procedures and critically examined their data. Studies were continually repeated as the staff and these workers themselves challenged the results. This conscientious and professional approach has contributed immensely to this volume.

Thanks should also be directed to the Pacific Northwest Red Cross Blood Center, Robert G. Pittenger, M.D., Director. This large blood center, which serves as the referral agency of its 85 component hospitals, initiated many serologic studies in referred problem cases. The immunohematology laboratory of this institution, under the capable direction of Mrs. Helen Nelson, M.T. (ASCP), made available interesting blood specimens and in many cases suggested the diagnosis which resulted in a subsequent clinical workup.

The final form of this volume has been derived from a preliminary text dominated by a "stream of consciousness" literary style. The observations presented here have been salvaged only through the aid of many strong souls who braved the initial manuscript. Dr. Alfred A. Amkraut, Dr. Maria Cordova, Dr. Robert D. Goldman, Dr. Robert D. Koler, Dr. Luis Sanchez-Medal, Dr. Marvin B. Rittenberg and Dr. D. Alarcón-Segovia have all made invaluable suggestions. My secretaries, Edith Kacalek and Rowena Tudor, undoubtedly deserve the greatest compassion. The innumerable typings and revisions were a challenge in tenacity. The author would still be laboring and this volume would still be unfinished without the help of all those mentioned above.

Dedication

To the physicians of the Pacific Northwest, whose concern for their patients
and interest in these diseases made this volume possible

Introduction

Major advances have been made in our knowledge of normal and aberrant immunologic mechanisms. The application of this knowledge to human disease has been one of the most exciting developments in modern medicine. Through such studies a new science of clinical immunology is rapidly emerging. The physician now has available for clinical application a series of powerful theoretical, diagnostic and therapeutic tools.

The incorporation of immunologic concepts into clinical medicine has not been easy. Physician training primarily orients the clinician toward the evaluation of disease processes on the basis of individual organs. When faced with pathophysiologic events which cross anatomic and functional barriers he is at a disadvantage. Immunologically mediated disease frequently will not appear within tidy anatomic divisions. Widespread, multisystem manifestations are common and frequently are the despair of the responsible physician. What is needed is the ability to study and to modulate a generalized body mechanism which may appear in a pathologic context through multiple target organs.

The concept of autoimmunization has played a prominent role in awakening our interest and in exposing the inadequacy of our knowledge of immunologic principles. There is no subspecialized phase of medicine that has not faced the problem of relating this hypothesis to its own cherished abnormalities. Autoimmune hemolytic anemia was the first human disease syndrome that was considered to result from an autoimmune pathogenesis. As such it is an excellent model system for the evaluation of this concept in terms of clinical significance. A vast literature spanning theoretical, experimental and clinical observations has developed in this area. Autoimmune hemolytic anemia appears as an ideal disease for the correlation and blending of immunologic and clinical studies. The object of this work is just such a correlation.

The task is difficult. This observer, as well as most investigators in clinical immunology, has suffered from a lack of communication. When discussing autoimmune hemolytic anemia with a clinician, pertinent concepts may be dismissed as coming from an "impractical immunologist." An attempt to outline the problem to the immunologist frequently fails. Relevant and important views are ignored as representing only the observations of a "clinician." This volume has been designed to function in the no man's land created by such narrow specialization.

The problem has been faced in the current publication by presenting the material in two separate but interrelated sections. The early chapters are devoted to delineating the complex clinical matrix loosely expressed under the term "autoimmune hemolytic anemia." As the clinical pattern unfolds, it becomes apparent that a single entity is not present. Rather, a complex group of syndromes may be defined and their distinctive characteristics quantitated. Such syndromes may be related only by a common end stage process in which an immune event involves the erythrocyte.

The later chapters are designed to review the theoretical and immunohematologic implications of this clinical viewpoint. The fundamental concepts of the self-recognition phenomenon and autoimmunization are presented in a simplified fashion. Although this abbreviated review may leave the immunologist unsatisfied, the intent is to supply the clinician with the necessary broad theoretical and semantic basis from which to approach immunologically mediated disease. An attempt has been made to analyze the autoimmune hemolytic anemias as a model system illustrating current concepts of autoimmunization. The various nonimmune, immune but not autoimmune, and autoimmune mechanisms are reviewed. A relatively detailed discussion of the serology of autoimmune hemolytic anemia is also presented. This encyclopedic section is necessary, although it may discourage the clinician. The autoimmune hemolytic anemias are documented through such serologic approaches. Mastery of this information is crucial to any thorough understanding of the disease process. Only in this fashion will the clinician learn the benefits and the limitations of the laboratory as an aid in his management of a patient. Throughout this volume the theoretical and the clinical material are liberally interchanged and used to support concepts and observations presented in the specific sections.

Any interpretive clinical investigation is dependent on the source and number of patients, the observer, the methods and the facilities available for detailed study. It is therefore pertinent and important to document the background upon which this work is based. The patients referred to were investigated, and the laboratory studies were performed, in the hospitals and clinics of the University of Oregon Medical School. Represented is a population distribution encompassing a large portion of the Pacific Northwest geographic area of the United States. Four critical aspects of these studies should be emphasized.

1. The approach to the patient was inclusive, rather than limited to only one phase of his illness. The patients presented were observed from the viewpoint of an internist and hematologist assuming responsibility for the care and management of their medical problem. Simultaneously with the clinical responsibilities, the necessary serologic and hematologic procedures were undertaken in the author's laboratory. These laboratory analyses ranged from the routine studies necessary for accurate medical management through a spectrum of research procedures under continual and detailed investigation. In this fashion a one-sided view emphasizing only the clinical state or the results of laboratory testing was avoided.

2. The clinical material reported was studied during the relatively short period of time between 1958 and 1966. This has resulted in a certain uniformity of diagnostic, therapeutic and investigational procedures. Both the clinical and the laboratory aspects of the autoimmune hemolytic anemias have changed drastically over the past two decades. The large volume of patients seen with these problems in recent years has permitted a telescoping of many recent observations. It has not been necessary to depend on impressions derived from cases seen in the past. This is not meant to minimize past observations. Rather, it emphasizes the advantage of building upon prior studies in order to follow accurately a large number of subjects. A confusing pattern of clinical and laboratory abnormalities may be more satisfactorily evaluated in this fashion.

3. Several detailed experimental studies were initiated during the same period of time. This has permitted the accumulation of clinical and laboratory data relatively free from the stigma of retrospective analysis. It is unfortunate that protocols are never complete enough and that an investigation cannot always anticipate the many significant reports that are published during a period of study. Accordingly, a retrospective approach can never be completely eliminated. This work therefore suffers, as others before it have, from a handicap. Several critical observations were unforeseen. As knowledge accumulated, expansion of the clinical study was carried out. In other instances significant relationships were not apparent until final analysis. As far as possible retrospective conclusions have been checked with recent observations.

4. The clinical background for the current publication is based on information obtained from the study of 234 patients with acquired hemolytic anemia and/or positive antiglobulin tests. All of these cases are examples of the warm acting type of autoimmune hemolytic anemia. A particular attempt has been made throughout the years to obtain adequate clinical data, laboratory studies and pertinent followups for this patient population. The statistical data that are presented are based primarily on this selected patient group. A substantial number of cases of autoimmune hemolytic anemia associated with cold acting erythrocyte autoantibodies were encountered during the same period of time. Unfortunately no attempt was made to segregate this group for either clinical or experimental purposes. Accordingly, statistical data are not available. Pertinent discussions of the relevant disease syndromes in this area therefore rely heavily on the literature and on selected cases with adequate records.

Contents

Part I
CLINICAL ASPECTS

Chapter 1

The Hemolytic Anemias—Historical Review and Classification

Current concepts of autoimmune hemolytic anemia are firmly rooted in past studies documenting and clarifying the hemolytic state. The autoimmune hemolytic anemias are merely one form of disease resulting from abnormal in vivo hemolysis. An understanding of this process therefore requires a broad perspective. Such a perspective is presented below from two aspects. An historical review appears necessary in order to chart the concepts which permitted emergence of autoimmune hemolytic anemia from other hemolytic diseases. In addition a brief examination of the hemolytic state as operating in all forms of hemolytic anemia is desirable. Only in this fashion will it be possible to clarify the fundamental differences among the various specific syndromes. Such an approach will supply the natural background from which firm and precise definitions may be derived and eventually applied to an accurate classification of autoimmune hemolytic anemia.

Historical Review

In its early aspects the history of hemolytic anemia is intimately associated with clarifying the interrelationship between jaundice, liver disease and diseases of the blood. Galen (1) in 150 A.D. deduced that not all cases of jaundice were necessarily related to liver disease. He describes a patient bitten by a viper whose "skin turned the color of a ripe leek." This probably represents the first description of an extracellular type of acquired hemolytic anemia. Dreyfus (2) quotes Galen as follows: "The spleen produces colors of this type, darker than those produced by the liver. They are difficult to explain, but easy to recognize if you have seen them often."

The concept that premature destruction of red blood cells might lead to a disease state and jaundice was first suggested by Vanlair and Masius (3) in 1871. These observers described a patient with anemia and marked splenomegaly without hepatomegaly. The patient suffered acute attacks of left upper quadrant pain and jaundice without acholia, and passed reddish brown urine. The attacks were intermittent, occurring every 2 to 3 weeks. Morphologic evidence of an erythrocyte abnormality was suggested by finding spherical dwarf cells or microcytes in the peripheral blood. "We propose to designate a morbid condition under the name of microcythemia whose principal characteristic resides, according to us, in a particular alteration of the blood which is manifested morphologically by the anomalous presence of a large number of red cells differing from ordinary cells, which we name, by virtue of their small dimension, microcytes."* Vanlair and Masius postulated that clinical jaundice could result from two different mechanisms, "mechanically by reabsorption or liver induced" and "paradoxical icterus." This latter group included the

---

* Quoted material in this paragraph translated by the author and Dr. Guy Laroye.

3

"blood induced icterus" where excessive amounts of colorant material is released from the blood cells and followed by the formation of bile which is deposited in the tissues. "There are at least a certain number of non-mechanical types of icterus which are caused by the exaggerated destruction of red cells and the transformation to bilirubin of released hematin." Little attention was paid to this remarkable publication and for almost 30 years hepatic disease, jaundice and hemolytic anemia became hopelessly intertwined.

Wilson (4, 5) in 1890 and 1893 called attention to "a condition in which an enlarged spleen, accompanied by a sallow or subicteric complexion, appears as an hereditary condition." He presented a genealogic chart encompassing four generations and documented icterus and splenomegaly in six family members. Subsequent autopsy studies performed on one of these patients "point to her death being really due to a rapidly progressing anemia, dependent upon an active hemolysis of splenic origin." The author suggested that this condition be termed "chronic splenic cachexia."

Studies at the turn of the century by Hayem and Minkowski made it apparent that jaundice associated with hemolytic anemia was distinct from hepatic disease. Hayem's paper in 1898 (6) distinguished the congenital form of hemolytic anemia from an acquired type which he called "chronic infectious splenomegalic icterus."† Minkowski in 1900 (7) and 1905 (8) described an hereditary condition characterized by chronic jaundice, urobilinuria, splenomegaly and siderosis of the kidney. Autopsy findings indicated that the liver was free of disease. Dreyfus (2) quotes Minkowski as follows. "Every symptom compels us to admit that this affection constitutes a peculiar anomaly of the metabolism of the blood pigment, perhaps following a primary alteration of the spleen." Minkowski was unable to document any blood abnormality.

----

† Translation by the author and Dr. Guy Laroye.

A possible mechanism of in vivo hemolysis was presented in 1904. Donath and Landsteiner (9) implicated a hemolytic substance in the serum as responsible for the disease of paroxysmal cold hemoglobinuria. This study now appears as the first documentation of an autoantibody resulting in or related to a specific autoimmune disease. The rarity of paroxysmal cold hemoglobinuria, however, prevented this observation from having vast general significance.

The French school of hematologists subsequently clarified the clinical findings of many of these symptom complexes. Their investigations documented the congenital and acquired forms of hemolytic anemia. Several publications called attention to the presence of erythrocyte autoagglutination (10–13). Chauffard (14) in 1907 expanded the concept of congenital hemolytic anemia and consolidated previous studies to present the osmotic fragility test system. In association with Troisier in 1908 (15) and Vincent in 1909 (16), Chauffard was among the first to describe autohemolysins in the serum of patients with acute acquired hemolytic anemia. He termed such cases "hemolysinic hemolytic anemia" (ictère hémolysinique, hémoglobinuria hémolysinique) and related the abnormal hemolysins to rapid in vivo hemolysis. Widel, with Abrami (17, 18) and with Abrami and Brulé (10–12, 19), presented a series of papers between 1907 and 1909 which emphasized and introduced the term acquired hemolytic anemia. Le Gendre and Brulé (13) described the rapid and profound anemia that could develop in such cases, in contrast to the more chronic appearing congenital varieties.

The acquired types of hemolytic anemia (ictères hémolytiques acquis) reported by these observers included severely symptomatic cases with marked anemia. They were often associated with various infections and intoxications (20). Cases of unknown etiology were also encountered. This latter group probably represents what is now called autoimmune hemolytic anemia. The publications from the French group stressed that autoagglutination of the erythrocytes was frequently seen.

Knowledge had advanced sufficiently by 1909 for Marcel Brulé (21) to present his thesis on "les ictères hémolytiques acquis," a remarkably thorough review of the entire subject.

These brilliant studies clearly distinguished hepatic jaundice and the jaundice resulting from premature and excessive destruction of erythrocytes. The hemolytic process was further differentiated to include both congenital and acquired forms. The observation that various agents could induce in vivo hemolysis and autoagglutination was made and emphasized in an etiologic relationship. The large amount of information available concerning the hemolytic anemias was summarized in the 12th session of the Congrès Français de Medicina which took place in Lyon in 1911 (22). The topic was the role of hemolysins in pathology, and papers were presented by many of the foremost physicians and pathologists of the day.

Several workers suggested that the spleen was somehow related to hemolytic anemia. The beneficial effect of splenectomy in acquired hemolytic anemia was noted by Micheli (23) in 1911, in Turin. The fundamental studies of Banti and his group (24–27) firmly documented the role of this organ in intravascular hemolysis. Banti, as part of his extensive investigation of splenic pathology, studied cases of acquired hemolytic anemia, and he emphasized splenic activity in this disease complex. In 1912 he introduced the term hemolytic splenomegaly (24). Banti noted that heteroimmune hemolytic serum, when transfused into splenectomized animals, led to less and slower hemolysis than that seen with normal animals. The spleens of animals undergoing hemolysis were found to be enlarged and congested. He implicated the splenic endothelial cells as erythrophagocytes and described agglutinated erythrocytes within the splenic pulp. Banti similarly showed that the Kupffer cells of the liver could have an erythrophagocytic function when intense hemolysis was present. Experimental splenectomy, as a therapeutic approach, was first carried out by the Italian group. These studies led to its eventual application in human syndromes

characterized by destruction of the blood elements.

This author is grateful to Dr. Luis Sanchez-Medal who made available his personal translations, transcriptions and summaries of many of the fundamental publications described above. These original studies were largely forgotten, which resulted in a loss of interest and cessation of experimental studies in acquired hemolytic anemia. Almost 30 years elapsed before general interest was reawakened. During this time a few interesting publications can be noted. In 1925 and again in 1930 Lederer (28, 29) described a total of six cases with severe anemia associated with an infectious disease. The cases were characterized by a rapid onset of anemia and rapid recovery following transfusions. Brill (30) reported a similar case in 1926. Lederer termed this syndrome "acute hemolytic (infectious) anemia." Apparently he was unaware of the prior French publications and did not do serologic studies. We can only assume that these cases of "Lederer-Brill anemia" were in actuality examples of autoimmune hemolytic anemia.

The loss of interest in acquired hemolytic anemia obliterated the clear distinction between congenital and acquired forms of hemolytic anemia established by the French investigators. Dacie (31) states that it was generally assumed in England that hemolytic anemia occurring in the adult was a latent form of hereditary spherocytosis. The lack of specific diagnostic procedures, the presence of spherocytes in both forms of hemolytic anemia and the unavailability of serologic testing made such a conclusion inevitable. This attitude is illustrated by the report of Dawson in 1931 (32). The congenital and acquired forms of hemolytic anemia were not distinguished, and Dawson stated that "in the sense that latent defects may be accentuated so as to become clinically manifest, hemolytic anemia can be acquired, but the defects themselves are inborn." This viewpoint was accepted by Vaughn (33). Doan and associates (34) strongly differed with this view. In 1934 they announced that "we believe that a sharper differentiation should be made between the various mechanisms responsible for the non-hereditary forms of hemolytic anemia, designating them as 'acquired,' 'atypical,' or 'pseudo' with full realization that these latter syndromes are fundamentally different. . . ."

In 1938 and 1940 the confusion between congenital and acquired hemolytic anemia was finally eliminated by the important studies of Dameshek and Schwartz (35–37). These workers reviewed the past literature thoroughly and documented the existence of an acquired form of hemolytic anemia. They were able to demonstrate that spherocytosis and increased osmotic fragility resulted during the development of such hemolytic anemias, both in man and in experimental animals. They demonstrated that abnormal hemolysins were present in the sera of three patients with acquired hemolytic anemia. An immunologic etiology for such forms of hemolytic anemia was suggested. These studies reawakened interest in acquired hemolytic anemia and laid the broad outline for our modern concepts of the clinical and serologic implications of autoimmune hemolytic anemia.

Serologic advances over the next two decades led to the development of diagnostic tools, working hypotheses as to etiology and pathogenesis and rational therapeutic procedures. These serologic studies were primarily an outgrowth of investigations involving the recently described rhesus or Rh blood group factor and its relationship to erythroblastosis fetalis.

In 1939 Levine and Stetson (38) postulated an immune mechanism as being etiologically related to erythroblastosis fetalis. They suggested that the transplacental passage of fetal erythrocytes into the maternal circulation produced maternal isoantibodies directed against fetal red blood cells. The subsequent passage of maternal isoantibodies through the placenta to the fetus resulted in premature death of fetal erythrocytes and in the clinical picture of erythroblastosis fetalis. At approximately the same time Landsteiner and Wiener (39) noted that rhesus monkey erythrocytes injected into guinea pigs resulted in antibody production. This antibody agglutinated some human erythrocytes as well as rhesus monkey erythrocytes. The antibody was termed antirhesus or Rh antibody. Landsteiner and Wiener postulated the existence of a blood group factor in human erythrocytes which they called the rhesus or Rh factor. Subsequent clinical studies (40, 41) indicated that the majority of cases of human erythroblastosis fetalis were due to the maternal development of such rhesus antibodies.

In 1944 Race (42) in England and Wiener (43) in the United States independently noted that there were two types of rhesus antibodies. Race conceived of immune agglutination as involving a two-step procedure. Figure 1 illustrates this concept. The rhesus antibodies which induced agglutination of erythrocytes suspended in saline were considered to be "complete antibodies," undergoing the two phases of the immune agglutination reaction. A new type of rhesus antibody was postulated and termed "incomplete antibody." This substance reacted with the erythrocyte surface in the first phase but

IMMUNE HEMAGGLUTINATION

Antibody + erythrocyte surface antigen

↓

Antibody fixed to erythrocyte surface antigen
(Stage I)

↓

Interaction of erythrocytes having fixed antibody
(Stage II)

↓

Lattice framework

↓

Hemagglutination

"*Complete*" erythrocyte antibody: Stage I and Stage II.
"*Incomplete*" erythrocyte antibody: Stage I only.

FIG. 1. The two-stage nature of immune hemagglutination.

was incomplete in that the second phase and agglutination did not result. Wiener, in a brilliant set of experiments, arrived at the same conclusion. He was able to demonstrate that antibody containing serum which did not lead to agglutination of saline suspended erythrocytes contained a rhesus antibody which fixed to the surface of the erythrocyte. This fixation blocked the subsequent action of a saline acting rhesus antibody. He termed this type of rhesus antibody a "blocking antibody."

The application of these concepts to patients involved in hemolytic syndromes now became a laboratory problem. Advances were dependent on the development of a simple and effective means to demonstrate the fixation of incomplete erythrocyte antibodies to the erythrocyte surface. Such a procedure became available in 1945 when Coombs and associates (44) demonstrated that an antiserum against human globulin would induce agglutination of erythrocytes coated with the incomplete variety of rhesus antibody. A similar technique to demonstrate the fixation of globulin molecules to cellular surfaces had been developed by Moreschi in 1908 (45, 46). However, incomplete antibodies were unknown at the time and general acceptance or use of this procedure never resulted. A direct antiglobulin test to demonstrate such antibodies fixed to the erythrocyte surface and an indirect antiglobulin test to reveal unbound antibodies in the plasma soon became available in most laboratories throughout the world. In 1946 Boorman and associates (47) applied the direct antiglobulin test in a study of various hemolytic anemias. They found a positive reaction indicating the fixation of incomplete antibodies to the erythrocyte in some patients with the "idiopathic" variety of hemolytic anemia. Negative results indicating an absence of such antibodies were found in the congenital and other forms of acquired hemolytic anemias studied. Confirmation of this initial observation was forthcoming from many laboratories. The presence of incomplete erythrocyte antibodies fixed to the erythrocyte surface became the pathognomonic sign of autoimmune hemolytic anemia. This test clearly distinguished the autoimmune from the congenital variety of hemolytic anemia. Currently, the presence of a positive direct antiglobulin test is considered by many to be synonymous with a definitive diagnosis of autoimmune hemolytic anemia. Although positive antiglobulin tests may occur in the absence of autoimmune hemolytic anemia, and autoimmune hemolytic anemia may occur with negative antiglobulin tests, there is little doubt that the antiglobulin reaction was the most important diagnostic tool developed. The use of enzyme procedures such as activated papain (48) and bromelin (49), following the original studies by Morton and Pickles (50), supplied valuable supplementary tests to demonstrate incomplete erythrocyte antibodies.

Extensive studies as to the nature of the globulin molecule coating the erythrocyte in autoimmune hemolytic anemia have been carried out. Most investigators accepted the antibody nature of this substance (51), as well as an etiologic relationship to the premature death of the erythrocyte. Accordingly, hemolytic anemia on the basis of an immunologic mechanism was presumed. Evans and his group expanded these observations to include idiopathic thrombocytopenic purpura and introduced the term "immunohemolytic anemia" (52). Young and associates (53) summarized the clinical picture of this syndrome. They accepted the antibody nature of the coating globulin and derived the term "autoimmune hemolytic anemia." The use of the term autoimmune hemolytic anemia implied acceptance of two fundamental concepts. If the disease syndrome was the result of an immune mechanism it differed from the types of immunohemolytic anemia previously known. In erythroblastosis fetalis and transfusion reactions the antibody responsible for premature destruction of the erythrocyte is produced by one individual and does not react with that individual's erythrocytes. Hemolytic anemia occurs only when the antibody is placed in contact with foreign erythrocytes containing the appropriate blood group substance. These antibodies are *isoantibodies,* and they illustrate the immune homeostatic mechanism described by Ehrlich under the term "horror autotoxicus" (54). For an individual to produce an antibody possessing the ability to destroy his own erythrocytes, the body's "regulatory contrivances" which prevent self-intoxication must be circumvented (see Chapter 13). The antibody produced would not be an isoantibody but rather could be termed *autoantibody,* indicating reactivity against the individual's own erythrocytes. The process of producing such an autoantibody may be termed *autoimmunization* and the hemolytic syndrome may be termed autoimmune hemolytic anemia. Through the extensive writings and teaching of Dameshek this concept of an autoimmune etiology for some types of acquired hemolytic anemia gradually obtained general recognition and application.

Not all investigators accepted an autoimmune concept to explain the fixation of gamma-globulin molecules to the erythrocytes in autoimmune hemolytic anemia. Witebsky (55) in particular was reluctant to draw the conclusion that the erythrocyte coating material demonstrated by the antiglobulin test was a true autoantibody. He considered it unproved that the erythrocyte could be involved in autoimmunization, with the implied breaking of the principle of horror autotoxicus. This reluctance to accept a positive antiglobulin test in autoimmune hemolytic anemia as proof of either autoantibody formation or autoimmunization led to the term "antiglobulin positive hemolytic anemia," as employed by Pirofsky in 1960 (56).

Current knowledge of the nature of the erythrocyte coating globulin characteristic of this form of immunohemolytic anemia leaves little doubt that an antibody is present. Weiner and associates (57) in 1953 reported the presence of such an antibody, with specificity of anti-hr″(e), occurring in a patient of blood group CDe/CDe and acquired hemolytic anemia. This initial observation of autoantibody specificity has been amply confirmed by other investigators. There is now general acceptance of both the antibody nature and autoimmune mechanism in this form of hemolytic ane-

mia. Many of the original objections to the concept of autoimmunization involving the erythrocyte have been withdrawn (58, 59). However, it has also become apparent that not all forms of acquired hemolytic anemia characterized by an antibody fixing to a patient's own erythrocytes represent true autoimmunity. Schulman (60, 61) demonstrated an innocent bystander role of erythrocytes which supply a reacting surface for unrelated immune complexes. Such studies emphasize the continual necessity of determining antigenic specificity before autoimmunization is accepted.

A rapid expansion of knowledge concerning autoimmune hemolytic anemia has developed with the availability of the antiglobulin test. Such knowledge is still accumulating. The amount of experimental, theoretical and therapeutic data appears almost impossible to cope with. All students of this subject are accordingly grateful for the brilliant summation and scholarly review of this subject by Dacie in 1954, revised in 1962 (31). This work has proved invaluable as a reference text and as a source of stimulating concepts with which to approach a rapidly changing field.

Classification of the Hemolytic Anemias

Hemolytic Anemia and a Hemolytic Component

Hemolytic anemia is an oddity in clinical medicine in that a precise definition of the condition is possible. It may be said that any syndrome associated with a shortening of the erythrocyte life span represents hemolytic anemia. This simple statement appears inadequate. The inherent complexity of these diseases is not related to the end stage of premature death of the erythrocyte; rather, variations in the pathophysiologic mechanisms responsible for early cell destruction introduce confusion. It is therefore important for the clinician to determine the exact mechanism responsible for the hemolytic state. An extension of this requires an evaluation of the magnitude of hemolysis and the role of such hemolysis in the clinical syndrome.

Several major difficulties exist in defining and understanding the hemolytic anemias. One problem results from the observation that the peripheral distribution of erythrocytes cannot be considered as separate from or independent of the bone marrow. An extreme example illustrating this relationship is the occurrence of severe hemolytic anemia without evidence of anemia. The peripheral blood picture, in reference to erythrocytes, represents a composite of the kinetics of erythrocyte death balanced by the rate of erythrocyte production. The bone marrow normally has the capacity to increase erythrocyte production approximately 6- to 8-fold (62). It is apparent that in the face of complete bone marrow compensation a severe hemolytic state with erythrocyte survival times shortened from the normal 120 days to 15 days could occur without overt anemia. Although this extreme state rarely occurs, lesser degrees of bone marrow hyperplasia frequently obscure the magnitude of the destructive process. The resulting peripheral blood count may then give only a limited approximation of the severity of the hemolytic affair. Crosby (63) has thoroughly reviewed this state of erythrocyte production in relation to the rate of destruction. His kinetic data should be reviewed by all students of hemolytic anemia.

The availability of precise serologic and radioisotope techniques designed to measure the life span of the erythrocyte has led to the study of erythrocyte survival in various clinical conditions. Considering the protean distribution and critical function of the erythrocyte, it is not surprising that a shortened red cell survival time has been documented in many common disease states. The significance of such premature erythrocyte death, however, varies greatly in individual cases. It is dependent on the underlying disease, the rate of destruction, the status of the bone marrow and other variables. Accordingly, although it is relatively simple to demonstrate the presence of premature destruction of erythrocytes, it frequently is much more difficult to decide whether the hemolytic state is significant and warrants the diagnosis of hemolytic anemia.

An evaluation of the importance of a hemolytic state is also complicated by the difficulty of considering anemia the result of a single isolated event. Anemia, as it is observed in an individual patient, is frequently not due to a single cause or pathophysiologic mechanism. Study of a patient with carcinoma of the stomach and anemia illustrates this observation. The anemia present may be due to a combination of multiple factors. These include acute blood loss, chronic blood loss, iron deficiency, protein deficiency associated with anorexia, an underlying state of pernicious anemia, a myelophthisic state due to bone marrow metastasis and a hemolytic component. In spite of the shortened red cell survival time in this example, it does not appear rational to call this state hemolytic anemia.

Even in less complex hematologic situations the hemolytic phase of a disease may be either well compensated or of little clinical significance. In this fashion ailments as diverse as aortic stenosis, iron deficiency anemia and various infectious diseases have well documented hemolytic components without hemolytic anemia as a major part of the clinical disease. The suggestion might be made to call such conditions hemolytic disease in contrast to hemolytic anemia, conforming to the terminology of sickle cell disease and sickle cell anemia. This does not appear particularly helpful. It should be emphasized that even in such conditions an increase in the rate of erythrocyte destruction, or a decrease in the ability of the bone marrow to increase erythrocyte production, may result in a full blown hemolytic anemia. This may occur without any fundamental change in the basic hemolytic problem. Accordingly, we may note the development of a severe, persistent mechanical hemolytic anemia when aortic valve prosthesis is employed to correct aortic stenosis. Other patients with a compensated form of hemolytic anemia may develop a fulminating hemolytic state when infection induces bone marrow depression.

Further difficulties in classification arise when a major abnormality exists which in itself may cause severe anemia. In such cases a hemolytic component is frequently a significant complicating factor. Pernicious anemia, the acute leukemias, thalassemia and liver disease are all examples of this combination of etiologic states with significant hemolytic components. In view of the clearly defined nature of the underlying disease they are not generally classified as hemolytic anemia.

For the purpose of this volume, the following terms are suggested and defined. Their use throughout this volume is restricted to the definitions given below.

Hemolytic component: a shortening of the erythrocyte survival time occurring in association with a clinical condition not dominated by hemolysis. The hemolytic component may be a *major* or a *minor* one depending on the degree of shortening of the erythrocyte life span and on the contribution that the hemolytic component makes to anemia and the disease state.

Hemolytic anemia: a disease state characterized by a shortening of the erythrocyte survival time and by marked evidence of hemolysis. This state may appear *compensated,* without anemia; *partially compensated,* with mild anemia; or *uncompensated* with moderate to severe anemia.

Employing this terminology, iron deficiency anemia frequently has a *minor hemolytic component* and pernicious anemia may contain a *major hemolytic component.* Aortic valve prosthesis surgery may convert the *minor hemolytic component* of aortic stenosis into an *uncompensated* mechanical *hemolytic anemia.* A patient with hereditary spherocytosis can present with either a *compensated* or *uncompensated hemolytic anemia.*

Major Categories of Hemolytic Anemia

The hemolytic anemias may be broadly classified into three major categories according to the underlying mechanism responsible for hemolysis. The role of the erythrocyte in the hemolytic affair forms the basis for this classification. In certain syndromes a defect in the erythrocyte leads to premature death of the cell and to hemolytic anemia. In other syndromes normal erythrocytes are present. However, some abnormality in the erythrocyte environment induces damage to the cell resulting in a shortening of its life span. This classical division of the hemolytic anemias now appears inadequate. It is apparent that in many cases a mixture or blending of these two states occurs, resulting in a hemolytic event. In such conditions an abnormality of the erythrocyte may exist; in addition, an environmental agent must also interact with such erythrocytes before hemolysis develops.

Intracellular Abnormalities

Hemolytic anemia resulting from an abnormality of the erythrocyte which leads to premature destruction of cells may be termed intracellular or intracorporeal hemolytic anemia. Table 1 lists the various specific entities which are included in this group of diseases. The cellular defects involved usually show a familial distribution. They may represent a genetically transferred abnormality of the erythrocyte membrane, the hemoglobin or one of the many enzymes necessary for maintenance of the physiologic state of the erythrocyte. The erythrocyte survival time is shortened. When these data are plotted on semilogarithmic paper a gradual curve becomes apparent when approximately 20 per cent of the labeled erythrocytes remain in the circulation. Labeled normal erythrocytes transfused into a patient suffering from an intracellular defect have a normal survival time. The patient's own cells, when labeled and transfused into a normal recipient, will have the characteristically shortened survival time.

Extracellular Abnormality

Hemolytic anemia resulting from the premature death of normal erythrocytes that are acted upon by an environmental factor may be termed extracellular or extracorporeal hemolytic anemia. In contrast to the intracellular syndromes, hemolytic anemia due to an extracellular abnormality does not generally appear to have a well defined genetic background. Frequently the term acquired hemolytic anemia is used to indicate this freedom from genetic influences. Table 2 lists the specific entities included in this classification. The erythrocyte survival time is also shortened in this group. In contrast to the graph of the patient with an intracellular defect, plotting the survival time on semilogarithmic paper reveals a straight line curve indicating a random destruction independent of the age of the erythrocyte. Figure 2 contrasts the erythrocyte survival time pattern found in the intracellular and extracellular abnormality groups. Labeled normal erythrocytes transfused into such a patient will also show an abnormal survival time. The patient's own cells, when labeled and transfused into a normal recipient, will have a survival time which approaches normal. An excellent review of the early studies involving investigations of such cross transfusion survival time has been presented by Estren and Dameshek (64).

Mixed Type

The mixed type of hemolytic anemia represents a group of hemolytic syndromes in which extracellular factors act on erythrocytes which have a cellular abnormality or special characteristic. Table 3 lists the precipitating causes which may initiate increased hemolysis in a patient whose erythrocytes are peculiarly susceptible to such agents. Although the erythrocytes may permanently carry the stigma of premature death, a hemolytic component or uncompensated hemolytic anemia generally does not appear unless a specific extracellular state is also present. Hemolytic crisis occurring upon intake of the fava bean by a patient whose erythrocytes are defective in the enzyme glucose 6-phosphate dehydrogenase illustrates a well defined syndrome. Less well understood are the episodes of hemolysis occurring during excessive walking, exposure to cold or slight changes in body pH, i.e., in cases of march hemoglobinuria, paroxysmal cold hemoglobinuria and paroxysmal nocturnal hemoglobinuria, respectively.

It should be emphasized that this mixed

TABLE 1. *Erythrocyte defects which may lead to premature death of erythrocytes and to hemolytic anemia*

Intracellular Hemolytic Anemia

I. Defect of erythrocyte membrane
   A. Hereditary spherocytosis
   B. Hereditary elliptocytosis
   C. Hereditary acanthocytosis
   D. Paroxysmal nocturnal hemoglobinuria
II. Defect of hemoglobin
   A. Certain hemoglobinopathies
   B. Combinations of abnormal hemoglobins
III. Defect of cellular enzymes
   A. Disorders of anaerobic glycolysis
      1. Pyruvate kinase deficiency
      2. Triosephosphate isomerase deficiency
      3. Diphosphoglycerate mutase deficiency
      4. Hexokinase deficiency
      5. Diphosphoglycerophosphate deficiency
   B. Disorders of the hexose monophosphate shunt
      1. Erythrocyte glutathione deficiency
      2. 6-Phosphogluconate dehydrogenase deficiency
      3. Glutathione reductase deficiency
      4. Glucose 6-phosphate dehydrogenase deficiency
         a. Negroid type
         b. Non-Negroid type
         c. High adenosine triphosphate, "American type"
   C. Methemoglobinemia formation
      1. Diphosphopyridine nucleotide-methemoglobin reductase deficiency
      2. Glutathione synthesis deficiency
      3. Diaphorase deficiency
   D. Erythropoietic porphyria
IV. Thalassemia group
   A. Thalassemia A and B, major and minor
   B. Combination thalassemia and abnormal hemoglobins
   C. Combination thalassemia B with increased pyruvate kinase, "Dutch type"

category represents an arbitrary classification. There is little doubt that extraerythrocyte factors frequently play an important role in the hemolytic anemias classically considered as resulting from a specific cellular defect. Hemolytic crisis in a patient with hemoglobin S-C disease, when the atmospheric pressure and oxygen are reduced as in air flight, is an example of such extracellular factors interacting with

TABLE 2. *Extracellular factors which may lead to premature death of normal erythrocytes and to hemolytic anemia*

Extracellular Hemolytic Mechanisms

  I. Physical agents
    A. Heat
    B. Ultraviolet irradiation
    C. Trauma: microangiotic hemolytic anemia
 II. Vegetable and animal agents
    A. Castor bean
    B. Snake venoms
III. Infectious agents
    A. Protozoa (malaria, etc.)
    B. Nonprotozoan blood parasites (Bartonella, etc.)
    C. Viruses (infectious mononucleosis, viral pneumonia, etc.)
    D. Bacteria (*Clostridium welchii, Salmonella typhi*, etc.)
 IV. Chemical agents—dose related*

Phenylhydrazine	Pheacetin	Methyl chloride
Trinitrotoluene	Dinitrobenzine	Allyl prophyldisulfide
Toluene	Aniline	Arsine
Benzine	Saponin	Lead
Nitrobenzine	Lecithin	Colloidal silver
Acetanilide	Promin	Water

  V. Antibodies—the immunohemolytic anemias
    A. Isoantibody immunohemolytic anemia
    B. Antiglobulin positive immunohemolytic anemia
    C. Autoimmune hemolytic anemia
        1. Clinical classification
           a. Idiopathic or primary type
           b. Symptomatic or secondary type
        2. Laboratory classification
           a. Warm acting antibody type
           b. Cold acting antibody type

* See Wintrobe, M. M.: *Clinical Hematology*, Ed. 5, p. 600. Lea & Febiger, Philadelphia, 1961.

an erythrocyte defect. In a similar fashion the extracellular hemolytic anemias no longer appear quite as independent of special erythrocyte characteristics as was once thought. There is excellent evidence that different populations of erythrocytes present differences of sensitivity to the action of various extracellular hemolytic agents. These variations may be dependent on cellular age, glycolytic enzyme reserve or genetic factors as yet unidentified. Doljanski and associates (65) present data suggesting that the peripheral blood has two populations of erythrocytes. Such cellular variations may influence hemolytic activity. Autoimmune hemolytic anemia may even be considered as an example of a mixed form of hemolytic anemia. The development of a warm acting autoantibody in a — — —/— — —(Rh null) pa-

tient, a cold acting anti-I autoantibody in an I negative individual and the Donath-Landsteiner antibody in a patient of blood group p or p^k would not lead to a hemolytic state. Host erythrocytes containing the appropriate antigen must be present for the extracellular antibody to exert its destructive effect. Yokoyama and associates (66) have reported hemolytic anemia in a female with an autoantibody of specificity Xg^a. The same antibody in a male would not result in hemolytic anemia. The possibility of a genetic predisposition for the development of acquired hemolytic anemia must also be considered. Such a state has been demonstrated experimentally with the NZB strain of inbred mice (67). In such cases, however, it is assumed that the genetic abnormality involves the antibody producing mechanism rather than the erythrocytes.

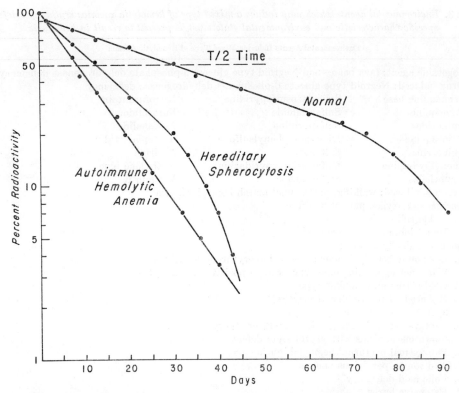

FIG. 2. Erythrocyte survival patterns seen in the normal, in a patient with an intracellular defect (hereditary spherocytosis) and in a patient with an extracellular defect (autoimmune hemolytic anemia). The erythrocytes have been labeled with chromium[51] and the results plotted on semilogarithmic paper. The survival time is usually expressed at the 50 per cent point (T/2 time).

The Immunohemolytic Anemias

Immunologic mechanisms have the greatest incidence and clinical significance in creating extracellular forms of hemolytic anemia. These immunohemolytic anemias have generally been divided into two types representing the production of either iso-antibodies or autoantibodies directed against erythrocytes. In Table 2, where the extracellular types of hemolytic anemia are classified, a third group termed anti-globulin positive hemolytic anemia has been added. This third type of immuno-hemolytic anemia appears necessary to clarify and maintain the term autoimmune hemolytic anemia. Throughout this volume immunohemolytic anemia is discussed within this classification. The following definitions are offered as an aid in utilizing this terminology.

Isoantibody immunohemolytic anemia: hemolytic anemia resulting from the action of an antibody produced by one individual and directed against the erythrocytes of another individual.

Antiglobulin positive immunohemolytic anemia: hemolytic anemia resulting from the action of an antibody or antibody-like globulin produced by an individual and damaging his own erythrocytes. The autologous globulin reacting with the erythrocytes is either not an antibody or is an antibody directed against exogenous material or host erythrocytes modified so as to appear exogenous.

Autoimmune immunohemolytic anemia: hemolytic anemia resulting from the action of an antibody produced by an individual and specifically directed against his own normal unmodified erythrocytic antigenic determinants.

TABLE 3. *Environmental agents which may induce a mixed type of hemolytic anemia; erythrocyte defect or specific characteristic and environmental state must be present to result in hemolysis*

Environmental Agents Inducing Mixed Type of Hemolytic Anemia

I. Vegetable agent: fava bean—non-Negroid type glucose 6-phosphate dehydrogenase deficiency
II. Drug induced: Negroid type glucose 6-phosphate dehydrogenase deficiency

Primaquine base	Salicylazosulfapyridine	Nitrofurantoin
Pamaquine	Sulfanilamide	Furazolidone
Quinocide	Sulfapyridine	Acetanalide
Chloroquine	Diaminodiphenylsulfone	Acetophenetidin
Quinacrine	Sulfoxone	Aspirin
Phenylhydrazine	Sulfamethoxypyridazine	Methylene blue
Naphthales	Sulfasoxizole	Vitamin K

III. Trauma induced: walking, paroxysmal march hemoglobinuria
IV. Decrease in oxygen partial pressure
   A. Sickle cell crisis
   B. Hemoglobin S-C disease crisis
V. Immunologically induced
   A. Isoimmunohemolytic anemia—specific erythrocyte antigen
   B. Warm acting autoimmune type—rhesus positive erythrocytes
   C. Cold acting autoimmune type
     1. Anti-I—I positive erythrocytes
     2. Anti-i—I negative erythrocytes
   D. Paroxysmal cold hemoglobinuria—P_1 or P_2 erythrocytes
VI. Unknown mechanisms with erythrocyte defect
   A. Paroxysmal nocturnal hemoglobinuria
   B. Addisonian pernicious anemia
   C. Folic acid deficiency
   D. Extensive burns
   E. Infections

The theoretical reasoning behind this classification is discussed in detail in Chapters 13 and 14. Table 4 presents an outline of the mechanisms involved in the three types of immunohemolytic anemia; the following discussion summarizes this viewpoint.

Isoantibody Immunohemolytic Anemia

Immunohemolytic anemia resulting from isoantibody formation is limited to a well recognized sequence of immunologic events. Isoantibody formation results from contact of a patient's antibody forming tissue with parenterally introduced foreign erythrocytes. There is no violation of the principles of self-recognition or horror autotoxicus. Rather, antibody formation occurs as a function of the normal immunologic homeostatic mechanism. Two major findings characterize this state. First, the antigenic material stimulating antibody formation is foreign to the organism producing the antibody. Second, the antibody produced does not react with the patient's own erythrocytes. Immunohemolytic anemia does not occur unless passive transfer of either antibody or antigen occurs. Accordingly, the erythrocytes of the individual producing the antibody are not involved in a hemolytic event. Clinically, passive transfer of antibody resulting in immunohemolytic anemia is seen in erythroblastosis fetalis or with a minor type of transfusion reaction (donor antibody reacting with recipient erythrocytes). Passive transfer of erythrocyte antigens leading to immunohemolytic anemia is seen with the usual major type of transfusion reaction (recipient antibody reacting with donor erythrocytes).

Antiglobulin Positive Immunohemolytic Anemia

The term antiglobulin positive hemolytic anemia has been used to designate a form of immunohemolytic anemia resulting from the production of antibody by an organism which leads to premature destruction of the organism's own erythrocytes. Antiglobulin positive immunohemolytic anemia is distinguished from autoimmune hemolytic anemia on the basis of specificity of the involved antibody. Two types of antibody specificity are concerned with the development of this form of immunohemolytic anemia. The antibody produced is either not directed against the erythrocyte or is directed against modified or denatured host erythrocyte antigenic material. Antibody formation does not represent a failure of horror autotoxicus or of the organism's capacity for immunologic self-recognition. The antibody produced, therefore, is not a true autoantibody, and the term autoimmune hemolytic anemia is to be avoided. Various environmental factors such as disease states, drugs, bacteria, bacterial products, viruses and physical factors may modify the erythrocyte surface so as to produce erythrocyte antigenic material "foreign" to the organism's immune apparatus. The creation of drug and chemical haptenes, the denaturation of surface antigens and the interaction of cross reacting antibodies are all theoretical possibilities. The function of the erythrocyte as an innocent bystander offering an adsorption surface for an immunologic event unrelated to the erythrocyte also leads to an antiglobulin positive immunohemolytic anemia. A drug such as penicillin or various bacterial products may be adsorbed to the erythrocyte. Antibodies directed against the drug or bacterial polysaccharides may then interact with these agents. During the process the innocent bystander erythrocyte may be damaged, leading to hemolytic anemia. In a similar fashion antibody-antigen immune complexes may be adsorbed to the erythrocyte surface, resulting in premature death of the erythrocyte. Complement appears to be involved in this adsorption-lysis phenomenon.

Autoimmune Hemolytic Anemia

The third type of immunohemolytic anemia, autoimmune hemolytic anemia, is the result of true autoantibody formation. In such cases an individual produces an antibody with specificity directed against

TABLE 4. *The immunohemolytic anemias: classification based on etiologic mechanisms*

The Immunohemolytic Anemias
I. Isoantibody immunohemolytic anemia
A. Passive antibody transfer type
1. Erythroblastosis fetalis
2. Minor type transfusion reaction
B. Passive antigen transfer type: major type transfusion reaction
II. Antiglobulin positive immunohemolytic anemia
A. Exogenous antigen
1. Cross reacting antibody
2. Innocent bystander erythrocyte
a. Adsorption of antigen
b. Adsorption of immune complex
B. Modified autologous antigen
1. Antigenic denaturation
2. Hapten formation
III. Autoimmune hemolytic anemia
A. Foreign clone formation
B. Immunodeficient individual
C. Forbidden clone proliferation
D. Termination of tolerance

his own unmodified erythrocytic antigenic substances. In order to satisfy the criteria for autoimmunization, a loss of immune self-recognition involving the erythrocyte must occur with a reversal of the state of normal immunologic unresponsiveness. Several mechanisms have been postulated as inducing such a state of autoantibody formation. These include the establishment of a new clone of cells leading to a graft-host reaction, the emergence of forbidden clones through genetic mechanisms, the presence of an immunodeficient individual and a termination of the normal state of immune tolerance. The uncovering of antigenic material previously unavailable for contact with the immune apparatus, i.e., a removal of immunologic quarantine, is difficult to classify. A true autoantibody could be formed in this fashion, although disruption of normal immune tolerance and self-recognition would not have occurred.

Idiopathic and Symptomatic Forms of Autoimmune Hemolytic Anemia

On the basis of clinical observations autoimmune hemolytic anemia may be further classified. Hemolytic anemia characterized by positive antiglobulin reactions is seen in two distinctly different clinical settings. It may appear spontaneously as an isolated and independent disease entity. Such forms have been termed *primary* or *idiopathic* autoimmune hemolytic anemia. Other cases of autoimmune hemolytic anemia occur in association with another disease process. These cases are referred to as *secondary* or *symptomatic* autoimmune hemolytic anemia (68). It should be emphasized that autoimmune hemolytic anemia may appear substantially in advance of its associated disease. This may result in an erroneous classification as a primary or idiopathic type. In addition, the presence of another pathologic state in a patient with autoimmune hemolytic anemia does not necessarily imply that a secondary form is present and that the two syndromes are related. The possibility of a fortuitous occurrence of two common disease processes must always be considered. The characteristics and relative distribution of the primary and secondary forms of autoimmune hemolytic anemia are discussed in Chapter 2.

Autoimmunity and Autoallergy

In 1906 Clemens von Pirquet (69) published his classical paper introducing a new term, "allergy." The coinage of a new term appeared necessary to describe the development of supersensitivity in the immunized organism. It appeared to von Pirquet that immunity and supersensitivity were closely related but different phenomena. He stated that "what we need is a new generalized term, which prejudices nothing but expresses the change in condition which an animal experiences after contact with any organic poison, be it animate or inanimate." Within this framework immunity was considered primarily as a protective mechanism. "The term immunity must be restricted to those processes in which the introduction of the foreign substance into the organism causes no clinically evident reaction, where, therefore, complete insensitivity exists. . . ." In contrast, "the vaccinated person behaves . . . in a different manner from him who has not previously been in contact with such an agent. Yet he is not insensitive to it. We can only say of him that his power to react has undergone a change." von Pirquet proposed that the term "allergy" be applied to describe this general concept of a changed reactivity.

Waksman (70) has listed a set of criteria which characterize allergic events. These include: (a) the allergic state is produced by sensitization with a specific antigen; (b) a latent period intervenes between sensitization and the appearance of the allergic state; (c) there is immunologic specificity in eliciting the allergic response; (d) the allergic response is always essentially the same in a given species, no matter what antigen is involved; (e) the allergic state tends to diminish and finally to disappear with the passage of time; (f) a secondary type of response occurs upon reexposure to the antigen; (g) the allergic state may be passively transferred; (h) disappearance of the allergic state, or desensitization, occurs upon introduction of the specific antigen. Waksman has emphasized that several of the diseases considered autoimmune fulfill many criteria which characterize allergic processes. He applied the above criteria to a series of diseases having excellent experimental animal model systems. These autoimmune syndromes are characterized by similar pathologic lesions and by lack of evidence of pathologically significant circulating autoantibodies, and they have many characteristics of delayed hypersensitivity. Such immunologically produced diseases were accordingly termed "autoallergic" diseases. The tissues involved included the central and peripheral nervous systems, the lens of the eye, the uvea, the testes, the thyroid and the adrenal gland.

Gell and Coombs (71) have expanded this viewpoint. They advocate a return to von Pirquet's original definitions and would consider any altered biologic state resulting from an immunologic mechanism as allergy. Using the term allergy in the sense that these workers suggest would not have any ". . . implied connotation as regards the production of *clinical* hypersensitivity or *clinical* immunity; it may entail either, or both simultaneously in the same individual. 'Hypersensitive' and 'immune' are descriptive terms only useful in indicating a clinical state, and are not mutually exclusive." Gell and Coombs suggest that "transplantation immunity" and "autoimmune disease" would be best designated as "transplantation allergy" and "autoallergy," respectively. Allergic events would include "autoallergic" hemolytic anemia, true immunity (protection), hypersensitivity reactions, transfusion reactions, erythroblastosis fetalis, homograft rejection, runt disease and actively acquired tolerance, among others that may be listed. An editorial in the New England Journal of Medicine (72) supports many of the points made by these investigators. This article, in a remarkably lucid presentation, discussed the influence of the terms "autoimmune" and "autoallergic" on the development of theoretical concepts in autoimmunization.

Dameshek (73) has objected to the use of the term "autoallergy." He emphasizes that "immunity has come a long way since 1906, and allergy has taken on a highly restricted meaning, having to do with wheezes, sneezes, and hives. Thus, immunity encompasses any condition in which, with the introduction of a foreign material in the body, a specific cellular response to it develops, with or without an observable reaction of 'supersensitivity' as Pirquet called it. Specificity is the important word, not protective." Employing Dameshek's rationale, the process should be termed "autoimmunity." The term "autoallergy" may possibly be employed to indicate various other forms of immunologic disorders. These would include conditions where exogenous antigens initiate an immunologic response. The subsequent involvement of additional tissues in a nonspecific fashion would appear to be a manifestation of the allergic event.

Semantics have again confused attempts to clarify the concepts of autoimmunization. A return to von Pirquet's meaning of the term allergy, as suggested by Gell and Coombs, would permit us to use "autoallergy" as a descriptive phrase. However, do we want to return to von Pirquet's

definitions? What purpose would be served by embracing a concept developed over 60 years ago and gradually modified as our knowledge increased? Currently "immune" is not used to signify a protective state and "allergy" is not used to encompass any detectable clinical response to an immunologic event. Employing these purely clinical terminologies would be a handicap rather than a help in approaching the immunologic aspects of tissue reactivity. The end stage effects of immunologic interactions are a critical phase of immunology. In fact a new science of clinical immunology is rapidly being developed to study such effects. There is little to suggest that the antibody response to antigenic material leading to protection or to clinically observed phenomena involves different mechanisms. With more precise tools it will undoubtedly be possible to show in vivo changes in all immunologic reactions. A logical extension of von Pirquet's concepts would then eventually result in the elimination of the term immunity. All immunologic reactions would then be "allergic," and what will have been accomplished?

Currently the term "immune" is loosely used to describe the specific sensitization of an organism by exposure to a specific antigenic substance. The end stage of either protection or supersensitivity does not enter into this usage. "Allergy" is used to describe a particular type of sensitization. A selected portion of the population, selected presumably on a genetic basis, shows an altered reactivity in their exposure to various common exogenous antigens. A particular type of immune response is involved with the production of a skin sensitizing antibody differing from the usual humoral and fixed tissue antibodies seen in other immune responses. This reaginic antibody may represent a specific class of immunoglobulins, the IgE class. Accepting this usage does not suggest that "autoallergy" is a preferable alternate term for "autoimmunity."

There may be some rationale for the employment of the term "autoallergy" with several types of hemolytic anemia characterized by positive antiglobulin tests. In this volume a group of such conditions has been removed from the autoimmune classification because true autoantibody formation is not present. These syndromes have been termed antiglobulin positive immunohemolytic anemia to differentiate them from the autoimmune group. The basic immunologic mechanism in such syndromes includes the response to exogenous antigens or to autogenous antigens which have been so modified as to appear foreign or exogenous to the immune apparatus. The end stage response of these conditions does have some resemblance to an allergic event. In particular, the innocent bystander role of the erythrocyte in adsorbing antigens such as penicillin and immune complexes deserves consideration as "autoallergic." This author would prefer not to classify them as "autoallergic" hemolytic anemia. The critical aspects of what we now term "allergy" involve an altered reactivity, an hereditary predisposition and the production of a specific type of antibody. None of these criteria is currently met in the antiglobulin positive immunohemolytic anemias. Accordingly, the argument concerning the employment of the term "autoallergic" in place of "autoimmune" does not serve a useful purpose other than that of emphasizing the marked semantic problem.

Application of the Concepts of Immunohemolytic Anemia

The immunohemolytic anemias, in particular the antiglobulin positive and autoimmune types, have assumed special significance in recent years. The diseases are common and easily available for detailed study. They can serve as a prototype or model system for an understanding of the process of autoimmunization. A clarification of the pathophysiology of autoimmune hemolytic anemia has particular value in understanding immunologic self-recognition, homotransplantation rejection and many confusing aspects of malignancies. The ease in obtaining erythrocytes and the development of precise immunohematologic techniques supply simple diagnostic tools permitting correlation of clinical observations with laboratory results.

The clinician encountering a patient with hemolytic anemia and positive direct antiglobulin tests must decide whether or not to label the process autoimmunization. This is an important decision and is not an exercise in semantics. Effective therapy in the future will certainly be dependent on determining the pathophysiologic mechanism. The importance of establishing an accurate etiologic diagnosis is already apparent. For example, it would be foolish to automatically treat such a patient with prolonged corticosteroid therapy, immunosuppressive drugs and/or splenectomy. Cure may result from simply stopping the administration of a drug such as penicillin, if a form of antiglobulin positive immunohemolytic anemia is present.

At the current level of our knowledge, autoimmune hemolytic anemia is common, whereas proven cases of antiglobulin positive hemolytic anemia are a rarity. Whether careful and detailed clinical and serologic studies will change this ratio in the future is unknown. Accordingly, throughout this volume the term autoimmune hemolytic anemia is used in the descriptive and interpretive sense outlined by Dameshek (74). Four criteria are to be met: (a) the patient's own erythrocytes give a positive antiglobulin test; (b) the adherent gammaglobulin has all of the characteristics of antibody protein; (c) it is injurious to the red blood cells, thus inducing their short survival time; (d) the abnormal globulin is produced in the patient's own body. These criteria satisfy both autoimmune hemolytic anemia and the antiglobulin positive hemolytic anemias. The clinician and investigator are encouraged to carry their studies the further steps necessary to delineate the role of autoimmunization in the specific cases they encounter.

In the clinical sections that follow the term autoimmune hemolytic anemia is employed to characterize the association of a hemolytic state and positive antiglobulin tests. Whenever possible, however, an attempt is made to analyze further the mechanisms suggesting either an antiglobulin positive or autoimmune pathogenesis. The reader is encouraged to study Chapters 13 through 15 in order to acquire the theoretical background necessary for such an analysis.

BIBLIOGRAPHY

1. Galen, C.: *Opera Omnia.* Vol. VIII, p. 356. Lipsiae, 1824.
2. Dreyfus, C.: *Some Milestones in the History of Hematology.* Grune & Stratton, Inc., New York, 1957.
3. Vanlair, C. F., and Masius, J. R.: De la microcythémia. Bull. Acad. Roy. Med. Belg. **5:** 515, 1871.
4. Wilson, C.: Some cases showing hereditary enlargement of the spleen. Trans. Clin. Soc. London **23:** 162, 1890.
5. Wilson, C., and Stanley, D.: Hereditary enlargement of the spleen (a sequel to some cases showing). Trans. Clin. Soc. London **26:** 163, 1893.
6. Hayem, G.: Sur une variété particulière d'ictère chronique. Ictère infectieux chronique splénomégalique. Presse Med. **6:** 121, 1898.
7. Minkowski, O.: Ueber eine hereditäre, unter dem Bilde eines chronischen Icterus mit Urobilinurie, Splenomegalie und Uierensiderosis verlaufende Affection. Verh. Kong. Inn. Med. **18:** 316, 1900.
8. Minkowski, O.: Die deutsche Klinik am Eingang des XX Jahrhunderts. **5:** 651, 1905.
9. Donath, J., and Landsteiner, K.: Ueber paroxysmale Hämoglobinurie. Munchen Med. Wschr. **51:** 1590, 1904.
10. Widal, F., Abrami, P., and Brulé, M.: Les ictères d'origine hémolytique. Arch. Mal. Coeur **1:** 193, 1908.
11. Widal, F., Abrami, P., and Brulé, M.: Autoagglutination des hématies dans l'ictère hémolytique. C. R. Soc. Biol. (Paris) **64:** 655, 1908.
12. Widal, F., Abrami, P., and Brulé, M.: Rétrocession des symptômes cliniques et des troubles hématiques au cours des ictères hémolytiques acquis. Bull. Soc. Med. Paris **28:** 73, 1909.
13. Le Gendre, P., and Brulé, M.: Ictère hémolytique congénital et ictère hémolytique acquis. Presse Med. **17:** 70, 1909.
14. Chauffard, M. A.: Pathogénie de l'ictère congénital de l'adulte. Sem. Med. **27:** 25, 1907.
15. Chauffard, M. A., and Troisier, J.: Anémie grave avec hémolysine dans le sérum; ictère hémolysinique. Sem. Med. **28:** 345, 1908.
16. Chauffard, M. A., and Vincent, C.: Hémoglobinurie hémolysinique avec ictère polycholique aigu. Sem. Med. **29:** 601, 1909.
17. Widal, F., and Abrami, P.: Types divers d'ictères hémolytiques non congénitaux, avec anémie. La recherche de la résistance globulaire par le procédé des hématies déplasmatisées. Bull. Soc. Med. Paris **24:** 1127, 1907.
18. Widal, F., and Abrami, P.: Hémolyse par fragilité globulaire et hémolyse par action plasmatique. C. R. Soc. Biol. (Paris) **63:** 346, 1907.
19. Widal, F., Abrami, P., and Brulé, M.: Dif-

férentiation de plusieurs types d'ictères hémolytiques par le procédé des hématies deplasmatisées. Presse Med. **15:** 641, 1907.
20. Widal, F., Abrami, P., and Brulé, M.: Pluralité d'origine des ictères hémolytiques: recherches cliniques et expérimentales. Bull. Soc. Med. Hop. Paris **24:** 1354, 1907.
21. Brulé, M.: Les ictères hémolytiques acquis (thesis). Paris, 1909.
22. Du Rôle des Hémolysines en Pathologia. Deuxième Question du XII Session du Congrès Français de Medicina, Lyon, 1911.
23. Micheli, F.: Unmittelbare Effekte der Splenektomie bei einem Fall von erworbenen hämolytischen splenomegalischen Ikterus, Typus Hayem-Widal. Wien. Klin. Wschr. **24:** 1269, 1911.
24. Banti, G.: La esplanomegalia hemolitica. Sem. Med. **32:** 265, 1912.
25. Banti, G.: La splenomegalia emolitica anemopoietica (anemia emolitica splenomegalica anemopoietica). Sperimentale **67:** 323, 1913.
26. Toti, E.: La milza nell'emolisida toluilendiamina. Sperimentale **67:** 379, 1913.
27. Banti, G.: Splénomégalie hémolytique anhémopoiétique: le rôle de la rate dans l'hémolyse. Sem. Med. **33:** 313, 1913.
28. Lederer, M.: A form of acute hemolytic anemia probably of infectious origin. Amer. J. Med. Sci. **170:** 500, 1925.
29. Lederer, M.: Three additional cases of acute hemolytic (infectious) anemia. Amer. J. Med. Sci. **179:** 228, 1930.
30. Brill, I. C.: Acute febrile anemia—a new disease? Arch. Intern. Med. (Chicago) **37:** 244, 1926.
31. Dacie, J. V.: *The Haemolytic Anaemias, Part II,* Ed. 2. Grune & Stratton, Inc., New York, 1962.
32. Dawson, B. E.: Hume lectures on hemolytic icterus. Brit. Med. J. **1:** 921, **2:** 963, 1931.
33. Vaughn, J. M.: *The Anaemias,* Ed. 2, p. 250. Oxford University Press, London, 1936.
34. Doan, C. A., Wiseman, B. K., and Erf, L. A.: Studies in hemolytic jaundice. Ohio Med. J. **30:** 493, 1934.
35. Dameshek, W., and Schwartz, S. O.: The presence of hemolysins in acute hemolytic anemia; preliminary note. New Eng. J. Med. **218:** 75, 1938.
36. Dameshek, W., and Schwartz, S. O.: Hemolysins as the cause of clinical and experimental hemolytic anemias. With particular reference to the nature of spherocytosis and increased fragility. Amer. J. Med. Sci. **196:** 769, 1938.
37. Dameshek, W., and Schwartz, S. O.: Acute hemolytic anemia (acquired hemolytic icterus, acute type). Medicine (Balt.) **19:** 231, 1940.
38. Levine, P., and Stetson, R. E.: An unusual case of intragroup agglutination. J. A. M. A. **113:** 126, 1939.
39. Landsteiner, K., and Wiener, A. S.: An agglutinable factor in human blood recognized

by immune sera for rhesus blood. Proc. Soc. Exp. Biol. Med. **43**: 223, 1940.

40. Levine, P., Katzin, E. M., and Burnham, L.: Isoimmunization in pregnancy, its possible bearing on the etiology of erythroblastosis fetalis. J. A. M. A. **116**: 825, 1941.

41. Levine, P., Vogel, P., Katzin, E. M., and Burnham, L.: Pathogenesis of erythroblastosis fetalis: statistical evidence. Science **94**: 371, 1941.

42. Race, R. R.: An "incomplete" antibody in human serum. Nature (London) **153**: 771, 1944.

43. Wiener, A. S.: A new test (blocking test) for Rh sensitization. Proc. Soc. Exp. Biol. Med. **56**: 173, 1944.

44. Coombs, R. R. A., Mourant, A. E., and Race, R. R.: A new test for the detection of weak and "incomplete" Rh agglutinins. Brit. J. Exp. Path. **26**: 255, 1945.

45. Moreschi, C.: Neue Tatsachen über die Blutkörperchenagglutination. Zbl. Bakt. **46**: 49, 1908.

46. Moreschi, C.: Beschleunigung und Verstärkung der Bakterienagglutination durch Antieiweissera. Zbl. Bakt. **46**: 456, 1908.

47. Boorman, K. E., Dodd, B. E., and Loutit, J. F.: Haemolytic icterus (acholuric jaundice) congenital and acquired. Lancet **1**: 812, 1946.

48. Löw, B.: A practical method using papain and incomplete Rh antibodies in routine Rh blood grouping. Vox Sang. **5**: 94, 1955.

49. Pirofsky, B., and Mangum, M. E.: Use of bromelin to demonstrate erythrocyte antibodies. Proc. Soc. Exp. Biol. Med. **101**: 49, 1959.

50. Morton, J. A., and Pickles, M. M.: Use of trypsin in the detection of incomplete anti-Rh antibodies. Nature (London) **159**: 779, 1947.

51. Dameshek, W.: Acquired hemolytic anemia. Physiopathology with particular reference to autoimmunization and therapy. In *Proceedings of the Third Congress of the International Society of Hematology*. William Heinemann, Ltd., London, 1951.

52. Evans, R. S., Takahashi, K., Duane, R. T., Payne, R., and Liu, C. K.: Primary thrombocytopenic purpura and acquired hemolytic anemia. Evidence for a common etiology. Arch. Intern. Med. (Chicago) **87**: 48, 1951.

53. Young, L. E., Miller, G., and Christian, R. M.: Clinical and laboratory observations on autoimmune hemolytic disease. Ann. Intern. Med. **35**: 507, 1951.

54. Ehrlich, P.: *Collected Studies on Immunity*, translated by C. Bolduan. John Wiley & Sons, Inc., New York, 1906.

55. Witebsky, E.: Historical roots of present concepts of immunopathology. In *Immunopathology, First International Symposium*, edited by P. Grabar and P. Miescher. Schwabe, Basel (Grune & Stratton, Inc., New York), 1959.

56. Pirofsky, B.: A new diagnostic test for antiglobulin positive (autoimmune) haemolytic anaemia. Brit. J. Haemat. **6**: 395, 1960.

57. Weiner, W., Battey, D. A., Cleghorn, T. E., Marson, F. G. W., and Meynell, M. J.: Serologic findings in a case of haemolytic anaemia, with some general observation on the pathogenesis of this syndrome. Brit. Med. J. **2**: 125, 1953.

58. Witebsky, E.: Acquired hemolytic anemia. Ann. N. Y. Acad. Sci. **124**: 462, 1965.

59. Pirofsky, B.: The structure and specificity of erythrocyte autoantibodies. Ann. N. Y. Acad. Sci. **124**: 448, 1965.

60. Schulman, N. R.: Mechanism of blood cell destruction in individuals sensitized to foreign antigens. Trans. Ass. Amer. Physicians **76**: 72, 1963.

61. Schulman, N. R.: Mechanism of cell destruction in individuals sensitized to foreign antigens and its implication in autoimmunity. Combined clinical staff conference at National Institutes of Health. Ann. Intern. Med. **60**: 506, 1964.

62. Crosby, W. H., and Akeroyd, J. H.: The limit of hemoglobin synthesis in hereditary hemolytic anemia; its relation to the excretion of bile pigment. Amer. J. Med. **13**: 273, 1952.

63. Crosby, W. H.: The hemolytic states. Bull. N. Y. Acad. Med. **30**: 27, 1954.

64. Estren, S., and Dameshek, W.: Current concepts of hemolytic anemias. Advances Intern. Med. **3**: 45, 1949.

65. Doljanski, F., Zajicek, G., and Naaman, J.: The size distribution of normal human red blood cells. Life Sci. **5**: 2095, 1966.

66. Yokoyama, M., Eith, D. T., and Bowman, M.: The first auto-Xg^a antibody in a female. Hawaii Med. J. **25**: 328, 1966.

67. Bielschowsky, M., Helyer, B. J., and Howie, J. B.: Spontaneous haemolytic anaemia in mice of NZB/Bl strain. Proc. Univ. Otago Med. Sch. **37**: 9, 1959.

68. Singer, K., and Dameshek, W.: Symptomatic hemolytic anemia. Ann. Intern. Med. **15**: 544, 1941.

69. von Pirquet, C.: Allergie. Munch. Med. Wschr. **30**: 1457, 1906. Translated by C. Prausnitz in *Clinical Aspects of Immunology*, edited by P. G. H. Gell and R. R. A. Coombs. F. A. Davis Company, Philadelphia, 1963.

70. Waksman, B. H.: *Experimental Allergic Encephalomyelitis and the "Auto-allergic" Diseases*. S. Karger, Basel, 1959.

71. Gell, P. G. H., and Coombs, R. R. A., editors: *Clinical Aspects of Immunology*. F. A. Davis Company, Philadelphia, 1963.

72. Autoimmune vs. isoimmune (editorial). New Eng. J. Med. **269**: 1381, 1963.

73. Dameshek, W.: Autoimmunity or dysgammaglobulinemia (correspondence). New Eng. J. Med. **270**: 639, 1964.

74. Dameshek, W.: Hemolytic anemia (reply to Letter to Editor). J. A. M. A. **176**: 252, 1961.

Chapter 2

General Clinical Concepts

The clinical material reported in this and subsequent chapters was obtained from analysis of 234 patients studied during the period from 1958 to 1966. All cases of hemolytic anemia were associated with warm acting erythrocyte autoantibodies. However, the classification of the various syndromes as autoimmune hemolytic anemia must be qualified. In most instances criteria suggested by Dameshek (1) have been met. These include a positive antiglobulin test and suggestive evidence that the coating globulin was produced by the host, resembled an antibody and was responsible for damage to the erythrocyte. These criteria are equally applicable to the antiglobulin positive and autoimmune varieties of hemolytic anemia. As such, the cases discussed probably represent a mixture of pathophysiologic mechanisms leading to hemolytic anemia in association with positive serologic tests. No attempt has been made to subdivide this group further into autoimmune and antiglobulin positive types. The term autoimmune hemolytic anemia is accordingly used with this reservation, conforming to current clinical usage. Whenever possible the etiology is discussed at a theoretical level in order to clarify this relationship.

General Clinical Observations

The information presented below has been derived from analysis of all cases studied. The statistical and clinical conclusions are therefore based on the entire group of patients and are valid only if a single disease entity is present. There is excellent evidence, primarily clinical, sug-gesting that this is not a sound or accurate approach. It is apparent that autoimmune hemolytic anemia includes many unrelated clinical syndromes. Thompson (2) and Dacie (3) have emphasized this point. The apparent similarity stems from a common end stage characterized by an immune reaction involving the erythrocyte. The underlying or associated disease process frequently dominates the clinical picture and colors statistical interpretations. The reader is therefore cautioned to temper the composite clinical observations reported below with more specific observations presented in subsequent chapters dealing with individual syndromes.

Incidence

The autoimmune hemolytic anemias are common. Dacie (3) reported 175 patients studied during a 14-year period at the Postgraduate Medical School of London. Dausset and Colombani (4) recorded 128 cases seen during a 9-year period at the Central Blood Bank in Paris. Swisher (5) indicates that 12 to 24 cases of the warm acting type of autoimmune hemolytic anemia are seen annually at the University of Rochester. Yunis and Bridges (6) mention 40 patients studied in 3 years at the University of Minnesota Hospital. Letman (7) states that 11 cases of autoimmune hemolytic anemia were seen in a 3½-year period in the county and city hospital of Odense, Denmark. This hospital receives all medical cases from a population of 230,000. An incidence of one case per year of autoimmune hemolytic anemia per 75,000 population can be calculated by extrapolating these data. Improved laboratory and clinical diagnostic procedures may appreciably raise this estimate.

Letman's study presents valuable data of comparative incidences of the various hemolytic anemias. Over a 5-year period of time 31 cases of hemolytic anemia were studied at the Odense hospital. Eighteen of these cases or 58 per cent were of the autoimmune variety. The remaining cases were scattered among hereditary spherocytosis (five cases), hereditary elliptocytosis, thalassemia major, nonspherocytic hemolytic anemia, paroxysmal nocturnal hemoglobinuria and others.

The relative frequency of encountering autoimmune hemolytic anemia is apparent in the present series of patients. Approximately 29 cases per year have been studied at our institution over an 8-year period. Such patients were obtained from a population distribution approximating 2.3 million, located in the Pacific Northwest of the United States. As such, the case density closely follows the incidence predicted by extrapolating Letman's data. An incidence of one case of autoimmune hemolytic anemia per 80,000 population may annually be anticipated. It should be noted that our population in this area has a high percentage of persons of Scandinavian ancestry. For example, the distribution of the D^u blood type (8) more closely resembles the distribution in Stockholm, as reported by Broman (9), than it does that of New York City. The fit of our data to those of Letman may therefore have some genetic significance.

Several distinctive features of the current series deserve emphasis. (a) Eighty-five hospitals in our population area are serviced by a central Red Cross blood center. Transfusion and typing problems from these hospitals are frequently referred to the central blood bank where initial serologic studies are performed. A close and fruitful relationship between the immunohematologic laboratories of this institution, the University of Oregon Medical School and various pathologists in our area has made available case material that otherwise could not be studied. (b) All hematologic patients seen at the University of Oregon Medical School undergo antiglobulin and enzyme studies as part of the routine hematologic workup. These serologic studies are carried out in the research immunohematology laboratory. Unexpected clinical states with positive serologic tests are frequently discovered, with the possibility of laboratory errors kept at a minimum. (c) Detailed research studies on various aspects of the hemolytic anemias were concomitantly initiated during this study. This created an atmosphere in which house staff, pathologists and clinicians searched for and were interested in the hemolytic syndrome. (d) A long standing program for diagnosis and therapy of the leukemias and lymphomas exists. Our institution therefore selects a large population of patients suffering from such conditions. The patient load is substantially greater than the hospital patient index for the area would normally permit. Selection of this type of patient has markedly increased our anticipated incidence of autoimmune hemolytic anemia, particularly of the secondary or symptomatic variety.

The reasons given above are not intended as an apology for the frequency with which we encounter autoimmune hemolytic anemia. Rather they are emphasized in order that the clinician may be aware of the relative commonness of this syndrome and of methods which may be employed to increase his exposure. The incidence of the various autoimmune hemolytic anemias is substantially greater than such "common" medical problems as acute rheumatic fever and acute glomerulonephritis. It is more common than all other combined causes of hemolytic anemia, with the exception of erythroblastosis fetalis. It is seen more frequently than such well recognized hematologic problems as pernicious anemia and the lymphomas. In comparison with other autoimmune disorders its frequency is at least equal to that of systemic lupus erythematosus, and it is more common than thyroiditis.

Age Distribution

Warm acting autoimmune hemolytic anemia may occur at any age. It differs from cold acting autoimmune hemolytic anemia. Dacie (3) has emphasized that cold acting syndromes, except paroxysmal cold hemoglobinuria, are extremely rare if they occur at all in the infant and the young. In his analysis of 125 patients with warm acting autoimmune hemolytic anemia an age distribution from 5 months to 78 years was noted. Swisher's study (5) of warm acting autoimmune hemolytic anemia apparently excluded children. An age range distribution from the 20's through the 70's was noted. In the groups of both Dacie and Swisher, the majority of patients appeared to be over 40 years of age.

The current series conforms to this diffuse age distribution. Figure 3 presents the ages and statistical data of 233 patients at the onset of autoimmune hemolytic anemia. A range of ages from 1 month to 87 years was seen. Of these patients, 170, or 73 per cent, were over 40 years of age. The peak incidence appeared between the ages of 60 to 70.

The underlying disease process has a marked effect on the age distribution. The 44 cases considered as idiopathic forms had a range of age similar to the entire group. Patients from the ages of 2½ to 79 years were seen. Of the patients 71 per cent were over age 40 with a peak incidence in the 50 to 70 age bracket. Secondary forms of hemolytic anemia varied greatly as to age at onset. Patients with chronic lymphocytic leukemia and autoimmune hemolytic anemia had an age distribution typical of the leukemic state. Of these patients 100 per cent were over 40 years of age. Cases of acute lymphocytic leukemia with autoimmune hemolytic anemia had an entirely different age distribution, which was again related to the underlying disease process. Of these patients 70 per cent were age 20 or younger. These observations emphasize that clinical features of autoimmune hemolytic anemia occurring in association with other diseases are frequently dominated by underlying pathologic states.

Autoimmune Hemolytic Anemia in the Young

Autoimmune hemolytic anemia is generally seen in adults. Its occurrence in the young is considered by many to be a rarity.

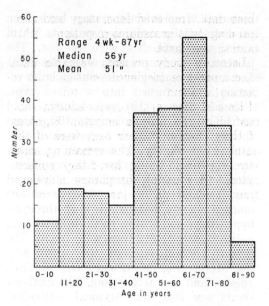

FIG. 3. The age distribution of 233 patients with autoimmune hemolytic anemia.

This is erroneous. A large literature is currently available describing this state in children (10–31). O'Connor and associates (10) reviewed the literature in 1956 and added 18 additional cases in children under age 5. Negri and associates (11) in 1960 summarized prior studies involving infants 13 months old or younger. In 1964 Malaguzzi Valeri and associates (12) reported 11 cases of autoimmune hemolytic anemia in the pediatric age. In several instances erythrocyte autoantibodies with rhesus specificity have been described. These include examples of anti-D (13, 14), anti-c (15) and anti-f (13).

Examples of this syndrome developing in infancy are of particular interest. The newborn is considered unable to produce significant IgG immunoglobulins until 3 months of age or older (32). The amount of IgG immunoglobulins normally produced usually is not significant until 6 months of age. In spite of this there are at least eight case reports of autoimmune hemolytic anemia presenting at age 3 months or less (4, 13, 16–21). The patients reported by Unger and associates (16) and Bakx and van Loghem (17) involved cold agglutinins, and an IgM immunoglobulin can be assumed. A possible relationship to maternal virus infections may have been present. In the remaining patients warm acting autoantibodies were present. The patient of Germain and associates (18) had a non-gamma-globulin-antiglobulin re-action which turned into a mixed type. Ritz and Haber (19) successfully eluted an IgG type of panhemagglutinin from the erythrocytes of their 6-week-old infant. A most remarkable case has been presented by Iafusco and Buffa (20). A 7-day-old in-fant, born from healthy parents, developed jaundice and pallor. At 10 days of age marked anemia, bone marrow erythrocytic hyperplasia and strong positive direct and indirect antiglobulin tests were found. The erythrocyte autoantibody was warm act-ing. Mother and infant had identical ABO, rhesus, Kell and MN typing. The mother's serum was free from atypical antibodies. The infant's death occurred soon after these initial studies.

The capacity of such infants to produce significant amounts of IgG erythrocyte autoantibodies deserves thorough investi-gation. These cases may have important etiologic connotations. The initiation of IgG immunoglobulin formation before, at or shortly after birth may relate to an aberration of the immune apparatus which prevents establishment or maintenance of normal immune tolerance.

In the present series 11 patients (4.7 per cent) with autoimmune hemolytic ane-mia were under age 10. Only two cases were 1 year old or less. The following his-tory summarizes the case of the youngest patient studied.

Case 1. A 4-week-old boy was seen for anemia and jaundice. Birth had been spon-taneous and uncomplicated after a 38-week gestation. The child weighed 7 pounds, and both mother and father were healthy. Jaundice was noted at birth. At 2 weeks of age an upper respiratory infection occurred and jaundice intensified. At 4 weeks of age petechiae, hep-atosplenomegaly, nystagmus and convulsions developed. The hemoglobin dropped from 12.5 gm. per cent to 9.5 gm. per cent in 4 days. Bilirubin was elevated to 8.0/12.8 mg. per cent. Proteinuria was found. At 5 weeks of age hemoglobin was 7.2 gm. per cent, white blood cells (WBC) were 39,000/mm.^{3}, thrombocytes

605,000/mm.^{3} and reticulocytes 25 per cent. Serologic tests for syphilis, albumin-globulin (A/G) ratio and spinal fluid were normal. Nucleated erythrocytes and spherocytes were seen in the peripheral blood. The bone marrow demonstrated erythrocytic hyperplasia. Several direct antiglobulin tests were positive. The liver was palpated 4 cm. and the spleen 2 cm. below the costal margin. Corticosteroid therapy was initiated with a progressive rise in hemo-globin. In spite of this, seizures continued. The urine and a renal biopsy demonstrated cyto-megalic inclusion bodies. Death occurred at 7 weeks of age from cytomegalic disease.

This patient illustrates the problem of autoimmune hemolytic anemia in infancy. Unfortunately, studies to delineate the na-ture of the autoantibody and antiglobulin reaction were not carried out. Either the infant was able to produce IgG immuno-globulins at an early age or else a warm acting IgM autoantibody was present. The placental passage of a potent iso- or autoantibody from the mother was ruled out. The association of cytomegalic disease with autoimmune hemolytic anemia has also been described by Zuelzer and asso-ciates (33). They have suggested that hemolytic anemia associated with diffuse virus infections in the pediatric age is un-related to autoantibody formation and correlates best with virus activity.

Sex

Both males and females may develop autoimmune hemolytic anemia. Swisher (5) noted a 60.5 per cent incidence of in-volved females in a relatively small series of patients. The idiopathic variety showed a marked selection with 71.4 per cent of the cases appearing in females. Sacks and associates (34) similarly noted a predomi-nance of females in the 147 cases of auto-immune hemolytic anemia they reviewed. Dacie (3) reported a predominantly female distribution of the warm acting autoim-mune hemolytic anemias. Of his series of 129 patients 58.1 per cent were females. Of the idiopathic group 65 per cent were females. Dausset and Colombani (4) noted that 61 per cent of patients with the idio-pathic variety were females, but 60 per cent of patients with secondary varieties of autoimmune hemolytic anemia were males. These figures differ from those of Lal and Speiser (35). They reported a female predominance of 55 per cent in idiopathic forms, and a 62.5 per cent incidence in secondary types of autoimmune hemolytic anemia.

The current series differs somewhat. No sex difference in the incidence of the warm acting type of autoimmune hemolytic anemia could be determined. The 234 patients studied were evenly distributed, with 117 cases occurring each in males and females. Marked differences in sex distribution were found, however, when the underlying pathologic state was considered. The idiopathic variety was more common in females. Of the 44 cases 63.6 per cent appeared in women. This female predilection was more obvious when cases of systemic lupus erythematosus were examined. Eighty per cent of these cases were in females. A male predominance was found when patients with reticuloendothelial neoplasia were analyzed. Males comprised 57.4 per cent of the cases of autoimmune hemolytic anemia complicating chronic lymphocytic leukemia. Similarly, 62.5 per cent of the cases of autoimmune hemolytic anemia complicating the lymphomas were in men. Table 5 summarizes the sex distribution in patients with warm acting autoimmune hemolytic anemia. It is apparent that the underlying pathologic state, rather than sex of the patient, is important in the development of autoimmune hemolytic anemia.

Pregnancy and the Autoimmune Hemolytic Anemias

No definitive conclusions could be drawn as to the influence of pregnancy on autoimmune hemolytic anemia. The present series is too limited in this regard. However, two patients became pregnant during remission states of their disease without exacerbation. In addition, two patients first manifested signs of their disease during pregnancy. Delivery was followed by transient remissions of the autoimmune syndrome. The following case illustrates the course of one such patient.

Case 2. A 24-year-old female in the 32nd

TABLE 5. *Sex distribution of 234 patients with warm acting autoimmune hemolytic anemia*

	Males		Females	
	No.	Per cent	No.	Per cent
All cases	117	50	117	50
Idiopathic variety	16	36.4	28	63.6
Secondary varieties				
Systemic lupus erythematosus	2	20	8	80
Chronic lymphocytic leukemia	27	56.3	21	43.7
The lymphomas	16	64	9	36

week of pregnancy entered with petechiae and gingival bleeding. Hepatosplenomegaly was present. The hematocrit was 35 per cent with a reticulocyte count of 3.2 per cent. Thrombocytes were 7,000/mm.[3] and the bone marrow was compatible with idiopathic thrombocytopenic purpura. Direct and indirect antiglobulin and bromelin tests were positive and elution revealed the presence of a panhemagglutinin. Kolmer and Kline tests were positive and detailed studies suggested a biologically false positive reaction. Multiple lupus erythematosus (LE) cell preparations were negative. Corticosteroid therapy was given without effect. The patient spontaneously delivered at 36-week gestation without difficulty. The infant appeared healthy with moderate to marked thrombocytopenia. Positive direct antiglobulin tests were present and persisted until 3 weeks of age. One month after delivery the patient's thrombocyte count had reached 225,000/mm.[3] but the positive antiglobulin test continued. Anemia persisted with an hematocrit of 30 per cent and a 3.7 per cent reticulocyte count. Over the next 5½ years the patient developed a typical picture of systemic lupus erythematosus with skin and mucous membrane lesions, nephropathy, fever, anemia, leukopenia, grand mal seizures and psychosis.

In the above patient an Evans' syndrome type of idiopathic autoimmune hemolytic anemia was initially diagnosed. Systemic lupus erythematosus subsequently became apparent. Pregnancy did not adversely affect the disease process. Delivery led to spontaneous remission of thrombocytopenia while positive antiglobulin tests persisted. The ability of antierythrocyte and antithrombocyte autoantibodies to traverse the placenta and affect the newborn should be noted. A similar case has been described by Burt and Prichard (36) and another by Seip (37). Wagner and Maresch (38), Wirtheimer (39), Mallarmé and associates (40), Jankelowitz and associates (41) and Swisher (5) all have studied pregnant females with autoimmune hemolytic anemia. Swisher mentions a patient in whom autoimmune hemolytic anemia underwent acute exacerbation with each subsequent pregnancy. He feels that pregnancy may initiate exacerbations of the disease in patients in whom it has been quiescent for many years. This has not been the experience in our current series.

Race

A racial basis for either predisposition toward or protection from autoimmune hemolytic anemia is not apparent. An adequate study in this area, however, has not been presented. The author's current series is too homogeneous to be of aid in analyzing this problem. The Negro is not free from development of autoimmune hemolytic anemia. Although our region has a relatively small Negro population, three cases, all of the secondary variety, were noted in Negroes. Small Chinese and Japanese populations are also present in our region. One patient of Japanese ancestry developed an idiopathic form of autoimmune hemolytic anemia. Lie-Injo and Pillay (42) have reported five cases in Asians and mention the occurrence of autoimmune hemolytic anemias in Indonesians and Chinese. They conclude that these syndromes are not rare in the tropics.

Genetic Predisposition

A familial predisposition apparently exists for the initiation of various human autoimmune diseases. This postulate is supported by observations concerning systemic lupus erythematosus (43, 44), rheumatoid arthritis (45), pernicious anemia (46, 47) and thyroiditis (48, 49). Genetic influences in the autoimmune hemolytic anemias are less clear. Until recently it was assumed that hereditary factors were not involved in the pathogenesis of this state. The development of the NZB

mice by Bielschowsky and associates (50) in 1959 offered an excellent model system which put in doubt the freedom from genetic factors. Hybridization studies by Howie and Helyer (51) have shown that a dominant genetic characteristic is involved which can be expressed in the heterozygous state and is not linked to sex, black coat color or a milk factor.

In his extensive review of 175 cases, Dacie (3) did not encounter a single familial example, and he specifically mentions a patient with autoimmune hemolytic anemia whose probable identical twin was unaffected by a similar disease. Other workers (52–59), however, have observed a familial occurrence of autoimmune hemolytic anemia. Eight families have been reported with two members suffering from this condition. In an unpublished study, Frank R. Schmid of Northwestern University School of Medicine, Chicago, Illinois, has investigated two identical twins with warm acting autoimmune hemolytic anemia. Fialkow and associates (59) described a patient with autoimmune hemolytic anemia, carditis and thyrotoxicosis. The mother of the proband had positive antiglobulin tests, and one sibling had developed polyarteritis nodosa. In addition, hypergammaglobulinemia, macroglobulinemia, rheumatoid factor, antinuclear factor and antibodies to cardiac and thyroid tissue were present in various close relatives.

In the present series a family with similar characteristics was encountered. Two sisters and a brother developed autoimmune hemolytic anemia. Their case histories are summarized below.

Case 3. A 49-year-old white female was seen in December 1953. The patient had been anemic for many years and at age 43 developed severe menorrhagia. Hemoglobin was found to be 36 per cent and dilation and curettage were performed, with oral iron therapy given. Pruritus, an erythematous rash and facial edema developed and disappeared with the cessation of iron therapy. These findings recurred on two occasions when iron was readministered. Hysterectomy was carried out at age 46 and 6 units of blood were transfused for profound anemia. Three years later marked anemia was noted and several transfusions were given. The hematocrit rapidly dropped and the patient was referred for hematologic consultation. Physical examination was entirely negative. Hemoglobin was 7.9 gm. per cent with a normal WBC. A 7.1 per cent reticulocyte count was found. Bone marrow aspiration revealed erythrocytic hyperplasia and a hypocellular pattern. Direct antiglobulin tests were strongly positive and a diagnosis of autoimmune hemolytic anemia was made. Hydrocortisone, 240 mg. daily, was given. During the next month symptomatic improvement occurred and the hemoglobin rose to 9.3 gm. per cent. Her clinical course was complicated by chronic, recurrent infections and hydrocortisone was gradually reduced. Over the next 6 months the hemoglobin dropped to 5.9 gm. per cent and persistent reticulocytosis occurred. Proteinuria was found and investigation revealed a total serum protein of 8.6 gm. per cent with a reversed A/G ratio. Serum electrophoresis demonstrated a sharp spike in the gamma zone which contained 5.06 gm. of protein and was typical of plasma cell myeloma. Cryoglobulins were not found. The urine was free of Bence-Jones protein. Repeat bone marrow examination was diagnostic of plasma cell myeloma. The hemolytic process persisted and splenectomy and liver biopsy were carried out. An infiltration of plasma cells in these two organs was noted. Four units of blood were transfused. Improvement of the hemolytic state did not occur. Hydrocortisone was discontinued and urethane was given. Hemolysis continued and the hemoglobin again dropped to 5.9 gm. per cent with a 6.1 per cent reticulocyte count. Jaundice became apparent. In spite of additional transfusions death occurred 11 months after diagnosis of autoimmune hemolytic anemia and 2 months after splenectomy. Autopsy revealed plasma cell myeloma, a hyperplastic bone marrow and an intraventricular hemorrhage.

Case 4. A 48-year-old white male, brother of the above patient, was seen in September 1955. At age 9 he had developed pneumonia and a pleural effusion and at age 14 rheumatic fever was diagnosed. At age 45 normal hematologic and urinary studies were made during an attack of dermatitis diagnosed as pityriasis rosea. Over the next 3 years a severe illness became apparent and was characterized by migratory polyarthritis, Raynaud's syndrome, high fever, acute pericarditis, pleuritis with pleural effusions, diabetes, proteinuria (4+), marked microscopic hematuria, anorexia, weight loss (35 pounds) and a progressive anemia which did not respond to hematinics. Multiple transfusions were given. Small doses of corticosteroids improved the severe arthritic disease. When the patient was first examined, pallor and weight loss were apparent. There was a maculopapular erythematous rash with raised centers over his back and chest. Two ulcers were noted in the buccal mucosa. Mild (1+) generalized lymphadenopathy was found. The liver was palpated at the costal margin. Generalized edema was present. The hemoglobin was 7.5 gm. per cent, reticulocyte count 0.5 per cent and erythrocyte sedimentation rate 122/144. Autoagglutination of the erythrocytes was noted. Direct antiglobulin and indirect trypsin tests were strongly positive. Bone marrow revealed an increased number of lymphocytes and benign plasmacytosis. Cryoglobulins were found in the serum and totaled 0.5 gm. per cent. After removal of the cryoglobulins, a total protein of 6.89 gm. per cent with 2.15 gm. of albumin was found. Serum electrophoresis of this specimen demonstrated an elevated alpha-2 globulin of 1.4 gm. per cent and a broad polyclonal elevation of the gamma-globulin which contained 27 per cent of the total protein. The urine showed 2+ proteinuria, an absence of Bence-Jones protein, glycosuria and microscopic hematuria. LE cell preparations and serologic tests for syphilis were negative. A diagnosis of systemic lupus erythematosus, cryoglobulinemia and autoimmune hemolytic anemia was made. A single dose of P^{32} was given and prednisone, 60 mg. daily, was started. The hemoglobin rapidly rose to 10.4 gm. per cent over the next 2 weeks. Marked renal insufficiency developed and the blood urea nitrogen rose to 65 mg. per cent. Eighty-five units of regular insulin were required daily to correct the severe diabetes, and prednisone therapy was accordingly decreased. Anemia rapidly recurred and multiple transfusions were given. The patient lapsed into uremic and hyperglycemic coma. Death occurred 5 weeks after the initial diagnosis of autoimmune hemolytic anemia.

Case 5. A 66-year-old white female, sister to the above two patients, was first seen in November 1962. Eleven months prior to this visit weight loss was first noted (35 pounds). Six months before admission anemia, pallor and jaundice were seen. Four blood transfusions were given. Anemia rapidly recurred and with it fatigue and congestive heart failure developed. Epistaxis, petechiae and purpura were present. Six weeks before admission, cross matches were found to be incompatible due to positive direct antiglobulin tests. Prednisone, 20 mg. daily, was given and the patient was referred for hematologic consultation. Physical examination revealed pallor, petechiae and epistaxis. A diffusely enlarged thyroid gland was found. Supraclavicular and inguinal lymphadenopathy was present without hepatosplenomegaly. The hemoglobin was 7.2 gm. per cent, the hematocrit 22 per cent, reticulocyte count 21.3 per cent, WBC 8,700/mm.³ and thrombocyte count 1,000/mm.³ Nucleated erythrocytes and spherocytes were found in the peripheral blood. The bone marrow revealed generalized hypocellularity. The erythrocyte sedimentation rate was 76/132 and the A/G ratio was 2.0/4.3 gm. per cent. Serum electrophoresis identified the gamma-globulin as a broad polyclonal elevation containing 29.1 per cent of the total protein. Cryoglobulins were noted in small amounts. Urinalysis was normal. Direct and indirect antiglobulin and bromelin tests were strongly positive and an erythrocyte autoantibody functioning as a panhemagglutinin was demonstrated. A diagnosis of an Evans' syndrome type of idiopathic autoimmune hemolytic anemia was made. Prednisone, 60 mg. daily, was started. After 2 weeks the hematocrit rose to 28 per cent with a 17.2 per cent reticulocyte count. Thrombocytes were only 3,700/mm.³ Six weeks after the start of prednisone remission was apparent with a hematocrit of 35 per cent, reticulocytes 1.5 per cent and thrombocytes 192,000/mm.³ Prednisone was gradually reduced to 5 mg. daily as a maintenance dose, after 15 weeks of therapy. At that time the hematocrit had reached 42.5 per cent and the thrombocyte count 100,000/mm.³ Symptomatic improvement occurred but edema and lower extremity muscular weakness was present. The patient developed moderate alopecia. She was then lost to followup and died 5 months later without an autopsy. Duration of illness from diagnosis of autoimmune hemolytic anemia was 11 months.

The clinical and laboratory findings obtained from the three siblings with autoimmune hemolytic anemia are presented in Table 6. There were two additional siblings in this family group. Both were available for study and each had a long history of anemia. Examination of the remaining brother revealed a peptic ulcer and severe hypochromic anemia. An additional sister was found to have mild hypochromic anemia. Karyotype studies in this sibling demonstrated a normal pattern. Neither of these two siblings had evidence of either a hemolytic state or dysproteinemia.

The current report adds another family with a predisposition toward developing autoimmune hemolytic anemia. Several aspects deserve emphasis. (a) Autoimmune hemolytic anemia with demonstrable erythrocyte autoantibodies was present in three siblings. (b) The course of disease in their cases differed from the course in those families in whom an inherited variant of the MNS blood group system was associated with positive antiglobulin tests (60–62) in the absence of hemolytic anemia. (c) The disease process did not occur in a close temporal relationship among the three siblings. Nine years elapsed between involvement of the first and the last siblings. (d) Employing the usual classification of autoimmune hemolytic anemia, different syndromes were present in the three family members. One sister had an Evans' syndrome type of idiopathic autoimmune hemolytic anemia. The remaining two siblings presented with a secondary or symptomatic variety of the disease. However, different associated pathologic states were noted, i.e., plasma cell myeloma in one sibling and systemic lupus erythematosus in the other. (e) Two siblings had complex clinical courses suggesting the presence of multiple immunologic abnormalities. Additional medical problems included rheumatic fever, diabetes, thrombocytopenia, thyromegaly, alopecia, myopathy and recurrent infections. (f) Dysgammaglobulinemia and hypergammaglobulinemia were apparent in all three siblings. One sister had a monoclonal gamma-globulin spike typical of plasma cell myeloma. A broad polyclonal elevation of gamma-globulin and moderate increases in alpha-2 and beta-globulins were seen in the remaining two siblings. Both of these patients had cryoglobulinemia.

The development of autoimmune hemolytic anemia in three siblings makes a fortuitous relationship unlikely. It is probable that genetic factors occupy an etiologic role. Dreyfus (58) has elegantly argued this point. The site of action and the nature of the genetic mechanism, however, are unknown and must be elaborated. Several investigators have suggested that autoimmune disease results from a genetically

TABLE 6. *Clinical and laboratory findings in three siblings with autoimmune hemolytic anemia*

Type of autoimmune hemolytic anemia	Case 3: Secondary (symptomatic)	Case 4: secondary (symptomatic)	Case 5: idiopathic (Evans' type)
Associated diseases	Plasma cell myeloma, recurrent infections, vascular hemorrhage, allergic to iron	Lupus erythematosus (arthritis, Raynaud's, pleuritis, pericarditis, renal insufficiency), diabetes, rheumatic fever	Enlarged thyroid, alopecia, steroid myopathy
Physical findings			
Lymphadenopathy	0	+	+
Hepatomegaly	0	±	0
Splenomegaly	0	0	0
Hematology			
Hemoglobin (gm.%)	7.9	7.5	7.2
Reticulocytes (%)	7.1	0.5	21.3
WBC/mm.^{3}	13,500	6,650	8,700
Thrombocytes/mm.^{3}	Normal	Normal	1,000
Bone marrow	Erythrocytic hyperplasia, plasma cell myeloma	Lymphocytosis and plasmacytosis	Generalized hypoplasia
Serum proteins			
Sedimentation rate (mm. 15/45 min.)	4/71	122/144	76/132
A/G ratio (gm.%)	2.2/6.4	2.15/4.74	2.0/4.3
Electrophoresis (gm. %)			
Albumin	2.2	2.1	2.0
Alpha-1	0.31	0.65	0.6
Alpha-2	0.41	1.40	0.9
Beta	0.62	0.86	1.0
Gamma	5.06 (monoclonal)	1.83 (polyclonal)	1.8 (polyclonal)
Cryoglobulins (gm. %)	Absent	0.5	Present
Urine studies			
Bence-Jones protein	Negative	Negative	Not done
Urine analysis	Normal	Proteinuria, glycosuria, hematuria	Normal
Serologic tests			
Syphilis	Negative	Negative	Negative
LE cell	Negative	Negative	Negative
Direct antiglobulin	Positive	Positive	Positive
Direct enzyme	Not done	Not done	Positive
Indirect antiglobulin	Not done	Not done	Positive
Indirect enzyme	Not done	Positive	Positive
Antibody elution	Not done	Not done	Panhemagglutinin found

mediated aberration of the immune apparatus. Burnet (63) postulated such a state as necessary to allow for a proliferation of "forbidden clones." Ziff (64) hypothesized that autoimmune disease results from a genetically controlled tendency to escape from immune tolerance. Leonhardt (44) suggested that a genetic abnormality

creates hyperproducers of antibodies. Fudenberg and associates (59, 65) feel that a
genetic predisposition is involved in a
tendency to break down immunologic homeostasis.

All of these concepts are applicable to
autoimmune hemolytic anemia. It has been
postulated that an aberrant immune apparatus, which prevents the establishment of
a normal immune homeostatic mechanism,
results in the development of autoimmune
hemolytic anemia, reticuloendothelial neoplasia and multiple immune abnormalities
(66). Such immunologically incompetent
individuals would be unable to efficiently
destroy cells modified by virus action or
somatic mutation. Single or multiple clones
of modified immunocompetent cells may
accordingly persist and replicate. These
cells, through a graft-host disease mechanism, may then produce multiple autoantibodies including erythrocyte autoantibodies.
Clinical syndromes of varying degrees of
complexity would result from this process.
The observation that immunologically incompetent rabbits develop autoimmune hemolytic anemia, a wasting disease and
amyloidosis supports this hypothesis (67).
Similar conditions apparently occur in the
human being. Schaller and associates (68)
have reported an infant with a familial
lymphopenic immune defect. This immunologically incompetent child developed
autoimmune hemolytic anemia, glomerulonephritis, hypergammaglobulinemia and
multiple infections. Two siblings also died
with lymphoid hypoplasia. The familial
predisposition seen in immunologically incompetent animals may not be primarily
related to genetic factors. Miller (69) has
suggested that vertical transmission of viruses in such animals may be the responsible mechanism. The studies of Mellors and
Huang with NZB mice (70, 71) support this
hypothesis.

It is important to determine at what
level of activity the hereditary influence is
expressed. Does it directly involve the
formation of erythrocytic autoantibodies?
Alternatively, is the abnormality related
to the establishment of an aberrant immune apparatus? The relative infrequency
of a familial production of erythrocyte

autoantibodies suggests that a simple, direct genetic relationship is unlikely. The
present report supports this. The three
siblings involved had different clinical
states, although erythrocyte autoantibodies
were present in all. One patient had an
idiopathic type of autoimmune hemolytic
anemia. The remaining two siblings had
secondary forms of the disease with dif-
erent associated pathologic states. This observation makes it unlikely that the familial abnormality is exclusively directed
toward erythrocyte autoantibody production.

Current data indicate that the hereditary defect does not specifically involve
erythrocyte immune homeostasis, but rather
influences a more fundamental aberration
of the immune apparatus. As such, neoplasia and multiple autoantibody formation may be anticipated (66, 72). Erythrocyte autoantibodies would appear to be
only one manifestation of the immunologically incompetent state. In our present
series most forms of autoimmune hemolytic anemia are of a secondary variety
(81.2 per cent). Associated abnormalities
include reticuloendothelial neoplasia and
various presumed autoimmune syndromes
such as thyroid and collagen disease, ulcerative colitis, pernicious anemia, etc. Of the
small group considered as idiopathic a significant number have a familial background
for the development of immunologically
mediated disease (see Chapter 4). A simple
retrospective historical analysis (73) demonstrated that 20 per cent of such patients
had family members involved in clinically
detectable autoimmune disease states. Further studies in this area are desirable.

Survival and Duration of Disease

Dacie (3) has analyzed a group of 85
patients with warm acting autoimmune
hemolytic anemia. Followup was available
for a period of at least 1 year. Fifty patients had the idiopathic variety of the
disease. A 46 per cent mortality was noted.
Of these patients 17 died within 2 years of
their illness and 19 patients survived for
5 years or more. Autoimmune hemolytic
anemia complicating neoplasia was present
in 17 cases with an 88 per cent mortality.

Other secondary forms presented a mortality of 45 per cent. In a later summary of the same group of patients, Dacie (74) recorded the death of 23 of his 50 patients. Death generally occurred within 2 years of diagnosis. Ten patients were "cured." These survival figures differed markedly from those seen in idiopathic cold hemagglutinin disease. Nine of 16 patients survived over 5 years. A more favorable prognosis is also seen in infants with autoimmune hemolytic anemia. A mortality of 28 per cent has been recorded for 29 children under age 13 months summarized from the literature (3).

In the author's series adequate followup was available at the time of analysis for 226 cases. Of this group 145 patients had died, leading to an overall mortality of 64.2 per cent. These raw data do not reflect either the survival or the prognosis of autoimmune hemolytic anemia. Length of followup and age at onset are only two factors which influence survival figures. As noted with sex and age statistics, the presence of an underlying disease influences the statistical data. This variation is of major importance in determining survival. It is therefore necessary for the reader to review the specific clinical discussions in subsequent chapters in order to derive meaningful mortality and survival figures. Several examples may be given at this time. Mortality of the idiopathic form of the autoimmune hemolytic anemias was only 38.1 per cent. Mortality of the secondary types of the autoimmune hemolytic anemias was approximately twice as great. This reflects in great part the influence of associated malignancies of the reticuloendothelium. A mortality of 85.4 per cent was seen in patients with associated chronic lymphocytic leukemia. Patients with all other forms of complicating leukemia had a 100 per cent mortality. When the various lymphomas and plasma cell myelomas were associated with autoimmune hemolytic anemia, a mortality of 91 per cent was observed. These figures differ markedly from these found in other secondary types of autoimmune hemolytic anemias. Infectious disease appearing at the onset of hemolytic anemia rarely leads to death. Complete

TABLE 7. *Mortality of patients with warm acting autoimmune hemolytic anemia: 226 patients studied with death occurring in 145*

	No. Dead/Total	Per Cent
All cases	145/226	64.2
Idiopathic variety	16/42	38.1
Secondary varieties	129/184	70.1
Chronic lymphocytic leukemia	41/48	85.4
The lymphomas	31/34	91.2
Other leukemias (27 acute)	29/29	100.0

hematologic remission frequently occurs with control of the underlying disease. Table 7 summarizes the observed mortality.

The 145 patients with autoimmune hemolytic anemia who have died presented a range of survival of 5 days to 215 months. Figure 4 charts the duration in months, and gives mean and median calculations as well. A skewed distribution is noted, emphasizing early death. Of the cases 26.9 per cent died within 3 months of the onset of autoimmune hemolytic anemia. By 1 year 60.0 per cent of all deaths had occurred. Only 11 patients, or 7.8 per cent, survived 5 years or longer before death occurred.

Eighty-one patients with autoimmune hemolytic anemia were still living at the time of statistical review. Analysis of this group is particularly difficult. Many patients had an acute onset of autoimmune hemolytic anemia which responded to treatment of the underlying associated disease, or to direct therapy of the hemolytic state, or to a combination of both therapies. Followup in many has been substantially greater than 5 years. Throughout this volume such patients are considered to be cases of quiescent hemolytic anemia in "remission." It may be equally true to consider the "remission" as complete cure. Continual followup is necessary before final classification. The possibility that such cases are forms of antiglobulin positive immunohemolytic anemia deserves investigation. "Cure" may represent removal of an immunologic sequence not primarily related to erythrocytes.

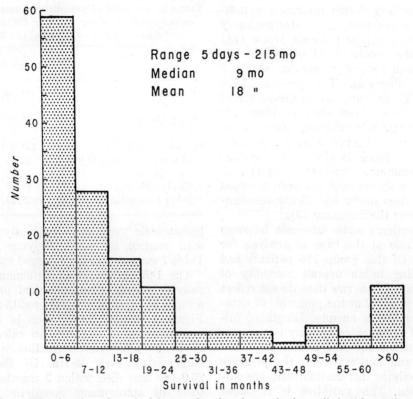

FIG. 4. The duration of survival in months of patients who have died with autoimmune hemolytic anemia (141 subjects are presented).

Signs and Symptoms

Presenting Symptoms

Autoimmune hemolytic anemia varies greatly in its presenting picture. Several factors are responsible for this variation. The majority of cases occur in association with an underlying disease. Frequently this additional pathologic state dominates the patient's complaints and obscures any specific effects of hemolytic anemia. For example, a patient may first be seen with complaints of bloody diarrhea, weakness, fatigue, anorexia and fever. A diagnosis of ulcerative colitis can be made. During routine hematologic investigation autoimmune hemolytic anemia may be documented as an unsuspected condition. Autoimmune hemolytic anemia may also be asymptomatic at time of diagnosis. A patient with chronic lymphocytic leukemia, under excellent control and in an asymptomatic state, is discovered to have a slowly falling hematocrit. Immunohematologic studies may then demonstrate autoimmune hemolytic anemia. Such variations of presenting complaints also occur in the idiopathic variety in which an underlying disease does not obscure the symptom complex. The rate of hemolysis and ability of the patient to compensate for and to become acclimated to the lowered blood count is important. One patient may be initially seen with a hematocrit of 15 per cent. Fatigue on exertion is his only complaint. Another patient may arrive with severe exhaustion, dyspnea, orthopnea and palpitations. A hematocrit of 30 per cent may be found in this patient.

The symptoms of patients initially seen with autoimmune hemolytic anemia may be divided into three basic groups. These include complaints referable to anemia, to the hemolytic state and to miscellaneous

TABLE 8. *Presenting symptoms of patients with autoimmune hemolytic anemia (AHA): 186 cases of a secondary variety (2°) and 44 cases of an idiopathic type (1°) analyzed*

	No. of Patients Seen Initially with Presenting Complaint								
Anemia	AHA type		Hemolysis	AHA type		Miscellaneous	AHA type	
	2°	1°		2°	1°		2°	1°
Weakness	164	39	Jaundice	31	17	Fever	77	8
Dizziness	98	17	Dark urine	3	3	Bleeding	17	6
Dyspnea	19	2	Hemoglobinuria	2	1	Weight loss	10	1
Congestive failure	10	1	Pruritus	1		Gastrointestinal complaints	10	3
Pallor	7	2				Cough	10	2
Edema	8	2				Anorexia	7	2
Angina	4	1				Arthralgia	2	2
Confusion	3	1						
Syncope		1						

causes. Table 8 lists the specific symptoms and their incidence in patients with idiopathic and symptomatic forms of autoimmune hemolytic anemia. In view of the diversity of underlying diseases associated with autoimmune hemolytic anemia, a complete listing of presenting symptoms would be encyclopedic. An attempt has therefore been made to select only those symptoms which may relate specifically to the hemolytic state.

Within the group of complaints referable to the anemic state, weakness was almost universal. It was noted in 87 per cent of patients. A linked series of complaints is frequent. These include weakness, dizziness, palpitations, dyspnea on exertion and an annoying pounding pulsation in the ears. All of these difficulties appear to be secondary to anemia and disappear as the hematocrit elevates. Edema, angina and frank congestive heart failure are not uncommon. Confusion and even syncope may occur.

Complaints directly related to the hemolytic state are frequently found. Jaundice is the most common and was noted by 48 patients or 21 per cent of the series. Pruritus, dark urine and hemoglobinuria may also be found.

A miscellaneous group of complaints which may be related to autoimmune hemolytic anemia is frequently encountered. Fever is prominent in this group; it was found in 81 patients or 35 per cent of the

cases. A variable number of complaints including petechiae and ecchymosis, anorexia, vomiting, weight loss, diarrhea, cough, etc., are also recorded.

It is difficult to separate those symptoms which are due to autoimmune hemolytic anemia from those which result from an underlying or an associated disease. The specific complaints noted by patients with the idiopathic variety of autoimmune hemolytic anemia supply an index. Table 8 lists such symptoms. It is of particular interest that jaundice occurred in 39 per cent of the idiopathic group, a substantially higher incidence than in the case of the secondary form. In contrast, fever was seen in 18 per cent of the idiopathic cases. This incidence is significantly lower than that found in the secondary types of autoimmune hemolytic anemia.

Physical Findings

Physical findings in autoimmune hemolytic anemia generally result from hemolysis or abnormalities of the reticuloendothelium. The physical diagnosis of anemia is remarkably difficult. The classic observation of pallor is generally unreliable. In the author's experience reliance on pallor to either diagnose or rule out the presence of anemia is almost useless. This observation is reflected in the current series, in which the presence of pallor was rarely observed. Jaundice was frequently seen, however,

TABLE 9. *Presenting physical signs in patients with autoimmune hemolytic anemia: 186 cases of the secondary variety (2°) and 44 cases of an idiopathic type (1°) analyzed*

Physical Abnormality	Percentage Seen with Abnormality	
	AHA type 2°	AHA type 1°
Splenomegaly	52	53
Hepatomegaly	48	32
Lymphadenopathy	37	23
Jaundice	16.7	38.7
Thyroid enlargement	10.8	9.0
Edema	5.4	6.8
Congestive failure	5.4	4.5
Pallor	4.3	4.5
Pleural effusion	2.2	
Ascites	2.2	
Pneumonia	2.2	
Abdominal mass	2.2	
Skin lesions	2.2	
Arthralgia	2.2	4.5
Mediastinal mass	1.1	
Splenic infarct	1.1	
Raynaud's phenomenon	0.5	

TABLE 10. *Degree of enlargement of various reticuloendothelial structures in patients with autoimmune hemolytic anemia (220 cases)*

Structure Palpated below Costal Margin	No. of Patients*						
	Spleen	Liver	Degree of lymphadenopathy				Hilar nodes
			1+	2+	3+	4+	
cm.							
At costal margin	10	5	39	27	14	10	3
Costal margin–2.9	27	26					
3.0–5.9	43	40					
6.0–8.9	15	22					
9.0–11.9	10	8					
12.0–14.9	2	2					
15.0–17.9	2	0					
18.0–20.9	3	2					
21 or greater	3	1					

* Only 57 patients had neither hepatosplenomegaly nor lymphadenopathy.

and was a valuable physical sign. Table 9 summarizes the various physical abnormalities noted.

Enlargement of various reticuloendothelial structures was common. Splenomegaly was present in approximately 50 per cent of both the idiopathic and secondary varieties of autoimmune hemolytic anemia. In general the spleen was firm, not tender and easily palpated. When measured in quiet respiration massive enlargement was rare. Palpated sizes of 21 cm. or larger were noted in only three cases. In 69 per cent of the cases the spleen was palpated less than 6 cm. below the costal margin. Accordingly, splenomegaly is only moderate in degree and spleen size appears to be less than that generally observed with chronic leukemias, hereditary spherocytosis and various inheritable lipid storage diseases. A splenic infarct was noted in two instances. Table 10 lists the degrees of splenomegaly found.

Hepatomegaly was common and more frequently observed in the secondary forms of autoimmune hemolytic anemias. The liver was generally firm and not tender. Massive enlargement was rare, and only five cases had liver enlargement greater than 12 cm. below the costal margin. As with splenic enlargement, hepatomegaly in the majority of cases was moderate and extended less than 6 cm. below the costal margin.

Lymphadenopathy was frequently documented. Differences in incidence were again observed with the secondary and idiopathic forms of autoimmune hemolytic anemia. Thirty-seven per cent of cases of the secondary variety and 23 per cent of the idiopathic types had palpable lymph nodes. The degree of enlargement was generally moderate, being recorded as 1+ or 2+ in most cases. These observations are also summarized in Table 10.

The large number of cases with an associated reticuloendothelial neoplasia makes an evaluation of the influence of autoimmune processes on the reticuloendothelium difficult. This difference of case material may explain Dacie's observation (3) that enlargement of lymph nodes does not usually occur in autoimmune hemolytic anemia. Enlargement of various reticuloendothelial structures appears as the most consistent abnormality found on physical examination. In general, splenomegaly, hepatomegaly and lymphadenopathy occur in association with each other. This is not inevitable. Individual and different combinations of such organ enlargement were noted. Only 26 per cent of all patients seen did not manifest enlargement of one or more of these reticuloendothelial structures.

Other physical findings were observed without any consistent regularity. Many were manifestations of the anemic state or of an underlying pathologic process. Congestive heart failure, pneumonia, various other infectious diseases, abdominal, mediastinal and thyroid masses, ascites, pleural effusions, hilar adenopathy, Raynaud's phenomenon and skin lesions were found. These observations are summarized in Table 9.

Incidence of Primary and Secondary Types of Autoimmune Hemolytic Anemia

Many reports of the relative incidence of idiopathic and secondary forms of autoimmune hemolytic anemia are available. Several of the pertinent observations are listed in Table 11. The publications of Dameshek and Komninos (75), Evans and Weiser (76) and Lal and Speiser (35) suggest that autoimmune hemolytic anemia is approximately evenly divided between idiopathic and secondary varieties. van Loghem and associates (77) noted that the

secondary variety was more common and was present in 55 per cent of the cases. A similar observation was made in the small series reported by Yunis and Bridges (6). Dausset and Colombani (4) and Dacie (3) have observed the reverse, with a substantially greater number of idiopathic cases. They reported an incidence of 70 per cent or higher of the idiopathic variety. Analysis of the 638 cases seen by these various investigators indicates an incidence of 57 per cent for the idiopathic form and 43 per cent for the secondary type.

The current series reported by this author is distinctly different. Of the 234 patients which have been studied, 44 patients or 18.8 per cent have been classified as having an idiopathic variety of autoimmune hemolytic anemia. The overwhelming number of cases (81.2 per cent) appeared in association with another pathologic abnormality sufficiently related to warrant a diagnosis of secondary autoimmune hemolytic anemia. It is important to examine the reasons for such a marked difference in this series, contrasted with those previously reported. Our patient population is characterized by many leukemia and lymphoma patients undergoing constant medical followup. This is reflected in a large number of cases of autoimmune

TABLE 11. *Comparative incidence of idiopathic (1°) and symptomatic (2°) forms of the autoimmune hemolytic anemias*

Series (reference)	Type of Antibody	Total Cases	AHA Type			
			1°		2°	
			No.	Per cent	No.	Per cent
Dameshek and Komninos (75)	Warm acting	43	21	50	22	50
Evans and Weiser (76)	Warm and cold acting	41	22	54	19	46
Lal and Speiser (35)	Warm acting	97	49	50	48	50
van Loghem and associates (77)	Warm and cold acting	122	55	45	67	55
Dausset and Colombani (4)	Warm and cold acting	128	93	73	35	27
Dacie (3)	Warm acting	129	89	70	40	30
	Cold acting	38	19	50	19	50
Yunis and Bridges (6)	Warm and cold acting	40	17	42.5	23	57.5
Total		638	365	57.2	273	42.8
Current series		234	44	18.8	190	81.2

hemolytic anemia associated with neoplasia of the reticuloendothelium. One hundred and fourteen patients have been studied. This represents an incidence of 48.7
per cent of the entire series or 60 per cent
of the secondary types. A deliberate search
for patients with autoimmune hemolytic
anemia has also been carried out. The routine employment of antiglobulin and proteolytic enzyme procedures in the investigation of any hematologic abnormality has
revealed a surprisingly large number of
positive results. The performance of the
immunohematologic tests in the research
laboratory and the employment of high
potency, broad spectrum antiglobulin serum
have also contributed greatly to the rate of
case discovery.

The type of antiglobulin serum employed
appears particularly important. Swisher
and associates (78) have used anti-gamma
and anti-C' antiglobulin sera in a similar
deliberate search for autoimmune hemolytic anemia. During a 6-year period they
found 188 antiglobulin positive cases, a
frequency greater than that in our current
series. Of these cases 107 had positive reactions graded as 1+ or higher. A high
incidence of the secondary type of autoimmune hemolytic anemia was noted. Of
the cases 32 per cent appeared as an idiopathic form and 73 per cent were of a
secondary type. Their cases were analyzed
for the presence of a rapidly falling hematocrit, chronic reticulocytosis, excessive
transfusion requirements and persistent
indirect bilirubinemia. By such criteria
it was determined that 91 per cent of the
idiopathic group and 42 per cent of the
secondary group had episodes of accelerated
hemolysis during the study. A similar lack
of correlation between positive antiglobulin tests and hemolysis was observed in
the current series.

Bohnen and associates (79) have reported the results of 17,000 direct antiglobulin tests performed in a 14-year
period; 178 patients with positive tests
were found. Only 13 patients or 7.3 per
cent of the series had idiopathic autoimmune hemolytic anemia. The remaining
92.7 per cent of the series had various

associated states. Unfortunately the data
of these authors do not suggest which patients had clinical hemolytic anemia, nor
do they indicate whether a classification
as a symptomatic form of autoimmune
hemolytic anemia is warranted. Many
examples of antiglobulin positive hemolytic anemia are included in their patient
group.

Swisher and associates (78) have drawn
some thought provoking conclusions from
their study. They suggest that two fundamentally different mechanisms for erythrocyte autosensitization exist. In one form
a true autoantibody is involved. This leads
to a positive anti-gamma-antiglobulin reaction. Complement is frequently involved,
resulting in an associated positive anti-C'
antiglobulin test. In contrast, many of the
secondary forms of autoimmune hemolytic
anemia only manifest anti-C' antiglobulin
reactions. It is suggested that such reactions result from unrelated antibody-antigen combinations fixing to an innocent
bystander erythrocyte. This latter group
would represent an immune but not autoimmune mechanism. In this volume such
reactions have been classified as antiglobulin positive hemolytic anemia. The distribution and the forms of secondary autoimmune hemolytic anemia noted in the
present series tend to support this hypothesis. In particular, the frequent association
of infectious disease with secondary forms
of autoimmune hemolytic anemia is striking (see Chapters 7 and 14).

Speiser (80) has presented a similar
study which also suggests two clinical patterns. This study was based on 540 patients
with positive antiglobulin reactions. Of
these patients, 220 had anemia as their
primary diagnosis, and presumably these
cases were considered to be idiopathic
autoimmune hemolytic anemia. The remaining 320 patients, or 60 per cent, had
secondary forms with various associated
diseases. Antiglobulin test results were
divided into strong and weak reacting
types. Approximately 65 per cent of the
secondary forms had weak reacting antiglobulin tests, and haptoglobin was absent
in 31 per cent of the group. In contrast,

only 47 per cent of the anemic form had weak antiglobulin reactions; 60 per cent of this primary type had absent haptoglobins.

In the current series many different underlying disease states were associated with autoimmune hemolytic anemia. Several pathologic conditions were present with a degree of regularity suggesting that a fortuitous occurrence was unlikely. Such conditions have previously been noted and include chronic lymphocytic leukemia, the lymphomas, other squamous neoplasia, systemic lupus erythematosus, various infectious diseases, including infectious mononucleosis, and ovarian cysts. The current series greatly expands this group. A listing of the clinical states associated with autoimmune hemolytic anemia in the present series is presented in Table 12. Each subgroup of this classification is expanded in detail at the start of the chapters discussing individual groups. The specific laboratory and clinical characteristics of the various associations are also presented in subsequent chapters. Several pertinent comments, however, must be made as to what determines a secondary type classification.

Classification of Autoimmune Hemolytic Anemia as a Secondary Type

The age range of patients with autoimmune hemolytic anemia makes it unlikely that many will be completely free of either past ailments or current medical problems at the onset of autoimmune hemolytic anemia. For example, either overt diabetes or diabetes developing concomitantly with corticosteroid therapy was commonly observed. In a similar fashion arteriosclerotic disease was frequently found in many patients presenting with autoimmune hemolytic anemia. Such associations have not been considered sufficiently striking to warrant diagnosis as etiologically related pathologic states. The assumption has been made that they represent the fortuitous occurrence of two relatively common disease states in the same patient. This assumption may not be correct. Several investigators (81) have suggested that diabetes represents a form of autoimmunization. If this should be true,

TABLE 12. *Primary and secondary types of warm acting autoimmune hemolytic anemia: 234 patients studied*

	No.	Per cent
I. Idiopathic (primary) type	44	18.2
II. Secondary (symptomatic) type	190	81.8
A. Neoplasia of the reticuloendothelium	114	48.7
1. The leukemias	77	32.9
a. Chronic lymphocytic	48	20.5
b. Others	29	12.4
2. The lymphomas	25	10.7
3. Plasma cell myeloma	9	3.8
4. Thymomas	3	1.3
B. Other malignancies	20	8.5
C. Benign cyst and tumor formation	16	6.8
D. Collagen and hypersensitivity diseases	35	15.0
E. Diseases of the thyroid	25	10.7
F. Infectious diseases		
1. Bacterial infections	53	22.6
2. Virus infections	21	9.0
3. Fungal infections	3	1.3
G. Diseases of the gastrointestinal tract	29	12.4
H. Miscellaneous group	21	9.0
1. Mechanical trauma, erythrocytes	9	3.8
2. Related to drugs	7	3.0
3. Iron deficiency	3	1.3
4. Myeloproliferative syndrome	1	0.4
5. Heterozygous pyruvate kinase deficiency	1	0.4

it will be necessary to reevaluate this association as a possible systemic autoimmune disease with two common manifestations.

Four main criteria were employed in the current series to diagnose a secondary form of autoimmune hemolytic anemia. (a) A relationship well recognized in past investigations was the first criterion. The development of autoimmune hemolytic anemia in patients with chronic lymphocytic leukemia or a lymphoma has automatically resulted in classification as a secondary form. The reverse clinical pattern is also accepted. The subsequent development of a disease such as systemic lupus erythematosus in a patient with autoimmune hemolytic anemia is considered to be evidence of a secondary relationship. Case 2 presented above illustrates such a sequence. (b) The second criterion was a regularity of association in the current series to the extent that a fortuitous relationship may be excluded. Pernicious anemia and various infectious diseases such as tuberculosis fall into this category. (c) An obvious association in the concomitant development of hemolytic anemia and of an additional pathologic state comprised the third criterion. Support for this association is frequently obtained by correction of the associated disease and simultaneous reversal of either the hemolytic state and/or the abnormal serologic test. Renal carcinoma, pernicious anemia, various infectious diseases and cases of drug toxicity illustrate this relationship. (d) The fourth criterion was the association of a disease state of presumed autoimmune etiology. Autoimmune hemolytic anemia may frequently appear as one part of a widespread systemic immunologic abnormality. The presence of an additional disease that is immunologically mediated suggests a significant relationship. Rheumatoid arthritis, serum sickness, thyroiditis, thymomas, ulcerative colitis, polyarteritis nodosa, pernicious anemia, scleroderma, systemic lupus erythematosus, etc., all fit into this category.

Autoimmune phenomena in the experimental animal and in the human being frequently result in extremely complex clinical states. Our terminology of disease is based on organ and system involvement. This anatomic orientation makes it difficult to classify disease syndromes that are dependent on physiologic abnormalities. Such diseases are manifest in multiple systems and cross many anatomic barriers. "Collagen diseases" (82) as a term was derived in an attempt to relate diseases of similar pathologic type to widespread protean clinical patterns. Even with this term, however, the anatomic boundary was maintained. Immunologically mediated disease presents a problem of classification never before contemplated. In the autoimmune syndromes clinical pictures are variable and are dependent on various host constituents functioning as target antigens

for multiple autoantibodies. Many of the disease patterns which result have previously been documented as specific entities. With multiple and simultaneous occurrences of such entities in one patient, the taxonomist is faced with a difficult task of classification. This is pertinent when the individual syndromes are possibly related through the same pathophysiologic mechanism. The classification of secondary types of autoimmune hemolytic anemia illustrates the problems encountered. The following two cases may be considered as examples.

Case 6. A 68-year-old white male was seen with urinary obstruction and benign prostatic hypertrophy. A nodular thyroid had been discovered at age 37. A retropubic prostatectomy was done. Four years later an enlarged nodular thyroid was again noted and diabetes was diagnosed. No therapy was given. Three years later the patient was seen with vomiting and jaundice. The hematocrit was 18 per cent and the reticulocyte count was 1.4 per cent. A megaloblastic bone marrow was found, no free acid could be demonstrated in the stomach secretions and a Schilling test revealed excretion of 0.3 per cent labeled vitamin B-12. The administration of intrinsic factor returned the Schilling test to normal. Six out of seven LE cell preparations were positive. Direct antiglobulin and bromelin test were positive on multiple occasions. Serologic tests for syphilis were positive. Vitamin B-12 and prednisone therapy were initiated. A reticulocyte response of 15.2 per cent occurred and was followed by a gradual return to normal hematocrit values. Prednisone was discontinued after 2 months and maintenance vitamin B-12 therapy was continued. The clinical course was complicated over the next year by pneumonia and recurrent pseudomonas cystitis. Hemolytic anemia did not occur. Thirty-four months after the start of anemia, an adenocarcinoma of the prostate was found and a large mediastinal mass was demonstrated by x-ray. Surgery was refused by the patient. Over the next 3 years the patient developed staphylococcus pneumonia and urinary obstruction which eventually led to death. Autopsy revealed adenocarcinoma of the prostate with invasion, a nodular adenomatous thyroid, a spindle cell type of thymoma and acute interstitial pancreatitis. Total course of disease dated from onset of antiglobulin positive state was 75 months; demonstrable thymoma was present for 41 months.

Exactly how should this patient be classified? This volume is concerned with autoimmune hemolytic anemia, so it is simple to list this case as a secondary type of autoimmune hemolytic anemia. But secondary to what? Is the development of the antiglobulin positive state related to one or all of the following: nodular adenomatous thyroid, pernicious anemia, systemic lupus erythematosus, adenocarcinoma of the prostate, spindle cell thymoma, pseudomonas cystitis, staphylococcus pneumonia and interstitial pancreatitis? The author has soothed his conscience and left out diabetes from these associated diseases.

Case 7. A 45-year-old white female was seen with complaints of photosensitivity, hyperpigmented skin and red urine. A diagnosis of porphyria cutanea tarda was made on the basis of diagnostic urine studies. Chelation therapy with ethylenediaminetetraacetic acid was followed by adenosine-5-monophosphoric acid. An episode of gout complicated this therapy. Corticosteroids were then initiated for persisting skin lesions. General alopecia and extreme fluid retention developed over the next 3 years. Hepatosplenomegaly was noted and marked hypoalbuminemia was found. Diffuse liver disease was present and skin lesions suggestive of scleroderma were found. This diagnosis was confirmed by skin biopsy. Marked bleeding occurred and the previous thrombocyte count of 292,000/mm.³ was now discovered to be 1,600/mm.³ Bone marrow examination was not diagnostic. Pleural effusions, ascites and pericarditis developed. LE cells were positive on two occasions. Oral infections and a lung abscess were now diagnosed. Positive direct antiglobulin tests were noted with an hematocrit of 29% and a reticulocytosis of 3.7 per cent. Lymphadenopathy, Raynaud's syndrome, azotemia and hypergammaglobulinemia developed. With corticosteroid therapy, thrombocytopenia, azotemia and anemia markedly improved. Followup is still continuing.

This patient may also be classified as a secondary form of autoimmune hemolytic anemia. But what is the underlying condition? Is it porphyria cutanea tarda, scleroderma, systemic lupus erythematosus, Evans' syndrome, liver disease (which could be called lupoid hepatitis) or is it related to a lung abscess?

These two cases, as well as many others in the current series, suggest that autoimmune hemolytic anemia may develop as one part of a multiple systemic immunologic abnormality. In order to classify the underlying or associated disease it is necessary to give equal significance to the various anatomically oriented diagnoses. Such a procedure has been carried out in the classification presented in Table 12. It is apparent that the percentage of involvement of such associated diseases is substantially over 100 per cent, reflecting multiple system involvement. It is tempting to avoid the entire problem and simply to create a new category entitled "diffuse autoimmune" or "diffuse immunologic" disease. This is not done for several reasons. Listing of associated diseases is valuable to the clinician as a listing of markers alerting him to the possible development of such syndromes. In addition, it is probable that all forms of autoimmune hemolytic anemia will fall into such a category. Our concept of idiopathic autoimmune hemolytic anemia may simply be illusory (73). With longer and more efficient followups the multisystem nature of the abnormality may become apparent. A logical extension of this view will be the elimination of the term "idiopathic" with the realization that only one facet of an immunologically mediated illness is present (73). It is possibly premature at this time to suggest that all cases of autoimmune hemolytic anemia represent a systemic immunologic disease, with associated diseases related to the same pathogenesis. The accurate separation of hemolytic anemia with positive serologic tests into autoimmune and antiglobulin positive types may eventually permit such a conclusion.

Clinical Pattern of Associated Diseases

If the concepts presented above are valid, a pattern of types of associated diseases underlying autoimmune hemolytic anemia should become apparent. Two different clinical states may be logically anticipated. In one form the associated disease would supply foreign antigens or create autologous antigens so modified as to appear foreign to the immune apparatus of the host. The erythrocyte may be involved directly in the modification or through a cross reacting system. It may be indirectly concerned as an innocent bystander offering a surface for an unrelated immune reaction. This group represents the previously hypothesized antiglobulin positive type of hemolytic anemia. It probably corresponds to the pure anti-C′ antiglobulin reaction group of secondary autoimmune hemolytic anemia described by Swisher and associates (78). Infectious diseases, drug reactions, trauma to the erythrocyte and ovarian cysts appear in the current series as major disease categories which may create hemolytic anemia through such mechanisms. Such states are not rare; 104 examples

were encountered in the current series. Table 13 summarizes the number and the types of cases which possibly may be placed in this category.

The second form of autoimmune hemolytic anemia may represent true autoimmunization. As such, evidence of systemic immunologic disease with multiple target organs may be anticipated. The best guide to this group is the presence of additional diseases which may involve immunologic mechanisms. Table 14 summarizes the associated diseases seen which currently may be placed in this category. Associated diseases characterized by either immunologic activity or a postulated immune etiology are frequently observed. In this series there were 114 examples of neoplasia of reticuloendothelial structures. The involvement of such neoplastic tissue in widespread immunologic diseases resembling graft-host disease has been postulated (66). Other diseases that have been considered as autoimmune are also frequently seen. These include thyroid disease, lupus erythematosus, pernicious anemia, rheumatoid arthritis, ulcerative colitis, scleroderma, etc. In all, 189 examples of immunologically dependent disease syndromes associated with secondary forms of autoimmune hemolytic anemia were found. It should again be emphasized that the number of patients classified in Tables 13 and 14 totals greater than 100 per cent. This reflects multiple system involvement.

TABLE 13. *Associated diseases in patients with symptomatic forms of autoimmune hemolytic anemia which may represent an antiglobulin positive type of mechanism*

Disease States	No. of Patients
Bacterial infections	53
Viral infections	21
Fungus infections	3
Trauma to erythrocytes	9
Drugs	7
Ovarian cysts	5
Iron deficiency	3
Folic acid deficiency	2
Pyruvate kinase deficiency	1
Total	104

TABLE 14. *Associated diseases in patients with autoimmune hemolytic anemia which have been previously postulated as involving immunologic mechanisms**

Disease States	No.	Disease States	No.
Lymphocytic leukemias	58	Ulcerative colitis	5
Monocytic leukemias	12	Scleroderma	3
Granulocytic leukemias	7	Idiopathic arthritis	3
Lymphomas	25	Sjögren's syndrome	1
Plasma cell myeloma	9	Polyarteritis nodosa	1
Thymoma	3	Serum sickness	1
Thyroid disease	25	Erythema multiforma	1
Lupus erythematosus	13	Erythema nodosa	1
Cirrhosis	8	Dermoid cyst	1
Rheumatoid arthritis	5	Mycosis fungoides	1
Pernicious anemia	5	Infectious hepatitis	1

* Total: 189 patients.

The 190 patients classified as having a secondary form of autoimmune hemolytic anemia have a total of 316 possibly significant associated diseases. Of these 189 appear immunologically oriented. In 104 instances an antiglobulin positive form of hemolytic anemia may have been created. Only 23 examples do not fit this pattern of two clinical categories. These include squamous cell malignancies, myeloproliferative syndromes and a parotid gland tumor. These cases may represent examples of a fortuitous occurrence of two unrelated syndromes. The possibility of subclinical bacterial or virus infections undetected in the usual hospital workup cannot be eliminated. Eventually these still unclassified associated diseases may be related to one or the other postulated patterns. For example, squamous cell malignancy may eventually be considered to represent failure of the immune self-recognition mechanism.

Summary

The current series presents a surprising predominance of secondary varieties of autoimmune hemolytic anemia. A confusing spectrum of associated diseases is present. Such conditions determine or influence many of the clinical characteristics of autoimmune hemolytic anemia. Superficially the associated diseases are heterogeneous and appear to defy analysis. They may be broadly grouped into nine separate categories which include over 50 specific disease entities. A more detailed analysis of these associated pathologic states suggests that they fall into either of two different etiologic categories. One type of associated disease pattern may lead to hemolytic anemia of an immune but not autoimmune type. This has been termed antiglobulin positive hemolytic anemia. The second type of associated disease has a common characteristic relating to an immunologic abnormality. In this group autoimmune hemolytic anemia appears as one of several syndromes reflecting a widespread systemic immunologic disease. These two groups are commonly considered together and are difficult to distinguish.

The end stage observation of an immunologic reaction involving and damaging the erythrocyte is similar. Further clinical and diagnostic procedures are needed to supplement the clinician's ability to clarify and document these two distinct pathophysiologic mechanisms.

BIBLIOGRAPHY

1. Dameshek, W.: Hemolytic anemia (reply to Letter to Editor). J. A. M. A. 176: 252, 1961.
2. Thompson, R. E.: Acquired hemolytic anemia. A review of 26 cases, including 5 of the hemolytic-uremic syndrome, with emphasis on the usefulness of steroids in therapy. Clin. Pediat. (Phila.) 6: 288, 1967.
3. Dacie, J. V.: The Haemolytic Anaemias, Part II, Ed. 2. Grune & Stratton, Inc., New York, 1962.
4. Dausset, J., and Colombani, J.: The serology and the prognosis of 128 cases of autoimmune hemolytic anemia. Blood 14: 1280, 1959.
5. Swisher, S. N.: Acquired hemolytic disease. Postgrad. Med. 40: 378, 1966.
6. Yunis, E. J., and Bridges, R. A.: Blood transfusion problems in autoimmune hemolytic anemias. Minnesota Med. 49: 759, 1966.
7. Letman, H.: Red cell destruction in the anaemias (thesis). Copenhagen, 1959.
8. Pirofsky, B., August, A., Nelson, H., and Pittenger, R.: Rapid mass anti-D (Rh₀) typing with bromelin. J. Lab. Clin. Med. 56: 911, 1960.
9. Broman, B.: Further observations on the Rh antigen Dᵘ. In Proceedings of the Fourth International Congress of the International Society of Hematology. Grune & Stratton, Inc., New York, 1954.
10. O'Connor, W. J., Vakiener, J. M., and Watson, R. J.: Idiopathic acquired hemolytic anemia in young children. Pediatrics 17: 732, 1956.
11. Negri, M., Pototschnig, C., and Maiolo, A. T.: L'anemia emolitica da autoanticorpi nello prima infanzia. Presentazione di im caso. Minerva Pediat. 12: 656, 1960.
12. Malaguzzi Valeri, O., Di Piero, G., and Carapella, E.: Considerazione su 11 casi di anemia emolitica autoimmune in età pediatrica. Riv. Ist. Sieroter. Ital. 39: 215, 1964.
13. Laski, B., Wake, E. J., Gunson, H., and Bain, H. W.: Idiopathic acquired anemia in two young infants. Amer. J. Dis. Child. 100: 524, 1960.
14. Gross, S., and Newman, D. J.: Autoimmune anti-D specificity in infancy. Amer. J. Dis. Child. 108: 181, 1964.
15. Di Piero, G., Mencarini, L., and Stegagno, G.: Anemia emolitica autoimmune con autoanticorpi anti-c in lattante. (Guarigione clinical dopo 23 mesi.) Rev. Clin. Pediat. 77: 305, 1966.
16. Unger, L. J., Wiener, A. S., and Dolan, D.:

Auto-hemolytic anemia in a newborn. Rev. Hemat. (Paris) **7**: 495, 1952.

17. Bakx, C. J. A., and van Loghem, J. J.: Acquired hemolytic anemia in a newborn. Vox Sang. **42**: 79, 1957.

18. Germain, D., Jeune, M., and Jouvenceaux, A.: Anémie hémolytique auto-immune à anti-corps chauds chez un nourrisson de trois mois (revêtement érythrocytaire non gamma-globulinique puis mixte). Med. Infant. (Paris) **72**: 501, 1965.

19. Ritz, N. D., and Haber, A.: Autoimmune hemolytic anemia in a six-week-old child. J. Pediat. **61**: 904, 1962.

20. Iafusco, F., and Buffa, V.: Autoimmune hemolytic anemia in a newborn infant. Pediatria (Napoli) **70**: 1256, 1962.

21. Gasser, C., and Holländer, L.: Anémie hémolytique acquise aiguë provoquée par des auto-anticorps, accompagnée de purpura thrombocytopénique, chez un nourrisson de 7 semaines. Rev. Hemat. (Paris) **6**: 316, 1951.

22. Denys, P., and van den Broucke, J.: Anémie hémolytique acquise et réaction de Coombs. Arch. Franc. Pediat. **4**: 205, 1947.

23. Larson, A.: Chronic idiopathic autoimmune hemolytic disease in childhood. Acta Paediat. (Scand.) **46**: 144, 1957.

24. Di Piero, G.: Su una nuova osservazione di anemia emolitica acquisata in eta pediatrica. Haematologica **44**: 989, 1959.

25. Cortesi, M.: A case of acute hemolytic anemia caused by auto-antibodies in an infant girl. Minerva Pediat. **13**: 1375, 1961.

26. Cabassa, N., Borgatti, L., and Lucci, R.: Autoimmune hemolytic anemia. Description of 2 cases in the 1st year of life. Arcisped. S. Anna Ferrara **15**: 397, 1962.

27. Bartolozzi, G., Pavari, E., and Guazzelli, C.: Anemia emolitica autoimmune in un lattante. Riv. Clin. Pediat. **72**: 249, 1963.

28. van Loghem, J. J., van der Hart, M., and van der Veer, M.: Verworven hemolytische Anemie met Auto-antistoffen bij Kinderen. Nederl. T. Geneesk. **108**: 438, 1964.

29. Rowecka-Trzebicka, K.: Nabytej niedokrwostôsci hemolitycznej na tie autoimmunizacji u 7-letniego chlopca. Pediat. Pol. **39**: 433, 1964.

30. Antonelli, G., and Vaccaro, R.: Considerazione sulla evoluzione dell'anemia emolitica auto-immune "protopatica" nell'età infantile. Clin. Pediat. (Bologna) **47**: 526, 1965.

31. Orsini, A., Rayband, C., Raoux, J. P., et al.: Anémie hémolytique par auto-anticorps chez un nourrisson. Pediatrie **20**: 865, 1965.

32. Stiehm, E. R., and Fudenberg, H. H.: Serum levels of immune globulins in health and disease: a survey. Pediatrics **37**: 715, 1966.

33. Zuelzer, W. W., Stulberg, C. S., Page, R. H., Teruya, J., and Brough, A. J.: The etiology and pathogenesis of acquired hemolytic anemia. Transfusion **6**: 438, 1966.

34. Sacks, M., Workman, J. B., and Jahn, E. F.: Diagnosis and treatment of acquired hemolytic anemia. J. A. M. A. **150**: 1556, 1952.

35. Lal, V. B., and Speiser, P.: Untersuchungen über Zusammenhänge zwischen erworbenen hämolytischen Anämien, klassischen Blutgruppen, Rhesusfactor, Geschlecht und Alter. Blut **3**: 15, 1957.

36. Burt, R. L., and Prichard, R. W.: Acquired hemolytic anemia in pregnancy. Obstet. Gynec. **10**: 444, 1957.

37. Seip, M.: Systemic lupus erythematosus in pregnancy with haemolytic anaemia, leucopenia and thrombocytopenia in the mother and her newborn infant. Arch. Dis. Child. **35**: 364, 1960.

38. Wagner, K., and Maresch, W.: Hämolytische Anämie und inkomplette Rhesus-Antikörper (anti-c) bei einer Schwangeren. Wien. Klin. Wschr. **67**: 856, 1955.

39. Wirtheimer, C.: Grossesse et anémie hémolytique. Bruxelles Med. **37**: 539, 1957.

40. Mallarmé, J., Auzépy, P., and Bercovici, J. P.: Un cas d'anémie hémolytique, acquise avec leucopénie et thrombopénie, de la grossesse. Nouv. Rev. Franc. Hemat. **5**: 765, 1965.

41. Jankelowitz, T., Eckerling, B., and Joshua, H.: A case of acquired hemolytic anemia associated with pregnancy. S. Afr. Med. J. **34**: 911, 1960.

42. Lie-Injo, L. E., and Pillay, R. P.: Idiopathic autoimmune hemolytic anemia in Malaya. Acta Haemat. (Basel) **31**: 282, 1964.

43. Pirofsky, B., and Shearn, M.: The familial occurrence of disseminated lupus erythrematosus. New York J. Med. **53**: 3022, 1953.

44. Leonhardt, T.: Familial studies in systemic lupus erythematosus. Acta Med. Scand. **176**: (suppl.): 416, 1964.

45. Fudenberg, H., German, J. L., and Kunkel, H.: The occurrence of rheumatoid factor and other abnormalities in families of patients with agammaglobulinemia. Arthritis Rheum. **5**: 565, 1962.

46. McIntyre, P. A., Hahn, R., Conley, C. L., and Glass, B.: Genetic factors in predisposition to pernicious anemia. Bull. Hopkins Hosp. **104**: 309, 1959.

47. Doniach, D., Roitt, I. M., and Taylor, K. B.: Autoimmunity in pernicious anemia and thyroiditis: a family study. Ann. N. Y. Acad. Sci. **124**: 605, 1965.

48. Hall, R., Owen, S. G., and Smart, G. A.: Evidence for genetic predisposition to formation of thyroid autoantibodies. Lancet **2**: 187, 1960.

49. Hung, W., and Winship, T.: Stroma lymphomatosa in mother and daughter with serologic and histologic evidence. J. Clin. Endocr. **23**: 465, 1963.

50. Bielschowsky, M., Helyer, B. J., and Howie, J. B.: Spontaneous hemolytic anemia in mice of the NZB/BL strain. Proc. Univ. Otago Med. Sch. **37**: 9, 1959.

51. Howie, J. B., and Helyer, B. J.: Autoimmune disease in mice. Ann. N. Y. Acad. Sci. **124**: 167, 1965.

52. Kissmeyer-Nielsen, F., Bent-Hansen, K., and

Kieler, J.: Immuno-hemolytic anemia with familial occurrence. Acta Med. Scand. **144:** 35, 1952.

53. Vajda, I., Aszodi, L., Hajdu, B., Stenszky, E., Barzo, P., and Howath, E.: Familial relationship in acquired hemolytic anemia. Magyar Belorv. Arch. **13:** 121, 1960.

54. Dobbs, C. E.: Familial auto-immune hemolytic anemia. Arch. Intern. Med. (Chicago) **116:** 273, 1965.

55. Cordova, M. S., Baez-Villaenor, J., Mendez, J. J., and Campos, E.: Acquired hemolytic anemia with positive antiglobulin test (Coombs' test) in mother and daughter. Arch. Intern. Med. (Chicago) **117:** 692, 1966.

56. Schwartz, R. S., and Costea, N.: Autoimmune hemolytic anemia; clinical correlations and biological implications. Sem. Hemat. **3:** 2, 1966.

57. Hennemann, H. H., and Krause, H.: Chronische Thrombozytopenie (Morbus werlhof) und Erworbene hämolytische Anämie bei zwei Schwestern. Deutsch. Med. Wschr. **89:** 1161, 1964.

58. Dreyfus, B.: Rôle probable d'un facteur héréditaire dans le déterminisme de certaines anémies hémolytiques par auto-anticorps. Nouv. Rev. Franc. Hemat. **4:** 669, 1964.

59. Fialkow, P. J., Fudenberg, H., and Epstein, W. V.: "Acquired" antibody hemolytic anemia and familial aberrations in gamma globulins. Amer. J. Med. **36:** 188, 1964.

60. Jakobowicz, R., Bryce, L. M., and Simmons, R. T.: The occurrence of unusual positive Coombs' reactions and M variants in the blood of a mother and her first child. Med. J. Aust. **2:** 245, 1949.

61. Jensen, K. G., and Freiesleben, E.: Inherited positive Coombs' reaction connected with a weak N-receptor (N₂). Vox Sang. **7:** 676, 1962.

62. Jeannet, M., Metaxas-Buhler, M., and Tobler, R.: Anomalie héréditaire de la membrane érythrocytaire avec test de Coombs positif et modification de l'antigène de groupe N. J. Suisse Med. **42:** 1508, 1963.

63. Burnet, F. M.: Theories of immunity. In *Conceptual Advances in Immunology and Oncology.* Hoeber Medical Division, Harper & Row, Publishers, New York, 1963.

64. Ziff, M.: Genetics, hypersensitivity and the connective tissue diseases. Amer. J. Med. **30:** 1, 1961.

65. Fudenberg, H.: Immunologic deficiency, autoimmune disease, and lymphoma: observations, implications and speculations. Arthritis Rheum. **9:** 464, 1966.

66. Pirofsky, B.: Autoimmune hemolytic anemia and neoplasia of the reticuloendothelium. With a hypothesis concerning etiologic relationships. Ann. Intern. Med. (Chicago) **68:** 109, 1968.

67. Kellum, M. J., Sutherland, D. E., Eckert, E.,

Peterson, R. D. H., and Good, R. A.: Wasting disease, Coombs positivity, and amyloidosis in rabbits subjected to central lymphoid tissue extirpation and irradiation. Int. Arch. Allerg. **27:** 6, 1965.

68. Schaller, J., Davis, S. D., Chung, Y., Lagunoff, D., Williams, C. P. S., and Wedgewood, R. J.: Hypergammaglobulinemia, antibody deficiency, autoimmune hemolytic anemia, and nephritis in an infant with a familial lymphopenic immune defect. Lancet **2:** 825, 1966.

69. Miller, J. F. A. P., Osoba, D., and Dukor, P.: A humoral thymus mechanism responsible for immunologic maturation. Ann. N. Y. Acad. Sci. **124:** 95, 1965.

70. Mellors, R. C., and Huang, C. Y.: Immunopathology of NZB/BL mice. V. Virus-like (filterable) agent separable from lymphoma cells and identifiable by electron microscopy. J. Exp. Med. **124:** 1031, 1966.

71. Mellors, R. C., and Huang, C. Y.: Immunopathology of NZB/BL mice. VI. Virus separable from spleen and pathogenic for Swiss mice. J. Exp. Med. **126:** 53, 1967.

72. Pirofsky, B., and Vaughn, M.: Addisonian pernicious anemia with positive antiglobulin tests; a multiple autoimmune disease syndrome. Amer. J. Clin. Path. **50:** 459, 1968.

73. Pirofsky, B.: Hereditary aspects of autoimmune hemolytic anemia; a retrospective analysis. Vox Sang. **14:** 334, 1968.

74. Dacie, J. V.: Prognosis in autoimmune hemolytic anemia. Aust. Ann. Med. **2:** 11, 1963.

75. Dameshek, W., and Komninos, Z. D.: The present status of treatment of autoimmune hemolytic anemia with ACTH and cortisone. Blood **11:** 648, 1956.

76. Evans, R. S., and Weiser, R. S.: The serology of auto-immune hemolytic disease: observations on forty-one patients. Arch. Intern. Med. (Chicago) **100:** 371, 1957.

77. van Loghem, J. J., van der Hart, M., and Dorfmeier, H.: Serologic studies in acquired hemolytic anemia. In *Proceedings of the Sixth International Congress of the International Society of Hematology.* Grune & Stratton, Inc., New York, 1956.

78. Swisher, S. N., Trabold, N., Leddy, J. P., and Vaughn, J.: Clinical correlations of the direct antiglobulin reaction. Ann. N. Y. Acad. Sci. **124:** 441, 1965.

79. Bohnen, R. F., Ultmann, J. E., Gorman, J. G., Farhangi, M., and Scudder, J.: The direct Coombs' test: its clinical significance. Ann. Intern. Med. **68:** 19, 1968.

80. Speiser, P.: Some remarks on human erythrocytic autoantibodies. Z. Immunitaetsforsch. **132:** 113, 1967.

81. Burch, P. R. J., Rowell, N. R., and Burwell, R. G.: Autoimmunity and chromosomal aberrations. Lancet **2:** 170, 1966.

82. Klemperer, P.: Concept of collagen diseases. Amer. J. Path. **26:** 505, 1950.

Chapter 3

General Laboratory Observations

The multisystem manifestations of immunologic disease create complex clinical and laboratory problems. The clinician must resort to the laboratory in order to document a heterogeneous collection of abnormalities. A summary of the laboratory observations encountered in a large collection of patients with autoimmune hemolytic anemia is presented below. The clinician should employ such data to interpret the confusing array of laboratory results seen during management of such patients. The results obtained reflect analysis of all patients studied with autoimmune hemolytic anemia in the current series. For the individual abnormalities characteristic of specific forms of autoimmune hemolytic anemia, the separate sections in subsequent chapters should be consulted.

The Peripheral Blood

The peripheral blood requires detailed and meticulous examination. The most important initial test in autoimmune hemolytic anemia is quantitation of the formed elements. An interpretation of the morphologic characteristics of the erythrocytes is equally crucial. Repeat studies of the peripheral blood are essential to evaluate the extent of disease, the effect of therapeutic regimes and evidence of either relapse or remission.

The Hematocrit

Some method of estimating red cell mass is necessary. Hemoglobin and erythrocyte count values are useful and are frequently employed. The hematocrit is well suited for this purpose. This procedure has a low incidence of technical error and is reproducible in the average diagnostic laboratory. Morphologic changes of erythrocytes will influence the hematocrit. For example, a substantial number of spherocytes will tend to reduce the hematocrit value. A large number of reticulocytes and/or macrocytes will have a reverse effect, elevating the hematocrit.

In the current series *initial* diagnostic hematocrit values were available in 218 patients. Figure 5 presents the figures obtained. A range of values from 9 per cent to 44.5 per cent was found. A moderate degree of anemia was the rule with a median hematocrit approximating 24 per cent. Seventeen cases had a severe anemic state with initial hematocrit values of 15 per cent or lower. Only seven patients were initially seen with normal hematocrit values of 39 per cent or higher.

Although the hematocrit may be only moderately depressed at the onset of hemolytic anemia, meticulous followup is necessary. A further reduction of the hematocrit may be anticipated. The hematocrit may rapidly fall. The term hemolytic crisis is frequently employed to describe this state. Relapse after remission may create an even more severe anemia than that initially found. When therapy is first started remission is induced after a variable period of time. During this time the hematocrit may progressively fall. Figure 6 presents the lowest hematocrit values obtained during the course of disease in 213 patients. Such an analysis clearly demonstrates that severe anemia is the rule in autoimmune hemolytic anemia. Forty-nine patients had

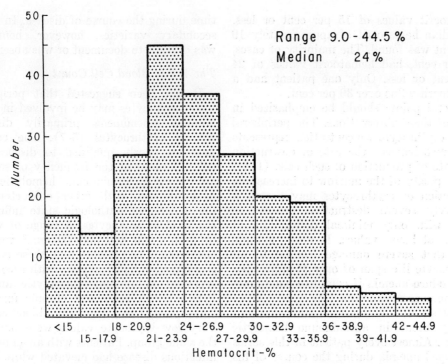

FIG. 5. The hematocrit obtained upon initial examination of 218 patients with autoimmune hemolytic anemia.

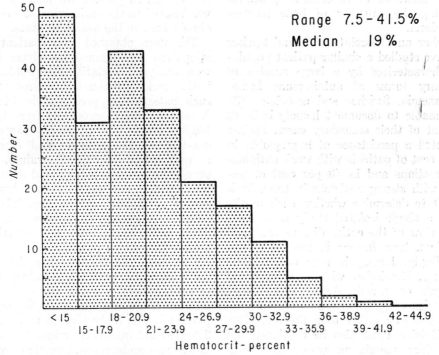

FIG. 6. The lowest hematocrit observed during the course of disease in 213 patients with autoimmune hemolytic anemia.

hematocrit values of 15 per cent or less. A median hematocrit of approximately 19 per cent was found. The majority of cases, 73 per cent, had hematocrit values of 24 per cent or less. Only one patient had a hematocrit value over 39 per cent.

Several points should be emphasized in view of these observations. The peripheral blood erythrocyte concentration represents a balance between the rate of destruction and rate of production of such cells (1, 2). The capacity of the marrow to increase its production of erythrocytes may permit a relatively severe destructive process to occur with only minimal deficiencies of peripheral blood values. It may be theorized that severe damage leading to an erythrocyte life span of only 15 days may not produce anemia if complete bone marrow compensation occurs. The current series indicates that this theorized state does not usually occur in autoimmune hemolytic anemia. Almost every patient in this series developed anemia during the course of his disease. This suggests either an inability of the bone marrow to compensate completely or the existence of destructive processes exceeding the capacity of bone marrow hyperplasia.

Swisher and associates (3) and Speiser (4) have studied a similar patient population characterized by a large number of secondary forms of autoimmune hemolytic anemia. Swisher and associates (3) were unable to document hemolysis in 42 per cent of their secondary cases. Speiser (4) noted a persistence of haptoglobin in 69 per cent of patients with weak antiglobulin reactions and in 40 per cent of patients with strong antiglobulin tests. It is difficult to determine whether such results reflect a single isolated study or a composite view of the entire disease course in a patient. The former is probably true. Accordingly, hemolysis may occur intermittently. Remission without evidence of hemolysis or anemia during the natural progression of autoimmune hemolytic anemia is the rule rather than the exception. The clinician must also be cautioned not to consider anemia as synonymous with hemolysis. In the current series anemia was almost universally present at some time during the course of disease. In many secondary varieties, however, hemolysis was difficult to document or was absent.

The White Blood Cell Count

It has been suggested that peripheral blood leukocytes may be involved in autoimmune phenomena primarily directed against erythrocytes (5–7). The current series is poorly qualified to discuss this point because of the frequency of secondary forms of autoimmune hemolytic anemia. As seen with other characteristics, the underlying pathologic state influences the level of leukocytes. A range of values between 1,000 and 590,000/mm.^{3} was encountered. The patients with these two extreme counts had leukemia with secondary types of autoimmune hemolytic anemia. Patients with acute and chronic forms of leukemia had very high white blood counts. Very low leukocyte values were found in the same group. Patients with an associated infectious disease had elevated white blood cell counts. Cases of systemic lupus erythematosus tended to have low white blood cell values. In general, the leukocyte count was related to the underlying disease more closely than to the hemolytic state.

The data obtained from patients with idiopathic autoimmune hemolytic anemia were analyzed to clarify this problem. The initial leukocyte counts obtained from 39 such patients are presented in Figure 7. A range of values extending from 1,400 to 108,000/mm.^{3} was obtained. More than one-half of the patients had essentially normal white blood cell values. However, significant elevations and depressions were noted. Six patients had leukocyte counts of 2,000/mm.^{3} or less. These occurred in a pattern of peripheral pancytopenia with hypoplastic or normal bone marrows. Seven patients had elevated white blood cell counts. Elevations ranging from 13,100 to 37,000/mm.^{3} were found in six. Leukocytosis reflected an increased number of neutrophilic granulocytes (five patients). The highest value was seen in a 2½-year-old infant. As might be expected at this age, an increased number of lymphocytes resulted in the leukocytosis. Bone marrow hyperplasia was generally present

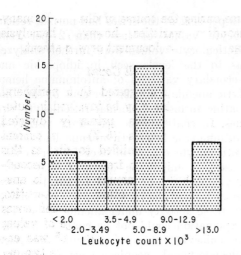

FIG. 7. The leukocyte count ($\times 10^3/mm.^3$) obtained upon initial examination of 39 patients with idiopathic autoimmune hemolytic anemia.

in these patients. The leukocytosis apparently reflected a total bone marrow response in the presence of severe anemic stress. The patient with a white blood count of 108,000/mm.³ represented a different category. An antiglobulin positive state with mild anemia developed during an acute allergic reaction secondary to penicillin. The elevated white blood count was due to an 88 per cent eosinophile count. It may seriously be questioned whether an idiopathic diagnosis is warranted in this patient.

Thrombocyte Values

In 1949 Evans and Duane (8) recorded the presence of thrombocytopenia in patients with autoimmune hemolytic anemia. This relationship was further documented in subsequent reports (9). It has since been confirmed repeatedly by many observers (10–17). The simultaneous occurrence of thrombocytopenia and autoimmune hemolytic anemia is now well recognized and is frequently referred to as "Evans' syndrome."

The extent and frequency of thrombocytopenia in the current series of patients with autoimmune hemolytic anemia were difficult to determine. Associated pathologic states, myelophthisic changes and chemotherapy all influenced the level of

thrombocytes. Accordingly, analysis was feasible only in patients without neoplasia of the reticuloendothelium. Adequate initial thrombocyte determinations were available in 77 such patients. Forty-six cases or 60 per cent had essentially normal values ranging from 100,000 to 300,000/mm.³ Thirteen patients had elevated thrombocyte values over 300,000/mm.³ In 11 cases there was marked depression of thrombocytes with values below 20,000/mm.³ A range of thrombocyte counts from less than 1,000 to over 1 million/mm.³ was seen.

An analysis of idiopathic and secondary varieties revealed marked differences in the two groups. Figure 8 summarizes these data. Thirty-one patients had the idiopathic form and 45 per cent were found to be thrombocytopenic; seven patients had thrombocyte values below 20,000/mm.³ One patient presented with idiopathic thrombocytosis and thrombocyte counts over 1 million/mm.³ Bean (18) has suggested that thrombocytosis may represent one facet of a systemic autoimmune disease. The possibility of a nonspecific bone marrow response under the stress of a hemo-

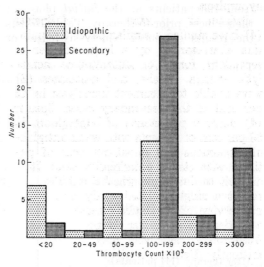

FIG. 8. The thrombocyte count ($\times 10^3/mm.^3$) obtained upon initial examination of 31 patients with idiopathic autoimmune hemolytic anemia and 46 selected patients with secondary varieties of autoimmune hemolytic anemia. Patients with an associated reticuloendothelial malignancy are excluded from analysis.

lytic state must also be considered. In contrast, only four patients or 9 per cent with secondary forms of autoimmune hemolytic anemia had thrombocyte counts below 100,000/mm.^{3} The two patients with thrombocyte values below 20,000/mm.^{3} were initially classified as having an idiopathic variety of Evans' syndrome. Systemic lupus erythematosus was eventually diagnosed in both (see Cases 2 and 7).

Reticulocyte Counts

In 1907 Chauffard (19) applied Ehrlich's stain to the peripheral blood of patients suffering from hemolytic anemia and discovered reticulocytes. Since this initial observation the measurement of reticulocytes in the peripheral blood has become a standard procedure in studying hemolytic anemia.

It is generally assumed that chronic and persistent reticulocytosis is inevitable in autoimmune hemolytic anemia. However, Crosby and Rappaport (20) reported the presence of reticulocytopenia and noted its association in aplastic states. The current series was analyzed with this observation in mind. Reticulocyte counts were obtained from 195 patients at the *initial* phase of their illness, prior to therapy. Table 15 lists the results obtained. Ninety-six cases or

49 per cent of the series had normal reticulocyte values of less than 2 per cent. Reticulocyte values were further analyzed as to the levels seen in idiopathic and secondary varieties of autoimmune hemolytic anemia. Only 26 per cent of the idiopathic forms had normal reticulocyte values. In contrast, the secondary variety of autoimmune hemolytic anemia had normal reticulocyte counts in over 50 per cent of cases. It might be assumed that either myelophthisic or chemotherapeutic processes limited the bone marrow's capacity to increase activity under anemic stress. This explanation could not be confirmed. When reticulocyte values of patients with reticuloendothelial neoplasia were examined *after* initiation of therapy, normal reticulocyte values persisted in only 17 per cent of cases. In over 83 per cent of the secondary varieties the ability of bone marrow to respond was noted. This response rate was comparable to that found in idiopathic forms.

It may surprise the clinician to note that 26 per cent of cases of idiopathic autoimmune hemolytic anemia initially had low to normal reticulocyte counts. In five, reticulocyte values were abnormally low, ranging from 0.0 to 0.3 per cent. These cases were initially misdiagnosed and con-

TABLE 15. *Reticulocyte counts seen in patients with autoimmune hemolytic anemia prior to and after initiation of therapy*

	Total Patients	<2%		2–4.9%		5–9.9%		>10%	
		No.	Per cent	No.	Per cent	No.	Per cent	No.	Per cent
Before therapy (195 patients)									
Idiopathic autoimmune type	35	9	25.7	8	22.9	8	22.9	10	28.6
Secondary type—neoplasia of reticuloendothelium	101	56	55.5	26	25.7	15	14.9	4	3.9
Secondary type—all others	59	31	52.5	13	22.0	9	15.3	6	10.2
Total	195	96	49.2	47	24.1	32	16.4	20	10.3
After therapy (144 patients)									
Idiopathic autoimmune type	25	4	16	4	16	5	20	12	48
Secondary type—neoplasia of reticuloendothelium	81	14	17.3	29	35.8	24	29.6	14	17.3
Secondary type—all others	38	2	5.3	9	23.7	9	23.7	18	47.4
Total	144	20	13.9	42	29.2	38	26.4	44	30.6

sidered as typical examples of aplastic anemia or pure erythrocytic aplasia. The hemolytic syndrome was unsuspected until routine transfusion therapy revealed a positive antiglobulin test. The clinical and theoretical implications of this patient group are discussed in Chapter 4.

Morphologic Changes of the Erythrocytes

A normochromic normocytic anemia is generally found in patients with autoimmune hemolytic anemia. Morphologic abnormalities of the erythrocytes, however, can distort this picture. A large number of spherocytes may suggest the presence of a microcytic anemia. A marked reticulocytosis will lead to macrocytosis and a macrocytic anemia may be suggested. A combination of these changes may result in the morphologic pattern of a "double population" of cells considered typical of hereditary spherocytosis.

In the current series no attempt was made to analyze retrospectively the peripheral blood smears of patients; rather, the initial interpretation of the laboratory technologist has been accepted in order to closely duplicate observations that the clinician will encounter in his own practice. The figures presented below may be higher than those seen in the average hospital. The technologists reporting the current series are particularly skilled in hematologic examinations. On the other hand, a retrospective analysis by a trained hematologist would be expected to increase substantially the reported observations.

Reports were available for 212 patients. Nucleated erythrocytes were noted in 72 cases or 34 per cent of the series. The immature red cells generally appeared at the metarubricyte (normoblast) level of maturity. Younger forms were occasionally found. Spherocytes were reported in 63 cases or 30 per cent of the series. The degree of spherocytosis may be quite marked. Lowman (21) has emphasized that the morphologic changes may even suggest the presence of hereditary spherocytosis. He has reported 11 cases of autoimmune hemolytic anemia, of which one-half were misdiagnosed as familial spherocytic types

because of spherocytosis. Macrocytes were only described in 14 cases or 7 per cent of patients. Seven of these patients had pernicious anemia or a folic acid deficiency. It is apparent that the term "macrocytes" in our laboratory is generally equated with "macrocytic anemia." Accordingly, this latter figure gives no index of the incidence of occasional macrocytes found in the blood smears of patients with autoimmune hemolytic anemia. Benitez (22) has emphasized that immunohemolytic anemias may present a predominantly macrocytic picture. Nucleated erythrocytes and spherocytes were generally observed in the same patients. Such individuals also presented with the most severe degree of hemolytic anemia.

No attempt was made to search for siderocytes. Remy (23) described one case of autoimmune hemolytic anemia with a 30 per cent siderocyte count in the peripheral blood. Douglas and Dacie (24) specifically searched for siderocytes in the peripheral blood smears of 19 patients. A range of siderocytes of 0.2 to 21 per cent was found; the average was 2 to 3 per cent. Dacie (17) has analyzed the significance of such findings.

Erythrophagocytosis may occasionally be found in peripheral blood preparations. Zinkham and Diamond (25) and deGruchy (26) have emphasized the value of buffy coat preparations in the study of this phenomenon. deGruchy noted erythrophagocytosis in five of eight patients with autoimmune hemolytic anemia. Additional reports of erythrophagocytosis are presented by Hargraves and associates (27), Landolt (28), Gasser and Holländer (10), Gasser (29), Sansone (30) and Pisciotta (31). It has been noted that in vitro incubation of blood samples generally increases the frequency with which erythrophagocytosis is observed. Both the monocyte and neutrophilic granulocyte are apparently involved in the phagocytic process; in general, the monocyte appears to be more active.

Agglutination and Hemolysis

Freshly drawn blood samples obtained from patients with warm acting autoimmune hemolytic anemia rarely reveal hemolysis. The author has encountered one case in which an attempt to label such cells with Cr^{51} led to complete hemolysis (Case 101). Acidification by the acid-citrate-dextrose solution used as the suspending medium appeared to be responsible for hemolysis.

Autohemagglutination, as the term is generally employed in the average laboratory, is extremely common. Unfortunately it is also commonly found in a vast variety of other hematologic and nonhematologic diseases. Rouleau formation rather than true agglutination is present in the great majority of cases. Although diagnostic significance has been ascribed to this phenomenon, it has appeared valueless for the author. For such an observation to have diagnostic significance in autoimmune hemolytic anemia it is crucial that a meticulous distinction be made between rouleau and agglutination. Stats and Wasserman (32) and Dacie (17) have listed the procedures that must be used in order to separate these two states, which may appear identical to the casual observer. Unless the laboratory reporting the presence of autohemagglutination conducts a specific and detailed examination of the blood in wet preparations, with saline dilutions and possibly phase contrast microscopy, it is best for the clinician to disregard such a report.

Plasticity of Erythrocytes

In 1959 Nicolau and associates (33) demonstrated that erythrocytes sensitized with incomplete anti-Rh_o(D) had an impaired ability to pass through filter paper. The loss of filtrability was considered to be the result of an alteration of erythrocyte plasticity. They investigated 17 patients with autoimmune hemolytic anemia and positive antiglobulin tests in an erythrocyte filtrability test system (34). Sixteen of these patients had an impaired plasticity. A high incidence of abnormal tests was seen in other hematologic disorders. It is suggested that plasticity alterations may represent a general phenomenon of erythrocyte pathology.

The Bone Marrow

Autoimmune hemolytic anemia is similar to other chronic hemolytic states with a balance established between the rate of destruction and the rate of production of erythrocytes. This balance will determine many of the clinical and laboratory characteristics of the disease. Anemic stress and anoxia are important stimuli increasing erythrocyte production in the bone marrow. Their effect may be limited in autoimmune hemolytic anemia by two factors. Myelophthisic, chemotherapeutic, infectious and azotemic states common to the secondary varieties will restrict the ability of the bone marrow to compensate. In addition, the effect of an erythrocyte autoantibody on erythrocyte precursors must also be considered. In a sense, we must determine when an erythrocyte becomes an erythrocyte, in immunologic terms. Is there a maturation or change of antigenic constituents during maturation of the cell? Do erythrocyte autoantibodies equally damage mature and immature erythrocytes? A more detailed consideration of this problem is presented in Chapter 4.

Bone marrow preparations were available from 162 patients at the approximate time of onset of the hemolytic syndrome. A tabulation of this group is presented in Table 16. A normal bone marrow was found only in 24 cases or 14.8 per cent of the series. Eighty-six cases or 53 per cent were classified as erythrocytic hyperplasia. In 69 cases or 42.6 per cent, generalized increased cellularity of the bone marrow was noted.

An abnormal bone marrow was almost universally found in the idiopathic variety of autoimmune hemolytic anemia. Only one case was considered normal. Of the cases 71.4 per cent had marked erythrocytic hyperplasia. It was noted that eight cases of the idiopathic variety, or 22.8 per cent, had an abnormal depression of erythrocyte precursors. In three of these cases almost no immature red cells were found, and the bone marrow was interpreted as pure erythrocytic aplasia. In four additional cases only occasional red cell precursors were identified, with the marrow suggesting aplastic anemia.

Remy and others (23, 35–40) have described morphologic abnormalities of erythrocyte precursors which resemble megaloblastic changes. Similar observations were commonly made in the current series. Of bone marrows examined, 25 cases or 15 per cent were classified as megaloblastic. This high incidence is partially explained by the concurrent presence of five cases of pernicious anemia and two cases of a folic acid deficiency. No clear explanation for megaloblastic changes in the others is available. Such changes may represent a relative lack of folic acid or of vitamin B-12 produced by intense and chronic erythropoietic activity characteristic of autoimmune hemolytic disease. Pernicious anemia and folic acid deficiency may occur in association with autoimmune hemolytic anemia (41) (see Chapter 9). Early and clinically undetected pernicious anemia or malabsorption syndromes may actually have been present in some of the cases with idiopathic megaloblastic changes.

Dacie (17) has reported that the amount of iron demonstrated by Perls's reaction is usually small. He suggests that this results from a rapid utilization of iron in the bone marrow. A reverse observation was made in the current series. Employing the Prussian blue reaction, an increased deposition of hemosiderin could be demonstrated in almost every instance it was searched for. Such a deposition of iron pigment can be anticipated in view of rapid death of cells without iron loss and increased gastrointestinal absorption of iron manifested by anemic patients. The therapeutic employment of iron and blood transfusions magnify this problem.

An increased plasma cell content in the bone marrow generally is not observed. Dacie (17) specifically mentions that the cold acting autoimmune hemolytic anemias do not reveal plasmacytosis. The bone marrow from 15 patients in the current series demonstrated significant plasmacytosis. It is striking, however, that no examples were seen in the idiopathic variety. All cases of plasmacytosis were observed in the second-

TABLE 16. *Bone marrow findings in 162 patients with autoimmune hemolytic anemia*

	Idiopathic Type	Secondary Type—Neoplasia of Reticuloendothelium	Secondary Type—All Others	Total	
				No.	Per cent
Total patients	35	74	53	162	
Total cellularity					
Increased	12	36	21	69	42.6
Decreased	6	6	2	14	8.6
Normal	17	32	30	79	48.8
Erythrocyte precursors					
Increased	25	27	34	86	53.1
Decreased	8	12	1	21	13.0
Normal	2	35	18	55	34.0
Granulocyte precursors					
Increased	4	39	3	46	28.4
Decreased	5	4	2	11	6.8
Normal	26	31	48	105	64.8
Megakaryocytes					
Increased	8	4	3	15	9.3
Decreased	7	5	2	14	8.6
Normal	20	65	48	133	82.1
Normal bone marrow	1	12	11	24	14.8
Increased plasma cells	0	10	5	15	9.3
Megaloblastic changes	7	7	11	25	15.4

ary form of autoimmune hemolytic anemia. Of this group, eight patients had plasma cell myeloma and the remaining seven examples occurred in patients with severe and chronic infectious disease.

Serologic Tests

Autoimmune hemolytic anemia may appear as one part of a systemic immune aberration. Accordingly, serologic tests are of great importance in the laboratory workup of any suspected case. Classification of autoimmune hemolytic anemia into different serologic types, depending on either warm acting or cold acting erythrocyte autoantibodies, creates a complex serologic picture. The frequency of associated diseases, particularly those involving immunologic mechanisms, further complicates serologic studies. The clinician should therefore not be surprised by the complex nature of serologic studies currently employed for the laboratory investigation of autoimmune hemolytic anemia. We have barely touched the surface. Diagnostic approaches will become more extensive and precise in the future. Routine studies now available include blood typing, serologic test for syphilis, lupus erythematosus (LE) cell testing, heterophile agglutinins, cold hemagglutinins, direct and indirect antiglobulin and proteolytic enzyme studies, etc. We may anticipate routine laboratory workups which will eventually include a search for rheumatoid factor, thyroid autoantibodies, parietal cell antibodies, deoxyribonucleic acid autoantibodies and a variety of tests still to be developed.

ABO and RH₀(D) Blood Grouping

Erythrocyte autoantibodies may have specificity directed toward known or postulated blood group antigens. It is therefore important to examine a large population of patients with autoimmune hemolytic anemia to determine if any selection occurs on the basis of blood type. Such studies have been carried out in the past with contradictory results. Employing relatively small series, Hunt and Lucia (42) and Clemens and Walsh (43) have noted a predilection for blood group O patients to develop autoimmune hemolytic anemia. Hunt and Lucia noted that 78 per cent of their 28 patients were blood group O. Clemens and Walsh reported 62 per cent of their 66 patients as blood group O. In larger

series reported by Lal and Speiser (44), Dunsford and Owen (45) and Dacie (17) no blood group differences from the normal population were found. Blood group O distributions of 39, 47.2 and 40 per cent, respectively, were encountered by these reporting groups.

In the current series, the ABO and Rh₀(D) blood types of 157 patients were available for analysis. Such blood typing studies were not performed in the author's laboratory; rather, they represent results obtained by the blood bank at the University of Oregon Medical School and by a number of other private hospitals. As such they present a blood typing experience comparable to that which may be expected outside the research laboratory. The results of this study as well as some of the past literature are summarized in Table 17. A large control population was available through the courtesy of Pittenger and Nelson at the Pacific Northwest Red Cross Blood Center, Portland, Oregon. Blood samples from 6814 normal donors were studied. Such donors represent the identical population from which cases of autoimmune hemolytic anemia were obtained. No significant differences in blood group O, A or B typing were observed between patients and normal donors. A significant increase in the number of patients typed as blood group AB was found. It is doubtful whether this increase has etiologic significance in development of autoimmune hemolytic anemia. Rather, it reflects the difficulties encountered in accurately typing patients with autoimmune hemolytic anemia. Such patients may be typed as AB, Rh₀(D)+.

TABLE 17. *Blood group distribution in autoimmune hemolytic anemia*

Source	Total Patients	Percentage having Blood Group Typing					
		O	A	B	AB	Rh₀(D)+	Rh₀(D)−
Dacie (17)	120	40	44	13.5	2.5		
Dunsford and Owen (45)	127	47.2	40.2	7.1	5.5	82.2	17.8
Controls (normal)	6000	45.4	43.3	8.6	2.7	82.1	17.9
Current series	157	43.4	40.1	9.5	7.0	84.0	16.0
Controls (normal)	6814	46.6	39.7	10.4	3.3	82.6	17.4

However, suspending the cells in normal serum without antibodies may also result in agglutination. The addition by manufacturers of albumin to various antisera, particularly antirhesus antisera, magnifies this problem. Accordingly, the clinician faced with a case of autoimmune hemolytic anemia typed as AB, $Rh_o(D)+$ should view this result with suspicion. Weiner and Nussey (46) and Githens and Hathaway (47) have reported this difficulty.

The 157 patients in the current series were also examined for the distribution of the $Rh_o(D)$ factor. No significant difference in $Rh_o(D)$ incidence was seen in patients with autoimmune hemolytic anemia, compared with our control population.

Serologic Tests for Syphilis

Positive serologic tests for syphilis, which appear to be biologically false reactions, have been occasionally reported in autoimmune hemolytic anemia (48–53). In the current series the results of serologic tests for syphilis were available for 141 patients. Seventeen of these were positive, an incidence of 11.9 per cent. This incidence is substantially greater than that seen in our usual hospital population (normal range: less than 3 per cent). No particular predilection was apparent for either idiopathic or secondary types of autoimmune hemolytic anemia. In three patients a definite history of luetic exposure was obtained. In four cases, representing 23.5 per cent of positive reactions, a biologically false positive serologic state was documented. All four of these cases were secondary varieties. Two patients had systemic lupus erythematosus and one patient was seen with Hodgkin's disease and hyperthyroidism, respectively. A marked difference as to sex was noted in the positive serologic reacting group. Only three of 68 males tested had positive serologic tests, an incidence of 4.4 per cent. Fourteen of 75 females, an incidence of 18.7 per cent, had positive reactions. Table 18 summarizes these data. A detailed investigation to rule out biologically false positive states should be carried out in patients with autoimmune

TABLE 18. *Results of serologic tests for syphilis in 143 patients with autoimmune hemolytic anemia*

	Total Tested	No. Positive	Per Cent Positive
Entire group	143	17	11.9
Incidence in females	75	14	18.7
Incidence in males	68	3	4.4
Idiopathic autoimmune type	26	3	11.5
History of luetic exposure	17	3	17.6
Biologically false positive reaction	17	4	23.5

hemolytic anemia and positive serologic tests. The possibility that such reactions are part of a systemic immunologic abnormality deserves strong consideration. Systemic lupus erythematosus should be searched for in every instance.

LE Cell Preparations

LE cell preparations from 57 patients were examined with positive results obtained in eight. All eight have been diagnosed as cases of systemic lupus erythematosus. It is difficult to interpret such LE cell testing. Discovery of a positive LE cell test in almost any patient with autoimmune hemolytic anemia would suggest classification as systemic lupus erythematosus. Two interpretations are possible. There may be many cases of systemic lupus erythematosus in the current series that are undiagnosed. Alternatively, systemic lupus erythematosus may not be a specific entity but may represent instead a symptom complex characterized by multiple autoantibody formation. Possibly all cases of autoimmune hemolytic anemia are examples of systemic lupus erythematosus within this definition. The inability of pathologists to unequivocally diagnose lupus erythematosus emphasizes this problem. A similar line of reasoning has been employed by Dameshek (54) in relating idiopathic thrombocytopenic purpura to systemic lupus erythematosus. The creation of a disease category termed "diffuse autoimmune" or "diffuse immunologic" disease may eventually be necessary to adequately describe this state.

Heterophile Agglutinin Studies

Heterophile agglutinin studies were infrequently performed in our series of patients with autoimmune hemolytic anemia. Such tests were carried out in only 16 instances. Diagnostic results with high titers (224 or higher) after adsorption with guinea pig or horse kidney antigen were found in three cases. The clinical state and morphologically abnormal lymphocytes warranted the diagnosis of infectious mononucleosis in all three. In the remaining 13, low titers in both unadsorbed and adsorbed specimens were obtained. The highest values in unadsorbed tests were 224 and 448, respectively. Adsorption studies in these two patients led to titers of 4 and 0, respectively.

Cold Agglutinin Titers

The current series is restricted to autoimmune hemolytic anemia developing in the presence of warm acting erythrocyte autoantibodies. It should not be assumed, however, that cold hemagglutinins are absent in the sera of such patients. A meticulous search for cold acting hemagglutinins will reveal their presence in almost every serum. Their significance, however, is highly dubious. Pathologically significant cold acting autoantibodies have high thermal levels (approaching 32°C.) and titers substantially over 500. In addition, a combination of both warm acting incomplete and cold acting complete erythrocyte autoantibodies may occur. Such a combination was seen in three cases. Cold hemagglutinin titers of 1024, 2048 and 5000 were found. Warm acting incomplete erythrocyte autoantibodies were identified by elution studies in the same patients.

Demonstration of the Autoantibody Fixed to the Erythrocyte

The diagnosis of autoimmune hemolytic anemia depends on the demonstration of an autoantibody fixed to the surface of the patient's erythrocytes. Three major techniques may be employed for this purpose: (a) suspension of the cells in colloid media containing large numbers of anisometric molecules; (b) the direct antiglobulin test; (c) various direct proteolytic enzyme tests. The warm acting autoantibodies are generally incomplete erythrocyte antibodies. Accordingly, spontaneous autoagglutination or autohemolysis is rarely observed. The employment of additional serologic procedures to demonstrate such antibodies is necessary. The theoretical and serologic rationale for these procedures is presented in detail in Chapter 18. Several general remarks are pertinent at this time.

The use of colloid anisometric suspension systems, when employed in classical serum or albumin techniques, with or without low speed centrifugation, are insensitive. They have little to offer except with rare and unusual autoantibodies. High speed centrifugation methods with albumin or polyvinylpyrrolidone are excellent for the demonstration of incomplete erythrocyte isoantibodies. The systematic utilization of such procedures in autoimmune hemolytic anemia has not been carried out. This appears to be a fruitful area for further research.

Only a limited number of enzyme preparations have been employed for detection of incomplete erythrocyte autoantibodies. Trypsin, papain and ficin erythrocyte pretreatment methods are not designed to demonstrate autoantibodies fixed to the erythrocyte surface. Activated papain may be employed in a direct procedure for this purpose. Unpublished studies in our laboratory indicate that this is an insensitive and poor technique. Ficin has not as yet been evaluated in this regard. Bromelin may be employed in a direct method to demonstrate such antibodies; the range of sensitivity and the pitfalls of this technique are discussed below.

The direct antiglobulin test is the procedure of choice to document the fixation of an autoantibody to the erythrocyte surface. This procedure is highly efficient. It should be emphasized, however, that both false positive and negative reactions occur. In addition, occasional erythrocyte autoantibodies will present negative reactions with antiglobulin serum prepared in the usual fashion. This experience is similar to that seen with incomplete erythrocyte isoantibodies (55, 56).

The results obtained with all test systems must be considered as only laboratory conclusions. Positive and negative reactions do not necessarily correlate with the clinical state of the patient or the degree of hemolysis observed. In some instances positive reactions may not even indicate the presence of erythrocyte autoantibodies. Accordingly, a positive test, even a positive antiglobulin test, should not be interpreted as diagnostic of autoimmune hemolytic anemia. The reverse is equally true. A negative antiglobulin test should not be considered as ruling out the presence of autoimmune hemolytic anemia.

The two techniques generally employed in a direct test system to detect erythrocyte autoantibodies are the antiglobulin and bromelin procedures (57). Such systems have been employed in duplicate during investigation of the current series.

The Direct Antiglobulin Test

Direct antiglobulin tests employing broad spectrum antiglobulin serum were performed on 232 patients at the time of diagnosis of autoimmune hemolytic anemia. In all but five, duplicate direct bromelin studies were simultaneously carried out. Positive direct antiglobulin tests were obtained in 202. Accordingly, failure of the antiglobulin procedure was noted initially in 12.9 per cent of the patients (30 cases). In 16 cases both the direct antiglobulin test and direct bromelin test were initially negative. Serologic confirmation of the diagnosis of autoimmune hemolytic anemia was obtained only during subsequent testing. In nine instances the direct antiglobulin test was negative while the proteolytic enzyme procedure was positive. In subsequent testing positive direct antiglobulin reactions were obtained in six of these nine patients. In one case elution revealed the autoantibody which could be demonstrated in an indirect antiglobulin procedure. The two remaining autoantibodies were repeatedly demonstrated by bromelin procedures but failed to give positive antiglobulin reactions. Similar examples of erythrocyte autoantibodies not demonstrated in the antiglobulin tests but documented with proteolytic enzymes have been reported by

TABLE 19. *Results of direct antiglobulin tests in 232 patients with autoimmune hemolytic anemia: patients tested at time of diagnosis and after therapy (results of the direct bromelin test in patients having negative antiglobulin tests are added)*

Procedures	No. Tested	No.	Per Cent
Initial testing			
Direct antiglobulin positive	232	202	87.1
Direct antiglobulin negative	232	30	12.9
No bromelin test	30	5	16.7
Direct bromelin negative	30	16	53.3
Direct bromelin positive	30	9	30.0
Subsequent testing			
Direct antiglobulin positive	164	98	59.8
Direct antiglobulin negative	164	66	40.2
Direct bromelin negative	66	47	71.2
Direct bromelin positive	66	19	28.8

Lemaire and associates (58), Payne and associates (59) and Baikie and Pirrie (36). Vetter (60) has reported an extensive study of the comparative sensitivity of direct antiglobulin and direct bromelin tests. In a large series of patients with hemolytic anemia, 80 were found to have positive direct bromelin tests. Failure of the direct antiglobulin test was noted in 16 of these patients. A similar experience was reported by Bedarida and Giraldi (61). In a detailed serologic investigation of 11 patients with autoimmune hemolytic anemia, three patients had negative direct antiglobulin tests in the face of positive bromelin reactions. Bromelin did not appear particularly sensitive when a non-gamma type of antiglobulin reaction was present.

In the present series positive direct antiglobulin reactions were obtained in 87 per cent of cases during the initial diagnosis of autoimmune hemolytic anemia. This figure was increased to 91 per cent positive serologic tests by employing the direct bromelin test in duplicate. With repeated application of the antiglobulin procedure during the course of the disease, and the employment of elution techniques, over 99 per cent of the current series had positive antiglobulin reactions. Table 19 summarizes these observations.

The strength of direct agglutination re-

TABLE 20. *Titer and degree of agglutination observed with antiglobulin serum in direct tests performed in patients with autoimmune hemolytic anemia*

Antiglobulin Serum: Degree of Agglutination					
0	Trace+	1+	2+	3+	4+
30	35	76	38	31	22

Dilutions of Antiglobulin Serum: End Point of Agglutination (1+)*			
1:1	1:4	1:16	1:64
85	54	29	20

* Prozone observed in five titrations.

actions obtained with antiglobulin serum ranges from trace to 4+ reactions in the current series. Reactions of 1+ were most commonly observed. A report of the intensity of antiglobulin reactions obtained on initial testing is presented in Table 20.

The direct antiglobulin test was routinely employed with a series of dilutions of antiglobulin serum. The antiglobulin serum was produced in our laboratory and had gamma and non-gamma activity, i.e., it was a broad spectrum antiserum. It should be realized that commercial antiglobulin serum is diluted from the original animal serum by the manufacturer for optimal reactivity. A similar dilution procedure was carried out in our laboratory in order to produce the basic reagent. This is simply referred to as antiglobulin serum. Dilutions, 4-fold, 16-fold and 64-fold, of this basic reagent were employed. The results of this study are also presented in Table 20. As might be expected, the end point of the antiglobulin reaction was generally observed with basic antiglobulin serum. In five cases, or 2.7 per cent of such serial dilution testing, a prozone phenomenon was encountered. This reaction, which is probably related to establishment of an equivalent zone of antibody and antigen, is significant. The reaction is characterized by weak or absent agglutination with the basic antiglobulin reagent. Further dilution of the antiglobulin serum in order to escape a zone of antibody excess leads to positive or intensified agglutination reactions. Such prozone reactions lead to the possibility of falsely reporting a negative antiglobulin test because of too "potent" (i.e., insufficiently diluted) antiglobulin serum. Our data suggest that such reactions occur in approximately one of 45 cases of autoimmune hemolytic anemia when the basic antiglobulin serum (undiluted commercial antiglobulin serum) is used in an undiluted state.

Attempting to relate the clinical course of patients to the intensity of the antiglobulin reaction is disappointing. Only a very crude correlation exists. As a general rule, stronger antiglobulin reactions were obtained in patients with a more severe degree of hemolytic anemia. However, numerous exceptions to this observation were noted. No predictability for either a therapeutic response or eventual survival was observed. The hematocrit appeared more reliable for documenting the severity of the hemolytic episode than did the antiglobulin reaction. The only value in quantitating the antiglobulin reaction by dilution or degree of positivity was discovery of the relatively uncommon prozone phenomenon.

Repeated antiglobulin tests were performed during the course of illness in 164 patients. Table 19 summarizes results obtained. In 98 cases or 60 per cent, direct antiglobulin tests remained positive. Persistence of positive reactions did not bear any relationship to severity of illness or therapeutic remission. It was not uncommon to record persistent positive antiglobulin tests after all evidence of hemolysis disappeared. In most cases positive reactions remained for over 6 months, and periods of 1 year or more after remission were not unusual. Negative direct antiglobulin and bromelin tests developed in 47 patients. Nineteen additional patients developed negative antiglobulin tests while the direct bromelin test remained positive. No clinical significance was apparent in this positive proteolytic enzyme and negative antiglobulin reaction state.

Although the antiglobulin test is easy to perform, it represents a complex immunologic procedure. It is the cornerstone for diagnostic studies of the hemolytic anemias. In view of its importance it is crucial that all those concerned with autoimmune hemolytic anemia have a working knowledge of the theoretical principles involved. Such a presentation is available in Chapter 18. Both false positive and false negative reactions may be encountered. The possible pitfalls of the antiglobulin reaction have been discussed by Muirhead (62), Mollison (63) and Revol and associates (64). False positive reactions may result from storage in the refrigerator (17), by exposure of erythrocytes in vitro to lipoid solvents (acetone, toluene, benzene, etc.) (65), cationic metals (chromic, ferric, etc.) (66), trypan blue (67) and other azodyes (68) and certain bacteria (69). Phenylhydrazine (70, 71) and lead poisoning (72–75) may create false positive antiglobulin reactions after in vivo exposure. Sutherland and colleagues (76) and Jandl (77) have demonstrated that reticulocytosis may result in false positive antiglobulin reactions. False negative reactions may be obtained because of incomplete washing, a prozone phenomenon, the use of contaminated or inactivated antiglobulin serum, poorly cleaned glassware and a variety of other technical flaws; forgetting to add antiglobulin serum appears to be the most common.

The Direct Bromelin Test

The direct bromelin test was employed to demonstrate erythrocyte autoantibodies fixed to the erythrocyte surface by Pirofsky (57) in 1960. Bedarida and Giraldi (61) and Vetter (60) confirmed the efficacy of this procedure. The initial optimism expressed in these reports no longer appears entirely justified.

In the present series direct bromelin tests were performed in 227 patients as part of the initial study of autoimmune hemolytic anemia. All tests were carried out in duplicate with the direct antiglobulin procedure. Table 21 summarizes the results of such testing. Positive reactions were obtained with both bromelin and antiglobulin procedures in 160 cases. Negative reactions in both tests were found in 16 patients. Accordingly, the bromelin test and antiglobulin test gave identical reactions in

TABLE 21. *Results of direct bromelin tests in 227 patients with autoimmune hemolytic anemia: patients tested at time of diagnosis and after therapy (results of direct antiglobulin tests in patients having positive and negative direct bromelin tests are added)*

Procedure	No. Tested	No.	Per Cent
Initial testing			
Direct bromelin positive	227	169	74.5
Direct antiglobulin positive	169	160	94.7
Direct antiglobulin negative	169	9	5.3
Direct bromelin negative	227	58	25.6
Direct antiglobulin positive	58	42	72.4
Direct antiglobulin negative	58	16	27.6
Identical direct bromelin and antiglobulin reactions	227	176	77.5
Subsequent testing			
Direct bromelin positive	164	82	50.0
Direct antiglobulin positive	82	63	76.8
Direct antiglobulin negative	82	19	23.2
Direct bromelin negative	164	82	50.0
Direct antiglobulin positive	82	35	42.7
Direct antiglobulin negative	82	47	57.3
Identical direct bromelin and antiglobulin reactions	164	110	67.1

Degree of Agglutination in Direct Bromelin Test				
Trace+	1+	2+	3+	4+
30	45	26	23	35

77.5 per cent of the cases of autoimmune hemolytic anemia. In nine additional cases the antiglobulin test failed and positive bromelin tests were found. In two, the antiglobulin test consistently failed to demonstrate the erythrocyte autoantibody. In 42 cases or 18.5 per cent of the series the bromelin test failed in the presence of positive antiglobulin tests. The best (or worst) that can be said for these results is that they were consistent. Twenty-eight of these cases were retested during the course of the disease and only five eventually gave positive reactions.

Agglutination in the direct bromelin reaction was graded as trace positive to 4+. Results from such quantitation are presented in Table 21. In general agglutination reactions paralleling those obtained with antiglobulin serum were found. Positive reactions of 4+ were more frequently noted in the bromelin procedure.

Repeated bromelin testing was performed in 164 patients during therapeutic remission and relapse. An equal number of cases, 82 in each instance, gave positive and negative reactions. In 110 patients the direct antiglobulin and direct bromelin tests gave identical reactions. In 19 cases, or 11.6 per cent, the antiglobulin test reverted to normal while the bromelin test remained positive. In 35 cases or 21.3 per cent, negative bromelin tests and positive antiglobulin tests were noted.

For an accurate performance of the direct bromelin test certain precautions are necessary (57). It should be emphasized that erythrocytes are not washed in this procedure (78), and serum factors may lead to false positive reactions (79). Cold acting hemagglutinins may be markedly potentiated by the action of bromelin. Accordingly, every positive reaction should be warmed to 37°C. to eliminate the possibility that a cold hemagglutinin in the patient's serum has led to the positive direct reaction. In addition, intense rouleau formation after centrifugation, particularly in the presence of dysproteinemic states, may be interpreted as agglutination. A serum control without bromelin should accordingly be tested in duplicate with each direct bromelin test.

Demonstration of Unbound Erythrocyte Autoantibodies

The direct antiglobulin test demonstrates erythrocyte autoantibodies fixed to the surface of host erythrocytes. A positive reaction is anticipated in every case of autoimmune hemolytic anemia. Autoimmune hemolytic anemia presumably can occur with negative direct antiglobulin reactions. In practice, however, the diagnosis is rarely made in such cases. Davidsohn and Spurrier (80) have reported five cases with negative direct antiglobulin tests and demonstrable unbound autoantibodies. Heni and Blessing (81) have reported a similar case. Such cases are now rare with the availability of direct enzyme testing.

The diagnosis of autoimmune hemolytic anemia is generally dependent on a positive direct antiglobulin test. This appears logical. The same rationale, however, does not apply to the demonstration of unbound erythrocyte autoantibodies. Sturgeon (82) and Denys and van den Broucke (83) independently demonstrated the application of the indirect antiglobulin test for this purpose.

Indirect Antiglobulin Test

The studies of Evans and Weiser (84), Evans and associates (85) and Hughes-Jones (86) strongly suggest that antibody bound to the erythrocyte surface is in dynamic equilibruim with free autoantibody in the serum. The ability to demonstrate unbound antibody reflects the sensitivity of the indirect procedure employed. The indirect antiglobulin test is generally used for this purpose. Evans and Weiser (84) noted positive indirect antiglobulin reactions in 63.4 per cent of the 41 cases they studied. van Loghem and associates (87) found that 59.5 per cent of their 38 cases had positive indirect antiglobulin reactions. Dacie's series of 79 patients (17) had positive indirect antiglobulin reactions in 37 or 47 per cent of the series. Dausset and Colombani (16) reported studies on 83 patients. They performed indirect antiglobulin testing on two groups, patients who had "recovered" and patients who later died. In the cured group positive indirect reactions were noted in only 18.5 per cent of the cases. In the group that later died positive indirect antiglobulin reactions were found in 52 per cent of the cases.

In the current series, the indirect antiglobulin test was employed as part of the initial serologic workup in 136 cases of autoimmune hemolytic anemia. Positive results were obtained in 61 cases or 44.8 per cent of the series.

Many observers (17) have noted that

clinical improvement frequently correlates with disappearance of a positive indirect antiglobulin test. The series of Dausset and Colombani (16) confirms such observations. The current series was analyzed in this regard. Serum specimens from 105 patients were tested throughout their clinical course with indirect antiglobulin procedures. Negative results were eventually obtained in 88 cases or 83.8 per cent of the series. As a general rule positive indirect antiglobulin tests were present and persisted in patients with severe hemolytic disease. Table 22 summarizes the results of such indirect tests.

Indirect Bromelin Test

Although the direct bromelin test was substantially less sensitive than the direct antiglobulin test, a reverse state was seen when an indirect procedure was employed. The bromelin procedure was markedly superior to the indirect antiglobulin test. A similar superiority of other proteolytic enzymes for indirect testing in autoimmune hemolytic anemia has been noted by Dausset and Colombani (16), Heller and associates (88) and Dacie (17).

The indirect bromelin test was performed as part of the initial serologic workup in 117 cases. Unbound erythrocyte autoantibody was demonstrated in 68 cases or 58.1 per cent of the series. The sensitivity of the indirect bromelin test became even more apparent in subsequent testing during the course of the disease. Positive results persisted in 33 of 95 patients tested, an incidence of 34.7 per cent. In several instances positive indirect bromelin tests were noted 5 or more years after therapeutic remission and negative conversion of indirect antiglobulin tests. Dacie and de-Gruchy (89) have reported a similar case.

Summary of Antiglobulin and Bromelin Testing

Several conclusions may be drawn on the basis of the above data. The most important diagnostic procedure for demonstrating erythrocyte autoantibodies fixed to the erythrocyte surface is the direct antiglobulin test. The sensitivity of this

TABLE 22. *Results of indirect antiglobulin and bromelin tests in patients with autoimmune hemolytic anemia*

Test Procedure	No. Tested	Per Cent Positive	Per Cent Negative
Initial testing			
Indirect antiglobulin	136	44.8	55.2
Indirect bromelin	117	58.1	41.9
Subsequent Testing			
Indirect antiglobulin	105	16.2	83.8
Indirect bromelin	95	34.7	65.3

procedure is markedly superior to that of the direct bromelin test. The reverse is apparent when tests to demonstrate unbound erythrocyte autoantibodies are considered. The indirect proteolytic enzyme technique is superior to the indirect antiglobulin test. Both antiglobulin and proteolytic enzyme tests should be employed on a routine basis in the initial workup and followup of any case of autoimmune hemolytic anemia. The combination of test procedures, both indirect and direct, minimizes technical errors not uncommonly encountered in the routine laboratory. In addition, no single test performed on a casual isolated basis possesses the ability to demonstrate all positive cases. It is true that duplicate testing would increase case discovery only in a limited fashion (4 per cent) in direct testing. In the current series of 232 patients nine cases were diagnosed employing the bromelin test. These would have been missed on the basis of a single antiglobulin test. In view of the clinical significance of such a diagnosis, the additional labor appears to be worth the extra effort.

The simple statement that the direct antiglobulin test was positive in over 99 per cent of cases of autoimmune hemolytic anemia must be clarified. An element of circular reasoning has entered into such statistics. An assumption of extreme sensitivity of the antiglobulin procedure is implied and may be unwarranted. At the current level of clinical experience, diagnosis of autoimmune hemolytic anemia is impossible without demonstrating an autoantibody bound to the erythrocyte surface.

The direct antiglobulin test is the most sensitive procedure available. Of cases currently diagnosed as autoimmune hemolytic anemia, 100 per cent are anticipated to have positive direct antiglobulin tests. Without such a positive reaction the diagnosis of autoimmune hemolytic anemia generally cannot be made. Data are not available to indicate the frequency of autoimmune hemolytic anemia in the absence of positive antiglobulin tests. Two or three such cases were found in the present series when the direct bromelin procedure documented the presence of erythrocyte autoantibodies. However, all investigators have encountered cases indistinguishable from autoimmune hemolytic anemia with the exception that serologic tests are consistently negative. The following protocol illustrates a typical example. How may such cases be classified? Improved serologic test procedures are necessary to deal with such problems.

Case 8. A 10-year-old white male was seen with a 4-year history of anemia and intermittent jaundice. Physical examination demonstrated scleral icterus, a liver palpated 4 cm. below the costal margin and a spleen 6 cm. below the costal margin. The hematocrit was 23 per cent and the reticulocyte count was 5.8 per cent. Bone marrow aspiration revealed erythrocyte hyperplasia. Direct and indirect antiglobulin and bromelin tests were negative. The patient's erythrocytes survived normally in a normal recipient. Compatible donor cells had a 3-day half-life survival time in the patient. Marked splenic sequestration and significant hepatic sequestration were present within 2 days of testing. The patient's mother, father and five siblings were studied without evidence of a hemolytic process. Corticosteroid therapy was initiated and led to a dramatic hematologic remission. Two attempts to withdraw such therapy resulted in return of hemolysis. Remission has been maintained for 4 years on 5 to 10 mg. of prednisone. Throughout this time multiple antiglobulin and bromelin tests have been negative.

Elution Studies

The elution of erythrocyte autoantibodies from the surface of erythrocytes is important in the study of autoimmune hemolytic anemia. By utilizing elution proce-

dures it is possible to accomplish the following: (a) prove that positive direct antiglobulin reactions are due to an erythrocyte autoantibody; (b) obtain the autoantibody in a form more amenable to detailed analysis; (c) document the presence of erythrocyte autoantibodies on the erythrocyte surface in patients with negative antiglobulin reactions; and (d) identify antigenic specificity of such autoantibodies. These optimistic criteria must be modified in view of the possibility of an Ogato phenomenon (90, 91) (see Chapter 17).

Elution procedures were carried out in 80 patients of the current series. The Weiner (92) alcohol ether procedure was generally used. In certain cases this procedure was supplemented by the heat technique of Landsteiner and Miller (93) and the digitonin method of Kochwa and Rosenfield (94). Positive eluates were obtained in 60 cases, an incidence of 75 per cent of successful elutions. This incidence of success is similar to that seen by Dacie (17). He reported successful elution in 69 per cent of 35 cases attempted. The degree of positivity of the direct antiglobulin test did not influence the success rate of elution in the current series. Table 23 summarizes the relationship of the degree of agglutination in the direct antiglobulin test to positive eluates. The potential value of this test procedure is apparent from these figures. Elution was performed in nine cases with negative direct antiglobulin reactions and 11 examples of trace positive agglutination. In 16 of these 20 cases elution procedures led to the successful demonstration of an erythrocyte autoantibody. It must be confessed, however, that in 15 of these 16 successful elutions stronger direct antiglobulin reactions had been previously recorded. In Chapter 17 the significance of elution procedures is discussed in more detail.

Specificity of Erythrocyte Autoantibodies

The importance and difficulty of identifying specificity of erythrocyte autoantibodies for erythrocytic antigenic determinants is discussed in Chapter 20. In the current series 57 eluates and 32 sera con-

TABLE 23. *Elution of erythrocyte autoantibodies in 80 patients with autoimmune hemolytic anemia*

	Total Patients	Degree of Agglutination in Direct Antiglobulin Test					
		Negative	Trace +	1+	2+	3+	4+
Autoantibody obtained (75%)	60	6	10	11	12	11	10
Autoantibody absent (25%)	20	3	1	11	4	1	0
Total	80	9	11	22	16	12	10

taining unbound warm acting erythrocyte autoantibodies were examined for such specificity. Particular attention was paid to eliminate any possibility that isoantibodies directed against nonhost erythrocytes were involved. The importance of this qualification has been emphasized by Whittingham and associates (95) and Croucher and associates (96). Eight warm acting erythrocyte autoantibodies (9 per cent) with erythrocyte antigenic specificity were found. In all instances the specificity was that of anti-hr″(e) and the hr″(e) agglutinogen was a normal antigenic constituent of host erythrocytes.

Premature Destruction of Erythrocytes

The development of methods to measure the life span of erythrocytes is an important area of research. Hemolytic anemia must involve premature destruction of erythrocytes. A technique to quantitate the extent of such destruction is highly desirable.

In 1919 Ashby (97) presented such a method. The procedure was dependent on transfusion of serologically compatible erythrocytes into a donor. Although the transfused erythrocytes were compatible, cells were chosen which were serologically foreign and could be distinguished by differential agglutination. Group O erythrocytes transfused into group A, B or AB recipients illustrates this approach. Group N cells transfused into group M recipients is also feasible. With appropriate antiserum the number of cells surviving after transfusion could be determined by counting erythrocytes remaining unagglutinated. Employing this method the normal average life span of the erythrocyte was found to be approximately 120 days.

In 1943 Dacie and Mollison (98) applied the Ashby technique to the study of hemolytic anemia. They demonstrated that normal erythrocytes survived normally in patients with hereditary spherocytosis. This was in contrast to patients with various acquired forms of hemolytic anemia whose systems rapidly destroyed transfused normal erythrocytes. Brown and associates (99) used the same procedure in two cases of autoimmune hemolytic anemia. Life spans of 7.8 and 13.1 days were obtained. The pattern of cell death suggested an exponential or random destruction of transfused erythrocytes independent of erythrocyte age. Loutit and Mollison (100, 101) confirmed and expanded these observations in subsequent publications. Selwyn and Hackett (102) performed the reverse experiment. They transfused antiglobulin positive erythrocytes obtained from patients with autoimmune hemolytic anemia into normal recipients and observed the survival of such cells. A distinct pattern was noted. Increased destruction of cells was seen for a 10- to 15-day period and was followed by a normal survival curve.

The Ashby technique employed in the studies mentioned above limited investigation to transfused cells. Methods were needed which would permit determination of the life span of erythrocytes within the host's own circulation. Such a method became available by employing radioactive chromium (Cr^{51}).

Chromium^{51} Survival Time

In 1950 Gray and Sterling (103, 104) demonstrated that human erythrocytes contained about 20 μg of chromium per 100 ml. Erythrocytes exposed to radioactive sodium chromate (Cr^{51}) rapidly absorbed the

TABLE 24. *The Cr⁵¹ half-life erythrocyte survival time (T/2) found in 35 patients with auto-immune hemolytic anemia*

T/2 Cr⁵¹ Erythrocyte Survival Time	No. of Patients
days	
0–1.9	0
2–5	7
5–10	10
11–15	10
16–20*	4
20–25	4
>25	0

* One patient postsplenectomy.

material. The chromium appeared to be bound to the globulin fraction of hemoglobin. Ebaugh and associates (105) demonstrated that elution of radioactive chromium would occur with a half-life approximating 70 days. The same approximate range of elution was noted by Read and associates (106) and Hughes-Jones and Mollison (107). Mollison (63) has discussed in detail the effect of chromium⁵¹ elution on the determination of the erythrocyte life span.

With the chromium⁵¹ life span technique, the half-life (point at which 50 per cent of labeled cells are destroyed: T/2 value) was found to range from 25 to 26 days by Read and associates (106), Mollison and Veall (108) and Donohue and associates (109). Values approaching 33 days were obtained by Necheles and associates (110) and Sutherland and McCall (111). Letman (112) found the average half-life span of chromium⁵¹ labeled erythrocytes to be 29.3 days, with a standard deviation of 2 days. This latter value closely approximates our own experience in which normal erythrocytes have a half-life survival of 28 days with a standard deviation of 2 days.

In the current series chromium⁵¹ survival time studies were performed in 35 patients using the patient's own erythrocytes in his own circulation. No normal values were found. The distribution of survival times is given in Table 24. The shortest half-life survival time was 2.2 days and the longest was 25 days. This range conforms to that found by Constantoulakis and associates (113). These investigators also state that a half-life survival time of less than 1 day in autoimmune hemolytic anemia is incompatible with life. In one case of the present series survival time studies were performed after splenectomy. A T/2 value of 18 days was found. In three instances survival time analysis was carried out both before and after corticosteroid therapy. Half-life survival times before therapy of 3.2, 9 and 12 days were converted to 20, 17 and 22.5 days, respectively, after therapy.

Body Surface Counting for Splenic Sequestration

In 1955 Korst and associates (114) and in 1956 Jandl and associates (115) introduced external scintillation counting to document sequestered chromium⁵¹ labeled erythrocytes in various body organs. The procedure was similar to the determination of Cr⁵¹ erythrocyte survival times. Erythrocytes were labeled with chromium⁵¹ and reinjected into the circulation. External scintillation counting over various organs was performed to quantitate the sequestration of such labeled erythrocytes. Jandl determined radioactivity over the midthorax and considered the value obtained to be that of peripheral blood. Radioactivity over the liver and spleen was then measured and expressed as a ratio of the thorax value. With this technique Jandl found that at the 50 per cent point (half-life) of erythrocyte destruction, liver sequestration ranged from 23 to 35 per cent of thorax values. Splenic radioactivity was slightly higher, ranging from 38 to 48 per cent of thorax radioactivity. Sequestration was considered significant when radioactivity values over the spleen and/or liver were substantially increased over those found at the thorax. Hughes-Jones and Szur (116) have reviewed the desired methods and possible pitfalls of external body scintillation counting.

In the current series body surface counting procedures were employed in 18 cases. Sequestration was not diagnosed unless splenic or hepatic-thorax ratios of 150 per cent or higher were obtained. Splenic sequestration was demonstrated in seven cases. In several instances marked sequestration over the liver was also noted. The significance of such sequestration in reference to splenectomy is discussed in Chapter 12.

Fragility of the Erythrocytes

Osmotic Fragility

Hereditary spherocytosis and acquired hemolytic anemia were confused for many years. Lowman (21) has emphasized the fact that this confusion may still persist. The presence of spherocytes in both states makes differentiation particularly difficult. The studies of Dameshek and Schwartz (117, 118) clarified this problem. They demonstrated that spherocytic changes of the erythrocyte would result from the action of heteroimmune and autoimmune erythrocyte antibodies. Osmotic fragility test systems designed to quantitate the spherocytic change may therefore be expected to have diagnostic value. The availability of the antiglobulin test, however, has almost eliminated the use of osmotic fragility testing in autoimmune hemolytic anemia.

Dacie (17) has noted the expected, i.e., that an increase of osmotic fragility generally parallels the degree of spherocytosis seen in warm acting autoimmune hemolytic anemia. In 22 cases osmotic fragility was normal in five and essentially normal in four additional patients. Splenectomy had no effect on osmotic fragility unless a therapeutic remission was induced. An incubated osmotic fragility test does not improve the sensitivity of the procedure. This differs from the observations of Young and Miller (119) in hereditary spherocytosis. Additional experience with osmotic fragility testing in the autoimmune hemolytic anemias is contained in the reports of Bakker-v. Aardenne and associates (120), Rossi and Bastistini (121) and Fiorina and associates (122). Negrini (123) has directly implicated the action of erythrocyte autoantibodies on the erythrocyte surface as creating the spherocytic state.

In the author's current series osmotic fragility was infrequently examined. Testing was performed in 17 cases and an abnormal increase in fragility was noted in five patients.

Mechanical Fragility

Ham and associates (124) have emphasized an additional effect of antibodies on the erythrocyte surface. They noted that erythrocytes exposed to antibodies had an increased fragility when subjected to mechanical trauma. There are few data available concerning this procedure in autoimmune hemolytic anemia. Such studies were not included in the present series. Young and associates (125) reported two patients with an increased mechanical fragility. Shaub and Maier (126) noted that five of six of their patients had an increased mechanical fragility. Bakker-v. Aardenne and associates (120) observed an increased mechanical fragility in three of five patients. These latter two groups noted that osmotic fragility and mechanical fragility did not necessarily coincide.

Urinary Findings

A surprisingly large number of cases in the current series were found to have abnormalities of the urine. However, the significance of this observation is questionable in view of the high incidence of associated pathologic states.

The complete urinalysis of 185 patients was available for review. Proteinuria was observed in 63 cases or 34 per cent of the group. The degree of proteinuria was generally slight, ranging from trace positive to 1+ in the majority of instances. In seven patients Bence-Jones protein could be identified. In five of these, an associated plasma cell myeloma was present. In the remaining two cases leukemic states were associated.

Evidence for infection characterized by excess bacteria and/or pus cells in the urine was found in 52 cases or 28 per cent of the series. Overt cystitis, pyelonephritis and cystitis and prostatitis were diagnosed by culture in 23 cases.

Hematuria, generally of a microscopic variety, was present in 11 cases. Hemo-

TABLE 25. *Results of various blood chemical analyses in patients with warm acting autoimmune hemolytic anemia*

Test Procedure	Total studied	Abnormal No.	Abnormal Per cent	Normal No.	Normal Per cent
Blood urea nitrogen	74	26	35.1	48	64.9
Uric acid	37	24	64.9	13	35.1
Protein bound iodine	14	5	35.7	9	64.3
Liver chemistries*					
Total serum bilirubin	120	66	55.0	54	45.0
Direct and indirect bilirubin	120	37	30.8	83	69.2
Direct bilirubin, alone	120	9	7.5	111	92.5
Indirect bilirubin, alone	120	20	16.7	120	83.3
Thymol turbidity	20	4	20.0	16	80.0
Cephalin flocculation	16	7	43.8	9	56.2

* Alk-Po₄, cholesterol, cholesterol esters, Bromsulphalein and prothrombin: normal except in patients with overt liver disease.

globinuria was distinctly unusual and was noted in only three patients.

The current series did not include routine analysis for either urinary urobilinogen or hemosiderin. Dacie (17) states that a moderate excess of urobilinogen is generally found and that occasionally bile pigment may also be noted. This observation was confirmed in many cases of the present series. Crosby and Dameshek (127) have reported that small amounts of hemosiderin are frequently found.

Glycosuria was a common observation. A surprisingly large number of latent diabetic states were discovered in repeated urine analysis performed in patients receiving corticosteroid therapy. No attempt was made to quantitate this observation with the degree of diabetes anticipated in the normal population matched as to age and sex.

A Schilling test based on the renal excretion of orally ingested cobalt⁶⁰ labeled vitamin B-12 was performed on 16 patients. An abnormally low value was obtained in five cases. In all five cases the diagnosis of pernicious anemia was made on the basis of a megaloblastic bone marrow, lack of free stomach acid, correction

of the abnormal Schilling test by the simultaneous administration of intrinsic factor (four cases) and reticulocytosis with correction of anemia after the parenteral administration of vitamin B-12 (41).

Biochemical Changes of the Blood

A large number of abnormalities were encountered in various biochemical determinations of the blood. In many cases the biochemical abnormalities could be directly attributed to pathologic states associated with autoimmune hemolytic anemia. This is not meant to minimize the significance of these abnormalities. Clinical and laboratory characteristics of autoimmune hemolytic anemia are heavily affected by such associated diseases. The eventual survival or death of the patient generally is dependent on the nature of this associated process. The pathologic environment upon which autoimmune hemolytic anemia is superimposed is of profound importance. The biochemical observations described below, as markers of this pathologic environment, are the best indications of the diversity and degree of abnormalities encountered. Table 25 summarizes the results obtained in various blood biochemical testing.

Blood Urea Nitrogen

A blood urea nitrogen determination was performed in 74 patients. Elevations over 25 mg. per cent were noted in 26 cases or 35 per cent of the series. The elevations were generally transient and normal values were obtained when clinical improvement occurred.

In spite of massive hemolysis which may develop during hemolytic crisis, acute renal failure is a rare complication. There are six case reports in the literature. Payne and associates (59), Bull and associates (128), Rappaport and Crosby (129), Recant and Hartcroft (130), Castleman (131) and Prager (132) have all reported patients with this picture. Such cases must be clearly differentiated from examples of the hemolytic-uremic syndrome seen in childhood (133). In such patients an autoimmune pathogenesis is still problematical.

Renal shutdown was unusual in the current series and only developed in two cases. The autoimmune hemolytic state was not recognized in one case and the patient developed acute renal failure following transfusions. The second case occurred postoperatively following aortic valve prosthesis insertion.

Uric Acid

The uric acid content of the blood was examined in 37 cases. An abnormal elevation over 5 mg. per cent was found in 24 patients or 65 per cent of the tested group. Sixteen of the 24 abnormal findings were noted in patients with malignancies of the reticuloendothelium. Such patients frequently have an elevated blood uric acid level which may correlate with the degree of production and death of malignant cells. Renal insufficiency and severe liver disease were each found in two additional patients. The possibility must be considered that some degree of uric acid elevation occurs as a result of the rapid formation and destruction of erythrocytes.

Protein Bound Iodine

A protein bound iodine determination was carried out in 14 cases; normal values were found in nine. Results suggestive of hypothyroidism were found in three cases and those suggestive of hyperthyroidism in two patients. These values are not unexpected in view of the frequency of thyroid disease in patients with autoimmune hemolytic anemia (see Chapter 10).

Liver Chemistries

No definitive pattern of abnormalities was found in a series of routine liver chemistry determinations. Alkaline phosphatase, Bromsulphalein, prothrombin time, cholesterol and cholesterol esters were all normal unless hepatic disease was concomitantly present. In view of the possibility that autoimmune hemolytic anemia reflects a dysglobulinemic state, it is pertinent to examine values obtained in cephalin flocculation and thymol turbidity tests. The cephalin flocculation test was performed in 16 cases, with normal results obtained in

nine. In seven cases 3+ or 4+ values were noted at 48 hours. Liver damage and infectious mononucleosis was present in many of these cases. The thymol turbidity test was carried out in 20 patients with abnormalities seen in only four. All four patients had liver disease.

Bilirubin

An elevation of serum bilirubin was one of the most consistent abnormalities noted in patients with autoimmune hemolytic anemia. Total serum bilirubin was determined in 120 patients. An elevated value was found in 66 cases or 55 per cent of the tested patients. In 57 the indirect bilirubin was increased above normal. In 20 the increased bilirubin was exclusively of an indirect variety. In 37 cases elevations of both direct and indirect serum bilirubin were found. In only nine patients was a mild elevation attributable exclusively to an increase in direct reacting bilirubin. In general, bilirubin elevations were not excessive unless liver disease was present. When the direct and indirect bilirubin values were elevated, the indirect type generally exceeded the direct reacting variety. With therapeutic remission rapid correction of direct reacting bilirubin was noted, followed by a more slowly decreasing indirect bilirubin value.

Serum Proteins

Total serum proteins were studied in 111 patients. Significant abnormalities were noted in 20 cases or 18 per cent of the tested group. In nine, values over 9 gm. per cent were obtained. In 11, values below 5.5 gm. per cent were found. In two of these, hypogammaglobulinemia with globulin values of 0.8 and 0.3 gm. per cent was present.

The presence of serum protein abnormalities became more apparent as detailed studies were performed. An increased globulin value creating a reversed albumin-globulin (A/G) ratio was seen in 23 out of 106 patients, an incidence of 21.7 per cent.

The sera of 64 patients with autoimmune hemolytic anemia were subjected to electrophoretic studies. Abnormalities were

TABLE 26. *Serum protein studies in patients with warm acting autoimmune hemolytic anemia*

Test Procedure	Patients Examined					
	Total tested	Abnormal		Normal	
		No.	Per cent	No.	Per cent
Serum proteins	111	20	18	91	82
Reversed A/G ratio	106	23	22	83	78
Serum electrophoresis	64	39	61	25	39
Polyclonal gamma peak	64	33	52	31	48
Monoclonal gamma peak*	64	4	6	60	94
Polyclonal alpha-2 peak	64	2	3	62	97

* All patients with myeloma.

	Polyclonal Gamma Peak: Per Cent of Total Protein					
	20-24	25-29	30-34	35-39	40-50	>50†
No. of patients	7	6	7	7	4	2

† 62 per cent and 73 per cent.

found in 39 cases or 61 per cent of the group. In four cases a monoclonal spike was noted in the gamma region; all four of these patients had plasma cell myeloma. In two cases an elevated polyclonal alpha-2 globulin peak was found. In 33 cases or 52 per cent of the tested series, the gamma-globulin content was greater than 20 per cent of the total protein. This increased gamma-globulin appeared as a broad polyclonal peak. In at least four instances the broad and diffuse elevation extended into the beta-globulin zone. The magnitude of the gamma-globulin elevation was variable. In six cases, more than 40 per cent of the total protein was gamma-globulin with values of 41, 41.4, 46, 48, 62 and 73 per cent, respectively. Table 26 summarizes the total protein, A/G ratio and electrophoretic studies.

Charbonnier and Dausset (134), Hennemann and Gillert (135) and Sussman and Sang (136) have all noted elevations of gamma-globulin in autoimmune hemolytic anemia. Christenson and Dacie (137) reported an analysis of 38 idiopathic and nine secondary cases of autoimmune hemo-

lytic anemia. Normal serum protein values were obtained in most, although a tendency toward an elevated gamma-globulin level was seen. Dacie (17) concluded that "there was no serum protein pattern characteristic of auto-immune hemolytic anemia of the warm-antibody type, but minor variations from the normal are not uncommon."

Results obtained in the current series indicate that a restatement of the status of serum proteins in autoimmune hemolytic anemia is necessary. The serum protein electrophoretic pattern obtained in patients with autoimmune hemolytic anemia is frequently abnormal. A characteristic although not diagnostic pattern is seen in over one-half of the cases. This abnormality consists of a broad elevation of gamma-globulin which may extend into the beta-globulin range. The gamma-globulin will frequently constitute over 20 per cent of total serum proteins and may be significantly higher. The electrophoretic elevation presents as a polyclonal peak and differs from monoclonal patterns found in plasma cell myeloma and cold hemagglutinin disease. The elevation of gamma-globulin may reflect the presence of associated disease states. These observations are compatible with the concept that erythrocyte autoantibodies may be only one manifestation of a multiple immunologic abnormality.

Pathologic Anatomy

There are no diagnostic lesions of autoimmune hemolytic anemia which may be documented by pathologic examination of organs or tissues. This disappointing observation emphasizes the importance of laboratory studies, particularly those of a serologic nature, in diagnosing these disease syndromes. It is not surprising that classic anatomic and pathologic approaches are of little value. Similar negative observations are frequently made in the presence of other immunologically mediated diseases. The anatomic diagnosis of serum sickness, anaphylactic shock, systemic lupus erythematosus and rheumatoid arthritis is also extremely difficult. Frequently the pathologist must resort to the clinical diagnosis and simply describe the various nonspecific anatomic changes. Autoimmune disease mediated through delayed hypersensitivity may have a common although nonspecific anatomic appearance. These changes have been outlined by Waksman (138). Similar changes have not yet been found in autoimmune syndromes characterized by humoral autoantibodies.

In autoimmune hemolytic anemia specific changes characteristic of the various associated diseases may be found. Anatomic changes reflecting the hemolytic stage, however, are nonspecific. These changes are generally limited to involvement of various reticuloendothelial structures.

The Bone Marrow

Changes found in the bone marrow are those which may be encountered in any chronic hemolytic state. Generalized cellular hyperplasia is frequently present and areas of bone marrow not normally active may show extreme cellularity. The long bones can be involved and fat tissue may be replaced by intense cellular proliferation. The increased cellularity generally reflects marked proliferation of erythrocyte precursors. Megaloblastic changes are not uncommon. Participation of other cellular elements in the proliferative response is frequently observed. Marked granulocytic and megakaryocytic activity may be found. Iron stains will usually reveal an intense deposition of hemosiderin.

The Spleen

The early observations of Banti (139) implicated the spleen as a major site for the hemolytic process. He carefully described splenic enlargement and congestion, and suggested that splenic endothelial cells function as erythrophagocytes. Agglutinated erythrocytes were identified within the splenic pulp. Dameshek and Schwartz (118) summarized this early literature and added their own observations. Rappaport and Crosby (129) have presented an extensive review of the pathologic changes they observed in 30 cases. The basic abnormalities were as follows: (a) enlargement to a mean value of 650 gm.; (b) congestion of the splenic pulp and sinuses; (c) hyperplasia of reticulum cells, endothelial

cells, plasma cells and macrophages; (d) infiltration by lymphocytes and macrophages; (e) hemosiderosis, primarily in endothelial cells; (f) extramedullary hematopoiesis; and (g) erythrophagocytosis. Maruyama (140) has also summarized the splenic histologic findings in experimental autoimmune hemolytic anemia. Dacie (17) pointed out that splenic pathology in autoimmune hemolytic anemia differs from that seen in hereditary spherocytosis. The distinguishing characteristics are reticulum cell hyperplasia and erythrophagocytosis in autoimmune hemolytic anemia.

The Liver

In Banti's original description of "hemolytic splenomegaly" (139) he noted that the Kupffer cells of the liver might manifest an erythrophagocytic function during intense hemolytic states. The result of this phagocytic activity is apparent by the excess deposition of hemosiderin in such cells. Hepatomegaly is frequently observed and usually appears to result from congestion. Extramedullary hematopoiesis may occasionally be found. Hemosiderosis is common and hemachromatosis may rarely be present. Various degrees of focal necrosis can occur.

Lymph Nodes

Hyperplasia of various lymph nodes is commonly observed, although the basic architecture of the node is preserved. Erythrophagocytosis is a common feature. Rappaport and Crosby (129) and Dacie (17) have described the uncommon occurrence of extramedullary hematopoiesis in lymph nodes.

General Changes

No specific abnormalities are noted. Excessive deposition of hemosiderin is common in many areas such as the kidney and thyroid gland. Renal tubular damage and a sclerotic thyroid may result when such iron deposits lead to tissue damage.

BIBLIOGRAPHY

1. Crosby, W. H., and Akeroyd, J. H.: The limit of hemoglobin synthesis in hereditary hemolytic anemia; its relation to the excretion

of bile pigment. Amer. J. Med. **13:** 273, 1952.

2. Crosby, W. H.: The hemolytic states. Bull. N. Y. Acad. Med. **30:** 27, 1954.

3. Swisher, S. N., Trabold, N., Leddy, J. P., and Vaughn, J.: Clinical correlations of the direct antiglobulin reaction. Ann. N. Y. Acad. Sci. **124:** 441, 1965.

4. Speiser, P.: Some remarks on human erythrocytic autoantibodies. Z. Immunitaetsforsch. **132:** 113, 1967.

5. Swisher, S. N.: Nonspecific adherence of platelets and leukocytes to antibody-sensitized red cells: a mechanism producing thrombocytopenia and leukopenia during incompatible transfusions. J. Clin. Invest. **35:** 738, 1956.

6. Wasastjerna, C.: Leukocyte-agglutinins in a case of chronic granulocytopenia and hemolytic anemia. Acta Med. Scand. **149:** 355, 1954.

7. Weinreich, J., and Müller, W.: Immunhämotologische Untersuchungen bei Panzytopenien. Acta Haemat. (Basel) **16:** 376, 1956.

8. Evans, R. S., and Duane, R. T.: Acquired hemolytic anemia. I. The relation of erythrocyte antibody to activity of the disease. Blood **4:** 1196, 1949.

9. Evans, R. S., Takahashi, K., Duane, R. T., Payne, R., and Liu, C. K.: Primary thrombocytopenic purpura and acquired hemolytic anemia. Evidence for a common etiology. Arch. Intern. Med. (Chicago) **87:** 48, 1951.

10. Gasser, C., and Holländer, L.: Anémie hémolytique acquise aiguë provoquée par des auto-anticorps, accompagnée de purpura thrombocytopénique, chez un nourrisson de 7 semaines. Rev. Hemat. (Paris) **6:** 316, 1951.

11. Loeb, V., Seaman, W. B., and Moore, C. V.: The use of thorium dioxide sol (thorotrast) in the roentgenologic demonstration of accessory spleens. Blood **7:** 904, 1952.

12. Crosby, W. H.: The clinical aspects of immunologic hemolytic anemia. Sang **26:** 3, 1955.

13. Chertkow, G., and Dacie, J. V.: Results of splenectomy in auto-immune acquired haemolytic anaemia. Brit. J. Haemat. **2:** 237, 1956.

14. Crosby, W. H., and Rappaport, H.: Autoimmune hemolytic anemia. I. Analysis of hematologic observations with particular reference to their prognostic value. A survey of 57 cases. Blood **12:** 42, 1957.

15. Harris-Jones, J. N., McLellan, D. N., and Owen, G.: Haemolytic anaemia following thrombocytopenic purpura. Brit. Med. J. **1:** 624, 1958.

16. Dausset, J., and Colombani, J.: The serology and the prognosis of 128 cases of auto-

immune hemolytic anemia. Blood **14:** 1280, 1959.

17. Dacie, J. V.: *The Haemolytic Anaemias, Part II,* Ed. 2. Grune & Stratton, Inc., New York, 1962.

18. Bean, R. H. D.: Thrombocytosis in autoimmune disease. Bibl. Haemat. **23:** 43, 1965.

19. Chauffard, M. A., and Fiessinger, N.: Ictère congénital hémolitique avec lésions globulaires. Bull. Soc. Med. Hop. Paris **24:** 1169, 1907.

20. Crosby, W. H., and Rappaport, H.: Reticulocytopenia in autoimmune hemolytic anemia. Blood **11:** 929, 1956.

21. Lowman, J. T.: Diagnostic confusion associated with spherocytes in Coombs positive acquired hemolytic anemia. Lancet **2:** 431, 1962.

22. Benitez, L. E. L.: Anemia immunohemolitica macrocitaria tipo Dyke-Young. Prensa Med. Argent. **50:** 1058, 1963.

23. Remy, D.: Cytomorphologische Besonderheiten (atypische Megaloblastose und Siderozyten) bei erworbener hämolytischer Anämie von Typ Loutit. Klin. Wschr. **30:** 947, 1952.

24. Douglas, A. S., and Dacie, J. V.: The incidence and significance of iron-containing granules in human erythrocytes and their precursors. J. Clin. Path. **6:** 307, 1953.

25. Zinkham, W. H., and Diamond, L. K.: *In vitro* erythrophagocytosis in acquired hemolytic anemia. Blood **7:** 592, 1952.

26. deGruchy, G. C.: The diagnosis and management of acquired haemolytic anaemia. Aust. Ann. Med. **3:** 106, 1954.

27. Hargraves, M. M., Herrell, W. E., and Pearman, R. O.: Erythrophagocytic anemia (Lederer's anemia?): report of a case with recovery. Proc. Mayo Clin. **16:** 107, 1941.

28. Landolt, R. F.: Akute hämolytische Anämie (Lederer-Brill) mit ausgedehuter Erythrozytenphagozytose im peripheren Blut. Helv. Paediat. Acta **1:** 335, 1946.

29. Gasser, C.: Akute erworbene hämolytische Anämien mit Immunkörpernachweis und Erythrozytenphagozytose im peripheren Blut. Schweiz. Med. Wschr. **82:** 42, 1952.

30. Sansone, G.: Anemie emolitiche acute idiopatiche a genesi autoimmunitario nell'infanza. Minerva Pediat. **9:** 270, 1957.

31. Pisciotta, A. V.: Clinical and laboratory correlation in severe autoimmune hemolytic anemia. Arch. Intern. Med. (Chicago) **104:** 264, 1959.

32. Stats, D., and Wasserman, L. R.: Cold hemagglutination—an interpretive review. Medicine (Balt.) **22:** 363, 1943.

33. Nicolau, C. T., Teitel, P., and Fotino, M.: Loss of filtrability of erythrocytes coated with incomplete antibodies. Nature (London) **184:** 1808, 1959.

34. Nicolau, C. T., Teitel, P., Fotino, M., Buto-ianu, E., and Taigar, S.: Alterations of erythrocyte plasticity in blood diseases (a three years' clinical experience with the erythrocyte filtrability test [E.F.T.]). Sangre (Barc.) **9**: 282, 1964.

35. Gruelund, S.: Megaloblastic hemolytic anemia. Acta Med. Scand. **239** (suppl.): 101, 1950.

36. Baikie, A. G., and Pirrie, R.: Megaloblastic erythropoiesis in idiopathic acquired haemolytic anaemia. Scot. Med. J. **1**: 330, 1956.

37. Rubio, F., and Burgin, L.: Hemolytic disease complicated by pernicious anemia. Report of 2 cases. Bull. Tufts New Eng. Med. Cent. **3**: 77, 1957.

38. Chanarin, I., Dacie, J. V., and Mollin, D. L.: Folic acid deficiency in haemolytic anaemia. Brit. J. Haemat. **5**: 245, 1959.

39. Conti, C., and Torlontano, G.: La megalo-blastosi delle malattie emolitiche. I. Suai effetti sulla eritropoiesi. Rass. Fisiopat. Clin. Ter. **32**: 665, 1960.

40. Willoughby, M. L. N., Pearce, M. A., Sharp, A. A., and Shields, M. J.: Megaloblastic erythropoiesis in acquired hemolytic anemia. Blood **17**: 351, 1961.

41. Pirofsky, B., and Vaughn, M.: Addisonian pernicious anemia with positive antiglobulin tests; a multiple autoimmune disease syndrome. Amer. J. Clin. Path. **50**: 459, 1968.

42. Hunt, M. L., and Lucia, S. P.: The occurrence of acquired hemolytic anemia in subjects of blood group O. Science **118**: 183, 1953.

43. Clemens, K., and Walsh, R. J.: Blood groups and acquired haemolytic anaemia. Aust. J. Sci. **17**: 136, 1954–1955.

44. Lal, V. B., and Speiser, P.: Untersuchungen über Zusammenhänge zwischen erworbenen hämolytischen Anämien, klassischen Blutgruppen, Rhesusfactor, Geschlecht und Alter. Blut **3**: 15, 1957.

45. Dunsford, I., and Owen, G.: Distribution of the ABO blood groups in cases of acquired haemolytic anaemia. Brit. Med. J. **1**: 1172, 1960.

46. Weiner, W., and Nussey, A. M.: Rhesus-typing in unsuspected acquired hemolytic anemia. Lancet **1**: 257, 1961.

47. Githens, J. H., and Hathaway, W. E.: Autoimmune hemolytic anemia and the syndrome of hemolytic anemia, thrombocytopenia and nephropathy. Pediat. Clin. N. Amer. **9**: 619, 1962.

48. Kracke, R. R., and Hoffman, B. J.: Chronic hemolytic anemia with autoagglutination and hypergammaglobulinemia; report of a fatal case. Ann. Intern. Med. **19**: 673, 1943.

49. Rubinstein, M. A.: Transient positive Wassermann test for syphilis in acute hemolytic anemia. J. Lab. Clin. Med. **33**: 753, 1948.

50. Rosenthal, M. C., Komninos, Z. D., and Dameshek, W.: Multiple antibody formation in autoimmune hemolytic anemia. New Eng. J. Med. **248**: 537, 1953.

51. Hennemann, H. H.: La formation d'anticorps multiples au cours d'anémies hémolytiques acquises. Rev. Belg. Path. **24**: 479, 1955.

52. Letman, H.: Auto-immune haemolytic anaemia. Danish Med. Bull. **4**: 143, 1957.

53. Jenkins, W. J., and Marsh, W. L.: Autoimmune haemolytic anaemia. Three cases with antibodies specifically active against stored red cells. Lancet **2**: 16, 1961.

54. Dameshek, W.: What is systemic lupus? (editorial). Arch. Intern. Med. (Chicago) **106**: 162, 1960.

55. Pirofsky, B., Nelson, H., Imel, T., and Cordova, M.: The present status of the antiglobulin and bromelin tests in demonstrating erythrocyte antibodies. Amer. J. Clin. Path. **36**: 492, 1961.

56. Dybkjaer, E.: Irregular blood group antibodies. A screening test including a two-stage papain technique. Danish Med. Bull. **13**: 188, 1966.

57. Pirofsky, B.: A new diagnostic test for antiglobulin positive (autoimmune) haemolytic anaemia. Brit. J. Haemat. **6**: 395, 1960.

58. Lemaire, A., Loeper, L., Boiren, M., and Dausset, J.: Anémie hémolytique aiguë avec auto-anticorps actifs seulement sur les hémanties traitées par un enzyme protéolytique. Bull. Soc. Med. Hop. Paris **70**: 997, 1954.

59. Payne, R., Spaet, T. H., and Aggeler, P. M.: An unusual antibody pattern in a case of idiopathic acquired hemolytic anemia. J. Lab. Clin. Med. **46**: 245, 1955.

60. Vetter, O.: Vergleichende Untersuchungen über den Coombs- und Bromelin-test zum Nachweis erythrozytärer Auto-antikörper. Z. Ges. Inn. Med. **10**: 439, 1963.

61. Bedarida, G., and Giraldi, A.: Il metodo della bromelina nella diagnosi delle anemie emolitiche autoimmuni. Riv. Emoter. Immunoemat. **9**: 310, 1962.

62. Muirhead, E. E.: The relationship of current transfusion practice to modern immunohematology. Ann. N. Y. Acad. Sci. **127**: 926, 1965.

63. Mollison, P. L.: *Blood Transfusion in Clinical Medicine*. Ed. 3. Charles C Thomas, Publisher, Springfield, Ill., 1961.

64. Revol, L., Lejeune, E., Brizard, C. P., Jouvenceaux, A., and Perrin, N.: Contribution a l'étude systématique des tests globulaires et sériques dans les syndromes hémolytiques (à propos d'une statistique de 2,400 examens). Sang **29**: 416, 1958.

65. Muirhead, E. E., and Groves, M.: Positive antiglobulin (Coombs) test of canine erythrocytes induced by lipid solvents *in vitro*. Amer. J. Clin. Path. **26**: 844, 1956.

66. Jandl, J. H., and Simmons, R. L.: The agglutination and sensitization of red cells by metallic cations: interactions between multivalent metals and red cell membranes. Brit. J. Haemat. **3**: 19, 1957.
67. Brown, D. V., Boehni, E. M., and Norlind, L. M.: Anemia with positive direct Coombs' test induced by trypan blue. Blood **18**: 543, 1961.
68. Norlind, L. M., Boehni, E. M., and Brown, D. V.: Positive direct Coombs' test induced by various azo dyes. Proc. Soc. Exp. Biol. Med. **119**: 970, 1965.
69. Weeden, A. R., Datta, N., and Mollison, P. L.: Adsorption of bacteria onto red cells leading to positive antiglobulin reactions. Vox Sang. **5**: 523, 1960.
70. Muirhead, E. E., Groves, M., and Bryan, S.: Positive direct Coombs test induced by phenylhydrazine. J. Clin. Invest. **33**: 1700, 1954.
71. Luginbühl, H.: Positiver Coombs-test bei experimentaller Phenylhydrazinanämie. Schweiz. Med. Wschr. **87**: 1251, 1957.
72. Sutherland, D. A., and Eisentraut, A. M.: The direct Coombs test in lead poisoning. Blood **11**: 1024, 1956.
73. Dunsford, I., and Grant, J.: *The Antiglobulin (Coombs) Test.* Charles C Thomas, Publisher, Springfield, Ill., 1960.
74. Watanabe, K.: Immunological study of experimental hemolytic anemia induced by lead acetate. 1. Incidence of Coombs positive erythrocytes in hemolytic anemia. Jap. Arch. Intern. Med. **8**: 469, 1961.
75. Watanabe, K.: Immunological study of experimental hemolytic anemia induced by lead acetate. 2. Immunological studies on Coombs positive erythrocytes in vitro and influences of various treatments given to the experimental animals on the incidence of Coombs positive erythrocytes. Jap. Arch. Intern. Med. **8**: 568, 1961.
76. Sutherland, D. A., Eisentraut, A. M., and McCall, M. S.: The direct Coombs test and reticulocytes. Brit. J. Haemat. **9**: 68, 1963.
77. Jandl, J. H.: The agglutination and sequestration of immature red cells. J. Lab. Clin. Med. **55**: 663, 1960.
78. Pirofsky, B.: The influence of a plasma factor on the erythrocyte antibody-antigen-bromelin reaction. Vox Sang. **5**: 442, 1960.
79. Pirofsky, B., August, A., Nelson, H., and Pittenger, R.: Rapid mass anti-D (Rh₀) typing with bromelin. J. Lab. Clin. Med. **56**: 911, 1960.
80. Davidsohn, I., and Spurrier, W.: Immunohematological studies in hemolytic anemia. J. A. M. A. **154**: 818, 1954.
81. Heni, F., and Blessing, K.: Die Bedeutung der Glutinine für die erworbenen hämolytischen Anämien. Dutsch. Arch. Klin. Med. **201**: 113, 1954.
82. Sturgeon, P.: A new antibody in serum of patients with acquired hemolytic anemia. Science **106**: 293, 1947.
83. Denys, P., and van den Broucke, J.: Anémie hémolytique acquise et réaction de Coombs. Arch. Franc. Pediat. **4**: 205, 1947.
84. Evans, R. S., and Weiser, R. S.: The serology of autoimmune hemolytic disease: observations on 41 patients. Arch. Intern. Med. (Chicago) **100**: 371, 1957.
85. Evans, R. S., Bingham, M., and Boehni, P.: Autoimmune hemolytic disease. Antibody dissociation and activity. Arch. Intern. Med. (Chicago) **108**: 60, 1961.
86. Hughes-Jones, N. C.: The antigen-antibody reaction. Brit. Med. Bull. **19**: 171, 1963.
87. van Loghem, J. J., van der Hart, M., and Dorfmeier, H.: Serologic studies in acquired hemolytic anemia. In *Proceedings of the sixth International Congress of the International Society of Hematology.* Grune & Stratton, Inc., New York, 1956.
88. Heller, I., Nelken, D., and Gurevitch, J.: Etudes sérologiques sur les anticorps anti-érythrocytaires, antileucocytaires et anti-plaquettaires dans différentes affections hématologiques. Sang **29**: 17, 1958.
89. Dacie, J. V., and deGruchy, G. C.: Autoantibodies in acquired haemolytic anaemia. J. Clin. Path. **4**: 253, 1951.
90. Ogata, T., and Matuhasi, T.: Problems of specific and cross reactivity of blood group antibodies. In *Proceedings of the Eighth Congress of the International Society of Blood Transfusion.* S. Karger, Basel, 1962.
91. Ogata, T., and Matuhasi, T.: Further observations on the problems of specific and cross reactivity of blood group antibodies. In *Proceedings of the Ninth Congress of the International Society of Blood Transfusion.* S. Karger, Basel, 1964.
92. Weiner, W.: Eluting red cell antibodies: a method and its application. Brit. J. Haemat. **3**: 276, 1957.
93. Landsteiner, K., and Miller, C. P.: Serologic studies on the blood of the primates. II. The blood groups in anthropoid apes. J. Exp. Med. **42**: 853, 1925.
94. Kochwa, S., and Rosenfield, R. E.: Immunochemical studies of the Rh system. I. Isolation and characterization of antibodies. J. Immun. **92**: 682, 1964.
95. Whittingham, S., Jakobowicz, R., and Simmons, R. T.: Multiple antibodies imitating the presence of a panagglutinin in the serum of a patient suffering from haemolytic anaemia. Med. J. Aust. **48**: 205, 1961.
96. Croucher, B. E. E., Crookston, M. C., and Crookston, J. H.: Delayed haemolytic transfusion reactions simulating auto-immune haemolytic anaemia. Vox Sang. **12**: 32, 1967.
97. Ashby, W.: Determination of length of life of transfused blood corpuscles in man. J. Exp. Med. **29**: 267, 1919.
98. Dacie, J. V., and Mollison, P. L.: Survival of

normal erythrocytes after transfusion to patients with familial haemolytic anaemia (acholuric jaundice). Lancet 1: 550, 1943.

99. Brown, G. M., Hayward, O. C., Powell, O. C., and Witts, L. J.: The destruction of transfused erythrocytes in anaemia. J. Path. Bact. 56: 81, 1944.

100. Loutit, J. F., and Mollison, P. L.: Haemolytic icterus (acholuric jaundice), congenital and acquired. J. Path. Bact. 58: 711, 1946.

101. Mollison, P. L.: The survival of transfused erythrocytes with special reference to cases of acquired haemolytic anaemia. Clin. Sci. 6: 137, 1947.

102. Selwyn, J. G., and Hackett, W. E. R.: Acquired haemolytic anaemia: survival of transfused erythrocytes in patients and normal recipients. J. Clin. Path. 2: 114, 1949.

103. Gray, S. J., and Sterling, K.: Tagging of red cells and plasma proteins with radioactive chromium. J. Clin. Invest. 29: 1604, 1950.

104. Sterling, K., and Gray, S. J.: Determination of circulating red cell volume in man by radioactive chromium. J. Clin. Invest. 29: 1614, 1950.

105. Ebaugh, F. G., Emerson, C. P., and Ross, J. F.: The use of radioactive chromium 51 as an erythrocyte tagging agent for the determination of red cell survival in vivo. J. Clin. Invest. 32: 1260, 1953.

106. Read, R. C., Wilson, G. W., and Gardner, F. H.: The use of radioactive sodium chromate to evaluate the life span of the red blood cell in health and certain hematologic disorders. Amer. J. Med. Sci. 228: 40, 1954.

107. Hughes-Jones, N. C., and Mollison, P. L.: The interpretation of measurements with Cr^{51}-labeled red cells. Clin. Sci. 15: 207, 1956.

108. Mollison, P. L., and Veall, N.: The use of the isotope Cr^{51} as a label for red cells. Brit. J. Haemat. 1: 62, 1955.

109. Donohue, D. M., Motulsky, A. G., Giblett, E. R., Pirzio-Biroli, G., Viranuvatti, V., and Finch, C. A.: The use of chromium as a red cell tag. Brit. J. Haemat. 1: 249, 1955.

110. Necheles, T. F., Weinstein, I. M., and LeRoy, G. V.: Radioactive sodium chromate for the study of survival of red blood cells. I. The effect of radioactive sodium chromate on red cells. J. Lab. Clin. Med. 42: 358, 1953.

111. Sutherland, D. A., and McCall, M. S.: The measurement of the survival of human erythrocytes by in vivo tagging with Cr^{51}. Blood 10: 646, 1955.

112. Letman, H.: Red cell destruction in the anaemias (thesis). Copenhagen, 1959.

113. Constantoulakis, M., Costea, N., Schwartz, R. S., and Dameshek, W.: Quantitative studies of the effect of red-blood-cell sensitization on in vivo hemolysis. J. Clin. Invest. 42: 1790, 1963.

114. Korst, D. R., Clatanoff, D. V., and Schilling, R. F.: External scintillation counting over the liver and spleen after the transfusion of radioactive erythrocytes. Clin. Res. Proc. 3: 195, 1955.

115. Jandl, J. H., Greenberg, J. S., Yonemoto, R. H., and Caste, W. S.: Clinical determination of the sites of red cell sequestration in hemolytic anemias. J. Clin. Invest. 35: 842, 1956.

116. Hughes-Jones, N. C., and Szur, L.: Determination of the sites of red-cell destruction using Cr^{51}-labeled cells. Brit. J. Haemat. 3: 320, 1957.

117. Dameshek, W., and Schwartz, S. O.: Hemolysins as the cause of clinical and experimental hemolytic anemias. With particular reference to the nature of spherocytosis and increased fragility. Amer. J. Med. Sci. 196: 769, 1938.

118. Dameshek, W., and Schwartz, S. O.: Acute hemolytic anemia (acquired hemolytic icterus, acute type). Medicine (Balto.) 19: 231, 1940.

119. Young, L. E., and Miller, G.: Differentiation between congenital and acquired forms of hemolytic anemia. Amer. J. Med. Sci. 226: 664, 1953.

120. Bakker-v. Aardenne. W. I. T., Verloop, M. C., and van Boetzelaer, G. C. D.: Osmotic and mechanical fragility of erythrocytes in patients with idiopathic and symptomatic hemolytic anemia. In Proceedings of the Sixth Congress of the European Society of Hematology. S. Karger, Basel, 1957.

121. Rossi, V., and Bastistini, N.: Studi sui rapporti tra fragilita osmotica e autoemolisi nelle anemie emolitiche autoimmuni. Arch. Maragliano Pat. Clin. 20: 183, 1964.

122. Fiorina, L., Prato, V., and Mazza, U.: Comportamento osmotico dell'eritrocita umano. V. L'eritrocita nella sferocitosi ereditaria e nelle anemie emolitiche acquisite autoimmuni. Arch. Sci. Med. (Torino) 118: 276, 1964.

123. Negrini, A. C.: Erythrocytic osmotic resistance in autoimmune idiopathic acquired hemolytic anemia, with special reference to relations between spherocytosis and osmotic fragility. Observations before and after therapy. Arch. Maragliano Pat. Clin. 16: 553, 1960.

124. Ham, T. H., Gardner, F. H., Wagley, P. F., and Shen, S. C.: Studies on the mechanism of hemolytic anemia and hemoglobinuria occurring in patients with high concentrations of serum cold agglutinin. J. Clin. Invest. 27: 538, 1948.

125. Young, L. E., Miller, G., and Christian, R. M.: Clinical and laboratory observations on autoimmune hemolytic disease. Ann. Intern. Med. 35: 507, 1951.

126. Shaub, F., and Maier, C.: Zur klinischen Bedeutung der mechanischen Resistenz der roten Blutkörperchen. Acta Haemat. (Basel) 15: 90, 1956.

127. Crosby, W. H., and Dameshek, W.: The significance of hemoglobinuria and associated hemosiderinuria, with particular reference to various types of hemolytic anemia. J. Lab. Clin. Med. **38**: 829, 1951.

128. Bull, G. M., Joekes, A. M., and Lowe, K. G.: Acute renal failure following intravascular hemolysis. Lancet **2**: 114, 1957.

129. Rappaport, H., and Crosby, W. H.: Autoimmune hemolytic anemia. 2. Morphologic observations and clinicopathologic correlation. Amer. J. Path. **33**: 429, 1957.

130. Recant, L., and Hartcroft, S. W.: Acute renal failure of obscure etiology. Amer. J. Med. **30**: 464, 1961.

131. Castleman, B.: Case records of the Massachusetts General Hospital. New Eng. J. Med. **267**: 612, 1962.

132. Prager, D.: Acquired auto-immune hemolytic anemia with acute renal insufficiency. Ann. Int. Med. **59**: 357, 1963.

133. Barnard, P. J., and Kibel, M.: The haemolytic-uraemic syndrome of infancy and childhood. A report of 11 cases. Cent. Afr. J. Med. **11**: 31, 1965.

134. Charbonnier, A., and Dausset, J.: Etude électrophorétique des protides sériques au cours des anémies hémolytiques avec autoanticorps incomplets chauds. Ann. Biol. Clin. (Paris) **11**: 22, 1953.

135. Hennemann, H. H., and Gillert, K. E.: Serum Labilitätsproben und electrophoretische Untersuchungen bei Erkrankungen mit positiven Coombs Test. Deutsch. Arch. Klin. Med. **201**: 158, 1954.

136. Sussman, L. N., and Sang, J. B.: Electrophoretic patterns in acute acquired hemolytic anemia. Proc. Soc. Exp. Biol. Med. **95**: 380, 1957.

137. Christenson, W. N., and Dacie, J. V.: Serum proteins in acquired haemolytic anaemia (auto-antibody type). Brit. J. Haemat. **3**: 153, 1957.

138. Waksman, B. H.: *Experimental Allergic Encephalomyelitis and the "Auto-allergic" Diseases*. S. Karger, Basel, 1959.

139. Banti, G.: Splénomégalie hémolytique anhémopoitique: le rôle de la rate dans l'hémolyse. Sem. Med. **33**: 313, 1913.

140. Maruyama, Y.: Histological studies on the experimental auto-immune hemolytic anemia. I. Histopathologic changes of the spleen. Jap. J. Allerg. **14**: 590, 1965.

Chapter 4

The Idiopathic Autoimmune
Hemolytic Anemias

Idiopathic or primary autoimmune hemolytic anemia is defined as hemolytic anemia characterized by positive antiglobulin tests in the absence of significant associated pathologic states. The criteria for "significance" of associated diseases are highly variable. Classification, accordingly, is constantly changing. The possibility that idiopathic or primary forms of autoimmune hemolytic anemia are purely illusory must be considered (1).

Types of Idiopathic Autoimmune Hemolytic Anemia

In the current series five different forms of idiopathic autoimmune hemolytic anemia may be segregated on the basis of differences observed in the peripheral blood and bone marrow. Table 27 presents a tentative classification and indicates the incidence of the various types seen.

Erythrocytic Type

The erythrocytic type is the most commonly observed form and represents the usual syndrome classified as idiopathic autoimmune hemolytic anemia. An isolated depression of erythrocytes is the prominent peripheral blood abnormality. The bone marrow is characterized by erythrocytic hyperplasia with or without an associated hypercellularity of other myeloid elements.

Evans' Syndrome Type

Evans' syndrome is a well recognized form of idiopathic autoimmune hemolytic anemia. In addition to anemia, marked thrombocytopenia is also observed in the peripheral blood. The bone marrow is generally hyperplastic. Erythrocytic hyperplasia and a normal to increased megakaryocytosis are characteristic abnormalities.

Pancytopenic Type

The pancytopenic type of autoimmune hemolytic anemia is characterized by anemia, thrombocytopenia and leukopenia. In spite of marked depression of the peripheral blood's formed elements, the bone marrow is essentially normal or has varying degrees of hyperplasia.

Aplastic Type

All three of the above syndromes are characterized by normal to hyperplastic changes in the bone marrow, in spite of deficiencies of peripheral blood formed elements. The aplastic type of autoimmune hemolytic anemia superficially appears similar to the pancytopenic type. Anemia, thrombocytopenia and leukopenia are prominent. However, bone marrow aspiration reveals marked hypoplasia of erythrocytic, thrombocytic and granulocytic precursors. Clinically, the picture may appear identical to aplastic anemia.

The Erythrocytic Aplasia Type

The erythrocytic aplasia type of autoimmune hemolytic anemia duplicates the more common erythrocytic type. Anemia appears

TABLE 27. *Classification and incidence of the various forms of idiopathic autoimmune hemolytic anemia*

Peripheral Blood Cell Depression Associated with:	No.	Per Cent
A. Normal or hyperplastic bone marrow	37	84.1
1. Erythrocytic type	30	68.2
2. Evans' syndrome type	5	11.4
3. Pancytopenic type	2	4.5
B. Hypoplastic bone marrow	7	15.9
1. Aplastic type	4 (5)*	9.1
2. Erythrocytic aplasia type	3	6.8
Total	44	100

* One patient was diagnosed as having an idiopathic form for 83 months until reticulum cell sarcoma developed.

as the only peripheral blood abnormality. Bone marrow aspiration, however, reveals a distinctly abnormal pattern. There are almost no erythrocytic precursors, although megakaryocytes and granulocyte precursors are well maintained.

The five types of idiopathic autoimmune hemolytic anemia described above may occasionally present blood values which blur the clear boundaries outlined. This blending of syndromes is particularly marked in the three forms characterized by hyperplastic or normal bone marrow examinations. It is not unusual for a patient with the erythrocytic type to have thrombocyte counts of 75,000 to 100,000/mm.^{3} The absence of bleeding and the moderate depression of thrombocytes in such cases do not warrant a diagnosis of Evans' syndrome.

Autoimmune hemolytic anemia is not a static clinical syndrome. Its clinical and laboratory features frequently change. This tendency introduces great difficulties in classification. The following case illustrates this problem.

Case 9. A 54-year-old female was seen with a virus form of pneumonia and treated with oral tetracycline. She improved but 1 month later developed a severe virus upper respiratory infection. Four weeks later extensive petechiae, purpura and ecchymoses were seen. Her hematocrit was 38 per cent and the thrombocyte count

below 10,000/mm.^{3}; clot retraction was absent in 24 hours. Bone marrow aspiration demonstrated an increased number of megakaryocytes, and idiopathic thrombocytopenia was diagnosed. She received 30 mg. of prednisone for 1 week and a prompt rise of thrombocytes was noted. Four months after thrombocytopenia, mild anemia occurred. Two months later the hematocrit had dropped to 30 per cent, a 14.5 per cent reticulocytosis was noted and the thrombocyte count was 250,000/mm.^{3} Direct and indirect antiglobulin and bromelin tests were positive. The autoantibody was identified as a panhemagglutinin. The bone marrow then demonstrated hyperplasia of the erythrocytic series. Renal function was normal and lupus erythematosus (LE) cell preparations were negative. Prednisone, 60 mg. daily, was started and an excellent therapeutic response occurred. Steroid therapy was gradually decreased, but the hematocrit fell when levels below 10 mg. per day were employed. The hematocrit was maintained at 32 per cent, using 15 mg. of prednisone daily. Eight months after the onset of hemolytic anemia, direct and indirect antiglobulin tests were negative although bromelin tests were strongly positive. Splenectomy is to be performed.

The author has classified this case as Evans' syndrome although the thrombocytopenia and autoimmune hemolytic anemia phases of the illness appear to be separated in time. It may be difficult to discriminate accurately among the three types of idiopathic autoimmune hemolytic anemia dependent on peripheral blood values. In contrast, the two forms characterized by depression of the bone marrow generally appear as unequivocal and distinct entities.

Classification of Autoimmune Hemolytic Anemia as an Idiopathic Type

The definition of idiopathic autoimmune hemolytic anemia given above is simple. Certain qualifications are necessary, however. Although autoimmune hemolytic anemia may occur in the complete absence of any other demonstrable disease, this is unusual. The clinician is frequently forced to make a decision as to relevancy of associated pathologic states before deciding on classification as an idiopathic or secondary variety. Guides for such a differentiation are outlined in Chapter 2.

The assumption of relevancy or irrelevancy of associated pathologic states is subject to discussion and modification. A patient with hyperthyroidism present before or after the development of autoimmune hemolytic anemia would have been classified as having an idiopathic form 10 years ago. Currently, the autoimmunologic implications of hyperthyroidism are sufficiently established to classify such cases as secondary varieties of autoimmune hemolytic anemia. The same rationale applies to associated thymomas, ulcerative colitis, pernicious anemia, etc.

An increasing experience with autoimmune hemolytic anemia also tends to change classification as to idiopathic or secondary associations. At the start of the current series active tuberculosis was considered an irrelevant, fortuitous associated state. Eight years later a clear cut association became apparent when six cases presenting this combination were analyzed. The temporal relationship of tuberculosis to the development of the hemolytic syndrome strongly suggested relevancy.

Even when an idiopathic variety of autoimmune hemolytic anemia can be unequivocally diagnosed, the clinician must be prepared to reverse this diagnosis. The subsequent development of associated pathologic states which can be etiologically related may then lead to diagnosis of a secondary form. The eventual diagnosis of systemic lupus erythematosus in a patient initially considered as having idiopathic autoimmune hemolytic anemia is a classic example of this situation. Such a patient has been presented in Case 2. Years may elapse before the associated clinical pattern becomes apparent. In addition, the clinician must realize that a pertinent associated disease can be present although diagnosis is impossible. The following case illustrates this sequence.

Case 10. A 72-year-old male entered with progressive heart failure. Jaundice was detected and mild hepatomegaly was present. An abdominal aneurysm was discovered on physical examination. The hematocrit was 20.5 per cent, reticulocytes 7.2 per cent and bilirubin 1.4/5.4 mg. per cent. A Cr^{51} half-life (T/2) survival time of 4.2 days, with splenic sequestration of 492 per cent, was demonstrated. Direct and indirect antiglobulin and bromelin tests were positive and elution obtained a panhemagglutinin. Prednisone therapy was initiated and an excellent therapeutic response noted. Maintenance prednisone was required to continue the remission. Severe abdominal and back pain gradually developed. Sixteen months after onset of hemolytic anemia, surgery to correct the abdominal aneurysm was carried out. During this procedure cholelithiasis and a carcinoma of the ascending colon were discovered, but not surgically treated. The patient expired 6 months later from an acute coronary occlusion.

In this case an initial diagnosis of idiopathic autoimmune hemolytic anemia was made. Classification was changed 16 months later to a secondary variety with the demonstration of a previously undiagnosed carcinoma of the colon.

A review of the current series of patients with autoimmune hemolytic anemia reveals a large number of cases originally classified as idiopathic autoimmune hemolytic anemia. Subsequently, many cases required reclassification as secondary forms. It is difficult to escape the extrapolation that an idiopathic form of autoimmune hemolytic anemia may not exist. Expansion of the number of diseases considered relevant to the development of autoimmune hemolytic anemia, and the subsequent diagnosis or development of pathologic states which are accepted as relevant, have greatly reduced the number of cases considered idiopathic. When this residual small group is viewed as possibly being involved in transient or subclinical disease states, such an extrapolation does not appear to be unwarranted. In many instances a familial predisposition to develop autoimmune syndromes may be documented by family studies (1).

Classification of autoimmune hemolytic anemia as idiopathic or secondary is not to be considered as an interesting exercise in semantics. Such classification has both clinical and theoretical significance. The diagnosis of idiopathic autoimmune hemolytic anemia may be impermanent. Such cases must be followed, treated and investigated as if the clinician were dealing with an "iceberg state." It must be assumed that only a small part of the entire pathologic process is within range of clinical evalua-

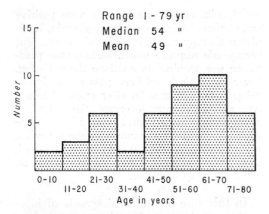

Range 1 - 79 yr
Median 54   "
Mean   49   "

Number

Age in years

FIG. 9. The age distribution of 44 patients with idiopathic autoimmune hemolytic anemia.

tion. The physician must be alert and conscientious in order to delineate as soon as possible the existence of relevant pathologic processes which may be amenable to therapy. In this fashion the disaster of developing autoimmune hemolytic anemia may be converted into a beneficial early clinical observation permitting a rapid diagnosis of correctable lesions. The large number of associated disease categories listed in Table 12 may serve as guideposts indicating the direction of necessary clinical investigations.

Questioning the accuracy of a diagnosis of idiopathic autoimmune hemolytic anemia is healthy. Through such studies the possible role of autoimmune hemolytic anemia as part of a generalized, systemic immunologic abnormality may become clear. The end stage process that we term autoimmune hemolytic anemia may be initiated by varied pathophysiologic mechanisms. Both autoimmune and immune but not autoimmune (antiglobulin positive) immunohemolytic processes are involved. This viewpoint may eventually permit construction of an accurate picture of autoimmune hemolytic anemia as it is related to clinical medicine.

Statistical Considerations

The information presented below is based on analysis of 44 cases of idiopathic autoimmune hemolytic anemia. The reader is encouraged to contrast the data with those obtained from the prior analysis of the entire group of patients with autoimmune hemolytic anemia.

Incidence

Most authors report the idiopathic variety as either the most common type of autoimmune hemolytic anemia or as equal in incidence to secondary forms. Exceptions to this general observation are contained in the reports of van Loghem and associates (2), who noted that 55 per cent of their 122 patients had a secondary type, Swisher and associates (3), who found that 68 per cent of 107 cases were of a secondary variety, and Speiser (4), who reported that 60 per cent of 540 cases were secondary forms. Yunis and Bridges (5) in a small series of 40 patients noted secondary forms in 57.5 per cent of cases. Bohnen and associates (6) reported an idiopathic form of autoimmune hemolytic anemia in only 13 of 178 patients having positive direct antiglobulin tests. It is unclear whether the remaining 92 per cent of the group had secondary forms of autoimmune hemolytic anemia. The current series documents the frequent occurrence of secondary types. Of 234 patients studied, only 44 cases or 18.2 per cent could be considered idiopathic. Accordingly, idiopathic autoimmune hemolytic anemia is relatively uncommon when contrasted with the entire group of autoimmune hemolytic anemias.

Age Distribution

Figure 9 presents the distribution of ages found in the 44 patients with idiopathic autoimmune hemolytic anemia. All age groups may be involved. A range of ages at onset of hemolytic anemia extending from 1 to 79 years was encountered. Of the series 31 cases or 71 per cent were over age 40. A peak incidence occurred in the 50- to 70-year age group.

Sex

Table 5 presents the sex distribution of patients with autoimmune hemolytic anemia. A definite preponderance of females in the idiopathic variety is noted. Of the series 63.6 per cent were females. This is in contrast to the entire series of patients with autoimmune hemolytic anemia where no influence of sex was noted. A 50 per cent incidence of involved females was found in the total series.

Genetic Predisposition

A genetic approach suggests that idiopathic forms of autoimmune hemolytic anemia may be illusory and may represent our limited ability to diagnose associated pathologic states. Support for this concept has been presented in Chapter 2 where the distribution of autoimmune hemolytic anemia in one family is discussed. The proband was diagnosed as idiopathic autoimmune hemolytic anemia, and two siblings were also found to have hemolytic anemia and positive antiglobulin tests. One sibling had plasma cell myeloma and the other had multiple abnormalities suggestive but not diagnostic of systemic lupus erythematosus. It is unlikely that the patient with the idiopathic variety had an isolated disease resulting from selective production of erythrocyte autoantibodies. The same pathologic process resulted in a broader clinical picture with easily documented associated diseases in the other two siblings.

Family histories of the 44 patients classified as having idiopathic autoimmune hemolytic anemia were analyzed in order to determine whether pertinent autoimmune syndromes were present in family members. It should be emphasized that a purely retrospective analysis was carried out (1). The information presented below was obtained from the initial history taken when no attempt was made to establish a genetic pattern. Eight additional patients were encountered with a significant history. The relationship and type of associated disease are summarized in Table 28.

The classification of family ailments as autoimmune introduces some difficulty. Many of these patients were not studied at our institution. A definitive diagnosis could not always be made even when family members were investigated by our group. This is noted in the case of Patient 8 of Table 28. The mother and one brother of this child had anemia, splenomegaly and jaundice in the absence of a demonstrable cause. The usual congenital forms of hemolytic anemia were ruled out. The observation that the patient and one other sibling had autoimmune abnormalities suggests a possible autoimmune relationship. The etiology of several of the conditions listed is debatable. However, selection was made on the basis of a high presumption of an immunologic pathogenesis as postulated by various authors. It is apparent that further study may deplete this list. The reverse is equally possible. Additional investigations may well expand the number and types of conditions generally accepted as being related to an autoimmune mechanism.

This retrospective study demonstrated that nine patients, or 20.4 per cent of the 44 cases of idiopathic autoimmune hemolytic anemia, had significant autoimmune family histories. It is possible that an earlier genetic orientation would have resulted in more efficient and thorough history taking and that it would have revealed a significantly higher incidence. This interpretation appears pertinent because five of the nine familial relationships were discovered in our own laboratory. The relationship became apparent because other family members had been or were subsequently referred for their individual medical problems. The clinician is accordingly urged to expand history and laboratory analysis to include other family members in order to clarify this very important point.

Survival and Duration of Disease

At the time of analysis 16 patients with idiopathic autoimmune hemolytic anemia had died, two were lost to followup and 26 were alive. Accordingly, a mortality rate of 38.1 per cent for the idiopathic form was obtained. This is substantially less than the mortality rate observed with the secondary varieties of autoimmune hemolytic anemia. Eleven of the 16 cases that died survived less than 2 years; six died in less than 1 year. Three cases survived more than 5 years. The range of survival prior to death extended from 2 weeks to 85 months. A median of 19 and mean of 29 months' duration before death were determined.

TABLE 28. *History of presumptive autoimmune disease in immediate family members of patients with idiopathic autoimmune hemolytic anemia (nine of 44 patients had pertinent histories)*

Patients with Autoimmune Hemolytic Anemia*			Immediate Family Members of Patient	
Case	Age	Sex	Involved relative	Presumptive autoimmune disease
1	66	F	Sister*	Autoimmune hemolytic anemia; plasma cell myeloma
			Brother*	Autoimmune hemolytic anemia; lupus erythematosus
2	61	F	Father*	Hodgkin's disease
3	19	M	Mother*	Chronic granulocytic leukemia; busulfan sensitivity
4	50	F	Father	Glomerulonephritis
5	62	F	Mother	Pernicious anemia
6	46	F	Sister	Pernicious anemia
			Aunt	Pernicious anemia
7	23	F	Sister	Stevens-Johnson syndrome
8	2.5	M	Mother*	Anemia, splenomegaly
			Brother*	Anemia, jaundice, splenomegaly
			Brother*	Thrombocytopenic purpura
9	53	F	Sister	Rheumatoid arthritis
			Sister	Lupus erythematosus
			Sister	Chronic granulocytic leukemia
			Grandnieces (4)	"Idiopathic" nephritis
			Grandniece*	Thrombocytopenic purpura; 4+ albuminuria

* Studied at our institution.

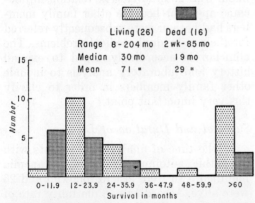

Living (26) Dead (16)
Range 8 - 204 mo 2 wk - 85 mo
Median 30 mo 19 mo
Mean 71 " 29 "

Survival in months

FIG. 10. The duration of survival in months of patients with idiopathic autoimmune hemolytic anemia. Sixteen patients who have died and 26 subjects still living are analyzed.

Of the 26 patients still living, all but one have been followed for over 12 months. Nine cases, or 32 per cent of the living group, have survived over 5 years. Four of these have survived for over 10 years with the longest period being 204 months. The mean

survival of patients still living is 70.8 months with a median of 29.5 months. Accordingly, the prognosis of idiopathic autoimmune hemolytic anemia is markedly superior to that of secondary varieties. Survival for 2 years suggests an excellent chance of maintaining long survival in excess of 5 years. Figure 10 summarizes the duration of survival of both the dead and still living patient groups.

Clinical Observations

Highly variable clinical patterns are presented by patients with idiopathic autoimmune hemolytic anemia. Such variations reflect the following: (a) the rate of destruction of erythrocytes, (b) the ability of the bone marrow to compensate by hyperplasia, (c) the rapidity of the drop of peripheral erythrocytes, and (d) the ability of the patient to acclimate to the lowered red cell mass. Marked extremes in these functions are found.

The symptoms of patients with idiopathic

autoimmune hemolytic anemia result from the anemic state, the hemolytic process and various miscellaneous causes. The incidence of the various symptoms is listed in Table 8 and is contrasted with that for the entire series of patients with autoimmune hemolytic anemia. Symptoms referable to the anemic state are most frequent and are almost universally found. They generally occur in a pattern characterized by weakness, fatigue, dizziness, shortness of breath on exertion and a pulsation or pounding in the ears. Similar symptoms are commonly observed in any anemic state. They are accordingly not diagnostic for autoimmune hemolytic anemia. In the elderly, various degrees of cardiac decompensation may be found. In most patients such symptoms develop gradually and progressively. The patient becomes acclimated to the lowered hematocrit with a variable degree of success. The explosive intensification of hemolysis, which is termed hemolytic crisis, is fortunately uncommon. In such patients hemolysis is violent and rapid and bone marrow compensation is limited or late. The patient has little or no opportunity to adjust to the rapidly dropping hematocrit. Such states are true medical emergencies and require immediate diagnosis and therapy. Jaundice and fever are frequently encountered. It is interesting that jaundice is more common in the idiopathic group, whereas fever is more frequently found in the secondary varieties of autoimmune hemolytic anemia.

The Erythrocytic Type of Idiopathic Autoimmune Hemolytic Anemia

Autoimmune hemolytic anemia characterized by a selective deficiency of peripheral erythrocytes and bone marrow erythrocytic hyperplasia is the most common form of idiopathic autoimmune hemolytic anemia. Of the current series, 30 of the 44 cases could be classified in this group.

Abnormalities discovered on physical examination were common in the erythrocytic type. Of these cases, 21 patients, or 70 per cent, had a palpable spleen at the onset or during the course of their disease. The spleen appeared firm and not tender, and massive enlargement was unusual. Hepatomegaly was less consistently found and was documented in 10 of the patients. Lymphadenopathy was the least common abnormality indicating involvement of the reticulo-endothelium. Only six patients, or 20 per cent, had palpable lymph nodes. The enlarged liver and palpable lymph nodes were generally firm, moderately enlarged and not tender. Jaundice was prominent and was noted by both the patient and examining physician. Fifteen patients or one-half of the series had clinical jaundice. Fever of a low grade variety was less commonly observed. Eight patients, or 27 per cent, had mild to moderate fever.

Anemia was the most prominent laboratory observation. A range of hematocrits extending from 13.5 to 40 per cent was found on initial examination. The mean and median hematocrit approximated 24 per cent. With continuation of the disease anemia became more prominent until therapeutic remission occurred. Followup hematocrits ranged from 11 to 32 per cent. In 77 per cent of the patients hematocrits were 24 per cent or lower. Approximately one-fifth of the series developed hematocrits of 15 per cent or less.

Reticulocytosis was usually evident at the initial examination. Only 12 per cent of cases had normal values. A marked elevation was not uncommon. A reticulocytosis of over 10 per cent was noted in 32 per cent of cases. This evidence of increased bone marrow activity became even more apparent after initiation of therapy. In all but one instance a further elevation of the reticulocyte count was found. In over 56 per cent of the cases a reticulocytosis exceeding 10 per cent was seen. Reticulocyte count values of 40 per cent or higher were not uncommon. Doan and associates (7) have reported a case of hemolytic anemia with a 100 per cent reticulocyte count.

The leukocyte count was normal in most patients. Transient leukopenia or leukocytosis were relatively unusual. In the majority, thrombocytes appeared in a normal range of 150,000 to 300,000/mm.^{3} Minor depressions ranging from 75,000 to 150,000/mm.^{3} were not uncommon. Spherocytes and

TABLE 29. *Statistical data obtained from 30 patients (20 females, 10 males) with an erythrocytic type of idiopathic autoimmune hemolytic anemia*

Test Procedure	Statistical Data			
	Total	Range	Mean	Median
Clinical data				
Age (years)	30	2.5–78	49	54
Survival, dead* (months)	9	0.5–85	38	18
Survival, alive* (months)	20	7–204	55	28
Laboratory data				
Initial hematocrit (%)	27	13.5–40	24.6	23.5
Lowest hematocrit (%)	26	11–32	20.7	20.5
Initial reticulocytes (%)	27	0.3–48	9.5	5.5
Therapeutic reticulocytes (%)	19	0.0–52	16.6	12.2
Initial WBC (10^3/mm.^{3})	26	2–108	9.1	5.85
Initial thrombocytes (10^3/mm.^{3})	23	15–1000	187	200

	Total	Increased	Decreased	Normal
Bone marrow aspiration				
Total cellularity	23	10	0	13
Erythrocyte precursors	23	22	0	1
Granulocyte precursors	23	4	0	19
Megakaryocytes	23	3	0	20
Megaloblasts	23	5	0	18

	Total	Spleen	Liver	Lymph nodes	Jaundice	Fever
Presenting signs						
Abnormal	30	21	10	6	15	8

* One patient was lost to followup.

nucleated erythrocytes were commonly observed.

Bone marrow examination almost always revealed abnormalities. A normal examination was reported in only one patient. Erythrocytic hyperplasia was the most common abnormality and was present in 22 of the 23 patients examined. In 10 cases generalized hypercellularity was also present. Increased granulocytic activity was reported in four specimens and three bone marrow samples had increased megakaryocytes. Megaloblastic changes were found in five bone marrow specimens. The statistical data obtained from analysis of the erythrocytic type of idiopathic autoimmune hemolytic anemia are summarized in Table 29.

The clinical pattern of patients with the erythrocytic type of idiopathic autoimmune hemolytic anemia was variable. It was diffi-

cult to predict the subsequent course from the initial workup. Wide extremes were found and included a rapid and progressive deterioration until death and long and relatively asymptomatic survivals. The following protocols illustrate some of the clinical patterns.

Case 11. A 62-year-old white male was investigated for generalized fatigue of unknown etiology. No diagnosis was made. Four years later he entered, complaining of weakness and dyspnea. The hematocrit was 20 per cent, and 26 units of blood were transfused over a 2-week period. Three months later the weakness and anemia had returned. Ten units of blood were given and the patient was transferred for diagnotic studies. The hematocrit was 37 per cent. Bronchopneumonia and jaundice were found. Over the next 5 days marked jaundice developed and splenomegaly became apparent. The hematocrit dropped to 11 per cent with a 5.6 per cent reticulocyte count noted. Thrombocytes and white blood cells (WBC) were mildly elevated. Cross matches for transfusion were all incompatible, and positive direct antiglobulin and bromelin tests were found. Elution studies revealed an anti-hr″(e) and the patient's erythrocytes were typed as hr″(e) positive. Prednisone therapy was started but the patient died within 12 hours. Autopsy revealed only splenomegaly with pulp congestion and hemosiderin and hyperplastic reticulum changes of the lymph nodes.

This case emphasizes the rapid and fulminating course that may occur in autoimmune hemolytic anemia. Over a 5-day period the hematocrit fell from 37 to 11 per cent. The diagnosable duration of disease was less than 5 months, and prior transfusion therapy obscured definitive studies. The inability to diagnose adequately the clinical problem led to a delay in therapy and to the patient's death.

Case 12. A 35-year-old female was referred because of complaints of fatigue. The hematocrit was 35 per cent and physical examination was normal. Various hematinics were used without success. Three months later low grade fever was noted. The hematocrit was 25 per cent and a reticulocyte count of 3.2 per cent was found. Bone marrow aspiration revealed erythrocytic hyperplasia. Serologic studies demonstrated positive direct antiglobulin tests. A chromium⁵¹ T/2 survival time of 9 days was obtained. Corticosteroid therapy was given, resulting in a reticulocytosis of 22 per cent and return toward a normal hematocrit. Corticosteroids were discontinued after 3 months, and the patient remained asymptomatic for over 3 years. Fatigue, jaundice and anemia then recurred. Corticosteroid therapy was initiated without a response. The hematocrit dropped to 17.5 per cent with a reticulocytosis of 31 per cent. Positive direct and indirect antiglobulin and bromelin tests were obtained. Splenomegaly was now apparent. A splenectomy was performed and was followed by a rapid therapeutic remission. Followup examination 11½ years after onset of disease, 7 years after splenectomy, revealed an asymptomatic patient with normal peripheral blood values and negative serologic studies.

This case emphasizes that idiopathic autoimmune hemolytic anemia is compatible with long and asymptomatic survival. An early diagnostic investigation and meticulous followup permitted accurate diagnosis with initiation of effective therapy. An important aspect of the successful result was the awareness that failure of therapy constitutes a medical emergency requiring other therapeutic procedures.

Case 13. A 22-year-old white female was investigated for anemia and jaundice. A diagnosis of "liver infection" was made and the patient treated with vitamin B-12. Pregnancy occurred 6 months later and anemia was again demonstrated. An hematocrit of 30 per cent with a 1.5 per cent reticulocyte count was found. Spherocytes and many nucleated erythrocytes were noted. Bone marrow aspiration revealed erythrocytic hyperplasia with megaloblastic changes. Therapy was not given. Two years later the patient complained of a left upper quadrant mass, fatigue, jaundice and dark urine. The hematocrit was 25 per cent with a 0.5 per cent reticulocyte count. Splenomegaly and jaundice were confirmed on physical examination. During the next year splenectomy was performed for persisting anemia. Two years later mild hepatomegaly was noted with a normal Cr⁵¹ T/2 survival time. The hematocrit was 30 per cent and a reticulocyte count of 3.2 per cent was found. The bone marrow still showed erythrocytic hyperplasia with megaloblastic changes. The patient remained essentially asymptomatic except for recurrent migratory arthritis over the next 7 years. Cholecystectomy for cholelithiasis was required at this time. Four years later the patient entered with colitis. Erythema nodosa was diagnosed and a family history of a Stevens-Johnson syndrome in a sister was obtained. The patient was found to have a diffusely enlarged thyroid gland. Physical examination was otherwise negative, and an hematocrit of 31 per cent with a reticulocyte count of 2.9 per cent was present. The direct antiglobulin test was weakly positive. Followup 17 years from the onset of her disease, and 13 years after splenectomy, demonstrated an essentially asymptomatic patient. An hematocrit of 37 per cent and a reticulocyte count of 2.2 per cent were found.

The course of the above patient again illustrates that long survivals are compatible with idiopathic autoimmune hemolytic anemia. In contrast with Case 12, however, it is apparent that an active disease process is still smouldering. The development of migratory polyarthritis, erythema nodosa and diffuse thyroid enlargement suggests that our series of idiopathic cases will again be reduced. It is apparent that significant associated pathologic states are present in this patient. The development of a Stevens-Johnson syndrome in one sibling also suggests a genetic influence in the development of a systemic immunologic disease. Meticulous followup in such cases is needed.

The Evans' Syndrome Type of Idiopathic Autoimmune Hemolytic Anemia

In 1949 Evans and Duane (8) called attention to the association of autoimmune hemolytic anemia and thrombocytopenia. They noted persistent thrombocytopenia in five of 11 patients with autoimmune hemolytic anemia. In one case purpura was present and in two an associated leukopenia was found. One patient was pregnant. Evans and Duane suggested that either the autoantibody responsible for hemolytic anemia had a broad range of activity which involved thrombocytes or an additional immune substance was present. They were inclined to the latter explanation in view of the lack of correlation between the degree of hemolysis and thrombocytopenia.

Evans and associates (9) expanded these observations in 1951. Eighteen patients with autoimmune hemolytic anemia were analyzed and normal thrombocyte and leukocyte counts were found in 10. The disease in this group corresponds to the erythrocytic type of idiopathic autoimmune hemolytic anemia discussed above. The eight cases with thrombocytopenia had varied clinical courses. Purpura was present in only four. Four patients of the total series had an associated leukopenia. Pregnancy was present in two patients. Evans and associates again suggested that a specific antibody directed against thrombocytes was the responsible agent.

Since these initial observations were made, many investigators have confirmed the existence of a syndrome characterized by autoimmune hemolytic anemia, thrombocytopenic purpura and bone marrow hyperplasia. Dausset and Colombani (10) noted the presence of such a syndrome in 11 of 83 cases of warm acting idiopathic autoimmune hemolytic anemia, an incidence of

13.2 per cent. Only one of these cases had leukopenia below 5,000/mm.[3] The authors also recognized that the temporal relationship between hemolytic anemia and thrombocytopenia varied. In five patients both states occurred simultaneously. In three instances idiopathic thrombocytopenia preceded the hemolytic anemia. In one of these thrombocytopenic purpura had been present for 16 years prior to the onset of hemolytic anemia. In three cases thrombocytopenia occurred after the development of hemolytic anemia. The longest interval separating this association was 17 months. Additional recent reports have been presented by Silverstein and Hech (11), Brunner and Frick (12) and Brunet and associates (13). Dacie (14) and Dacie and deGruchy (15) have also reported the occurrence of hemolytic anemia in patients previously splenectomized for idiopathic thrombocytopenic purpura.

Several authors have suggested that the association of thrombocytopenia and autoimmune hemolytic anemia has a poor prognosis. Crosby (16) and Crosby and Rappaport (17) noted a mortality rate of 31 per cent in 16 patients with autoimmune hemolytic anemia. Seventeen patients with associated thrombocytopenia and autoimmune hemolytic anemia had a mortality rate of 71 per cent. Chertkow and Dacie (18) and Dacie (14) also emphasize the poor prognosis of Evans' syndrome.

In the current series five of the 44 idiopathic forms had associated thrombocytopenia with hyperplastic bone marrows. This incidence of 11.3 per cent closely simulates the experience of Dausset and Colombani (10), particularly if their one case with leukopenia is excluded. The secondary varieties of autoimmune hemolytic anemia have been excluded from this tabulation. Such an exclusion was not performed in the original reports of Evans and associates (8, 9). This may explain their observation of a 44.4 per cent incidence. Cases of systemic lupus erythematosus and tuberculosis of the spleen are specifically mentioned by these workers as being present in their patients. The relationship of systemic lupus erythematosus to Evans' syndrome is particularly striking. Cases 2 and 7 in this series illustrate this occurrence.

Three females and two males in the present series conform to the criteria of an Evans' syndrome type of idiopathic autoimmune hemolytic anemia. No particular age dependency was noted, with a range of 1 to 65 years seen. Two of these patients have died. One case with a simultaneous occurrence of hemolytic anemia and thrombocytopenia survived 15 months. The other patient developed thrombocytopenia at age 1, and 3 years later hemolytic anemia was diagnosed. Death occurred 3½ years after the hemolytic process was documented. The surviving three cases have been followed for the relatively short periods of 8, 12 and 17 months, respectively.

Two patients had the simultaneous development of hemolytic anemia and thrombocytopenia. In the remaining three cases thrombocytopenia preceded the development of hemolytic anemia. The time between development of thrombocytopenia and subsequent occurrence of hemolytic anemia was 6, 7 and 51 months, respectively. Case 9 describes one of these patients.

Physical findings were not remarkable. Hepatosplenomegaly was present in two patients. Lymphadenopathy was noted in one additional case. Jaundice was prominent in two and fever in one patient. Petechiae, purpura, hematomas and other bleeding phenomena were common, and were recorded in four of the five cases.

The hematocrit was moderately depressed in all cases and an elevated initial reticulocyte count was found in three. Reticulocytosis was found in all patients after therapy was started. The initial thrombocyte count was markedly depressed below 30,000/mm.[3] in all cases. Values below 10,000/mm.[3] were found in three patients. A return to normal thrombocyte values was noted in two patients after corticosteroid therapy. The leukocyte count was normal in four of the five patients. An initial WBC of 1,800/mm.[3] in one case spontaneously returned to normal levels without specific therapy. Nucleated erythrocytes and spherocytes were commonly found in the peripheral blood smears.

Bone marrow erythrocytic hyperplasia was described in three cases, and normal erythrocytic activity was recorded in the remaining two. Increased megakaryocytes were documented in three and normal to lowered numbers were seen in two cases. Megaloblastic changes of erythrocytic precursors were noted in two patients. The various statistical determinations are summarized in Table 30.

Evans and Duane in 1949 (8) questioned whether a single autoantibody or two autoantibodies with specificities directed against erythrocytes and thrombocytes respectively were involved in this syndrome. The current series does not settle this problem. The original observation of a lack of correlation between hemolysis and thrombocytopenia can, however, be confirmed. This suggests that two different antibodies are involved. Experimental reports of Matoth and associates (19) and Kumar and Saraya (20) further indicate that distinct and separate antibodies are concerned. It has been noted, however, that various blood group antigens, including rhesus factors, may be present in thrombocytes. Accordingly, it is equally possible that one autoantibody could be responsible for both hemolytic anemia and thrombocytopenia.

The possibility that autoimmune hemolytic anemia appears as part of a widespread immunologic disease characterized by multiple autoantibody formation also suggests that separate autoantibodies may be present. The following case of Evans' syndrome reinforces this suggestion.

Case 14. A 1-year-old white female was investigated for purpura. Hepatosplenomegaly was demonstrated. The hematocrit was 30 per cent, reticulocytes were 1.2 per cent and thrombocytes were 29,000/mm.[3] The bone marrow was normal except for increased megakaryocytes. Steroid therapy was initiated with an excellent therapeutic response. However, thrombocytopenia and purpura recurred whenever corticosteroid therapy was discontinued. Two years later splenectomy was carried out and followed by a transient elevation of thrombocytes. Direct antiglobulin tests were negative. Continual steroid administration was required. One year later positive direct antiglobulin tests were obtained. Such serologic tests remained consistently positive

TABLE 30. *Statistical data obtained from five patients (three females, two males) with an Evans'
syndrome type of idiopathic autoimmune hemolytic anemia*

Test Procedure	Total	Statistical Data		
		Range	Mean	Median
Clinical data				
Age (years)	5	1–65	40	45
Survival, dead (months)	3	12–75	34	15
Survival, alive (months)	2	8–17	25	25
Thrombocytopenia prior to hemolytic anemia (months)	3	6–34	16	7
Laboratory data				
Initial hematocrit (%)	5	19–30	25.4	26
Lowest hematocrit (%)	5	19–30	25.4	26
Initial reticulocytes (%)	3	1.0–14.5	5.6	1.2
Therapeutic reticulocytes (%)	4	5.2–36.4	17.4	14.1
Initial WBC (10^3/mm.^{3})	5	1.8–12	7.7	8.7
Initial thrombocytes (10^3/mm.^{3})	5	0.5–16	8.3	10

		Increased	Decreased	Normal
Bone marrow aspiration				
Total cellularity	5	0	2	3
Erythrocyte precursors	5	3	1	1
Granulocyte precursors	5	0	1	4
Megakaryocytes	5	3	2	0
Megaloblasts	5	2	0	3

		Spleen	Liver	Lymph nodes	Jaundice	Bleeding
Presenting signs						
Abnormal	5	2	2	1	2	4

on direct and indirect antiglobulin testing; the bromelin tests were negative. Elution revealed a panhemagglutinin in the antiglobulin procedure. Anemia and reticulocytosis were minimal. The patient's course was complicated by repeated episodes of purpura and infections. Edema did not appear as a problem. At age 5 chickenpox occurred and the thrombocytes increased to 1,310,000/mm.^{3} without steroid therapy. Thrombocyte counts remained elevated for 2½ months. Bleeding and thrombocytopenia then recurred and required corticosteroid therapy. One year later severe bleeding developed in spite of adequate thrombocyte replacement therapy. A circulating anticoagulant was discovered and antihemophiliac globulin levels of less than 1 per cent were found. It was felt that an antihemophiliac A autoantibody was present. This substance persisted and a hemorrhagic death occurred 75 months after the onset of thrombocytopenia and 41 months after the first positive antiglobulin test.

Three major observations can be derived from this case. A widespread immunologic disease with multiple autoantibody formation is suggested. Although the possibility exists that a single autoantibody was responsible for both thrombocytopenia and hemolytic anemia, this is unlikely. Thrombocytopenia was present for 3 years with negative antiglobulin tests and no evidence of hemolysis. A possible abnormal propensity to form autoantibodies is also evident with the terminal production of a circulating autoantibody directed against antihemophiliac globulin A. A cross reacting antibody, produced in response to transfusion therapy and assuming an allotypic status of antihemophiliac globulin, would provide an equally satisfactory explanation. An important clinical point is illustrated in the above case. The patient's course was dominated by thrombocytopenic purpura. Hemo- lytic anemia appeared as an interesting laboratory finding rather than as a contrib- utory factor to the clinical status. Such a dichotomy between laboratory findings and clinical manifestations are quite common in Evans' syndrome. Clinical variations re- sulting from the relative importance of bleeding phenomena and hemolytic anemia are marked and should be anticipated.

The Pancytopenic Type of Idiopathic Auto- immune Hemolytic Anemia

In 1908 Chauffard (21) reported a patient with acquired hemolytic anemia character- ized by a serum hemolysin, purpura and leukopenia. Wiseman and Doan (22) noted the association of hemolytic anemia, spleno- megaly and pancytopenia in a syndrome they called "primary splenic neutropenia." They considered that splenic hypertrophy might increase the capacity to destroy cel- lular elements of the blood. Fisher (23) also noted the presence of pancytopenia in ac- quired hemolytic anemia. He suggested that such a state could occur by the production of autoantibodies directed against all cellu- lar elements. Dameshek and Estren (24) re- ported pancytopenia occurring as part of "hypersplenic" hemolytic anemia. A hor- monal inhibition of cellular elements was presumed to result from splenic hyper- trophy. An excellent therapeutic response to splenectomy was noted. In the description by Evans and Duane (8) of thrombocyto- penia and hemolytic anemia, leukopenia was also noted in some cases. An autoanti- body etiology was postulated and the terms immunohemolytic anemia and immunopan- cytopenia were derived. Additional descrip- tions of this association were published by Moeschlin and associates (25, 26) and Bernard and associates (27) in 1954. The latter publication reported the presence of leukoagglutinins. Müller and Weinrich (28, 29) studied 27 cases of hemolytic anemia complicated by pancytopenia. In three cases antibodies directed against erythrocytes, thrombocytes and leukocytes were found. Positive antiglobulin reactions, three weak and three strong, were seen in this patient group. Leukoagglutinins were found in 12 cases and thrombocyte antibodies were

found in eight cases. The overwhelming ma- jority had had prior transfusions. Matoth and associates (19) and Baumgartner (30) also demonstrated the association of leuko- agglutinins and thrombocyte antibodies. Dausset and Brecy (31) employed the anti- globulin consumption test to identify leuko- agglutinins and thrombocyte antibodies in patients with idiopathic pancytopenia. Im- mune pancytopenia occurring in association with systemic lupus erythematosis has been reported by Goudsmit and van Loghem (32) and Müller and Redojícíc (33).

In the current series pancytopenia with a normal to hyperplastic bone marrow and idiopathic autoimmune hemolytic anemia was a rare occurrence. Only two such cases were seen. Insufficient data are available to present a meaningful clinical summary. Ac- cordingly, the two cases are briefly sum- marized below.

Case 15. A 79-year-old white female was in- vestigated for anemia. No diagnosis was made and she was transfused with 3 units of blood to an hematocrit of 37 per cent. Iron and vitamin B-12 therapy were administered. One month later weakness and jaundice were noted. The hematocrit was 21.5 per cent, reticulocytes were 1.5 per cent, thrombocytes were markedly de- pressed and the leukocyte count was 2,900/mm.^{3} Total bilirubin was 4.5 mg. per cent (mostly indirect variety) and direct and indirect anti- globulin and bromelin tests were positive. Re- peated LE cell preparations were negative. A cold hemagglutinin with a titer of 512 was found. Bone marrow examination revealed marked erythrocytic hyperplasia with other cellular ele- ments normal. The spleen was 10 cm. below the costal margin and the liver was 8 cm. down. Transfusions were started but discontinued be- cause of severe reactions. The hematocrit dropped to 18 per cent. Corticosteroids were given and a reticulocyte count of 17.3 per cent was obtained in 4 days. Thrombocytes remained markedly depressed but bleeding did not occur. Leukocytes ranged from 1,380 to 2,200/mm.^{3} The hematocrit gradually rose to 34 per cent. Relapse of the hemolytic state occurred whenever predni- sone was decreased below 30 mg. daily. The pa- tient died 20 months after the onset of disease with massive hepatosplenomegaly as the only pertinent finding.

Case 16. A 44-year-old white male was in- vestigated because of petechiae and purpura. Fatigue and anemia were noted and were unresponsive to hematinics. Physical examination was negative. The hematocrit was 16.5 per cent with reticulocytes 2.3 per cent. Thrombocytes were 5,000/mm.³ and WBC 2,500/mm.³ A normal to hypercellular bone marrow was found. A 4-month trial of corticosteroids was unrewarding, with the patient requiring 12 units of blood to maintain his hematocrit above 15 per cent. Antiglobulin and bromelin tests were normal. Androgen therapy was initiated and a therapeutic response occurred within 6 weeks. The hematocrit stayed at levels over 30 per cent and reticulocyte counts ranged from 1.5 to 5.6 per cent. Thrombocytes were consistently below 30,000/mm.³ and a WBC below 4,000/mm.³ was maintained. Forty-one months after therapeutic remission, relapse occurred in spite of maintenance androgen therapy. The hematocrit dropped to 18 per cent with a reticulocytosis of 4.4 per cent. The bone marrow was unchanged. The WBC was 1,800/mm.³ and the thrombocyte count was below 10,000/mm.³ Petechiae and purpura recurred. The direct antiglobulin test was now positive and a Cr^{51} T/2 survival time of 22.8 days was found without splenic sequestration. No response to corticosteroid and androgen therapy was obtained. Thirty-nine units of blood were transfused during this 1-year period of therapeutic trials. Splenectomy was carried out with a pathologic diagnosis of "hypersplenism." In the 3 years following splenectomy the patient has maintained hematocrits of 25 to 30 per cent without transfusions and with a persistence of low grade reticulocytosis. The leukopenia and thrombocytopenia without bleeding have persisted. Followup is continuing 87 months since the onset of disease.

These two cases are so dissimilar that different pathophysiologic mechanisms are probably involved. In one case massive hepatosplenomegaly was seen. In the other, the liver and spleen could not be palpated. Bleeding was present in one case and not in the other. A dramatic therapeutic response to corticosteroid therapy was seen in one case, and a complete failure was seen in the second patient. It is apparent that further clinical observations in the pancytopenic type of idiopathic autoimmune hemolytic anemia must be obtained before this syndrome is clarified.

The Aplastic Type of Idiopathic Autoimmune Hemolytic Anemia

Idiopathic autoimmune hemolytic anemia associated with pancytopenia and a normal to hyperplastic bone marrow were relatively rare occurrences in this series. A superficially similar syndrome was not infrequently found, however. Such forms of idiopathic autoimmune hemolytic anemia also presented with pancytopenia. An entirely different bone marrow picture was observed. In all cases a marked depression of myeloid cellular elements existed, leading to a diagnosis of aplastic anemia.

This association has previously been recognized by many workers and termed "aplastic crisis." Such cases have been reported by Linke (34), Davis and associates (35), Bonham Carter and associates (36), Wagner (37), Bowman (38), Seip (39), Veras and Manios (40), Martoni and Musiani (41), Lees (42), Burston and associates (43) and Pirofsky (44). The syndrome is characterized by rapid and marked bone marrow depression, depressed or absent reticulocytosis, pancytopenia, a rapidly falling hematocrit and a transient course. A precipitating event leading to bone marrow depression, such as an infectious process, may frequently be found. The classic features of this state involve an explosive onset and rapid recovery. A more prolonged clinical picture is possible (36, 41, 42, 44). Bousser and associates (45) reported a case of aplastic anemia which persisted for 5 months until spontaneous remission occurred. A typical autoimmune hemolytic anemia subsequently developed. Pirofsky (44) has emphasized the chronic nature of this syndrome which may closely simulate aplastic anemia.

In the current series five cases of idiopathic autoimmune hemolytic anemia with pancytopenia and an aplastic bone marrow pattern were found. Two males and three females were involved. Their ages ranged from 30 to 62 years. Hemolytic anemia and an aplastic bone marrow were simultaneously discovered in all patients. Two patients are dead, two are living, and one was lost to followup. The two living patients have survived 92 and 96 months, respectively, since the onset of disease. One patient died within 2 weeks and the other 87 months after the start of disease. Each of two patients had splenomegaly, hepatomegaly and lymphadenopathy. Jaundice and fever were present in one patient. Bleeding phenomena were noted in four of the five cases.

The laboratory findings were striking. A moderately severe anemia was present in all cases; the hematocrit ranged from 9 to 25 per cent. Reticulocyte counts of 0 per cent were noted in three cases. Two patients had initial reticulocyte counts of 0.2 and 1.4 per cent. Leukopenia was universal and ranged from 500 to 4,500/mm.[3] The thrombocytes were described as rare in three cases and quantitated as 2,000 and 39,000/ mm.[3] in the remaining two. Spherocytes were seen in three cases and peripheral blood nucleated erythrocytes in two patients. The leukocyte differential revealed granulocytopenia with lymphocyte counts ranging from 75 to 96 per cent of total white cells. Total serum bilirubin was not elevated in the three cases tested. Multiple

LE cell preparations were negative in all five patients.

The bone marrow findings were similar in all five cases. A marked reduction of cellularity was noted. This depression involved erythrocytic precursors, the granulocytic series and megakaryocytes. A diagnosis of aplastic anemia was initially made in all five patients on the basis of the peripheral blood and bone marrow examination. Table 31 summarizes the clinical and laboratory data for these cases.

Several striking clinical characteristics were observed. Only one case conformed to the commonly described pattern of an aplastic crisis.

Case 17. A 40-year-old white female developed weakness and Jacksonian epilepsy. Seven years later a carcinoma of the uterus was diagnosed and removed. At age 50 surgical removal

TABLE 31. *Statistical data obtained from five patients (three females, two males) with an aplastic type of idiopathic autoimmune hemolytic anemia*

Test Procedure	Statistical Data			
	Total	Range	Mean	Median
Clinical data				
Age, years	5	30–62	51	56
Survival, dead* (months)	2	0.5–87		
Survival, alive* (months)	2	92–96		
Laboratory data				
Initial hematocrit (%)	5	9–30	20.9	21
Lowest hematocrit (%)	5	9–25	18	20
Initial reticulocytes (%)	5	0–1.4	0.3	0.1
Therapeutic reticulocytes (%)	5	0.2–5.9	2.4	4.1
Initial WBC (10^3/mm.[3])	5	0.5–4.5	1.76	1.2
Initial thrombocytes (10^3/mm.[3])	5	2–39	20	20

	Increased	Decreased	Normal
Bone marrow aspiration			
Total cellularity	5	0	5	0
Erythrocyte precursors	5	0	5	0
Granulocyte precursors	5	0	5	0
Megakaryocytes	5	0	5	0
Megaloblasts	5	0	0	5

	Spleen	Liver	Lymph nodes	Jaundice	Bleeding
Presenting signs					
Abnormal	5	2	2	2	1	4

* One patient was lost to followup.

of a meningioma was carried out. Mesantoin therapy was given for one week and Dilantin therapy was then substituted and maintained. Thirteen months later she was investigated for pallor, weakness, jaundice and severe epistaxis. The spleen was not felt, but 1+ lymphadenopathy and a liver palpated 10 cm. below the costal margin were demonstrated. Fever was persistent but mild. The hematocrit was 9 per cent and multiple reticulocyte counts ranged from 0.0 to 0.2 per cent. Only rare thrombocytes could be found. The WBC ranged from 5,000 to 1,700/mm.^{3}. The bone marrow demonstrated marked aplasia, hemosiderosis and only rare erythrocytic precursors. Cross matches for transfusion were incompatible, and positive antiglobulin and bomelin tests were obtained. Five transfusions were given with multiple reactions. The patient lapsed into coma. Corticosteroids were started but the patient died 14 days later without a therapeutic response. The patient's total course was 2 weeks.

The above case illustrates the explosive nature of autoimmune hemolytic anemia associated with an aplastic bone marrow. It may be questioned whether this patient should be classified as idiopathic in view of transient Mesantoin and continual Dilantin therapy. Such drugs may induce an aplastic bone marrow. The autoimmune state may be either an incidental or etiologically related complication of aplastic anemia. This point deserves emphasis when the remaining four cases in this series are examined. In three of these, a recent (less than 4 months previously) exposure to Butazolidin, Chloromycetin and Achromycin, respectively, occurred prior to development of the hemolytic state. Accordingly, four of the five patients with autoimmune hemolytic anemia and an aplastic bone marrow were in contact with potent marrow depressive agents in a time relationship compatible with the development of bone marrow hypoplasia.

Four patients in this series did not present with an explosive or rapid onset typical of an aplastic crisis. The disease process in these patients gradually became evident and assumed a chronic nature. The following case illustrates this pattern.

Case 18. A 56-year-old white male was investigated because of fatigue and epistaxis. Mild anemia, leukopenia and thrombocytopenia approximating 75,000/mm.^{3} were found. No diagnosis was made. No therapy was given. One year later hematuria developed. Physical examination revealed hepatosplenomegaly and axillary adenopathy. The hematocrit was 20 per cent, reticulocytes were 0.0 per cent and the WBC ranged from 640 to 3,000/mm.^{3} Thrombocytes were rarely seen. LE cell preparations and bilirubin were normal. Bone marrow aspiration revealed a marked depression of cellularity, and aplastic anemia was diagnosed. An attempt to transfuse the patient led to incompatible cross matches. Positive direct and indirect antiglobulin and bromelin tests were found. Corticosteroid therapy was started and a reticulocyte response to 4.6 per cent was obtained in 2 days. The hematocrit gradually rose to normal levels, although leukopenia and thrombocytopenia without bleeding persisted. Hepatosplenomegaly and lymphadenopathy disappeared. Maintenance prednisone therapy, 7.5 mg. daily, was continued. The patient's course was complicated by staphylococcus pneumonia and recurrent bronchopneumonia. Followup is continuing 96 months since the onset of disease and 82 months after the therapeutic remission.

The remaining three cases in this series had a similar chronic course with a variable period of time between onset of complaints and diagnosis. The fulminating characteristics described in the literature and seen in Case 17 were not found. In one case the patient was followed as a classic example of aplastic anemia by two different hematologists. Diagnosis of aplasia was based on four different bone marrow examinations taken over a 3-month period of time. This patient developed reticulum cell sarcoma after 83 months of autoimmune hemolytic anemia. Her protocol is presented as Case 38.

Diagnosis is difficult when hemolytic anemia is complicated by pancytopenia and an aplastic bone marrow. In all five cases of the current series an initial diagnosis of aplastic anemia was made. Autoimmune hemolytic anemia was not suspected. Serologic investigations which indicated the presence of autoimmune hemolytic anemia were performed only when incompatible cross matches were found. The internist who requested consultation because of an inability to obtain compatible blood for Case 18 summarized the position of the clinician. He appeared dubious when the diagnosis of autoimmune hemolytic anemia was made. He said, "How can such a diagnosis be made with pancytopenia and an aplastic bone marrow, in the absence of erythrocytic hyperplasia, reticulocytosis, and hyperbilirubinemia?" Only through serologic studies and an immediate therapeutic response to corticosteroid therapy was this diagnosis justified. The clinician is therefore urged to employ antiglobulin and proteolytic enzyme tests as a routine procedure in all cases of aplastic anemia.

It is difficult to explain the two entirely different clinical patterns characteristic of autoimmune hemolytic anemia and an aplastic bone marrow. The following can be suggested. A patient with autoimmune hemolytic anemia is dependent on increased production of erythrocytes in order to maintain the peripheral erythrocyte blood count. A precarious balance between destruction and production is established. Any inhibition of the bone marrow's capacity to compensate through erythrocytic hyperplasia will suddenly magnify overt evidence of the hemolytic process. This will lead to an explosive clinical state characterized by fulminating anemia. An aplastic crisis is an appropriate description of this event. The seriousness of this state can be gauged by the observation of Crosby and Rappaport (46) that reticulocytopenia at the time of intense hemolysis has a high mortality, even in the face of bone marrow erythrocytic hyperplasia. Bone marrow depression in such patients may be transient if it reflects conditions such as an infectious disease. Accordingly, aplastic crisis is generally short lived. The patient will not survive if it persists.

A chronic pancytopenic state may also develop. If the hemolytic process is mild or if the aplastic state develops prior to or simultaneously with autoimmune hemolytic anemia, the explosive characteristic of this syndrome can be lost. A new homeostasis balancing the production and destruction of erythrocytes is established. This leads to chronic but progressive anemia. The entire process is prolonged in time and closely simulates typical aplastic anemia. Such events, in the author's experience, are more common than the dramatic appearance of aplastic crisis.

The exact etiologic relationship of autoimmunization to aplastic anemia still must be clarified. The immunologic implications are discussed below and suggest that immunologic events may result in an aplastic bone marrow. There are excellent experimental examples of this sequence in heteroimmune systems. Can the reverse happen? The observation that four of the five cases in the current series were exposed to marrow depressing drugs is suggestive. The case presented by Bousser and associates (45) also suggests that aplastic anemia may occur first and be followed by autoimmune hemolytic anemia. One such example of aplastic anemia followed by a secondary autoimmune hemolytic component was seen in this series.

Case 19. A 59-year-old white female developed virus pneumonia followed by myocarditis. Anemia was noted and was treated with transfusions. Two years later multiple infections occurred. Her hematocrit was 18 per cent, reticulocytes were 0.0 per cent, WBC were 3,000/mm.³ and thrombocytes were 60,000/mm.³. Bone marrow aspiration revealed a hypoplastic pattern and the diagnosis of aplastic anemia was made. Antiglobulin and bromelin tests were negative. Corticosteroids were given without success. Androgen therapy was initiated with a gradual return to normal. Forty months later a radical mastectomy was performed for a breast tumor. Hodgkin's disease was diagnosed from the pathologic specimen. Local radiation therapy was given. Three months later massive hepatosplenomegaly and 2+ lymphadenopathy were found. The hematocrit was 37 per cent and reticulocytes were 2.1 per cent. The WBC was 2,700/mm.³ and thrombocytes were 82,000/mm.³. The antiglobulin test was negative and the bromelin test was strongly positive. Vinblastine and chlorambucil therapy was given. Two weeks later the hematocrit had dropped to 28 per cent, the WBC to 1,600/mm.³ and thrombocytes to 21,000/mm.³. The antiglobulin test was now positive, as was the bromelin test. Following chemotherapy the hematocrit gradually rose to 34.5 per cent. Nine days later the patient suddenly developed fatigue and jaundice. The hematocrit was found to be 14 per cent. The patient died as corticosteroid therapy and transfusions were started.

In this patient a well documented episode of aplastic anemia was successfully treated, only to be followed 3½ years later by Hodgkin's disease. Rapid death occurred, caused by autoimmune hemolytic anemia. It may legitimately be questioned whether the prior aplastic anemia was related to subsequent reticuloendothelial malignancy and/or autoimmune hemolytic anemia.

The Erythrocytic Aplasia Type of Autoimmune Hemolytic Anemia

In 1954 Eisemann and Dameshek (47) called attention to a previously undescribed type of autoimmune hemolytic anemia. A selective depression of erythrocyte precursors in the bone marrow was a distinctive feature. Eisemann and Dameshek reported that splenectomy led to reticulocytosis and they suggested that erythrocytic aplasia had resulted from "hypersplenism."

Ross and associates (48) in 1954 also observed the association of autoimmune hemolytic anemia and pure bone marrow erythrocytic aplasia. They studied one patient with profound anemia, absent reticulocytes, positive antiglobulin tests, a shortened Cr^{51} survival time and selective depression of erythrocytic precursors in the bone marrow. This patient had a thymoma which was surgically removed. No effect was noted on the erythrocytic aplastic state. Repeated transfusion therapy led to the eventual development of hemochromatosis.

In the current series three patients were studied with characteristics similar to those described above. Two females and one male were involved. Ages ranging from 53 to 77 years were noted. Two patients died after a disease duration approximating 3 years. One patient is living with a disease duration of 78 months. The clinical and laboratory characteristics of these patients are summarized in Table 32.

A characteristic laboratory pattern was observed in all cases. Profound anemia was present with an absence of reticulocytes. No depression of leukocytes or thrombocytes was observed. Bone marrow aspiration revealed a normal to increased cellularity of granulocyte precursors and megakaryocytes. Erythrocyte precursors were extremely rare and only occasional cells could be found after extensive examination. In all cases positive antiglobulin and proteolytic enzyme studies were obtained. In one case a thymoma was subsequently discovered. Surgical removal did not improve the erythrocytic aplasia, the reticulocytopenia or the anemia. In a second case, no response to steroids or to androgen therapy was obtained, and the patient died with extensive hemochromatosis in spite of deferoxamine therapy. This case was particularly interesting as anemia was initially associated with a hyperplastic bone marrow and a pattern of erythrocyte maturation arrest. This persisted for 2 years until pure erythrocyte aplasia was observed. The third case responded to steroid therapy. A carcinoma of the colon was removed 4 years after the onset of hemolytic anemia. The case history of one patient with erythrocytic aplasia is presented below.

Case 20. A 59-year-old white male developed a rash on two successive occasions after contact with a weed killer. Two months after the last exposure, fatigue, dyspnea and syncope developed. These symptoms became progressively more severe. Four months after first exposure to the toxin, hematologic evaluation revealed an hematocrit of 8 per cent, a reticulocyte count of 0.0 per cent, WBC of 7,900/mm.³ and thrombocytes of 225,000/mm.³. The direct antiglobulin test was negative but the direct bromelin test was 3+. Bone marrow aspiration revealed pure erythrocytic aplasia. Physical examination and chest x-rays were negative. Androgen therapy was given without success, and multiple transfusions were employed. Ten months after the onset of disease and 6 months after the last negative chest x-ray, a mediastinal mass was discovered by x-ray. Liver biopsy revealed hemosiderosis. Thymectomy was performed and a spindle cell thymoma was removed. Both the direct antiglobulin and bromelin tests were now positive. The anemia, complete reticulocytopenia and bone marrow erythrocytic aplasia continued. Corticosteroid therapy was given without a therapeutic response. The patient required 2 units of blood every 2 weeks to maintain hematocrit values of 15 per cent. Nine months after thymectomy both direct and indirect anti-

TABLE 32. *Statistical data obtained from three patients (two females, one male) with an erythrocytic aplasia type of idiopathic autoimmune hemolytic anemia*

Test Procedure	Statistical Data			
	Total	Range	Mean	Median
Clinical data				
Age (years)	3	53–77	63	59
Survival, dead (months)	2	36–38		
Survival, alive (months)	1	78		
Laboratory data				
Initial hematocrit (%)	3	9–28	17	14
Lowest hematocrit (%)	3	8–18	13.3	14
Initial reticulocytes (%)	3	0.0	0.0	0.0
Therapeutic reticulocytes (%)	3	0.0–5.8	2.9	2.9
Initial WBC (10^3/mm.^{3})	3	3.2–8.2	5.8	6.0
Initial thrombocytes (10^3/mm.^{3})	3	170–225	198	200
		Increased	Decreased	Normal
Bone marrow aspiration				
Total cellularity	3	0	0	3
Erythrocyte precursors	3	0	3	0
Granulocyte precursors	3	2	0	1
Megakaryocytes	3	1	0	2
Megaloblasts	3	0	0	3

		Spleen	Liver	Lymph nodes	Jaundice	Fever
Presenting signs						
Abnormal	3	1	1	1	0	0

globulin and bromelin tests were positive and a panagglutinating erythrocyte autoantibody could be documented. Death occurred 38 months after the onset of erythrocytic aplasia and autoimmune hemolytic anemia and 29 months after demonstration and removal of the thymoma.

The diagnosis of an idiopathic variety of autoimmune hemolytic anemia may also be questioned in this case. Exposure to a toxic agent occurred immediately prior to the development of erythrocytic hypoplasia. This patient appears similar to one with a thymoma observed by Ross and associates (48). Removal of the tumor in both patients did not influence the erythrocytic aplasia. In the patient of Ross and associates the antiglobulin test and Cr[51] survival time eventually returned to normal. This sequence did not occur in our patient. Korn and associates (49) have also reported the association of immune deficiencies, aplastic anemia and thymoma.

Summary of Hypoplastic Bone Marrow Syndromes

A diagnosis of autoimmune hemolytic anemia suggests a pattern of reticulocytosis, hyperplastic bone marrow and, more specifically, erythrocytic hyperplasia. It is well recognized that catastrophic fulminating hemolysis may occur in a transient, abrupt pattern. This can be associated with bone marrow depression. Such episodes are termed aplastic crises and are considered rare. Most clinicians are unaware of a chronic syndrome resulting from the association of autoimmune hemolytic anemia with various degrees of bone marrow depression. In the current series eight examples, or 18.2 per cent of the 44 cases of idiopathic autoimmune hemolytic anemia, presented with either complete depression of myeloid elements or selective erythrocytic aplasia.

Hyperplasia of the bone marrow, and particularly erythrocytic hyperplasia, is generally explained by assuming bone marrow compensation under the stress of anemia and anoxia. Such an explanation carries the tacit assumption that mature erythrocytes are targets for erythrocyte autoantibody action and that erythrocyte precursors are exempt from the adverse effect of immune interaction. No such assumption is warranted. It is possible that during maturation of erythrocytes new antigenic components are produced and supply the target for erythrocytic autoantibodies. There is no evidence to support this concept, however. Experimental studies suggest that antigenic determinants on erythrocyte precursors can react with erythrocyte autoantibodies. Steffen (50), Pisciotta and Hinz (51) and Yunis and Yunis (52) have all demonstrated that erythrocyte autoantibodies can interact with nucleated erythrocytes. Rossi and associates (53) and Sacchetti and associates (54) have shown that even rubriblasts may be agglutinated and may manifest cellular damage after exposure to erythrocyte autoantibodies.

Autoimmune hemolytic anemia should therefore be considered as a disease involving both peripheral blood erythrocytes and bone marrow erythrocytic precursors. With this concept several variables enter into the eventual production of either hypoplastic or hyperplastic bone marrow patterns. The avidity and amount of autoantibody in relation to the total antigenic environment are important. The total number of mature erythrocytes greatly exceeds available erythrocyte precursors. Mature cells will bind the bulk of erythrocyte autoantibody with limited autoantibody production, or antibodies of low avidity. This peripheral blood cell involvement is clearly shown with our usual serologic procedures. Damage to such cells may also be demonstrated by survival time studies. The lesser number of erythrocyte precursors, with a substantially smaller amount of available antigenic determinants, will show a proportionally lesser degree of involvement. The unavailability of either serologic tests or survival time procedures for bone marrow elements makes it impossible to demonstrate nucleated erythrocyte involvement in this process. The ability of uninvolved or minimally involved erythrocyte precursors to respond to anemic stress will result in rapid compensation and increased mitosis of nucleated erythrocytes. This may completely obscure the premature death of a small number of marrow cells. Erythrocytic hyperplasia of the bone marrow will accordingly be observed. With a large amount of available autoantibody and/or antibodies with great avidity, a substantial number of erythrocyte precursors may reflect the destructive immune process. This will result in varying degrees of erythrocyte precursor damage, leading to hypoplasia or even erythrocytic aplasia. Yamamoto (55, 56) has presented an experimental system demonstrating the effect of antierythroblastic antibodies on peripheral blood and bone marrow cells. Kontek (57) also postulates the presence of an immunologic factor leading to irreversible bone marrow failure and hemolysis.

Pancytopenia and bone marrow aplasia may also be considered within this postulated sequence. Leukoagglutinins and thrombocyte antibodies have been documented in some cases of pancytopenia (19, 27–33). Such autoantibodies may affect the peripheral blood and bone marrow elements in a manner identical to that postulated for the erythrocyte series. The many variations encountered clinically and documented in the current series become understandable with this concept. Kumar and Saroya (20) have shown that rabbit anti-guinea pig antiserum specific for cellular elements may lead to selective depression of the individual cells. A mixture of antisera directed against erythrocytes, thrombocytes and leukocytes results in pancytopenia and bone marrow hypoplasia. A similar clinical conclusion was reached by Matoth and associates (19).

It is not necessary to postulate three separate autoantibodies in pancytopenia. There is excellent evidence to suggest that warm acting erythrocyte autoantibodies are primarily directed against the rhesus blood group of erythrocytes (see Chapter 20). Blood group substances, including rhesus agglutinogens, are probably present in granulocytes, thrombocytes and their precursors. Accordingly, a single autoantibody could produce pancytopenia, with or without bone marrow aplasia, through the same sequence of events as described above for erythrocytes. Brody and Beizer (58) have demonstrated common antigens on erythrocytes and lymphocytes from patients with chronic lymphocytic leukemia. Erythrocyte autoantibodies may react with both cell lines.

It is therefore possible in autoimmune hemolytic anemia for antibody formation, either multiple or single, to result in leukopenia, thrombocytopenia or pancytopenia with hypoplastic or hyperplastic bone marrows. This immunologic explanation is an expansion of the original views of Fisher (23) and Evans and Duane (8). It appears to be compatible with the laboratory variations seen and the blending of characteristics of the five types of syndromes described above.

Other explanations are possible. Bone marrow depression may be caused by unrelated factors. Infectious diseases are frequently encountered in patients with autoimmune hemolytic anemia. Bone marrow depression secondary to infection should particularly be considered in the fulminating type of aplastic crisis. A high exposure rate of patients with hypoplastic marrows to various marrow depressing agents was noted in this series. This suggests either that aplastic anemia may be etiologically related to autoimmune hemolytic anemia, or that hemolytic anemia creates a bone marrow particularly susceptible to such toxic agents. Recent data (59) documenting the development of somatic mutations and leukemia in patients recovering from bone marrow depression suggest an additional mechanism. A graft-host disease picture may result from such "foreign" clone formation. This pattern of a malignancy following a prior aplastic state was encountered in Cases 19 and 38. An entirely different pathogenesis is suggested by the occurrence of a thymoma in one patient. The possibility must be considered that we are dealing primarily with an immunologic deficiency resulting in systemic immunologic diseases.

The subdivision of idiopathic autoimmune hemolytic anemia into five syndromes should not suggest five entirely different disease processes. An examination of the entire series and of the individual syndromes does not reveal distinguishing characteristics on the basis of age, sex, physical examination and survival time. Such a subdivision, however, is valuable for the clinician. It emphasizes the variations which may be encountered because of different degrees of peripheral blood and bone marrow involvement. If the suggested immunologic sequences are valid, the clear distinctions defined above will be blurred and obscured by various combinations of abnormalities. These distinctions will also have varying degrees of permanence. The possibility of other mechanisms should not be ignored. The evaluation of these postulates must await the accumulation of further case material and experimental studies.

BIBLIOGRAPHY

1. Pirofsky, B.: Hereditary aspects of autoimmune hemolytic anemia; a retrospective analysis. Vox Sang. **14:** 334, 1968.
2. van Loghem, J. J., van der Hart, M., and Dorfmeier, H.: Serologic studies in acquired hemolytic anemia. *Proceedings of the Sixth Congress of the International Society of Hematology.* Grune & Stratton, Inc., New York, 1956.
3. Swisher, S. N., Trabold, N., Leddy, J. P., and Vaughn, J.: Clinical correlations of the direct antiglobulin reaction. Ann. N. Y. Acad. Sci. **124:** 441, 1965.
4. Speiser, P.: Some remarks on human erythrocytic autoantibodies. Z. Immunitaetsforsch. **132:** 113, 1967.
5. Yunis, E. J., and Bridges, R. A.: Blood transfusion problems in auto-immune hemolytic anemia. Minnesota Med. **49:** 759, 1966.
6. Bohnen, R. F., Ultmann, J. E., Gorman, J. G., Farhangi, M., and Scudder, J.: The direct Coombs test: its clinical significance. Ann. Intern. Med. **68:** 19, 1968.
7. Doan, C. A., Curtis, G. M., and Wiseman, B. K.: Hemolytopoietic equilibrium and emergency splenectomy. J. A. M. A. **105:** 1567, 1935.
8. Evans, R. S., and Duane, R. T.: Acquired hemolytic anemia. I. The relation of erythrocyte antibody to activity of the disease. II.

The significance of thrombocytopenia and leukopenia. Blood **4**: 1196, 1949.

9. Evans, R. S., Takahashi, K., Duane, R. T., Payne, R., and Liu, C. K.: Primary thrombocytopenic purpura and acquired hemolytic anemia. Evidence for a common etiology. Arch. Intern. Med. (Chicago) **87**: 48, 1951.

10. Dausset, J., and Colombani, J.: The serology and the prognosis of 128 cases of autoimmune hemolytic anemia. Blood **14**: 1280, 1959.

11. Silverstein, M. N., and Hech, F. J.: Acquired hemolytic anemia and associated thrombocytopenic purpura: with special reference to Evans' syndrome. Proc. Mayo Clin. **37**: 122, 1962.

12. Brunner, H. E., and Frick, P. G.: Simultaneous thrombopenic purpura and autoimmune hemolytic anemia. Deutsch. Med. Wschr. **87**: 1002, 1962.

13. Brunet, P., Najean, Y., and Bernard, J.: Etude de dix cas d'association d'anémie hémolytique idiopathique immunologique et de purpura thrombopénique. Sem. Hop. Paris **40**: 294, 1964.

14. Dacie, J. V.: *The Haemolytic Anaemias, Part II*, Ed. 2. Grune & Stratton, Inc., New York, 1962.

15. Dacie, J. V., and deGruchy, G. C.: Auto-antibodies in acquired haemolytic anaemia. J. Clin. Path. **4**: 253, 1951.

16. Crosby, W. H.: The clinical aspects of immunologic hemolytic anemia. Sang **26**: 3, 1955.

17. Crosby, W. H., and Rappaport, H.: Autoimmune hemolytic anemia. I. Analysis of hematologic observations with particular reference to their prognostic value. A survey of 57 cases. Blood **12**: 42, 1957.

18. Chertkow, G., and Dacie, J. V.: Results of splenectomy in autoimmune acquired haemolytic anaemia. Brit. J. Haemat. **2**: 237, 1956.

19. Matoth, V., Elian, E., Nelken, D., and Nevo, A. C.: Specificity of lytic factors for erythrocytes, leukocytes, and platelets in a case of pancytopenia. Blood **11**: 735, 1956.

20. Kumar, S., and Saraya, A. K.: Experimental production of bone marrow aplasia by immunological means. Acta Haemat. (Basel) **27**: 306, 1962.

21. Chauffard, M. A.: Sem. Med. **28**: 345, 1908. Quoted by Letman, H.: Red cell destruction in the anaemias (thesis). Copenhagen, 1959.

22. Wiseman, B. K., and Doan, C. A.: Primary splenic neutropenia; a newly recognized syndrome closely related to congenital hemolytic icterus and essential thrombocytopenic purpura. Ann. Intern. Med. **16**: 1097, 1942.

23. Fisher, J. A.: The cryptogenic acquired haemolytic anaemias. Quart. J. Med. **16**: 245, 1947.

24. Dameshek, W., and Estren, S.: *Spleen and Hypersplenism*. Grune & Stratton, Inc., New York, 1948.

25. Moeschlin, S., Siegenthaler, W., Gasser, C., and Hässig, T. A.: Immunopancytopenia associ-

ated with incomplete cold hemagglutinins in a case of primary atypical pneumonia. Blood **9**: 214, 1954.

26. Moeschlin, S., Meyer, H., Israels, L. G., and Tarr-Gloor, E.: Experimental agranulocytosis. Its production through leukocyte agglutination by antileukocytic serum. Acta Haemat. (Basel) **11**: 73, 1954.

27. Bernard, J., Dausset, J., Malinvaud, G., and Lesneur, G.: Anémies, leucopénies, thrombopénies immunologiques; association d'anticorps dirigés contre les trois lignées cellulaires du sang. Bull. Soc. Med. Hop. Paris **70**: 651, 1954.

28. Müller, W., and Weinreich, J.: Immun-pancytopenien. Klin. Wschr. **34**: 505, 1956.

29. Weinreich, J., and Müller, W.: Immunhämatologische Untersuchungen bei Panzytopenien. Acta Haemat. (Basel) **16**: 376, 1956.

30. Baumgartner, W.: Klinik der erworbenen hämolytischen Anaemie. Helv. Med. Acta **23**: 324, 1956.

31. Dausset, J., and Brecy, H.: Test direct de consommation de l'antiglobuline sur les leucocytes et les plaquettes de certains malades atteints de pancytopénies idiopathiques. Vox Sang. **3**: 197, 1958.

32. Goudsmit, R., and van Loghem, J. J.: Studies on the occurrence of leukocyte antibodies. Vox Sang. **3**: 58, 1953.

33. Müller, W., and Redojícíc, B.: Vorkommen leukocytenagglutinierender und thrombocytärer Antikörper bei einem Fall von akutem Lupus erythematosus disseminatus. Klin. Wschr. **34**: 577, 1956.

34. Linke, A.: Klinische und experimentelle Beobachtungen über aplastische Krisen der Erythropoese bei hämolytischen Anämien. Verh. Deutsch. Ges. Inn. Med. **58**: 724, 1952.

35. Davis, L. J., Kennedy, A. C., Baike, A. G., and Brown, A.: Haemolytic anaemia of various types treated with ACTH and cortisone. Glasgow Med. J. **33**: 263, 1952.

36. Bonham Carter, R. E., Cathie, I. A. B., and Glasser, C.: Aplastische Anämie (chronische Erythroblastophthise) bedingt durch Autoimmunisierung. Schweiz. Med. Wschr. **84**: 1114, 1954.

37. Wagner, K.: Durch inkomplete Autoantikörper bedingte akute febrile, haemolytische aregeneratorische Anämie. Acta Haemat. (Basel) **14**: 313, 1955.

38. Bowman, J. M.: Acquired hemolytic anemia. Use of replacement transfusion in a crisis. Amer. J. Dis. Child. **89**: 226, 1955.

39. Seip, M.: Aplastic crisis in a case of immuno-hemolytic anemia. Acta Med. Scand. **153**: 137, 1955.

40. Veras, S., and Manios, S.: Anémie hémolytique acquise par auto-immunisation ayant présenté dans son évolution une aplasie érythroblastique aiguë. Arch. Franc. Pediat. **13**: 1096, 1956.

41. Martoni, L., and Musiani, S.: Anemia emolitica

acquisata idiopatica autoimmune complicata di mieloaplasia eritoblastica in un lattante di 6 mesi. Clin. Pediat. **38**: 483, 1956.

42. Lees, M. H.: Case of immune aplastic haemolytic anaemia with thrombocytopenia. Brit. Med. J. **1**: 110, 1960.

43. Burston, J., Husain, O. A. N., Hutt, M. S. R., and Tanner, E. I.: Two cases of autoimmune haemolysis and aplasia. Brit. Med. J. **1**: 83, 1959.

44. Pirofsky, B.: Serologic and clinical findings in autoimmune hemolytic anemia. Series Haemat. **9**: 47, 1965.

45. Bousser, J., Christol, D., Dausset, J., Rampon, S., Jallut, H., and Méry, J. P.: Episode érythroblastopénique prolongé ayant marqué le début d'une anémie hémolytique chronique avec auto-anticorps. Sang **26**: 804, 1955.

46. Crosby, W. H., and Rappaport, H.: Reticulocytopenia in autoimmune hemolytic anemia. Blood **11**: 929, 1956.

47. Eisemann, G., and Dameshek, W.: Splenectomy for "pure red-cell" hypoplastic (aregenerative) anemia associated with autoimmune hemolytic disease. Report of a case. New Eng. J. Med. **251**: 1044, 1954.

48. Ross, J. F., Finch, S. C., Street, R. W., and Strieder, J. W.: The simultaneous occurrence of benign thymoma and refractory anemia. Blood **9**: 935, 1954.

49. Korn, D., Gilderman, A., Cage, G., Nathanson, D., and Strauss, A. J. L.: Immune deficiencies, aplastic anemia and abnormalities of lymphoid tissue in thymoma. New Eng. J. Med. **276**: 1333, 1967.

50. Steffen, C.: Untersuchungen über den Nachweis sessiler Antikörper an Knockenmark- zellen bei erworbener hämolytischer Anämie. Wien. Klin. Wschr. **67**: 224, 1955.

51. Pisciotta, A. V., and Hinz, J. E.: Occurrence of agglutinins in normoblasts. Proc. Soc. Exp. Biol. Med. **91**: 356, 1956.

52. Yunis, J. J., and Yunis, E.: Cell antigens and cell specialization. I. A. study of blood group antigens on normoblasts. Blood **22**: 53, 1963.

53. Rossi, V., Diena, F., and Sacchetti, C.: Demonstration of specific and nonspecific agglutinogens in normal bone marrow erythroblasts. Experientia **13**: 440, 1957.

54. Sacchetti, C., Diena, F., and Rossi, V.: Comportamento degli eritroblasti nella anemia emolitica acquisata. Haematologica **42**: 895, 1957.

55. Yamamoto, M.: Experimental studies on immunological mechanisms of aplastic anemia. 1. Effects of antierythroblastic antibody on peripheral blood and bone marrow. Jap. J. Allerg. **14**: 55, 1965.

56. Yamamoto, M.: Experimental studies on immunological mechanisms of aplastic anemia. 2. On a few characteristics of antierythroblastic antibody. Jap. J. Allerg. **14**: 72, 1965.

57. Kontek, M.: Ostra, odwracalna nievydolnosc szpiku z komponenta hemolityezna (na tle immunologicynynn?). Wiad. Lek. **18**: 1263, 1965.

58. Brody, J. I., and Beizer, L. B.: The cross reactivity of lymphocyte and red cell antibodies. J. Lab. Clin. Med. **63**: 819, 1964.

59. Brauer, M. J., and Dameshek, W.: Hypoplastic anemia and myeloblastic leukemia following chloramphenicol therapy. New Eng. J. Med. **277**: 1003, 1967.

Chapter 5

The Leukemias and Autoimmune Hemolytic Anemia

The association of autoimmune hemolytic anemia with the leukemias has been well recognized for many years. An awareness of this relationship has stimulated the development of several important theoretical concepts relating immunologic events to malignancy (1, 2). In spite of this there is little material published regarding the specific clinical features of such combined syndromes. The following two chapters explore the patterns of disease presented in the association of neoplasia of the reticuloendothelium and autoimmune hemolytic anemia.

Reticuloendothelial Neoplasia and Autoimmune Hemolytic Anemia

In the current series of cases of autoimmune hemolytic anemia, there is a large number of secondary forms. This high incidence reflects in part an inordinate number of patients having neoplasia of the reticuloendothelium. This frequency of association may not present a true picture of the population distribution of primary and secondary forms of autoimmune hemolytic anemia. Our hematologic patient load is selected so that cases of leukemia, lymphoma and plasma cell myeloma are seen in numbers greatly in excess of that normally anticipated. In addition, this selected population has been closely followed clinically and in the laboratory for many years, with a consistency which may not be compatible with average medical care or investigation.

An association of autoimmune hemolytic anemia with neoplasia of the reticuloendo-thelium was seen in 113 patients (114 neoplastic examples). This represents an incidence of 48.3 per cent of our total series or 59.5 per cent of the secondary varieties. All forms of leukemia and the lymphomas are involved in this association. Table 33 lists the number of cases encountered with the various neoplasias.

Many other investigators have noted the propensity of patients with neoplasia of the reticuloendothelium to develop autoimmune hemolytic anemia. Published series, however, vary greatly in the relative incidence given for this relationship. Case selection and the population of patients undergoing hematologic investigation appear to be the factors responsible for the discrepancy. An analysis of the series presented by Dameshek and Komninos (3), van Loghem and associates (4), Dausset and Colombani (5), Evans and Weiser (6), Dacie (7), Crosby and Rappaport (8), Yunis and Bridges (9), Speiser (10) and Bohnen and associates (11) is presented in Table 34 and contrasted with the current series. These workers reported a total of 1324 cases of autoimmune hemolytic anemia with 744 cases of a second variety. Malignancies of the reticuloendothelium were present in 258 patients or 19.5 per cent of the total series. Reticuloendothelial neoplasia was involved in 35 per cent of the secondary forms of autoimmune hemolytic anemia. Within these mean figures, marked variations are seen. The incidence of this relationship is reduced by the large series of Speiser and of Bohnen and associates. The diagnosis in Speiser's series

(10), however, was that of the initial medical examination. It may be supposed that additional examples of reticuloendothelial neoplasia were discovered by further detailed investigation. In the study of Bohnen and associates (11) the criteria for diagnosis of autoimmune hemolytic anemia are unclear. In the series of Dameshek and Komninos (3) 44 per cent of cases of autoimmune hemolytic anemia, and 82.6 per cent of secondary varieties, were related to malignancies of the reticuloendothelium. In contrast, the numerically similar series of Evans and Weiser (6) suggests that associated malignancies of the reticuloendothelium are relatively uncommon in autoimmune hemolytic anemia. These authors observed a 7.3 per cent incidence in their entire series, and a 15.8 per cent incidence in secondary forms.

Chronic Lymphocytic Leukemia

Anemia is a frequent complication in patients with chronic lymphocytic leukemia. As early as 1906 the possible etiologic role of hemolysis in creating this anemic state was suggested. Hirschfeld (12) and Pappenheim (13), in related publications, both rec-

TABLE 33. *Association of autoimmune hemolytic anemia and neoplasia of the reticuloendothelium: 113 patients involved in a series of 234 with autoimmune hemolytic anemia*

Type of Neoplasia	No. Patients
The leukemias	77
Chronic lymphocytic	48
Acute lymphocytic	10
Acute monocytic	12
Acute and chronic granulocytic	7
The lymphomas	25
Hodgkin's disease	13
Lymphosarcoma	7
Reticulum cell sarcoma	4
Giant follicular lymphoma	1
Plasma cell myeloma	9*
Thymoma	3*
Total patients	113
Percentage of total series (113/234)	48.3

* One patient had both plasma cell myeloma and thymoma.

TABLE 34. *Association of neoplasia of the reticuloendothelium in 1324 patients with autoimmune hemolytic anemia: survey of the literature*

Investigator	Total Patients	Total, Secondary Type	Neoplasia of Reticuloendothelium		
			No.	Per cent of total	Per cent of Secondary type
Dameshek and Komninos (3)	43	23	19	44.2	82.6
Crosby and Rappaport (8)	57	23	16	28.0	69.6
van Loghem and associates (4)	122	67	28	23.0	41.8
Dausset and Colombani (5)	128	45	28	21.9	62.2
Yunis and Bridges (9)	40	23	8	20.0	34.8
Speiser (10)	540	320	100	18.5	31.3
Bohnen and associates (11)	178	165	31	17.4	18.8
Dacie (7)	175	59	25	14.3	43.4
Evans and Weiser (6)	41	19	3	7.3	15.8
Total	1324	744	258	19.5	34.7
Current series	234	190	113	48.3	59.5

ognized that hemolysis may be an important mechanism. The latter investigator suggested that toxic materials released by tumor tissue were hemolytic. Some experimental support for this concept was obtained in analyzing extracts of leukemic leukocytes. Most early investigators were aware of a myelophthisic element in the leukemias. In spite of the possibility of a hemolytic component they felt that myelophthisis was the most common cause of the anemic state. Paschkis (14) published in 1927 the first clear report of acquired hemolytic anemia developing in a patient with chronic lymphocytic leukemia. Jaffe (15) in 1935 challenged the prevalent concept that a myelophthisic state was the major mechanism leading to anemia. He again emphasized the importance of hemolysis in the leukemias. Since that time hemolytic anemia occurring in association with chronic lymphocytic leukemia has been described with regularity. Of all forms of reticuloendothelial neoplasia, chronic lymphocytic leukemia shows the highest incidence of

complicating autoimmune hemolytic anemia. Its frequency of occurrence is such that
a fortuitous juxtaposition of these two
common disease states is unlikely. There is
general agreement that some fundamental
relationship exists between these syndromes.

*Incidence of Autoimmune Hemolytic Ane-
mia in Chronic Lymphocytic Leukemia*

Although the association of autoimmune
hemolytic anemia and chronic lymphocytic
leukemia is well known, statistical data are
meager. Accurate incidence figures for autoimmune hemolytic anemia complicating
chronic lymphocytic leukemia are not available.

Bigley and associates (16) reviewed 350
cases of chronic lymphocytic leukemia studied from 1941 through 1960. They noted
that 34 per cent of patients were anemic
on initial examination and that 22 per cent
had a nonhemolytic variety of anemia. Of
this leukemic population, 24 per cent eventually developed hemolytic anemia. Wasserman and associates (17) reported that 15.5
per cent of 58 consecutive cases of chronic
lymphocytic leukemia had hemolytic anemia. Miale (18) states that approximately
25 per cent of cases of chronic lymphocytic
leukemia developed hemolytic anemia.
Wintrobe (19) suggests an incidence of 18
per cent for hemolytic anemia developing in
chronic lymphocytic leukemia. Dameshek
and Gunz (20) estimate that 20 per cent of
chronic lymphocytic leukemia patients develop hemolytic anemia. Seaman and associates (21) studied 212 cases of chronic
lymphocytic leukemia and noted one case of
hemolytic anemia per 231 months of leukemic life. Sixty examples were present, an
incidence of 28 per cent. Four years later
Osgood (22) reanalyzed the same patient
group and found that 78 cases then had
hemolytic anemia, an incidence of 36 per
cent. This represented one case of hemolytic
anemia for 217 months of leukemic duration.

The above reports illustrate the problems
involved in determining the incidence of
autoimmune hemolytic anemia in chronic
lymphocytic leukemia. The authors have
generally employed simple clinical and laboratory tools to implicate the hemolytic

state. A transfusion requirement in excess of
that required with bone marrow aplasia, in
the absence of overt blood loss, frequently
is the sole indication of hemolysis. Such criteria may lead to substantial errors. It is
not unusual to demonstrate asymptomatic
gastric or duodenal ulcers in such patients.
This is particularly prevalent if corticosteroid therapy has been given. Undetected
gastrointestinal bleeding may simulate a
hemolytic state in a substantial number of
these cases. In contrast, a dependence on
transfusion requirements for diagnosis certainly prevents discovery of compensated or
mild hemolysis. This inaccuracy is further
complicated either by an associated myelophthisic state or by an inability of the
bone marrow to respond adequately to the
anemic state. Wasserman and associates
(17) have termed this latter situation
"hemopathic" hemolytic anemia.

The data presented above may have little
relationship to the incidence of autoimmune
hemolytic anemia. Few studies have dis-
criminated between immunohemolytic anemia and a hemolytic state resulting from
nonimmune mechanisms. Wasserman and
associates (17) noted that five of their nine
cases had positive antiglobulin tests. Two
patients had negative tests, and antiglobulin tests were not performed in two other
cases. Data presented by Bigley and associates (16), Seaman and associates (21) and
Osgood (22) give no indication of the relative numbers of cases with positive or negative antiglobulin tests. Osgood in particular
treats these two groups as the same. "We
have used the term 'antiglobulin-positive
type' to characterize this group of related
cases even though some of these have negative Coombs or bromelin tests."

The assumption that hemolytic anemia
complicating chronic lymphocytic leukemia
results from only one mechanism is unwarranted. Hemolytic anemia may develop
through the toxic effects of various hemo-
lyzing and agglutinating materials released
from leukemic leukocytes (23). It may be
initiated by hyperactivity of an enlarged
spleen and other reticuloendothelial organs.
In addition, there is no reason to suppose
that all cases of autoimmune hemolytic
anemia are discovered by antiglobulin test-

TABLE 35. *Age and sex distribution of 48 patients with chronic lymphocytic leukemia (CLL) and autoimmune hemolytic anemia (AHA)*

Series	Total Patients	Age in Years			Sex	
		Range	Mean	Median	Male	Female
		years			*%*	
CLL + AHA (current series)					56	44
Onset of CLL	48	37–82	62	64		
Onset of AHA	48	43–82	64	66		
CLL 1941–1954 (control)	212	27–92		62	68	32
CLL + AHA (Rosenthal and associates (27))	20	47–78	62	60	75	25
CLL + AHA (Kyle and associates (26))	16	49–80	63	60	62.5	37.5

ing. More sensitive test procedures may permit a more accurate demonstration of erythrocyte autoantibodies. An immunohemolytic anemia cannot be assumed, however, unless positive antiglobulin or proteolytic tests are obtained. In spite of this, identical episodes of recurrent hemolytic anemia may develop in the same patient, with positive antiglobulin tests on one occasion and negative results on another (24).

The hemolytic state may appear at any time during the clinical course of chronic lymphocytic leukemia. Its reported incidence will accordingly be partially dependent on the length of followup. This suggests that increased survival time resulting from efficient therapy will increase the risk of developing autoimmune hemolytic anemia. The only accurate way to determine the incidence of such hemolytic states is to follow all patients serologically until death. This is exceedingly difficult. Long survivals characterize chronic lymphocytic leukemia, and a 20- to 30-year projected study is necessary.

A firm figure of the incidence of autoimmune hemolytic anemia associated with chronic lymphocytic leukemia is not available. A working estimate of 25 per cent of patients with chronic lymphocytic leukemia eventually developing autoimmune hemolytic anemia is a conservative approximation of our current patient population.

Incidence of Chronic Lymphocytic Leukemia in the Autoimmune Hemolytic Anemias

The proportion of patients with autoimmune hemolytic anemia that have associated chronic lymphocytic leukemia is more easily determined. The patient population undergoing hematologic examination will greatly modify the relationship. Dameshek and Komninos (3) noted a 39.5 per cent incidence of chronic lymphocytic leukemia in autoimmune hemolytic anemia. Dausset and Colombani (5) and Evans and Weiser (6) found an incidence of 10 and 7.3 per cent, respectively. Wasserman and associates (17) and Swisher (25) encountered an incidence of 31 and 32.1 per cent, respectively of chronic lymphocytic leukemia in cases of secondary autoimmune hemolytic anemia. The current series falls within these extremes. Forty-eight cases of autoimmune hemolytic anemia in association with chronic lymphocytic leukemia were encountered. Accordingly, chronic lymphocytic leukemia was present in 20.5 per cent of patients with autoimmune hemolytic anemia and in 25.3 per cent of the secondary varieties. This association is therefore extremely common, and a diagnosis of autoimmune hemolytic anemia requires an evaluation to rule out concomitant chronic lymphocytic leukemia.

Age and Sex Distribution

Autoimmune hemolytic anemia complicating chronic lymphocytic leukemia is primarily a disease of the elderly. A range of ages from 36.5 to 81.5 years was found. The mean age of the 48 patients was 62 years with a median of 64 years. Autoimmune hemolytic anemia frequently develops after the onset of chronic lymphocytic leukemia. This is clearly shown in Table 35. These observations are in agreement with values

TABLE 36. *Relationship between time of onset of chronic lymphocytic leukemia (CLL) and autoimmune hemolytic anemia (AHA)*

Series	Total Patients	Simultaneous Onset of CLL and AHA		Duration of CLL Before Onset of AHA		
		No.	Per cent	Range	Mean	Median
				months		
Current series	48	17	35.4	2–154	41	29
Wasserman and associates (17)	9	4	44.4	12–72	38	36
Rosenthal and associates (27)	20	9	45	6–60	34	36
Kyle and associates (26)	16	5	31.3	3–168	40	30
Total	93	35	37.6	2–168	38	33

obtained by analyzing the 16 cases presented by Kyle and associates (26) and the 20 cases of Rosenthal and associates (27).

The influence of age in the association of autoimmune hemolytic anemia with chronic lymphocytic leukemia was examined. A large series of patients with chronic lymphocytic leukemia has been under continual study at our institution from 1941. Through 1954, 212 consecutive cases of chronic lymphocytic leukemia had been encountered. The population was similar to that of the current series in population and geographic distribution, racial background, therapy and followup investigation. In fact, several current cases of autoimmune hemolytic anemia had an onset of leukemia placing them in this group. No essential differences in age distribution are noted between this control series and the group with complicating autoimmune hemolytic anemia.

In the current series 56 per cent of cases of chronic lymphocytic leukemia and autoimmune hemolytic anemia occurred in males and 44 per cent occurred in females. This sex distribution significantly differs from a consecutive population of patients with chronic lymphocytic leukemia. The control population of 212 cases of lymphocytic leukemia had a female incidence of only 32 per cent. Accordingly, males are more frequently involved than females in chronic lymphocytic leukemia with or without autoimmune hemolytic anemia. The development of autoimmune hemolytic anemia, however, reveals a predilection for the female, who is more susceptible to such autoimmune complications.

Duration of Leukemia in Relation to Onset of Autoimmune Hemolytic Anemia

Autoimmune hemolytic anemia may be simultaneously diagnosed with chronic lymphocytic leukemia or it may be discovered at any time in the subsequent course of leukemic disease. It is rare for patients with autoimmune hemolytic anemia eventually to develop chronic lymphocytic leukemia. In the current series, 17 cases or 35.4 per cent had a simultaneous discovery of both conditions. In the remaining 31 cases chronic lymphocytic leukemia existed for varying times before autoimmune hemolytic anemia developed. A duration range of prior chronic lymphocytic leukemia from 2 to 154 months was noted in these cases. The median duration of time was 29 months and the mean was 41 months. This implies that followup examinations of patients with chronic lymphocytic leukemia must include serologic and hematologic procedures designed to document the onset of a complicating autoimmune hemolytic anemia. The clinical and laboratory status of the leukemic process appears to be unrelated to the eventual development of autoimmune hemolytic anemia. The clinician, therefore, must periodically investigate the patient, irrespective of stabilization or fluctuation of chronic lymphocytic leukemia.

The reports of Wasserman and associates (17), Rosenthal and associates (27) and Kyle and associates (26) were analyzed in a similar fashion. Table 36 summarizes the relative times of onset of the leukemic and hemolytic processes encountered by these workers. Differences between the current series and these reports are not outstanding.

The Presence of Chronic Subleukemic Lymphocytic Leukemia

Gauld and associates (28) and Bethel (29) reported that 15 to 20 per cent of cases of chronic lymphocytic leukemia are of a subleukemic variety. An incidence of 19 per cent for the subleukemic state was reported by Bigley and associates (16) in their series of 350 patients with chronic lymphocytic leukemia. The subleukemic state is defined as a peripheral white blood cell count under 15,000/mm.³ in the presence of a bone marrow typical of chronic lymphocytic leukemia. The series of Bigley and associates provides an accurate control group to determine the influence of the subleukemic state on the association of autoimmune hemolytic anemia. Similar patient populations and methods of study were involved in that series and in the one currently reported. Many of the cases of the present series were included in the report of Bigley and associates.

Of the 48 cases of autoimmune hemolytic anemia associated with chronic lymphocytic leukemia, 13 patients or 27 per cent of the series appeared to have a subleukemic variety. This significantly differs from the anticipated 19 per cent incidence of subleukemic lymphocytic leukemia. Accordingly, a slightly increased risk of eventually developing autoimmune hemolytic anemia is present in the subleukemic variety of chronic lymphocytic leukemia.

Survival Data

Autoimmune hemolytic anemia complicates the management of patients with chronic lymphocytic leukemia and it may influence their survival. An evaluation of this influence is dependent on having a control series undergoing identical diagnostic and therapeutic procedures. Such a patient population is available in the 212 cases of chronic lymphocytic leukemia reported by Osgood (30). In this series 181 patients had died at time of analysis. A mean survival of 76 months since the onset of leukemia was found; the median was 64 months.

In the current series of patients with autoimmune hemolytic anemia and chronic lymphocytic leukemia, 41 of the 48 patients had died at time of analysis. A mean survival of 47 months from the onset of leukemia was obtained. The median was 36 months. The seven living patients were similarly analyzed. A mean duration of 59 and a median of 49 months of leukemia were found. Accordingly, autoimmune hemolytic anemia is a serious complication of chronic lymphocytic leukemia which leads to a shorter survival. Autoimmune hemolytic anemia complicating a subleukemic state creates even shorter survival times. The median is less than half that seen in a control population of patients with chronic lymphocytic leukemia. The autoimmune state is only partially responsible for the shorter survival. Patients with uncomplicated forms of the subleukemic variety also have a shorter survival than do those with the leukemic variety of chronic lymphocytic leukemia.

The disastrous impact of autoimmune hemolytic anemia is even more apparent when cases with a simultaneous onset (diagnosis?) of autoimmune hemolytic anemia and chronic lymphocytic leukemia are analyzed. A mean survival from the onset of combined disease of 20 months, with a median of 12 months, was obtained. Accordingly, such patients survived only one-fifth of the duration of a similar population with uncomplicated chronic lymphocytic leukemia.

The duration of autoimmune hemolytic anemia prior to death was also determined. The 41 patients who died had autoimmune hemolytic anemia for periods ranging from 0.5 to 74 months. A mean duration of survival after the onset of autoimmune hemolytic anemia of 20 months was found; the median for this group was 15 months. The subgroups with a subleukemic pattern and a simultaneous onset of autoimmune hemolytic anemia were similarly analyzed. No statistically significant differences in duration of autoimmune hemolytic anemia prior to death were noted. Accordingly, a subleukemic state and the simultaneous onset of autoimmune hemolytic anemia shorten the anticipated survival of patients with chronic lymphocytic leukemia. This occurs without appreciably affecting survival after the de-

TABLE 37. *Survival data obtained from patients with chronic lymphocytic leukemia (CLL) and autoimmune hemolytic anemia (AHA)*

Patient Group	No./Total	Duration of Disease					
		Chronic lymphocytic leukemia			Autoimmune hemolytic anemia		
		Range	Mean	Median	Range	Mean	Median
			months			*months*	
Control series, dead	181/212		76	64			
Current series							
Dead, total	41/48	0.5–228	47	36	0.5–74	20	15
Living, total	7/48	24–101	58	49	17–101	37	24
Subleukemic, dead	10/13	7–95	42	30	1–62	16	11
Simultaneous onset of CLL and AHA, dead	15/17	0.5–56	20	12	0.5–56	20	12

velopment of hemolytic anemia. Such data strongly suggest that death primarily reflects the development of autoimmune hemolytic anemia, rather than the leukemic status. Survival of a patient with chronic lymphocytic leukemia after the development of autoimmune hemolytic anemia is limited, with mean and median durations of substantially less than 2 years. Table 37 summarizes the survival data.

Presenting Symptoms

In secondary forms of autoimmune hemolytic anemia it is difficult to separate symptoms referable to the underlying disease from those related to autoimmune hemolysis. This difficulty was apparent in the present report of patients with chronic lymphocytic leukemia. Of these patients 45 complained of weakness, 23 of dizziness, eight of fever and three of subcutaneous or other hemorrhagic phenomena. These complaints are similar to those encountered in cases of uncomplicated chronic lymphocytic leukemia. Marked contrasts in the clinical states were observed. In some patients severe anemia was obvious, with weakness, dizziness, palpitations, otic pulsations and varying degrees of cardiac decompensation. Other patients were essentially asymptomatic and the autoimmune state was only discovered on routine hematologic and serologic testing.

Rosenthal and associates (27) felt that the hemolytic state initiated the eventual diagnosis of chronic lymphocytic leukemia in nine of their 20 patients. The association

of these two conditions may result in a severe syndrome forcing the patient to seek medical consultation earlier. It should be emphasized, however, that the presenting symptoms are those of anemia and are not diagnostic of an autoimmune hemolytic process. Bigley and associates (16) reported significant anemia in 34 per cent of cases of chronic lymphocytic leukemia at initial examination. Accordingly, symptoms of anemia are not sufficient to diagnose immune hemolysis. This is not meant to minimize the significance of anemia and its resulting symptoms. Twenty-five per cent of patients with chronic lymphocytic leukemia eventually develop autoimmune hemolytic anemia. This diagnosis must always be considered when chronic lymphocytic leukemia and anemia are seen together.

Presenting Physical Signs

Abnormalities discovered during physical examination were common in the 48 patients with an associated autoimmune hemolytic anemia and chronic lymphocytic leukemia. In general the abnormalities were referable to enlargement of various reticuloendothelial structures. Splenomegaly, hepatomegaly and lymphadenopathy were extremely common. Only 9 per cent of patients did not have such organomegaly at the time of onset of hemolysis. The incidence of reticuloendothelial hypertrophy is substantially greater than that found in either the total secondary or idiopathic types of autoimmune hemolytic anemia. This strongly suggests that organ enlargement reflects the chronic lymphocytic leukemic state rather than autoimmune hemolytic anemia. A high incidence of splenomegaly in the erythrocytic type of idiopathic autoimmune hemolytic anemia minimizes the value of this conclusion. Table 38 summarizes these data.

A similarly high incidence of hepatosplenomegaly and lymphadenopathy was noted by Kyle and associates (26) and Rosenthal and associates (27). In the current series the degree of splenomegaly and hepatomegaly was mild to moderate, with massive enlargement uncommon. This conforms to the experience of Kyle and associates. The patients of Rosenthal and associates presented more marked splenomegaly. Enlargement to the umbilicus was noted in almost all cases.

Differences were observed in the current series from those of Kyle and associates (26) and Rosenthal and associates (27) in two areas. In the series of Rosenthal and colleagues, all patients had pallor and jaundice. In the series of Kyle and associates all patients had pallor and approximately 12 of 16 had jaundice. In the current series pallor was uncommon and only occasionally significant. Clinically detected jaundice was rare. Only two of the 48 cases initially had this abnormality. This is in marked contrast to the observation of overt jaundice in 50 per cent of cases of the erythrocytic form of idiopathic autoimmune hemolytic anemia. This difference may partially reflect early diagnosis in the current series. Many of these patients were discovered during routine continual followup examinations of long term patients with chronic lymphocytic leukemia.

Laboratory Observations

Anemia was almost universal in this patient group. The mean hematocrit observed on initial examination for hemolytic anemia was 25.9 per cent with a median of 26.5 per cent. The severity of the anemic process became more apparent with repeated examinations. A range of hematocrits from 10 to 36 per cent was seen, with a median and mean of 20 per cent.

Reticulocyte counts on initial examina-

TABLE 38. *Physical findings on initial examination in patients with autoimmune hemolytic anemia: patients with associated chronic lymphocytic leukemia (CLL) compared with secondary types, idiopathic types and idiopathic erythrocytic types*

Autoimmune Hemolytic Anemia Type	Total Patients	Abnormalities			
		Spleen	Liver	Nodes	Jaundice
		%			
All idiopathic types	44	53	32	23	38.7
Idiopathic erythrocytic type	30	70	33	20	50
All secondary types	186	52	48	37	16.7
Secondary to CLL type	48	77	55	71	4.2

tions were of little aid in indicating hemolysis. Reticulocyte counts ranged from 0.0 to 27.8 per cent. Of patients with chronic lymphocytic leukemia and autoimmune hemolytic anemia, 56 per cent had reticulocyte levels below 2 per cent at diagnosis of hemolytic anemia. This lack of initial reticulocytosis differs from the experience reported by Rosenthal and associates (27) and by Kyle and associates (26). It more closely resembles the observations of Crosby and Rappaport (8). It is tempting to ascribe this "hemopathic" hemolytic anemic state to marrow depression secondary to myelophthisic or chemotherapeutic influences. All patients in this series received either P[32], chlorambucil or triethylene melamine therapy. Chemotherapeutic marrow depression is unlikely, however. The bone marrow was able to respond when corticosteroid therapy was initiated. A mean reticulocytosis of 6.6 per cent, with a median of 4.4 per cent, followed such therapy. Only 14 per cent of patients had reticulocyte counts below 2.0 per cent. Accordingly, in a significant number of cases the bone marrow is unable to compensate for the hemolytic state prior to therapy. This observation is similar to that reported by Hyman and Harvey (31) for disseminated malignant disease.

Peripheral white blood cell counts did not appear significant in indicating either onset or response of the hemolytic state. Values obtained reflected the form of leukemia and ranged from 1,300 to 405,000/mm.[3] It was difficult to determine whether the autoimmune process influenced thrombocyte values. Fifteen of the 45 patients had values below 50,000/mm.[3] on initial hemolytic diagnosis. Nineteen patients were essentially normal. Eleven patients were mildly thrombocytopenic with counts ranging from 50,000 to 150,000/mm.[3]

Erythrocyte morphologic abnormalities were common. Seven patients each had significant nucleated erythrocytes and spherocytes in the peripheral blood.

Bone marrow examinations in 28 patients were available at the approximate time of onset of autoimmune hemolytic anemia. Increased lymphocytes compatible with the leukemic diagnosis were noted in 25 cases. Erythrocytic hyperplasia was seen in nine patients. Decreased erythropoiesis was reported in six cases, with a normal erythrocytic series in 13. The bone marrow values correlated with the degree of reticulocytosis observed.

Bilirubin determinations were performed in 16 patients at the onset of hemolytic anemia, and were elevated in seven. In six of these, the indirect bilirubin was abnormal. In all, bilirubin levels were moderate.

Total protein and albumin-globulin ratio values were available in 16 patients and were found to be normal in 11. Total proteins were low in three and elevated in one patient. A reversal of the albumin-globulin ratio was noted in one case. Serum electrophoresis was performed in six cases. A normal value was found in one patient and a monoclonal spike due to macroglobulins was found in another. The remaining four cases had an abnormal broad polyclonal elevation in the gamma region.

Blood urea nitrogen determinations were performed in 13 cases. An abnormal elevation over 25 mg. per cent was found in six. Serum uric acid levels were determined in nine patients. In five, abnormal values over 5 mg. per cent were obtained. The laboratory results are summarized in Table 39.

Clinical Patterns

Autoimmune hemolytic anemia in association with chronic lymphocytic leukemia

can appear in any clinical setting. A rapidly falling hematocrit, reticulocytosis, bone marrow erythrocytic hyperplasia and clinical jaundice in chronic lymphocytic leukemia should immediately suggest autoimmune hemolytic anemia. However, the clinician will miss the majority of cases of autoimmune hemolytic anemia if he waits for this classical picture. The most efficient method to diagnose this combined syndrome is the routine application of antiglobulin and proteolytic enzyme tests in all cases of chronic lymphocytic leukemia. Such procedures should be carried out on initial examination and periodically thereafter. Failing this, the clinician must initiate the necessary serologic approach whenever anemia appears during the course of chronic lymphocytic leukemia.

Clinical variations seen in the association of these two disease states are marked. A fundamental clinical principle must be recognized. The development and the course of autoimmune hemolytic anemia appear to be independent of the degree of leukemic activity. A patient developing the combined syndrome may be essentially asymptomatic, in excellent leukemic control, or involved in an active leukemic process. Superimposed on this leukemic variation are variations resulting from the degree of hemolysis. The autoimmune hemolytic state may be found as a curious laboratory observation without clinical significance. In contrast, it may also appear as a severe fulminating process. The following case illustrates one clinical pattern.

Case 21. A 75-year-old female was noted to have leukocytosis on a routine blood count. Bone marrow examination was performed and a diagnosis of chronic lymphocytic leukemia was made. Four months later she was seen at our laboratory where the diagnosis was confirmed. Fatigue was her only complaint and 1+ generalized lymphadenopathy was the only physical abnormality. The hematocrit was 33 per cent, the reticulocyte count was 0.8 per cent, white blood cells (WBC) were 57,000/mm.[3] and thrombocytes were 143,000/mm.[3] Repeat bone marrow aspiration confirmed chronic lymphocytic leukemia and documented a normal erythrocytic series. Routine serologic studies revealed strong positive antiglobulin and bromelin tests. Chlorambucil therapy was initiated and maintained the WBC

TABLE 39. *Laboratory studies performed at time of diagnosis of hemolytic anemia in 48 patients with chronic lymphocytic leukemia and autoimmune hemolytic anemia*

Test Procedure	Total	Statistical Data		
		Range	Mean	Median
Hematologic studies				
Initial hematocrit (%)	47	14–41	25.9	26.5
Lowest hematocrit (%)	47	10–36	20.0	20.0
Initial reticulocytes (%)	43	0–27.8	2.9	1.4
Therapeutic reticulocytes (%)	35	0.1–31	6.6	4.4
Initial WBC (10^3/mm.^{3})	47	1.3–405		
Initial thrombocytes (10^3/mm.^{3})	45	0–296		
		Increased	Decreased	Normal
Bone marrow aspirations				
Total cellularity	28	19	2	7
Erythrocyte precursors	28	9	6	13
Lymphocytes	28	25	1	2
Megakaryocytes	28	3	2	23
Megaloblasts	28	3	0	25
		Abnormal		Normal
Biochemical tests				
Total bilirubin (mg.%)	16	7		9
Total protein (gm.%)	16	5		11
Serum electrophoresis	6	5		1
Blood urea nitrogen (mg.%)	13	6		7
Serum uric acid (mg.%)	9	5		4

below 20,000/mm.^{3} The hematocrit persisted at 31 per cent without a reticulocytosis. Six months after therapy was started the serologic tests reverted to negative without change in the patient's hematologic status. She remained essentially asymptomatic except for continually recurring herpes simplex stomatitis. Gammaglobulin therapy was given monthly for over 2 years. Maintenance chlorambucil therapy was given. Thirty-six months after negative conversion of serologic tests, positive antiglobulin tests were again found without hematologic changes. Two months later a large mass on the thigh was noted. Biopsy revealed leukemia. The patient progressively deteriorated. Over a 2-month period her hematocrit dropped to 18 per cent, with normal WBC and reticulocyte counts. Prednisone, 60 mg. per day, was started. Radiation to the spleen was given for 4 days before death without effecting the hemolytic process. Herpes viremia occurred and extensive moniliasis was present. The patient died 50 months after the onset of leukemia and 45 months after the onset of autoimmune hemolytic anemia.

In this patient autoimmune hemolytic anemia appeared as a laboratory observation without influencing the clinical course. The syndrome was easily diagnosed serologically but did not require therapy for over 3½ years. Eventually, however, both autoimmune hemolytic anemia and chronic lymphocytic leukemia became active, leading to rapid deterioration and death.

Case 22. A 57-year-old male was investigated because of generalized lymphadenopathy. Lymph node biopsy was interpreted as lymphosarcoma, but bone marrow aspiration was typical of chronic lymphocytic leukemia. The spleen was not felt, the liver was 3 cm. below the costal margin and 2+ lymphadenopathy was present. The hematocrit was 45 per cent and the WBC was 16,700/mm.^{3} Thrombocytes and reticulocytes were normal. Chlorambucil therapy was given with an excellent clinical response. The liver and spleen were not palpated and lymph nodes were only minimally enlarged. Fourteen months after start of therapy, the hematocrit was 43 per cent with a 1.1 per cent reticulocyte count. The WBC had risen to 31,000/mm.[3] and chlorambucil therapy was increased. Five months later the patient was in acute distress. He had developed a peroneal nerve paralysis, and jaundice was noted. The hematocrit was 14 per cent, the WBC was 64,000/mm.[3] and direct antiglobulin tests were positive. Prednisone therapy was initiated. In spite of 12 transfusions over the next 3 weeks, acute pulmonary edema developed with the hematocrit persisting at 12 per cent. Death occurred with pulmonary embolization. Total duration of leukemia was 20 months with hemolytic anemia present for 3 weeks.

In contrast with Case 21, the above patient had relatively weak serologic tests, although fulminating hemolytic anemia was present. Activity of the leukemic process was mild, and death resulted primarily from uncontrolled hemolysis. A review of both cases at the onset of either leukemia or hemolytic anemia would not predict the subsequent course or therapeutic response.

Case 23. A 62-year-old female was investigated for weakness and jaundice. The spleen was felt 6 cm. below the costal margin. Liver size was normal and lymphadenopathy was not found. The hematocrit was 18 per cent with a reticulocyte count of 28 per cent. Indirect bilirubin values were elevated. The WBC was 5,650/mm.[3] and the bone marrow aspiration was typical of chronic lymphocytic leukemia. A superimposed erythrocytic hyperplasia was noted. Lupus erythematosus cell preparations were negative. Prednisone therapy was given with reduction of splenomegaly and progressive rise of the hematocrit to 30 per cent. Prednisone therapy was continued at 10 mg. per day for 2 years and then discontinued. Anemia recurred and splenic irradiation was employed with improvement. Nine months later the spleen was 10 cm. below the costal margin, the liver was 6 cm. down and inguinal lymph nodes were enlarged. Fever and splenic tenderness developed. The hematocrit dropped from 30 to 16 per cent in 1 month with a reticulocyte count of 6.0 per cent. Direct and indirect antiglobulin and bromelin tests were strongly positive. Prednisone, 60 mg. daily, was initiated, followed by reticulocytosis and rapid reduction in the size of the liver and spleen. The hematocrit stabilized at approximately 30 per cent, and maintenance prednisone therapy was employed. Thirty-seven months later the hematocrit precipitously dropped and the spleen was 14 cm. and the liver was 5 cm. below the costal margins. Antiglobulin and bromelin tests

were then negative. Splenic irradiation, 340 r, was given in nine treatments, with stabilization of the hematocrit and reduction in splenic size and tenderness. In spite of maintenance prednisone therapy, splenic pain recurred 1 year later. The hematocrit had dropped from 35 to 27 per cent, and the reticulocyte count was 2.6 per cent. Splenic irradiation, 325 r, in six treatments was given. Hemolysis decreased and the hematocrit rose. The patient is currently receiving maintenance prednisone, 30 mg. daily, with the hematocrit at 31 per cent, reticulocytes at 3.2 per cent and a spleen palpated 11 cm. below the costal margin. Followup is continuing 101 months since the simultaneous onset of chronic lymphocytic leukemia and autoimmune hemolytic anemia.

Several interesting points are illustrated in the above case. Patients may survive for long periods after the onset of autoimmune hemolytic anemia. In spite of impressive clinical and laboratory evidence of hemolysis, this patient has had several excellent therapeutic responses. In the two patients described previously the laboratory evidence of severe hemolysis was minimal and existed for only a short time. Therapeutic responses did not occur and death resulted. It is apparent that the therapeutic response and laboratory abnormalities do not necessarily correlate in autoimmune hemolytic anemia. One further clinical observation must be emphasized. In Cases 21 and 22 leukemia dominated the clinical picture until hemolytic anemia and death occurred. In Case 23 the leukemic state was never a problem in medical management. Chronic lymphocytic leukemia has now been diagnosed for 8½ years and specific chemotherapy has not been given. The clinical dissociation of hemolytic anemia and leukemia is further illustrated in the next protocol.

Case 24. A 62-year-old female developed herpes zoster. On routine investigation a WBC of 181,500/mm.[3] was discovered in a pattern typical of chronic lymphocytic leukemia. The spleen was palpated 2 cm. and the liver 3 cm. below the costal margin. Lymphadenopathy, 2+, was found. The hematocrit was 35 per cent. P[32] therapy was given. In 6 weeks the liver and spleen were no longer felt. Over the next 89 months P[32] was administered intravenously every 12 weeks. Leukemic activity could not be documented. The WBC was below 15,000/mm.[3] and the hematocrit was over 35 per cent. The hematocrit suddenly dropped to 27 per cent with a 1.1 per cent reticulocyte count. The WBC was 1,900/mm.^{3} and thrombocytes were 18,000/mm.^{3} Antiglobulin and bromelin tests were negative. P^{32} therapy was discontinued and prednisone, 60 mg. daily, was given. The hematocrit continued to fall, reaching 22.5 per cent over the next 6 weeks. Leukopenia and thrombocytopenia persisted. There was no hepatosplenomegaly. The direct antiglobulin test was then positive. Over the next 2 months, in spite of prednisone therapy, the hematocrit fell to 20 per cent with a reticulocytosis of 5.7 per cent. The antiglobulin test remained positive. Congestive heart failure and death occurred 94 months after the onset of the leukemic state and 4 months after complicating autoimmune hemolytic anemia developed.

The above patient was in excellent leukemic control for over 7 years. Autoimmune hemolytic anemia developed and led to death in 4 months without any change in leukemic status. The two diseases appeared as if they were unrelated syndromes fortuitously occurring in the same patient.

The four cases presented above illustrate only a few of the clinical and laboratory variations which are encountered in patients with chronic lymphocytic leukemia and autoimmune hemolytic anemia. On the basis of the 48 cases reviewed, the following clinical impressions and observations deserve emphasis:

(a) Autoimmune hemolytic anemia may occur at any time during the course of chronic lymphocytic leukemia. It may be discovered simultaneously with chronic lymphocytic leukemia or it may develop after many years of preexisting leukemia. Autoimmune hemolytic anemia existing prior to leukemia is discussed in detail at the end of Chapter 6.

(b) The clinical status of chronic lymphocytic leukemia appears to be unrelated to the development of autoimmune hemolytic anemia. Although autoimmune hemolytic anemia is frequently seen in the presence of active leukemia, the reverse is equally true. Patients with quiescent chronic lymphocytic leukemia may suddenly develop autoimmune hemolytic anemia after many years.

(c) Dameshek (32) has emphasized that radiation or chemotherapy may initiate the onset or clinical evidence of autoimmune hemolytic anemia in patients with chronic lymphocytic leukemia. The theoretical rationale of this viewpoint is discussed in Chapter 15. The current series does not clarify this problem. Almost every patient received radiation or chemotherapy upon initial examination and had continual therapy throughout the course of his disease. It should be pointed out, however, that 35 per cent of the patients in the current series, and many patients reported by Wasserman and associates (17), Rosenthal and associates (27) (45 per cent) and Kyle and associates (26) (31 per cent), had a simultaneous diagnosis of autoimmune hemolytic anemia and chronic lymphocytic leukemia. In such patients therapeutic regimens cannot be implicated as disturbing immune homeostatic balances and leading to overt autoimmune hemolytic anemia.

(d) The clinical picture of the combined autoimmune hemolytic anemia and chronic lymphocytic leukemia syndrome may be dominated by the leukemic state, the hemolytic state or a combination of both conditions. This implies that autoimmune hemolytic anemia may appear as a laboratory observation without influencing clinical management. It also indicates that the onset of autoimmune hemolytic anemia does not imply activity of the leukemic state requiring extensive or precipitous antileukemic therapy. It is frequently necessary to treat these two parts of the syndrome separately in the same patient. One word of caution is indicated. The initiation of corticosteroid therapy will generally create profound leukocytosis in patients with chronic lymphocytic leukemia. The clinician treating a leukemic patient on the basis of WBC levels may make the error, in the face of such leukocytosis, of rapidly increasing chemotherapy. With control of the hemolytic process and reduction of corticosteroids, marrow depression may develop from an overdose of long acting chemotherapeutic agents.

(e) This author is unable to document any clinical or laboratory criteria which may be employed as prognostic signs indicating the eventual effect of autoimmune hemolytic anemia. This lack of prognostic information applies both to the activity and the duration of survival of chronic lymphocytic leukemia. All cases must be treated as serious with an anticipated shortening of survival. The ability of corticosteroid therapy to induce remission appears most important. A lack of therapeutic response to corticosteroids generally heralds death. An excellent therapeutic response, however, does not guarantee that relapse will not occur or that it will be responsive to the identical therapy.

Autoimmune Hemolytic Anemia in Other Leukemic States

The early literature clearly suggests that hemolytic anemia may complicate various acute leukemias and chronic granulocytic leukemia. These observations have frequently been ignored. A tacit assumption is made by most clinicians that autoimmune hemolytic anemia occurs only during the course of chronic lymphocytic leukemia. This assumption is erroneous. In the current series autoimmune hemolytic anemia was diagnosed in 29 patients with leukemias other than the chronic lymphocytic form. Acute lymphocytic, acute monocytic and acute and chronic granulocytic types were all discovered.

Several reasons exist for the misconception that such forms of leukemia are not susceptible to association with autoimmune hemolytic anemia. Many textbooks and clinics have accepted the premise that autoimmune hemolytic anemia does not occur in such states. This teaching limits the number of investigations performed to determine whether an autoimmune hemolytic process is present. The problem is further magnified because severe anemia is prominent in these forms of leukemia. Almost all patients have developed anemia during the course of their disease. This development is frequently accepted as part of the natural history and its presence does not stimulate investigations designed to discover associated etiologies.

The serologic reactions obtained in patients with other types of leukemia may be substantially weaker than those seen in chronic lymphocytic leukemia. They may be missed or misinterpreted in the routine laboratory. In the current group of 29 cases, trace positive antiglobulin reactions were found in eight cases and 1+ reactions were seen in 12. The direct bromelin test appeared even less sensitive. Negative reactions were found in seven, trace positive reactions in 10 and 1+ reactions in seven cases.

Most investigators dealing with large patient populations have encountered the combined syndrome in leukemic types other than chronic lymphocytic leukemia. Its relative rarity, however, forces the clinician to relegate it to a rare or uncommon status. Classification as uncommon, when compared with chronic lymphocytic leukemia, is accurate. However, large numbers of leukemic patients are now undergoing continual therapy and followup. Survival in these forms of leukemia is increasing. The development of autoimmune hemolytic anemia in such patients is not rare, and such states will be found if searched for.

The Acute Leukemias

Jaffe (15) in 1935 emphasized that the anemia found in acute leukemia appeared hemolytic more often than myelophthisic. Tudhope (33) found a shortened erythrocyte survival time in most cases of acute leukemia. Nathan and Berlin (34), Wetherley-Mein and associates (35), Whitelow and associates (36) and Bowie and associates (37) also noted that many, but not all, cases of acute leukemia presented a shortened erythrocyte survival time. In spite of this, hemolytic anemia with positive antiglobulin tests occurring in association with the acute leukemias is rarely reported. Frumin and Kohn (38) reported one example in acute granulocytic leukemia. Evans and Weiser (6) mention one case of acute lymphocytic leukemia associated with autoimmune hemolytic anemia. Wasserman and associates (17) encountered two cases of "acute blastic" leukemia. Dausset and Colombani (5) found one example in acute lymphocytic leukemia and two examples in undefined malignancies of the blood. Bile and associates (39) noted one example of an acute granulocytic type with associated chloromas. In Dacie's series (7) four cases of "other leukemias" are mentioned. Cassell and Chaplin (40) had two acute leukemic patients in their series of 26 patients with autoimmune hemolytic anemia.

Acute Lymphocytic Leukemia

Ten cases of acute lymphocytic leukemia with hemolytic anemia and positive antiglobulin tests are included in the current series. Seventy per cent occurred in males. A range of ages from 3 to 71.5 years, with a median of 15 years, was found. In three patients autoimmune hemolytic anemia was simultaneously diagnosed with the acute

leukemic state. In the remaining seven, acute leukemia occurred first and existed for a variable period before autoimmune hemolytic anemia developed. A mean duration of 8.4 months and a median of 4 months of preexisting leukemia were encountered. All 10 of these patients have died. Short survivals were noted. Autoimmune hemolytic anemia was present for a median of 4 months and a mean of 12 months before death.

The presenting symptoms and physical signs at the onset of autoimmune hemolytic anemia are summarized in Table 40. Symp-

TABLE 40. *Statistical data obtained from 10 patients (three females, seven males) with acute lymphocytic leukemia (ALL) and autoimmune hemolytic anemia (AHA) (all patients had died at time of analysis)*

Test Procedures	Total	Statistical Data		
		Range	Mean	Median
Clinical data				
Age (years)	10	3–72		15
Duration of ALL before AHA* (months)	7	1–31	8	4
Survival (months)	10	0.2–61	18	8
Duration of AHA (months)	10	0.2–54	12	4
Laboratory data				
Initial hematocrit (%)	10	14–34	24.3	22.5
Lowest hematocrit (%)	9	9–25	18.5	20
Initial reticulocytes (%)	10	0–4.4	1.2	0.5
Therapeutic reticulocytes (%)	7	0–8.9	4.1	4.2
Initial WBC (10^3/mm.^{3})	10	1–590		
Initial thrombocytes (10^3/mm.^{3})	9	4–200	82	35

		Increased	Decreased	Normal
Bone marrow aspiration				
Total cellularity	6	5	0	1
Erythrocyte precursors	6	0	0	6
Lymphocytes	6	6	0	0
Megakaryocytes	6	0	0	6
Megaloblasts	6	0	0	6

		Weakness	Dizziness	Fever	Bleeding
Presenting symptoms					
Abnormal	8	8	7	5	1

		Spleen	Liver	Lymph nodes	Jaundice
Presenting signs					
Abnormal	9	6	9	7	0

* Three patients had simultaneous diagnosis of ALL and AHA.

toms were present in all patients. Hepatosplenomegaly and/or lymphadenopathy were observed in all patients.

Marked anemia was characteristic of this group. A median hematocrit of 22.5 per cent was found at the onset of hemolytic anemia. During the course of disease anemia became more profound. Reticulocytosis at onset of hemolytic anemia was uncommon. A range extending from 0.0 to 4.4 per cent was seen, with a median of 0.5 per cent. The capacity of the bone marrow to respond was not permanently inhibited. After initiation of therapy, reticulocytosis occurred with a median of 4.2 per cent. The WBC was variable and reflected the leukemic state. A range of values extending from 1,000 to 590,000/mm.³ was noted. Thrombocyte counts similarly varied. A median of 35,000/mm.³ and a mean of 82,000/mm.³ were determined. Bone marrow examinations at the onset of hemolytic anemia were available in six cases and a normal erythrocytic series was noted in all.

Clinical Patterns

The statistical data presented above suggest that autoimmune hemolytic anemia has few typical features when associated with acute lymphocytic leukemia. A lack of reticulocytosis before therapy and an absence of bone marrow erythrocytic hyperplasia are characteristic. These observations emphasize the difficulty of diagnosing the state if serologic studies are not carried out.

Case 25. A 15-year-old white male suddenly developed fever, severe bilateral ear pain, aphasia and diplopia. Physical examination revealed petechiae, purpura, retinal hemorrhages and a few shotty lymph nodes. The hematocrit was 21.5 per cent with a reticulocyte count of 0.5 per cent. Thrombocytes were less than 20,000/mm.³ and the white count was 590,000/mm.³ with morphologic evidence of acute lymphocytic leukemia. Cross matching of blood for transfusion was incompatible and positive direct antiglobulin tests were obtained. Intravenous corticosteroids were given and 4 units of fresh plastic bag blood were transfused. Death occurred 3 days later from multiple intracranial hemorrhages. A total duration of leukemia and hemolytic anemia of 5 days could be documented.

The above protocol illustrates a fulminating case of acute lymphocytic leukemia, complicated by positive antiglobulin tests. The associated autoimmune hemolytic anemia, however, had little to do with the rapidly fatal course. Death appeared as the result of severe thrombocytopenia and bleeding.

Case 26. A 71-year-old white male suddenly developed severe anemia 2 weeks after cholecystectomy. The liver was felt 4 cm. below the costal margin, with the spleen and lymph nodes not palpated. The hematocrit was 14 per cent, the reticulocyte count was 0.0 per cent, the WBC was 2,600/mm.³ and thrombocytes were 44,000/mm.³ Bone marrow aspiration was diagnostic of acute lymphocytic leukemia. An attempt to transfuse the patient revealed incompatible cross matches. Antiglobulin and bromelin tests were strongly positive. Prednisone, 60 mg. per day, was given without a reticulocyte response but with a steady rise of the hematocrit to 31 per cent. When prednisone was decreased to 30 mg. per day hemolysis recurred. Full doses of prednisone were again given in conjunction with 6-mercaptopurine. In spite of incompatible cross matches a total of 8 units of blood were transfused. The hematocrit stabilized at 30 per cent. The patient subsequently refused all transfusion therapy and corticosteroids. Death occurred 11 months after the simultaneous onset of both acute lymphocytic leukemia and autoimmune hemolytic anemia.

In this patient hemolytic anemia dominated the patient's clinical course, whereas leukemic activity was minimal. The absence of reticulocytosis and jaundice did not suggest hemolytic anemia in this patient. Cross match procedures employed in an attempt to transfuse the patient gave the first indication of an autoimmune abnormality. This led to the discovery of positive antiglobulin and enzyme tests and to the diagnosis of autoimmune hemolytic anemia. A limited therapeutic response to corticosteroid therapy was noted. In contrast with Case 25, autoimmune hemolytic anemia was compatible with a relatively long survival.

Acute Monocytic Leukemia

Autoimmune hemolytic anemia as a complication of acute monocytic leukemia is rarely mentioned in the literature. This is surprising in view of the well recognized association of autoimmune hemolytic anemia with Hodgkin's disease. Malignancy of the monocyte series has been associated with Hodgkin's disease by several observers on the basis of morphologic characteristics. Accurate analysis is complicated by the use of different standards in different laboratories for the diagnosis of acute monocytic leukemia. In our laboratory a diagnosis of acute monocytic leukemia is made when malignant monocytes of an early age are found in increased numbers in the peripheral blood and/or bone marrow. These cells are generally peroxidase positive, with granules appearing larger but fewer in number than those seen in immature granulocytes. Mature granulocytes are readily found in the peripheral blood. Leukocyte alkaline phosphatase determinations on such cells are generally normal. Auer bodies may or may not be demonstrated.

Twelve cases of autoimmune hemolytic anemia in association with this form of acute leukemia were seen in the current series. In six, a subleukemic pattern was found. A marked predilection for the female was observed in contrast with the male preponderance generally seen in acute leukemias. Ten patients or 83 per cent of the series were females. Elderly patients were generally involved in this process. A median age of 58 and a mean of 55 years were observed. In five patients hemolytic anemia and acute leukemia were simultaneously diagnosed. In five additional cases acute leukemia occurred prior to autoimmune hemolytic anemia. The median duration of prior leukemia was 4 months. In two cases autoimmune hemolytic anemia antedated the onset of the leukemic state. Preexisting autoimmune hemolytic anemia for 11 months and 203 months was recorded. This duration is sufficiently long that a concomitant but undiagnosed acute leukemia is unlikely.

Survival data clearly demonstrate the poor prognosis of autoimmune hemolytic anemia in association with acute monocytic leukemia. A median survival of 6 months with a mean of 7 months was obtained. Hemolytic anemia, excluding the two preexisting states, had a median duration of 6 months with a mean of 5 months before death occurred.

The presenting symptoms and physical findings at the onset of autoimmune hemolytic anemia are summarized in Table 41. Only three of the 12 cases did not have either splenomegaly, hepatomegaly or lymphadenopathy.

Hematologic data also indicate the severity of disease. During the course of illness the median hematocrit was only 15 per cent. Mild reticulocytosis before initiation of therapy was common. After therapy, however, reticulocytosis was the rule, with a median reticulocyte count of 5.5 and a mean of 9.6 per cent. Both leukocyte and thrombocyte counts reflected the leukemic state. Nucleated erythrocytes and spherocytes were found in nine of the 12 cases. Bone marrow examination at the onset of hemolytic anemia was not particularly helpful in establishing the hemolytic state. Erythrocytic hyperplasia was found in only four of the nine examinations. Erythrocytic hypoplasia was seen in three cases.

Clinical Patterns in Acute Monocytic Leukemia

Case 27. A 71-year-old white male was noted to have mild anemia. Six months later a severe urinary tract infection occurred. The spleen and liver were both felt 8 cm. below the costal margins and 2+ axillary adenopathy was found. The hematocrit was 21 per cent with a 4.0 per cent reticulocyte count. The WBC was 295,000/mm.^{3} and the blood smear was diagnostic for acute monocytic leukemia. Lupus erythematosus cells, osmotic fragility and iron concentrations were normal. The antiglobulin test was positive. 6-Mercaptopurine therapy was initiated, with a progressive drop of the white count. Eight units of blood were transfused over the next 2 months. In spite of this the hematocrit dropped to 15 per cent. Four more units of blood were transfused. During this time the antiglobulin test was positive on four separate occasions and negative on six occasions. Although hepatosplenomegaly grew progressively less and the WBC stabilized at approximately 25,000/mm.^{3}, hemolytic anemia persisted. Seven further transfusions were necessary. The patient died 6 months after the simultaneous diagnosis of acute monocytic leukemia and autoimmune hemolytic anemia.

TABLE 41. *Statistical data obtained from 12 patients (10 females, two males) with acute monocytic leukemia (AML) and autoimmune hemolytic anemia (AHA) (all patients had died at time of analysis)*

Test Procedures	Total	Statistical Data		
		Range	Mean	Median
Clinical data				
Age (years)	12	18–79	55	58
Duration of AML before AHA* (months)	5	1–14	5	4
Duration of AHA before AML* (months)	2	11–203		
Duration of AHA after AML (months)	10	0.25–10	5	6
Survival with AML (months)	12	0.25–17	7	6
Laboratory data				
Initial hematocrit (%)	12	10–33.5	22.6	21.5
Lowest hematocrit (%)	12	10–24	16	15
Initial reticulocytes (%)	10	0.1–6.4	2.9	1.8
Therapeutic reticulocytes (%)	7	0.0–36.2	9.6	5.5
Initial WBC (10^3/mm.^{3})	12	1.8–295		
Initial thrombocytes (10^3/mm.^{3})	11	1.6–200	66	50

		Increased	Decreased	Normal
Bone marrow aspiration				
Total cellularity	9	7	1	1
Erythrocytic precursors	9	4	3	2
Monocytes	9	6	0	3
Megakaryocytes	9	0	0	9
Megaloblasts	9	3	0	6

		Weakness	Dizziness	Fever	Bleeding
Presenting symptoms					
Abnormal	12	12	9	7	2

		Spleen	Liver	Lymph nodes	Jaundice
Presenting signs					
Abnormal	12	4	5	7	3

* Five patients had simultaneous diagnosis of AML and AHA.

Case 28. A 67-year-old white female was investigated for fatigue and congestive heart failure. The liver was felt 10 cm. below the costal margin, but the spleen and lymph nodes were not enlarged. The hematocrit was 10 per cent with a 0.4 per cent reticulocyte count. The WBC was 3,900/mm.^{3} Bone marrow examination revealed hypercellularity, acute monocytic leukemia and erythrocytic hyperplasia with megaloblastic changes. Direct and indirect antiglobulin and bromelin tests were positive. Seven transfusions were given and 6-mercaptopurine therapy was started. In spite of this the hema-

tocrit stayed at 12.5 per cent. Prednisone therapy was initiated without a therapeutic response. During this period antiglobulin tests were positive on three occasions and negative on two testings. The patient died 12 days later of a hemorrhagic infarct after three additional transfusions. Her total course of associated autoimmune hemolytic anemia and acute monocytic leukemia was less than 1 month.

Both of these cases illustrate the severe clinical sequences that are encountered when acute monocytic leukemia and autoimmune hemolytic anemia are seen together. A therapeutic response for either condition seldom occurs. If responses do develop, they are frequently of short duration. Additional patients with acute monocytic leukemia associated with autoimmune hemolytic anemia are presented as Cases 37 and 39.

The marked variation in antiglobulin testing is striking. In nine of the 12 cases multiple antiglobulin tests were performed. In eight of these, variations from negative to 2+ reactions were found in the same patient, in periods of time as short as 1 week. (Positive reactions/total tests in individual patients: 3/9, 1/2, 7/10, 3/8, 1/2, 3/7, 3/5, 4/10). The presence or absence of positive antiglobulin reactions did not correlate with clinical activity. The clinician, therefore, must not rely on a single negative antiglobulin test to rule out an associated autoimmune hemolytic anemia. This confusing laboratory observation deserves further detailed investigation.

The Granulocytic Leukemias

The association of granulocytic leukemia and autoimmune hemolytic anemia has been recognized in the past as an uncommon occurrence. Brill (41) in 1924 described hemolytic anemia occurring in a patient with granulocytic leukemia. In Paschkis' 1927 report (14) acquired hemolytic anemia as a complication of both chronic lymphocytic leukemia and chronic granulocytic leukemia is clearly described. Jonsson and associates (42), Marchal and Duhamel (43), Stats (44), Meacham and Weisberger (45), Young and associates (46) and Wasserman and associates (17) have also reported cases of granulocytic leukemia associated with hemolytic anemia in the face of negative serologic tests. Schunk and Lehman (47) presented a case of congenital chronic granulocytic leukemia with hemolytic anemia and positive antiglobulin tests. Videbaek (48) encountered two cases of chronic granulocytic leukemia, hemolytic anemia and positive antiglobulin tests. Frumin and Kohn (38) noted one case of acute granulocytic leukemia and autoimmune hemolytic anemia; the autoantibody was demonstrated in albumin and antiglobulin tests.

Hennemann (49) noted one positive test in 10 patients. Cassell and Chaplin (40) reported an example of chronic granulocytic leukemia with positive antiglobulin reactions. Dacie (7) mentions one case of a subacute myelomonocytic leukemia with positive antiglobulin reactions. Pirofsky (24) reported six examples of their association in 137 cases of autoimmune hemolytic anemia.

In the current series autoimmune hemolytic anemia was associated with granulocytic leukemia in seven cases. Four cases of a chronic variety, one case of a chronic form that had converted into an acute type and two cases of acute granulocytic leukemia are included. A female predominance was noted with four of the seven cases occurring in women. An elderly population was generally involved. In three patients autoimmune hemolytic anemia and granulocytic leukemia were simultaneously diagnosed. In four cases granulocytic leukemia was first present. After a median duration of 29 months autoimmune hemolytic anemia developed.

Patients with the combined syndrome lived a mean of 29 months and a median of 36 months after the onset of the leukemic state. The two cases of acute granulocytic leukemia survived 1.5 and 5 months, respectively. The duration of hemolytic anemia in the total group of patients ranged from 1.5 to 41 months. The patients survived a median of 8 and a mean of 12 months after hemolytic anemia. The clinical data and the presenting symptoms and signs at the onset of hemolytic anemia are summarized in Table 42.

Anemia was universally present at the onset of autoimmune hemolytic anemia. The magnitude of this abnormality became more apparent with followup examinations. A mean hematocrit of 18 and a median of 17 per cent were found. Mild reticulocytosis was common at the onset of autoimmune hemolytic anemia. A further reticulocyte response was apparent after therapy. Thrombocytopenia was uncommon. The WBC was compatible with the leukemic state. Nucleated erythrocytes were demonstrated in five patients. Bone marrow preparations were available only in the two acute

TABLE 42. *Statistical data obtained from seven patients (four females, three males) with granulocytic leukemia (GL) and autoimmune hemolytic anemia (AHA) (all patients had died at time of analysis)*

Test Procedures	Total	Statistical Data		
		Range	Mean	Median
Clinical data				
Age (years)	7	27–72	54	55
Duration of GL before AHA* (months)	4	2–57	34	29
Survival (months)	7	1.5–65	29	36
Duration of AHA (months)	7	1.5–41	12	8
Laboratory data				
Initial hematocrit (%)	7	17–30	23	23
Lowest hematocrit (%)	7	11–26	18	17
Initial reticulocytes (%)	7	0.2–6.8	2.9	2.6
Therapeutic reticulocytes (%)	6	0.0–12.9	5.7	2.5
Initial WBC (10^3/mm.^{3})	7	1.4–288	2.9	200
Initial thrombocytes (10^3/mm.^{3})	7	51–536	224	200

	Weakness	Dizziness	Fever	Bleeding
Presenting symptoms				
Abnormal	7	6	1	1

	Spleen	Liver	Lymph nodes	Jaundice
Presenting signs				
Abnormal	5	5	5	0

*Three patients had simultaneous diagnosis of GL and AHA.

cases. Erythrocytic hyperplasia was noted in one and erythrocytic hypoplasia in the other.

Clinical Patterns in Granulocytic Leukemia

The few cases available make it difficult to project any typical clinical pattern of autoimmune hemolytic anemia associated with chronic granulocytic leukemia. The following protocol appears to be representative of our experience with this syndrome.

Case 29. A 51-year-old white female was investigated because of mild fatigue. Physical examination was negative except for a thyroid nodule. The hematocrit was 44 per cent and the WBC 23,170/mm.^{3} Bone marrow examination was diagnostic for chronic granulocytic leukemia. Over the next 9 months the hematocrit dropped to 24 per cent with normal reticulocyte values. The WBC rose to 52,000/mm.^{3} Intravenous P^{32} therapy was initiated. The hematocrit rose to 37 per cent and a 6.4 per cent reticulocytosis developed. The WBC was main-

tained below 25,000/mm.^{3} The patient became asymptomatic, and intermittent P^{32} therapy was continued for 16 months. At this point weakness and fatigue returned. The hematocrit dropped to 30 per cent with a 2.9 per cent reticulocyte count. Pneumonia, pulmonary embolization and rapid liver enlargement occurred. The spleen was palpated 3 cm. below the costal margin and the WBC rose to 37,000/mm.^{3} The hematocrit progressively dropped to 23 per cent. Direct antiglobulin and bromelin tests were positive. Prednisone therapy was initiated, with a rapid rise of the hematocrit. The spleen and liver were no longer palpable. Eight months later severe abdominal pain occurred and a splenic infarct was diagnosed; the spleen was enlarged 6 cm. below the costal margin. The antiglobulin and bromelin tests had reverted to normal, but anemia persisted in spite of continual prednisone therapy. Forty-five transfusions were necessary during this 9-month period. Splenic irradiation totaling 302 r was given without halting the hemolytic process. The antiglobulin and bromelin tests were again strongly positive, and 20 additional transfusions were given over the next 3 months. Death occurred 44 months after diagnosis of chronic granulocytic leukemia and 15 months after autoimmune hemolytic anemia. Autopsy revealed a hemorrhagic thyroid adenoma as well as the leukemic condition.

The above patient presented a clinical pattern not unlike that seen with chronic lymphocytic leukemia. The leukemic process was well controlled at onset of autoimmune hemolytic anemia. Over the next 15 months, until death, the hemolytic state dominated the clinical picture. Although a severe disease process was apparent, the leukemic state never flared into violent activity. Therapy was directed primarily toward hemolysis, although the leukemic process was still evident.

Case 30. A 61-year-old white male was investigated for fatigue, anemia, black stools and evidence of hemolytic anemia. Physical examination was negative. The peripheral white blood cell count was 21,000/mm.³ and suggested acute granulocytic leukemia. Bone marrow aspiration confirmed this diagnosis and also revealed erythrocytic hypoplasia. One month later physical examination was still normal. The hematocrit was 26 per cent and the reticulocyte count was 0.4 per cent. The WBC was 21,000/mm.³ Direct antiglobulin and bromelin tests were both 2+. 6-Mercaptopurine therapy was started. Two weeks later the hematocrit dropped to 17 per cent with 0.0 per cent reticulocytes. Prednisone, 60 mg. per day, was given in conjunction with 6-mercaptopurine. In spite of 25 transfusions anemia persisted and reticulocyte counts (five examinations) remained at 0.0 per cent. The antiglobulin test remained positive. The patient died 5 months after the onset of the leukemic state and 3 months after autoimmune hemolytic anemia had developed.

This case emphasizes the poor prognosis of autoimmune hemolytic anemia developing in a patient with granulocytic leukemia. Erythrocytic hypoplasia and lack of therapeutic response to corticosteroids and immunosuppressive drugs are particularly ominous signs. The inability of the bone marrow to compensate for the hemolytic state is almost inevitably followed by death.

Summary

A remarkable association exists among the various forms of leukemia and autoimmune hemolytic anemia. This relationship is most apparent in chronic lymphocytic leukemia. Approximately 25 per cent of such patients eventually develop autoimmune hemolytic anemia.

Although this complication is not as apparent in other forms of leukemia, it is not rare. Diagnosis of autoimmune hemolytic anemia in patients with leukemia other than the chronic lymphocytic variety may be difficult. Atypical aspects of a superimposed hemolytic syndrome are common. The ability of the bone marrow to compensate by erythrocyte hyperplasia and reticulocytosis is frequently lost. Adequate corticosteroid therapy may initiate the restoration of this bone marrow function. Serologically, antiglobulin testing is variable and positive reactions may be weak or only moderately strong.

Development of autoimmune hemolytic anemia is a grave prognostic sign in all forms of leukemia. Survival of patients with the simultaneous diagnosis of chronic lymphocytic leukemia and autoimmune hemolytic anemia is only one-fifth that of a comparable group of patients with uncomplicated chronic lymphocytic leukemia. A lack of bone marrow response to corticosteroid therapy is particularly ominous. A persistent failure to respond usually results in death.

Neither the onset nor therapeutic response of autoimmune hemolytic anemia correlates with the degree of leukemic activity. It frequently appears as if two separate processes are occurring in the same patient. In spite of this, the survival of patients with both syndromes is substantially less than that seen for patients with either syndrome alone.

BIBLIOGRAPHY

1. Schwartz, R. S.: Immunologic disorders in malignant lymphomas. In *Proceedings of the Fifth National Cancer Conference.* J. B. Lippincott Company, Philadelphia, 1964.
2. Pirofsky, B.: Autoimmune hemolytic anemia and neoplasia of the reticuloendothelium. With a hypothesis concerning etiologic relationships. Ann. Intern. Med. **68:** 109, 1968.
3. Dameshek, W., and Komninos, Z. D.: The present status of treatment of autoimmune hemolytic anemia with ACTH and cortisone. Blood **11:** 648, 1956.

4. van Loghem, J. J., van der Hart, M., and Dorfmeier, H.: Serologic studies in acquired hemolytic anemia. *Proceedings of the Sixth International Congress of the International Society of Hematology.* Grune & Stratton, Inc., New York, 1956.

5. Dausset, J., and Colombani, J.: The serology and the prognosis of 128 cases of autoimmune hemolytic anemia. Blood **14:** 1280, 1959.

6. Evans, R. S., and Weiser, R. S.: The serology of autoimmune hemolytic disease. Observations on forty-one patients. Arch. Intern. Med. (Chicago) **100:** 371, 1957.

7. Dacie, J. V.: *The Haemolytic Anaemias, Part II,* Ed. 2. Grune & Stratton, Inc., New York, 1962.

8. Crosby, W. H., and Rappaport, H.: Autoimmune hemolytic anemia. I. Analysis of hematologic observations with particular reference to their prognostic value. A survey of 57 cases. Blood **12:** 42, 1957.

9. Yunis, E. J., and Bridges, R. H.: Blood transfusion problems in auto-immune hemolytic anemia. Minnesota Med. **49:** 759, 1966.

10. Speiser, P.: Some remarks on human erythrocytic autoantibodies. Z. Immunitaetsforsch. **132:** 113, 1967.

11. Bohnen, R. F., Ultmann, J. E., Gorman, J. G., Farhangi, M., and Scudder, J.: The direct Coombs test: its clinical significance. Ann. Intern. Med. **68:** 19, 1968.

12. Hirschfeld, H.: Ueber Leukanämie. Folia Haemat. (Leipzig) **3:** 332, 1906.

13. Pappenheim, A.: Bemerkungen über Leukanämie in Anschull an vorstehende Mitteilung von Hans Hirschfeld. Folia Haemat. (Leipzig) **3:** 339, 1906.

14. Paschkis, K.: Über atypische häemolytische Anämien. Z. Klin. Med. **105:** 301, 1927.

15. Jaffe, R. H.: The nature of the anemia in acute leukemia. Arch. Path. (Chicago) **20:** 725, 1935.

16. Bigley, R. H., Koler, R. D., Pirofsky, B., and Osgood, E. E.: A comparison of chronic leukemic lymphocytic leukemia, chronic subleukemic lymphocytic leukemia, and lymphocytic sarcoma. Cancer Chemother. Rep. **16:** 231, 1962.

17. Wasserman, L. R., Stats, D., Schwartz, L., and Fudenberg, H.: Symptomatic and hemopathic hemolytic anemia. Amer. J. Med. **18:** 961, 1955.

18. Miale, J. B.: *Laboratory Medicine—Hematology,* Ed. 2. The C. V. Mosby Company, St. Louis, 1962.

19. Wintrobe, M. M.: *Clinical Hematology,* Ed. 5. Lea & Febiger, Philadelphia, 1961.

20. Dameshek, W., and Gunz, F.: *Leukemia,* Ed. 2. Grune & Stratton, Inc., New York, 1964.

21. Seaman, A. J., Koler, R. D., Pirofsky, B., and Osgood, E. E.: Incidence and treatment of acquired hemolytic anemia complicating chronic lymphocytic leukemia. *Proceedings*

of the Sixth International Congress of the International Society of Hematology. Grune & Stratton, Inc., New York, 1956.

22. Osgood, E. E.: Antiglobulin-positive hemolytic anemias. Arch. Intern. Med. (Chicago) **107:** 313, 1961.

23. Pirofsky, B.: Studies on the hemolysin and agglutinin of leukemic leukocytes. Blood **12:** 620, 1957.

24. Pirofsky, B.: Serologic and clinical findings in autoimmune hemolytic anemia. Series Haemat. **9:** 47, 1965.

25. Swisher, S. N.: Acquired hemolytic disease. Postgrad. Med. **40:** 378, 1966.

26. Kyle, R. A., Kiely, J. M., and Stickney, J. M.: Acquired hemolytic anemia in chronic lymphocytic leukemia and the lymphomas. Arch. Intern. Med. (Chicago) **104:** 61, 1959.

27. Rosenthal, M. C., Pisciotta, A. V., Komninos, Z. D., Goldenberg, H., and Dameshek, W.: The autoimmune hemolytic anemia of malignant lymphocytic disease. Blood **10:** 197, 1955.

28. Gauld, W. R., Innes, J., and Robson, H. N. A.: Survey of 647 cases of leukemia, 1938–1951. Brit. Med. J. **1:** 585, 1953.

29. Bethel, F. H.: Leukemia: the relative incidence of its various forms and their response to radiation therapy. Ann. Intern. Med. **18:** 757, 1943.

30. Osgood, E. E.: Treatment of chronic leukemias. J. Nucl. Med. **5:** 139, 1964.

31. Hyman, G. A., and Harvey, J. L.: Studies on anemia of disseminated malignant neoplastic disease. I. The hemolytic factor. Blood **9:** 911, 1954.

32. Dameshek, W.: Theories of autoimmunity. In *Conceptual Advances in Immunology and Oncology.* Hoeber Medical Division, Harper & Row, Publishers, New York, 1963.

33. Tudhope, G. R.: The survival of red cells and the causation of anaemia in leukaemia. Scot. Med. J. **4:** 342, 1959.

34. Nathan, D., and Berlin, N. I.: Studies of the rate of production and life span of erythrocytes in acute leukemia. Blood **14:** 935, 1959.

35. Wetherley-Mein, G., Epstein, I. S., Foster, W. D., and Grimes, A. J.: Mechanisms of anaemia in leukaemia. Brit. J. Haemat. **4:** 281, 1958.

36. Whitelaw, D. M., Evelyn, K. A., Solvonuk, P. F., and Tang, E.: Studies of erythrocyte survival in acute leukaemia. Canad. Med. Ass. J. **80:** 944, 1959.

37. Bowie, E. J. W., Kiely, J. M., Tauxe, W. N., and Stickney, J. M.: The anemia of leukemia. J. Nucl. Med. **3:** 423, 1962.

38. Frumin, A. M., and Kohn, A.: Autoimmune hemolytic disease in acute leukemia. Arch. Intern. Med. (Chicago) **95:** 326, 1955.

39. Bile, G., deBiasi, R., and Ventruto, V.: Anemia emolitica autoimmune in corso di cloroma. *Proceedings of the Seventh International*

Congress of the International Society of Hematology. Il Pensiero Scientifico, Rome, 1960.

40. Cassell, M., and Chaplin, H.: Studies on anti-eluate sera. II. Comparison of a conventional antiglobulin serum with three anti-eluate sera in the study of 70 patients with acquired hemolytic anemia. Vox. Sang. **5**: 43, 1960.

41. Brill, N. E.: Chronic hemolytic icterus complicated by a myeloid leukemia. Med. Clin. N. Amer. **8**: 153, 1924.

42. Jonsson, U., Hansen-Pruss, O. C., and Rundles, R. W.: Hemolytic anemia in myelogenous leukemia with splenectomy. Blood **5**: 920, 1950.

43. Marchal, G., and Duhamel, G.: L'anémie hémolytique dans les leucémies. Sang **21**: 254, 1950.

44. Stats, D.: The sedimentation differential agglutination test. I. Method of the test. II. Observations on the destruction and production of red cells, with special reference to myeloblastic leukemia and comparison with the results of the radioactive phosphorus method. Blood **5**: 950, 1950.

45. Meacham, G. G., and Weisberger, A. S.: Early atypical manifestations of leukemia. Ann. Intern. Med. **41**: 780, 1954.

46. Young, L. E. Platzer, R. F., and Laurence, J. S.: Unusual anemia associated with chronic myeloid leukemia. Acta Haemat. (Basel) **5**: 345, 1951.

47. Schunk, G. J., and Lehman, W. L.: Mongolism and congenital leukemia. J. A. M. A. **155**: 250, 1954.

48. Videbaek, A.: Auto-immune haemolytic anaemia in some malignant systemic diseases. Acta Med. Scand. **171**: 463, 1962.

49. Hennemann, H. H.: Leukämiestudien (IV). Hämolytische Syndrome bei Leukämien, zugleich ein Beitrag zur Fehldiagnose: Hämolytische Anämie mit leukämoider Reaktion oder myeloische Leukose. Z. Ges. Inn. Med. **11**: 436, 1956.

Chapter 6

The Lymphomas and Autoimmune Hemolytic Anemia

The early descriptions (1–4) of hemolytic anemia complicating the leukemic state have been amply confirmed. The leukemias and lymphomas both appear as malignancies of reticuloendothelial structures. It is not surprising therefore that an association of autoimmune hemolytic anemia with the lymphomas has also been observed.

In 1927 Holler and Paschkis (5) reported two cases of Hodgkin's disease complicated by hemolytic anemia. Since that initial observation many individual reports have confirmed the fact that symptomatic or secondary hemolytic anemia may occur in all forms of lymphoma. This association is now universally recognized. Acceptable medical practice currently requires consideration of a possible underlying lymphoma in any case of autoimmune hemolytic anemia of obscure origin. In the present series autoimmune hemolytic anemia was found to be associated with a lymphoma in 25 patients. This represents an incidence of 10.7 per cent of the total series and 13.2 per cent of secondary varieties.

The frequency of associated lymphomas in the current series of patients with autoimmune hemolytic anemia is not particularly impressive. This observation is pertinent when considered in relation to the assumption that such associations are common. The present series is dominated by a high incidence of secondary varieties of autoimmune hemolytic anemia. The patient population was selectively weighted with a large proportion of patients having leukemia and lymphomas. Large numbers of lymphoma cases were studied in the 8 years spanned by the current series. In this perspective it must be concluded that the association of autoimmune hemolytic anemia with lymphoma is uncommon, in spite of the number of cases presented below.

Hodgkin's Disease

In 1927 Holler and Paschkis (5) reported two cases of hemolytic anemia complicating Hodgkin's disease. This relationship was confirmed in reports by Davidson (6) of three cases, Watson (7) with two cases and Davis (8) and Marchal and associates (9) each reporting two cases. Reports of single cases of Hodgkin's disease associated with hemolytic anemia were also common in the early literature. Many of the early publications are summarized by Singer (10), Marchal (11) and Paraf and Dausset (12). Marchal and associates (9) were so impressed with this phenomenon that they suggested hemolysis as the sole mechanism for the anemia seen in Hodgkin's disease. By 1941 the relationship was sufficiently recognized that Singer and Dameshek (13) included Hodgkin's disease as a major category in their classification of symtomatic forms of hemolytic anemia.

Frequency and Mechanism of Hemolytic Anemia in Hodgkin's Disease

Hemolytic anemia in Hodgkin's disease has classically been considered to result from an increased erythrophagocytic function of histiocytes and monocytes. The studies of Jensen (14), Waggener and as-

118

sociates (15), Giannopoulos and Bergsagel (16), Veeger and associates (17) and Cline and Berlin (18) indicated that erythrocyte survival times were generally lowered in Hodgkin's disease. Giannopoulos and Bergsagel described a moderate increase in erythropoiesis and a marked increase of iron stores.

The frequency of hemolytic anemia as a complication of Hodgkin's disease is still to be determined accurately. Gall and Mallory's series (19) of 618 cases of lymphoma and leukemia surprisingly did not reveal any examples of hemolytic anemia. Goia (20) noted four instances of hemolytic anemia in 90 cases of Hodgkin's disease. Wasserman and associates (21) found hemolytic anemia in eight of 104 consecutive cases of Hodgkin's disease. In contrast, Matthias (22) felt that a hemolytic complication was present in all patients in the terminal stage of their disease.

The possibility of an autoimmune etiology for the hemolytic anemia complicating Hodgkin's disease was considered soon after the antiglobulin test became available. Grueland (23) in 1947, Brown and Maynell (24) and Trinick (25) in 1949, and Von Sulzer (26) and Rundles and Barton (27) in 1952 all reported cases with positive antiglobulin tests.

The incidence of positive antiglobulin tests in Hodgkin's disease associated with hemolytic anemia is difficult to determine. In the series of Wasserman and associates (21) which included eight hemolytic cases (out of 104 consecutive patients with Hodgkin's disease), positive antiglobulin tests were found in two of six tested. Hennemann (28) found one positive antiglobulin reaction in 52 patients. Grobbelaar (29) reported three positive antiglobulin reactions in seven patients with Hodgkin's disease. Both warm and cold acting autoantibodies were found. In the group of Kyle and associates (30) of seven patients, positive antiglobulin tests were found in three of six tested. Dausset and Colombani (31) encountered two cases in their large series. Crosby and Rappaport (32) reported four cases of Hodgkin's disease in their series of 57 cases of autoimmune hemolytic anemia. All four cases had positive antiglobulin

tests. Bousser and associates (33) and Videbaek (34) have reported more than single cases. Matthias (22) has reported the highest incidence of positive antiglobulin tests in Hodgkin's disease; in his series 12 of 50 patients had positive serologic reactions.

Eisner and associates (35) have presented a large series of patients with associated autoimmune hemolytic anemia and Hodgkin's disease. Direct antiglobulin tests were performed in 219 cases of Hodgkin's disease. Positive antiglobulin tests were obtained in six patients (3 per cent). Their analysis was based on this group and on four additional patients with the combined syndrome. Unfortunately, single antiglobulin tests were performed in most patients with Hodgkin's disease and anemia. An accurate incidence of the autoimmune state is therefore not available. Eisner and associates concluded that autoimmune hemolytic anemia is an infrequent complication of Hodgkin's disease.

Analysis of Present Series

In the current series 13 cases of autoimmune hemolytic anemia were found in association with Hodgkin's disease. A predominantly male distribution was seen, with only four cases in females. This 69 per cent incidence of involved males is similar to the sex distribution reported for all cases of Hodgkin's disease in a series reported by Scott (36). Scott's series had a male distribution of 73 per cent and may be considered as a control group of random patients with Hodgkin's disease for analysis. Several of the patients in the current study were included in Scott's analysis. The sex distribution differs markedly from that observed by Eisner and associates (35). Their 10 patients with the combined syndrome showed only a 40 per cent occurrence in males.

Patients with Hodgkin's disease of all age groups developed autoimmune hemolytic anemia. Four cases in the current series were under age 16, with the youngest 6 years old. The mean and median ages of patients were in the mid 40's. This distribution did not differ substantially from that of the control group reported by Scott. A younger population was reported by Eisner and associates as having the combined syndrome. A median and mean age approximating 35 years was found in their patient series.

In three patients Hodgkin's disease and autoimmune hemolytic anemia were simultaneously diagnosed. In the remaining 10 cases Hodgkin's disease preceded autoimmune hemolytic anemia. A median of 19 months and a mean of 33.8 months of preexisting Hodgkin's disease were found. The series of Eisner and associates presented a longer history of preexisting Hodgkin's disease. Only one case had a simultaneous onset of autoimmune hemolytic anemia and Hodgkin's disease. A median duration of 38 months of Hodgkin's disease preceded the development of autoimmune hemolytic anemia in the remaining nine patients. This is twice as long as the median value found in the current study.

In the 12 cases who have died in the current series, a median duration of survival of 25 months from the onset of Hodgkin's disease was found. The one surviving case has had Hodgkin's disease for 252 months. It is apparent that the current series involves a different patient population from that reported by Eisner and associates. Survivals substantially longer than those anticipated in any unselected group of patients with Hodgkin's disease were seen. Duration of Hodgkin's disease ranged from 22.5 to 265 months in their cases. Eight patients have died in their series. A median of 52 and a mean of 73 months for duration of Hodgkin's disease may be calculated from their data.

The median duration of hemolytic anemia in the 12 patients of the present series that have died was 7 months. One patient is living 120 months after diagnosis of autoimmune hemolytic anemia. These results again differ markedly from those reported by Eisner and associates. The clinical data and laboratory observations at the onset of hemolytic anemia are presented in Table 43. Calculations made from the data of Eisner and associates (35) and of Scott (36) are also included.

Moderate anemia was present in all cases at the time of diagnosis of autoimmune hemolytic anemia. The severity of anemia was less pronounced than that seen in leukemic cases. This pattern was maintained when the lowest hematocrit values obtained during the course of hemolytic disease were examined. Initial reticulocytosis was low grade but not uncommon. Therapy usually resulted in a more marked reticulocyte response. The initial white blood cell count (WBC) was variable with five patients having values below 4,000/mm.^{3} and three patients with counts above 10,000/mm.^{3} Thrombocytopenia was not a problem although it was noted in two patients. Nucleated erythrocytes and spherocytes were found in three cases. Bone marrow examinations were performed in 12 patients. The only abnormality noted was erythrocytic hyperplasia in five specimens.

Clinical Patterns

The clinical picture of Hodgkin's disease associated with autoimmune hemolytic anemia differed from the relationship observed in the leukemias. In 12 of the 13 cases autoimmune hemolytic anemia occurred during heightened activity of the underlying malignancy. Similar observations were made by Matthias (22). Ranløv and Videbaek (37) observed an even more positive relationship between activity of Hodgkin's disease and autoimmune hemolytic anemia. They reported a patient with cyclic episodes of hemolytic anemia synchronous with Pel-Ebstein febrile episodes. The development of hemolytic anemia in a well stabilized patient, as was frequently observed in chronic lymphocytic leukemia, was not seen. Activity of the two disease states usually occurred in parallel.

The superimposition of autoimmune hemolytic anemia on active Hodgkin's disease usually led to a stormy and complex clinical course. The fulminating nature of such a combination has been described in Case 19. The following protocol is typical of the clinical pattern seen in most patients.

Case 31. A 16-year-old white male developed fatigue and cervical adenopathy. Lymph node biopsy revealed Hodgkin's disease. A mediastinal mass was noted and radiation therapy was given. The patient remained asymptomatic for 11 months. Fatigue, cough, fever, pruritus, back pain and generalized adenopathy then occurred. Four months later the thyroid became diffusely

TABLE 43. *Statistical data obtained from 13 patients (four females, nine males) with Hodgkins' disease (HD) and autoimmune hemolytic anemia (AHA)*

Test Procedures	Total	Statistical Data		
		Range	Mean	Median
Clinical data, age (years)				
Current series	13	6–81	41	46
Scott's series (36) (control HD)	188	6–92	40	
Series of Eisner and associates (35)	10	12–65	34	35
Duration of HD before AHA (months)				
Current series*	10	3–132	34	19
Series of Eisner and associates (35)†	9	0.5–132	47	38
Survival with HD, dead (months)				
Current series	12	4–72	29	25
Series of Eisner and associates (35)	8	23–207	73	52
Duration of AHA, dead (months)	12	1–39	12	7
Laboratory data				
Initial hematocrit (%)	13	21.5–35	28	27
Lowest hematocrit (%)	13	13.5–35	21.4	18
Initial reticulocytes (%)	13	0.5–14.6	2.9	1.7
Therapeutic reticulocytes (%)	10	1.1–26	6.3	4.2
Initial WBC (10^3/mm.^{3})	12	2.1–20	8	7.7
Initial thrombocytes (10^3/mm.^{3})	13	21–491	195	200

		Increased	Decreased	Normal
Bone marrow aspiration				
Total cellularity	12	2	2	8
Erythrocyte precursors	12	5	0	7
Leukocytes	12	1	1	10
Megakaryocytes	12	1	2	9
Megaloblasts	12	0	0	12

		Weakness	Dizziness	Fever	Bleeding
Presenting symptoms					
Abnormal	12	12	9	7	2

		Spleen	Liver	Lymph nodes	Jaundice
Presenting signs					
Abnormal	12	4	5	7	3

* Three patients; simultaneous diagnosis of HD and AHA.
† One patient; simultaneous diagnosis of HD and AHA.

enlarged and the liver and spleen could be felt at the costal margins. The hematocrit was 34 per cent with a 2.4 per cent reticulocyte count. Nitrogen mustard therapy was given intravenously and followed with maintenance oral chlorambucil. Three months later the hematocrit had dropped to 27 per cent with a 2.8 per cent reticulocyte count. Direct antiglobulin and bromelin tests were positive. Repeat nitrogen mustard was given intravenously and prednisone was started.

The antiglobulin test remained positive and the hematocrit dropped to 18 per cent; reticulocytes were maintained at 2 per cent. Oral moniliasis and ascites developed. Five blood transfusions were given. Vinblastine therapy was initiated. The severe anemia persisted. Prednisone therapy was continued and, in sequence, cyclophosphamide and vincristine were employed. Bacterial septicemia and extensive moniliasis were then documented. Nine additional transfusions were necessary to maintain the hematocrit in the low 20's. Death occurred 27 months after the onset of Hodgkin's disease and 8 months after the start of autoimmune hemolytic anemia.

A major difference is apparent between the current series of patients with Hodgkin's disease and autoimmune hemolytic anemia and that reported by Eisner and associates (35). In the present series development of autoimmune hemolytic anemia was an extremely poor prognostic sign. The clinical course was severe and death generally occurred with persisting hemolytic anemia. In the series of Eisner and associates hemolytic anemia was transient and apparently did not influence the natural course of Hodgkin's disease. In none of the observed deaths was hemolytic anemia related to the terminal event. Differences as to age, sex distribution, duration of preexisting Hodgkin's disease and duration of survival from the onset of Hodgkin's disease are noted between the two groups. No explanation for these differences can be offered other than the small numbers involved in these two patient populations.

Lymphosarcoma

Dameshek and Schwartz (38) have emphasized the importance of abnormal lymphocytes in autoimmune hemolytic anemia. This lymphoproliferative aspect is supported by the frequency with which autoimmune hemolytic anemia occurs in association with chronic and acute lymphocytic leukemia.

A similar relationship between lymphosarcoma and autoimmune hemolytic anemia can be anticipated. Case reports in the early literature describing this relationship have been published by Singer and Dameshek (13), Introzzi and associates (39), Davis (8), Stats and associates (40), Aubert and Brendemoen (41), Dustin and Drochmans (42), Fisher and associates (43), Rosenthal and associates (44), Wasserman and associates (21), Kyle and associates (30), Crosby and Rappaport (32) and Dausset and Colombani (31). Both cold and warm acting erythrocyte autoantibodies have been described. In a series of 1269 cases of lymphosarcoma (including reticulum cell sar-

coma and giant follicular lymphoma) reported by Rosenberg and associates (45), no routine attempt was made to discover hemolytic states. However, seven cases with severe hemolysis were discovered. The antiglobulin test was positive in two patients. Negative antiglobulin tests were found in 84 cases, usually in patients investigated because of jaundice and anemia.

Analysis of Present Series

In the current series autoimmune hemolytic anemia associated with lymphosarcoma was encountered in seven patients. The criteria employed for diagnosis of lymphosarcoma deserve elaboration. Biopsy and tissue examination, with a pathology report of lymphosarcoma, was required in all cases. However, a diagnosis of lymphosarcoma was not accepted until bone marrow and peripheral blood examinations were reviewed. Lymphocytosis in the bone marrow and/or peripheral blood resulted in a diagnosis of chronic lymphocytic leukemia irrespective of the tissue report. This differentiation is important, particularly in reference to the chronic subleukemic lymphocytic leukemia group previously discussed. Many of these patients, such as Case 22, were initially considered to have lymphosarcoma on the basis of tissue pathologic examinations. The patients presented below had a tissue diagnosis of lymphosarcoma with a bone marrow and peripheral blood picture free from abnormal or excessive lymphocytes.

Three males and four females had lymphosarcoma and autoimmune hemolytic anemia. Lymphosarcoma was present prior to the onset of autoimmune hemolytic anemia in all patients. A mean and median duration of approximately 50 months of preexisting lymphosarcoma was found. This long duration of prior lymphosarcoma suggests that autoimmune hemolytic anemia develops during the end stage of disease. Extremely short survivals after development of autoimmune hemolytic anemia are a factor which supports this view. In the six patients who have died the duration of autoimmune hemolytic anemia ranged from 1 week to 9 months. A median of only 3 months and a mean of 4 months for survival after the onset of hemolytic anemia were obtained. The one surviving patient has had lymphosarcoma for 24 months, with an associated hemolytic anemia for 21 months.

Autoimmune hemolytic anemia appears to develop preferentially in patients with long-standing lymphosarcoma. The study by Bigley and associates (46) of 46 patients with lymphosarcoma represents a control series in terms of diagnostic and therapeutic procedures. A mean survival of 54 months from the onset of lymphosarcoma was found in this group. Thirty-three patients had died and their mean survival was 46 months. In contrast, the six patients with an associated autoimmune hemolytic anemia who have died survived for a mean of 64 months from the onset of lymphosarcoma. Such data suggest that the development of autoimmune hemolytic anemia in patients with lymphosarcoma may be a function of duration of disease. Prolonged survival increases the risk of superimposed autoimmune hemolytic anemia. Although the occurrence of autoimmune hemolytic anemia in a patient with lymphosarcoma is ominous, many such patients survive longer than the mean survival duration of a random population of patients with lymphosarcoma. This reflects the end stage nature of the complicating autoimmune hemolytic anemia.

Anemia was present in all cases at the time of onset of autoimmune hemolytic anemia. It appeared moderately severe with a mean hematocrit of 23 per cent. Reticulocytosis was not prominent at the onset of disease. After therapy, however, an elevated reticulocyte count was characteristic, with a mean value of 8 per cent. Thrombocytopenia was variable and a mild tendency toward leukopenia was apparent. Nucleated erythrocytes and spherocytes were observed in the peripheral blood in three cases. Erythrocytic hyperplasia in the bone marrow was noted in three of the five cases examined.

The presenting symptoms and signs at the onset of autoimmune hemolytic anemia are tabulated in Table 44 with the statistical and laboratory observations. In two of the patients neither hepatomegaly, splenomegaly nor lymphadenopathy was present at the onset of hemolytic anemia.

Clinical Patterns

A characteristic disease pattern was seen in the seven patients who developed autoimmune hemolytic anemia as a complication of lymphosarcoma. In general, a long history of preexisting lymphosarcoma was obtained. Autoimmune hemolytic anemia appeared as a severe complication and was frequently followed by short survivals.

Case 32. A 49-year-old white male developed progressive back and leg pains. Nine months later a laminectomy was performed and lymphosarcoma was diagnosed on biopsy of a tumor. He was treated with radiation and nitrogen mustard. The patient remained asymptomatic for 46 months, at which time a cervical cord tumor was demonstrated. He was again treated with radiation and nitrogen mustard. Recurrence was apparent in 4 months and vincristine was given with excellent results. Toxicity necessitated discontinuation of this therapy. Lymphadenopathy developed and chlorambucil was started. Three months later hepatosplenomegaly was noted. Three and one-half months later the hematocrit had dropped to 24 per cent with a 4.2 per cent reticulocyte count. Erythrocytic hyperplasia was noted in the bone marrow. Antiglobulin and bromelin tests were negative but became positive 1 month later. These positive serologic tests persisted throughout the remaining clinical course. Prednisone therapy was initiated and reticulocyte values as high as 6.7 per cent developed. In spite of this, anemia continued, requiring blood transfusions. Extensive oral moniliasis developed. Hepatosplenomegaly continued. Death occurred with bronchopneumonia and an hematocrit of 21.8 per cent. Total course of lymphosarcoma was 72 months, with a terminal autoimmune hemolytic anemia of 3.5 months.

In this patient a longstanding quiescent lymphosarcoma became active. Autoimmune hemolytic anemia developed during the progressive and relentless course of the lymphoma. The patient survived this complication for only a short period.

In the other patients in this series a similar pattern was seen. A preexisting lymphosarcoma of long duration was generally present prior to the onset of autoim-

TABLE 44. *Statistical data obtained from seven patients (four females, three males) with lymphosarcoma (LS) and autoimmune hemolytic anemia (AHA)*

Test Procedures	Total	Statistical Data		
		Range	Mean	Median
Clinical data				
Age (years)	7	49–71	60	62
Duration of LS before AHA (months)	7	3–144	52	50
Survival with LS, dead (months)				
Current series	6	7–144	64	60
Series of Bigley and associates (46) (control LS)	33	2.5–127	46	
Duration of AHA, dead (months)	6	0.2–9	4	3
Laboratory data				
Initial hematocrit (%)	7	12–32	23	24
Lowest hematocrit (%)	7	10–32	21	21.8
Initial reticulocytes (%)	6	0.7–4.2	2.2	1.8
Therapeutic reticulocytes (%)	6	0.8–30	8.0	4.3
Initial WBC (10^3/mm.^{3})	6	2.1–13	4.5	3.0
Initial thrombocytes (10^3/mm.^{3})	5	21–387	148	50
		Increased	Decreased	Normal
Bone marrow aspiration				
Total cellularity	5	0	0	5
Erythrocyte precursors	5	3	0	2
Leukocytes	5	0	0	5
Megakaryocytes	5	0	0	5
Megaloblasts	5	0	0	5

		Weakness	Dizziness	Fever	Bleeding
Presenting symptoms					
Abnormal	7	6	2	1	0
		Spleen	Liver	Lymph nodes	Jaundice
Presenting signs					
Abnormal	7	3	4	2	1

mune hemolytic anemia. However, activity of the lymphoma did not necessarily correlate with the onset of the hemolytic state. In one patient lymphosarcoma had been present for 144 months and had been quiescent for 11 years when autoimmune hemolytic anemia developed. Death occurred in less than 1 week in a severe hemolytic state without evidence of lymphoma activity. Autopsy revealed lymphosarcoma localized in the lower abdomen, pelvis and kidneys. The liver and spleen were not involved in the lymphomatous process. This lack of relationship between activity of lymphoma and onset of autoimmune hemolytic anemia is similar to that observed with chronic lymphocytic leukemia.

Reticulum Cell Sarcoma

Reports of reticulum cell sarcoma complicated by hemolytic anemia are not uncommon. Scott and Robb-Smith (47), Krah (48) and Sievers and Harwerth (49) initially published examples of this association. Paraf and Dausset (12) reported an additional case and reviewed eight other examples of the combination. Giroud and associates (50) reported the development of reticulum cell sarcoma in a patient with paroxysmal cold hemoglobinuria. Individual cases have been reported by Widmann (51) and Boulet and associates (52). Both cold and warm acting erythrocyte autoantibodies have been described.

The frequency of this association is not clear. In Dausset and Colombani's series (31), five of the 35 cases of secondary autoimmune hemolytic anemia appeared in patients with reticulum cell sarcoma. Crosby and Rappaport (32) mention one case in their series of 23 secondary forms. Five of Dacie's series (53) of 250 patients with autoimmune hemolytic anemia had an associated reticulum cell sarcoma.

Immunohematologists are not the only group troubled by semantic difficulties. Pathologists have had a similar problem and this is particularly apparent in the classification of lymphomas. In many instances reticulum cell sarcoma is not differentiated from lymphosarcoma. A clear division between reticulum cell sarcoma and Hodgkin's sarcoma is frequently not possible. In other series the lymphomas are simply discussed as a homogeneous group. In some cases a category of "leukemia and lymphoma" represents the only differentiation. This problem of terminology undoubtedly has contributed to the obscure incidence of autoimmune hemolytic anemia complicating reticulum cell sarcoma.

Analysis of Present Series

In the current series the association of autoimmune hemolytic anemia and reticulum cell sarcoma was observed in four patients. Three males and one female were involved. All patients had died at time of analysis. In one case autoimmune hemolytic anemia existed for 83 months before reticulum cell sarcoma occurred. In the remaining three cases reticulum cell sarcoma preceded the development of autoimmune hemolytic anemia. A mean of 20 months and median of 26 months of preexisting reticulum cell sarcoma were found.

Survival of patients with reticulum cell sarcoma and autoimmune hemolytic anemia was short. A mean and median of approximately 20 months for duration of reticulum cell sarcoma was observed. Autoimmune hemolytic anemia was present before death for 1, 6 and 9 months, respectively, in three patients. In one patient autoimmune hemolytic anemia existed for 87 months, with reticulum cell sarcoma present in the last 4 months of life.

The laboratory studies and clinical data at onset of autoimmune hemolytic anemia are presented in Table 45. It is apparent that the association of autoimmune hemolytic anemia with reticulum cell sarcoma represents a serious disease. In this regard it closely resembles Hodgkin's disease rather than lymphosarcoma. This distinction is not necessarily related to the influence of autoimmune hemolytic anemia. Hodgkin's disease and reticulum cell sarcoma without autoimmune hemolytic anemia both have a poorer prognosis than lymphosarcoma.

Clinical Patterns

An insufficient number of cases are available in the current series to permit a valid presentation of clinical patterns. The one example of autoimmune hemolytic anemia terminating in reticulum cell sarcoma is described as Case 38. A more typical clinical pattern is seen in the following protocol.

Case 33. A 52-year-old white male developed inguinal adenopathy. Lymph node biopsy revealed reticulum cell sarcoma. The peripheral blood and bone marrow were normal. The biopsy wound became infected. During therapy a mediastinal mass, hepatomegaly and femoral lymphadenopathy became apparent. The patient received nitrogen mustard therapy with an excellent response. A massively enlarged liver was reduced to 6 cm. below the costal margin. Six months later jaundice developed and surgical exploration revealed reticulum cell sarcoma of the head of the pancreas. A return of lymphadenopathy 3 months later required additional nitrogen mustard therapy. Severe bone pain in the cervical region developed and 2000 r of radiation therapy were administered to cervical vertebrae. A continuation of bone pain and lymphadenopathy necessitated nitrogen mustard therapy 5 months later. This was again employed in 7 months and chlorambucil was added. One month later severe fatigue and

TABLE 45. *Statistical data obtained from four patients (one female, three males) with reticulum cell sarcoma (RCS) and autoimmune hemolytic anemia (AHA) (all patients had died at time of analysis)*

Test Procedures	Total	Statistical Data		
		Range	Mean	Median
Clinical data				
Age (years)	4	44–63	52	47
Duration of RCS before AHA* (months)	3	6–28	20	26
Survival with RCS (months)	4	4–35	20	21
Duration of AHA* (months)	3	1–9	5	6
Laboratory data				
Initial hematocrit (%)	4	19–27	24.1	25.7
Lowest hematocrit (%)	4	15–23	18.7	17.8
Initial reticulocytes (%)	4	0–3.1	1.7	0.5
Therapeutic reticulocytes (%)	3	5.9–8.0	6.7	6.3
Initial WBC (10^3/mm.^{3})	4	2.1–5.4	3.8	3.5
Initial thrombocytes (10^3/mm.^{3})	4	50–343	192	175

		Increased	Decreased	Normal
Bone marrow aspiration				
Total cellularity	3	0	1	2
Erythrocyte precursors	3	1	1	1
Leukocytes	3	0	1	2
Megakaryocytes	3	0	1	2
Megaloblasts	3	0	0	3

		Weakness	Dizziness	Fever	Bleeding
Presenting symptoms					
Abnormal	4	4	2	1	0

		Spleen	Liver	Lymph nodes	Jaundice
Presenting signs					
Abnormal	4	3	2	2	0

* One patient had AHA for 83 months prior to the development of RCS. This time was not added to AHA duration data.

pallor were present. The liver was 20 cm. below the costal margin, multiple lymph nodes and bone lesions were present and pleural and pericardial effusions could be demonstrated. The previous hematocrit of 44.5 per cent had dropped to 19 per cent, with a 3.1 per cent reticulocyte count. Antiglobulin and bromelin tests were positive. Prednisone, 40 mg. per day, was given, with a progressive rise of the hematocrit. This reached 40 per cent in 6 weeks, with a reticulocyte count of 6.3 per cent. Activity of the lymphoma continued. X-ray therapy to the mediastinum and vincristine therapy were sequentially given. The hematocrit dropped to 24 per cent in spite of continuing prednisone. Death occurred 35 months after the onset of

reticulum cell sarcoma and 9 months after the onset of autoimmune hemolytic anemia.

Giant Follicular Lymphoblastoma

Only infrequent reports of the association of giant follicular lymphoma and autoimmune hemolytic anemia are available. The semantic problems mentioned above are also present with this pathologic diagnosis. This may partially explain the infrequency of described cases.

Reports of this association have been presented by Evans and Doan (54) (seven cases), Wasserman and associates (21),

Rosenthal and associates (44) and Crosby and Rappaport (32). Dausset and Colombani (31) encountered two such cases in the 35 secondary varieties of autoimmune hemolytic anemia that they investigated. Kyle and associates (30) reported three cases, with negative antiglobulin tests in the two patients tested. Dacie (53) reported only one case in his 250 patients with autoimmune hemolytic anemia.

In the current series the combined syndrome of giant follicular lymphoma and autoimmune hemolytic anemia was found in one patient.

Case 34. A 66-year-old white male developed inguinal adenopathy. Lymph node biopsy revealed giant follicular lymphoma. Generalized lymphadenopathy and a liver palpated 2 cm. below the costal margin were noted on physical examination. Peripheral blood and bone marrow examinations were normal. Nitrogen mustard therapy was given with excellent results. Relapse occurred and required a further course of nitrogen mustard therapy in 14 months and again 10 months later. Maintenance chlorambucil therapy was started on this latter occasion. Remission with chlorambucil was maintained for 75 months. Relapse then occurred and nitrogen mustard was given for the fourth time. Chlorambucil therapy was maintained; remission resulted. Six months later the patient returned with severe fatigue and bone pain. Physical examination was negative except for pallor. The hematocrit had dropped to 15 per cent with a 0.6 per cent reticulocyte count. Bone marrow aspiration and examination were normal. Direct and indirect antiglobulin and bromelin tests were strongly positive, and elution revealed a panhemagglutinin. Prednisone therapy was given without a therapeutic response. Osteolytic lesions with severe bone pain were present and did not respond to radiation, cyclophosphamide or vincristine. Multiple transfusions were employed. Death occurred 110 months after the onset of giant follicular lymphoma and 3 months after the diagnosis of autoimmune hemolytic anemia.

In the above case autoimmune hemolytic anemia developed during marked activity of the malignancy. It is unfortunate that further biopsies were not obtained and that autopsy was refused. The character of lymphomatous disease changed drastically in this patient. It is probable that conversion to reticulum cell sarcoma,

Hodgkin's disease or lymphosarcoma occurred. The development of autoimmune hemolytic anemia may possibly be related to a change in the state of the underlying malignancy.

Plasma Cell Myeloma

It has been amply confirmed that lymphocytic proliferation is frequently present in autoimmune hemolytic anemia. This observation has led to the concept that modified host immunocompetent cells may produce antibodies against various host constituents. A human clinical syndrome similar to experimental graft-host disease may then develop. The same logic can be employed for describing the effects of abnormal plasma cells on immune homeostasis. Plasma cells produce humoral antibody and immunoglobulins. Accordingly, it may be anticipated that malignancies of plasma cells would have a high rate of association with positive antiglobulin tests.

There are certain differences between lymphoproliferative and plasma proliferative states which modify this postulated association. Serum electrophoretic studies in autoimmune hemolytic anemia are frequently abnormal, with a polyclonal type of gamma abnormality. This suggests that multiple proteins are formed in an abnormal fashion. In plasma cell myeloma the characteristic abnormality is monoclonal, suggesting that a single clone is actively producing a single paraprotein. Several investigators (55–57) have reported an exception to this rule by documenting the production of two myeloma paraproteins from a single clone in a patient with plasma cell myeloma. This fundamental difference between lymphoproliferative and plasma cell proliferative syndromes has received added support from the studies of allotypic typing of proteins and L chains. The Gm typing and L chains of paraproteins generally appear as a single type. This is most obvious in cold acting erythrocyte autoantibodies (58, 59). In contrast, warm acting erythrocyte autoantibodies present a mixture of kappa and lambda L chains (60, 61). This suggests that more than one cell clone is involved in the production of warm acting erythrocyte autoantibodies.

Frequency and Mechanism of Hemolytic Anemia in Plasma Cell Myeloma

Anemia is common in patients with plasma cell myeloma. Several workers have stated that a hemolytic phenomenon may be responsible. Cline and Berlin (62) demonstrated a shortened half-life survival of erythrocytes in nine of 11 anemic myeloma patients. An immunohemolytic pathogenesis, however, is not generally assumed. The shortening of erythrocyte survival time may be attributed to sludging of erythrocytes or to the effect of azotemia or erythrophagocytosis.

The clinical experience of encountering positive antiglobulin tests in patients with plasma cell myeloma is highly variable. In Dausset and Colombani's series (31) of 128 cases of autoimmune hemolytic anemia, three patients had plasma cell malignancies. Forster and Moeschlin (63) described a case with possible plasma cell leukemia and positive antiglobulin reactions. Cassell and Chaplin (64) had three patients with plasma cell myeloma in their 29 cases of autoimmune hemolytic anemia. Two patients with this association were reported by Massei and Pallone (65) and Pirofsky (66). Single examples of this association have been noted by Hennemann and associates (67), Videbaek (34), Bohrod and Bottcher (68), Wright and associates (69), Frenger and associates (70) and Yamada (71). Dacie (53) noted one patient with plasmacytomas and positive antiglobulin reactions in his series of 250 cases of autoimmune hemolytic anemia. Matthias (22) found positive antiglobulin reactions in five of 21 patients with plasma cell myeloma.

Diagnosis of Associated Autoimmune Hemolytic Anemia

The diagnosis of autoimmune hemolytic anemia associated with plasma cell myeloma is a difficult task. Anemia is frequently found in this disease and its presence does not necessarily suggest the development of autoimmune hemolytic anemia. Serologically, accurate diagnosis is particularly precarious. Paraproteins may induce intense rouleau formation suggesting hemagglutination. The direct and indirect bromelin tests are almost worthless because of this state. These procedures depend on agglutination occurring after the patient's serum, in the presence of bromelin, reacts with patient or test erythrocytes. The paraprotein may induce such intense rouleau formation after centrifugation that agglutination cannot be evaluated. Controls performed without bromelin generally reveal a similar degree of pseudoagglutination. The antiglobulin test, which is performed after test cells are washed free from serum proteins, is a more satisfactory procedure. However, this author has seen pseudoagglutination persist after centrifugation, even after the usual washing procedure. Elution and identification of the autoantibody appear to be the only satisfactory technique. Even this approach may be invalid if the Ogada phenomenon functions with paraproteins.

Analysis of Present Series

An association between autoimmune hemolytic anemia and plasma cell myeloma has conflicting theoretical implications. Its documentation in the past literature is highly variable. It is extremely difficult to demonstrate erythrocyte autoantibodies accurately with current serologic procedures. In spite of these obstacles this association was found in nine patients of the current series. Plasma cell myeloma and autoimmune hemolytic anemia occurring in the same patient, therefore, does not appear uncommon. Its frequency exceeded that observed with either lymphosarcoma, reticulum cell sarcoma or giant follicular lymphoma. This incidence possibly reflects a high exposure to this disease at our institution. Plasma cell myeloma is probably seen more frequently than any of the lymphomas.

A marked female predilection was observed in the current series. Six of the nine patients were females. This incidence is substantially higher than in the sex distribution found in a random group of patients with plasma cell myeloma. The female incidence of plasma cell myeloma at our institution has been reported as 42 per cent (14 out of 33 cases) by Osgood (72).

The age distribution of patients with the combined syndrome corresponded to that generally found with plasma cell myeloma. Osgood's series, which may be used as a control for this study, had a median age of 62 years, which is identical with the current series.

In four patients plasma cell myeloma and autoimmune hemolytic anemia were simultaneously diagnosed. In two cases autoimmune hemolytic anemia preceded the development of a plasma cell malignancy. Hemolytic anemia existed for 29 and 48 months, respectively, before neoplasia was diagnosed. This length of time makes it unlikely that myeloma was actually present but undiagnosed. In three cases plasma cell myeloma occurred before autoimmune hemolytic anemia. A median duration of 17 months of preexisting myeloma was documented. Eight of the nine patients have died. Survival duration of myeloma in these cases had a median value of only 11 months. This represents almost a 50 per cent shortening of survival compared with the control series. Hemolytic anemia had a somewhat longer duration due to the two preexisting cases of autoimmune hemolytic anemia. A mean of 23 and median of 12 months were found.

Clinical and laboratory data obtained from this patient group are presented in Table 46. In addition to the usual complaints of weakness and dizziness, fever was present in four cases and bone pain developed in eight cases. Hepatosplenomegaly and lymphadenopathy were common. Only three patients did not develop reticuloendothelial organ enlargement. Jaundice was frequent and was found in four cases. Anemia was moderately severe at the time of diagnosis and progressed with development of the disease. Reticulocytosis before therapy was common and increased after therapy. Neither the WBC nor thrombocyte levels were abnormal in any consistent patterns. Nucleated erythrocytes and spherocytes were found in three cases. The bone marrow was abnormal in all cases. In seven of the eight, malignant plasma cells were found

and were diagnostic of plasma cell myeloma. In the remaining case node biopsy revealed a plasmacytoma and autopsy eventually revealed plasma cell myeloma. Erythrocytic hyperplasia was noted in three cases and megaloblastic changes in one.

Proteinuria was demonstrated in seven of the eight examined cases, and Bence-Jones protein was identified in five. Total protein and/or albumin-globulin (A/G) ratio studies were available for analysis in eight of the nine patients. In two the total proteins were 10.4 and 13.9 gm. per cent, respectively. A/G ratios in the remaining six patients were 4.1/1.6 (plasmacytoma case) and 3.4/6.9, 3.9/5.6, 3.7/5.0, 2.3/11.9 and 2.5/16.7 gm. per cent, respectively. The serum electrophoretic pattern was reviewed in five cases. A gamma spike characteristic of a monoclonal myeloma pattern was found in all five.

Clinical Patterns

Several unusual clinical patterns were observed in patients having plasma cell myeloma and autoimmune hemolytic anemia. Two patients each initiated their disease state with autoimmune hemolytic anemia. The hemolytic state was present for 29 and 48 months, respectively, before a plasma cell malignancy became apparent. One of these patients presented with a plasmacytoma, thyroid hyperplasia and a thymoma (Case 36). Two siblings of one patient (Case 3) subsequently developed autoimmune hemolytic anemia. Rather than plasma cell myeloma, the two siblings had an Evans' syndrome (Case 5) and systemic lupus erythematosus (Case 4) as associated diseases. The combined syndrome became apparent in another patient after removal of a dermoid cyst. One patient had sufficient malignant plasma cells in the peripheral blood to warrant a diagnosis of acute subleukemic plasma cell leukemia. Accordingly, five of the nine examples of plasma cell malignancy associated with autoimmune hemolytic anemia had unusual clinical variations from the pattern generally seen in plasma cell myeloma. The following case illustrates one of these.

TABLE 46. *Statistical data obtained from nine patients (six females, three males) with plasma cell myeloma (PCM) and autoimmune hemolytic anemia (AHA)*

Test Procedures	Total	Statistical Data		
		Range	Mean	Median
Clinical data				
Age (years)	9	43–84	62	63
Duration of PCM before AHA* (months)	3	10–33	20	17
Survival with PCM, dead (months)				
Current series	8	2–54	21	11
Osgood's series (72) (control PCM)	33	1.3–82	30	20
Duration of AHA, dead (months)	8	1.5–58	23	12
Laboratory data				
Initial hematocrit (%)	9	19–25	21.4	22
Lowest hematocrit (%)	9	14–23	18.7	19
Initial reticulocytes (%)	8	0.8–13	4.7	4.3
Therapeutic reticulocytes (%)	6	2.9–8.5	5.4	4.4
Initial WBC (10³/mm.³)	9	1.7–14	6.7	4.5
Initial thrombocytes (10³/mm.³)	7	34–200	129	157

		Increased	Decreased	Normal
Bone marrow aspiration				
Total cellularity	8	2	0	6
Erythrocyte precursors	8	3	2	3
Leukocytes	8	0	1	7
Megakaryocytes	8	0	1	7
Megaloblasts	8	1	0	7
Plasma cells	8	7	0	1

		Weakness	Dizziness	Fever	Bone pain
Presenting symptoms					
Abnormal	9	8	7	4	8

		Spleen	Liver	Lymph nodes	Jaundice
Presenting signs					
Abnormal	9	5	5	4	4

* Four patients had simultaneous diagnosis of PCM and AHA. Two patients had AHA prior to PCM.

Case 35. A 43-year-old white female had surgical removal of a dermoid cyst. This was followed by pneumonia, which recurred on several occasions. Herpes zoster and mild bone pain developed in association with severe anemia. This did not respond to hematinics and the patient received over 50 transfusions during the next 3½ years. Severe bone pain then became apparent and the patient was seen in consultation. The spleen was found to descend into the pelvis and 2+ axillary nodes were found. The hematocrit was 23 per cent and the reticulocyte count was 0.3 per cent. The bone marrow was diagnostic of plasma cell myeloma and erythrocytic hypo-

plasia was noted. The A/G ratio was 2.5/16.7 and a monoclonal gamma spike was found on electrophoresis. Proteinuria, 2+, was present with Bence-Jones protein absent. NSC-1026 therapy was started. The clinical course was complicated by repeated infections. Severe anemia persisted and required seven transfusions. Multiple transfusion reactions were noted. Investigation revealed positive direct antiglobulin tests. The spleen descended 2 cm. below the costal margin and the liver 4 cm. Urinary tract infection and repeated pneumonia developed. The patient went into coma during an episode interpreted as endotoxin shock, but recovered.

Cyclophosphamide therapy was initiated without response and was followed by L-sarcolysine. Local x-ray therapy was given to areas of severe bone pain and destruction. No therapeutic response occurred. During this year, transfusions were required approximately every 2 weeks to maintain the hematocrit at 20 per cent. The antiglobulin test remained positive on the six occasions tested. Prednisone therapy was initiated with the hematocrit at 18 per cent and reticulocyte count at 0.6 per cent. No therapeutic response occurred. The patient died 4 months later with severe infections, while requiring frequent transfusions. Total duration of the severe anemic state was 54 months. It appeared that plasma cell myeloma had occurred simultaneously with autoimmune hemolytic anemia.

The severity of this combination may be appreciated when it is considered that this case represents our longest survival of a patient with plasma cell myeloma and autoimmune hemolytic anemia. Additional examples of this combination are presented as Cases 3, 36 and 40.

Thymoma

A malignant process has been present in the previously discussed examples of autoimmune hemolytic anemia associated with neoplasia of the reticuloendothelium. Malignancy does not appear to be critical, however. Benign neoplasia of the reticuloendothelium may also be associated with the development of autoimmune hemolytic anemia. Infectious mononucleosis is an example of this association which is discussed in Chapter 7. Thymoma is another benign neoplasia which has recently assumed importance in reference to the immune apparatus. The theoretical rationale for a relationship of the thymus to autoimmune hemolytic anemia is reviewed in Chapter 22.

The association of thymoma with autoimmune hemolytic anemia has been previously noted by Ross and associates (73), Janbon and associates (74), Halperin and associates (75), Jacox and associates (76) and Mongan and associates (77). The improvement of hemolytic anemia and systemic lupus erythematosus following surgical or radiation thymectomy, as noted by Wilmers and Russell (78) and Richmond and associates (79), also supports the concept that a relationship may exist between autoimmune hemolytic anemia and thymomas.

Analysis of Present Series

In the current series the association of a thymoma with autoimmune hemolytic anemia was noted in three patients. Complex clinical patterns were present, preventing the derivation of any specific clinical syndrome. Only one characteristic appeared typical among these three patients. In all cases a disease process was initiated without evidence of a thymoma. Hemolytic anemia was associated with the disease state at the time of onset in two of the three patients. In the third, autoimmune hemolytic anemia was diagnosed 3 months later. The thymoma became apparent relatively late in the clinical course. Durations of 10, 26 and 34 months elapsed from the onset of disease until a recognized mediastinal mass indicated the presence of a thymic lesion. In one patient thymectomy was performed without correcting either hemolytic anemia or an associated erythrocytic aplasia.

One case presented a confusing picture of pernicious anemia, positive lupus erythematosus (LE) cells, positive antiglobulin tests, diabetes, thyroid adenoma, multiple infections, adenocarcinoma of the prostate, interstitial pancreatitis and a thymoma (Case 6). A second patient entered with a history of two exposures to a toxic weed killer and a pattern of bone marrow erythrocytic aplasia. Autoimmune hemolytic anemia was diagnosed 3 months later. A thymoma subsequently developed and was surgically removed (Case 20). The third example of autoimmune hemolytic anemia with an associated thymoma is described below.

Case 36. A 63-year-old white female was investigated because of fatigue and swelling of her jaw. Anemia, leukopenia, splenomegaly and lymphadenopathy were noted. No definite diagnosis was made. Six months later she was seen in consultation because of fever. The spleen and liver were both 4 cm. below the costal margin and a thyroid adenoma was noted. The hematocrit was 25 per cent with a 6.8 per cent reticulocyte count. The WBC was 2,700/mm.³ Bone marrow aspiration revealed erythrocytic hyperplasia. Antiglobulin and bromelin tests were positive. Elution studies revealed a panhemagglutinin. A search for LE cells was negative and serologic tests for syphilis were positive. Prednisone, 60 mg. daily, was given with a progressive rise of the hematocrit to 31 per cent. Splenomegaly and leukopenia disappeared. A urinary tract infection was discovered 5 months later and prednisone was decreased to 15 mg. daily. An hemolytic crisis occurred. Increasing prednisone led to a therapeutic response. Six months later prednisone was again reduced, and again hemolytic crisis occurred. With maintenance prednisone for the next 10 months the hematocrit reached 39 per cent. Diabetes and cutaneous bleeding in the presence of normal thrombocytes developed during this period of time. The liver was enlarged 9 cm. below the costal margin. Prednisone was reduced to 10 mg. daily in anticipation of splenectomy, and the hematocrit dropped to 25 per cent. A large mediastinal mass became apparent 26 months after the onset of hemolytic anemia. Antiglobulin and bromelin tests remained positive. Severe back pain developed. Adenopathy in the mandibular and axillary areas was noted. Biopsy 29 months after the onset of autoimmune hemolytic anemia revealed a plasmacytoma. The A/G ratio was 4.1/1.6 and urinalysis was normal. L-sarcolysine therapy was added to prednisone with relief of bone pain and disappearance of lymph nodes. The patient died 5 months later with an hematocrit of 22 per cent and severe bone pain. Autopsy revealed a thymoma and plasma cell myeloma. Total course of hemolytic anemia was 34 months, of thymoma 8 months and of diagnosable plasma cell myeloma 5 months.

A complex clinical pattern was present in the above patient. The association of autoimmune hemolytic anemia and thymoma was complicated by the eventual development of a malignancy of the plasma cell series. Thyroid disease, diabetes and multiple infections were all noted. Table 47 summarizes some of the pertinent data obtained from the three patients with a thymoma.

The Relationship between Reticuloendothelial Neoplasia and Autoimmune Hemolytic Anemia

A relationship exists between malignancies of the reticuloendothelium and im-munologic abnormalities. Evidence for this is apparent from two sources. First, neoplasia of reticuloendothelial tissue is frequently complicated by autoimmune phenomena. Most often this takes the form of autoimmune hemolytic anemia. The extent of this relationship is seen upon analysis of the 234 cases of autoimmune hemolytic anemia presented in this volume. Of these cases, 113 patients, or 48.2 per cent of the series, had a secondary form of autoimmune hemolytic anemia related to various neoplastic changes of the reticuloendothelium. Second, patients with such neoplastic growths do not appear to have a normal capacity for initiating immune responses. This deficiency is characterized by a marked susceptibility to severe bacterial and viral infections. It may even entail an inability to produce normal delayed hypersensitivity (80).

The remarkable association of neoplastic transformation of immunocompetent cells and autoimmune hemolytic anemia has stimulated many experimental and speculative studies (81). The majority of such studies have been based on the observation that neoplasia of reticuloendothelial tissue generally occurs either prior to or simultaneous with the immunologic abnormality. This has resulted in the concept that autoimmune hemolytic anemia may be etiologically related to a population of immunocompetent cells foreign to the host and capable of initiating graft-host disease* (38, 82–84).

Ahrengot (85) first suggested that the development of autoimmune hemolytic anemia in a patient with a teratoma might be related to the production and survival of a population of genetically modified cells. Greene (82, 83) postulated a similar relationship in the leukemias and speculated that such malignancies would establish a clone of cells foreign to the host. Dameshek and Schwartz (38) and Kaplan

* Runt disease (graft-host, GVH, secondary, wasting, allogenic or homologous disease): a syndrome which develops when foreign immunocompetent cells survive and proliferate in a host. Such cells do not recognize the host as "self" but rather as foreign, and they initiate immunologic reactions against host tissues.

TABLE 47. *Statistical data obtained from three patients (one female, two males) with a thymoma and auto-immune hemolytic anemia (AHA) (all patients had died at time of analysis)*

Test Procedures	Total	Statistical Data		
		Range	Mean	Median
Clinical data				
Age (years)	3	59–75	67	66
Duration of AHA before thymoma (months)	3	10–34	23	26
Survival from onset of AHA (months)	3	34–75	49	38
Survival from onset of thymoma (months)	3	8–41	26	28
Laboratory data				
Initial hematocrit (%)	3	9–25	17.3	18
Lowest hematocrit (%)	3	8–22	16	18
Initial reticulocytes (%)	3	0–6.8	2.5	0.6
Therapeutic reticulocytes (%)	3	0–15.2	7.4	6.9
Initial WBC (10^3/mm.^{3})	3	2.7–8.2	4.9	3.7
Initial thrombocytes (10^3/mm.^{3})	3	165–225	197	200

	Total	Weakness	Dizziness	Fever	Bleeding
Presenting symptoms					
Abnormal	3	3	3	1	0

	Total	Spleen	Liver	Lymph nodes	Jaundice
Presenting signs					
Abnormal	3	1	1	1	1

	Case 20	Case 36	Case 6
Other observations			
Peripheral blood, spherocytes	0	+	+
Peripheral blood, nucleated (red blood cells)	0	+	+
Serologic tests for syphilis	0	+	+
LE cell tests	0	0	+
Bone marrow aspiration	Erythrocytic aplasia	Erythrocytic hyperplasia	Megaloblastic
Other associated diseases	Exposure to chemical toxin	Thyroid, diabetes, plasma cell myeloma, infections	Pernicious anemia, systemic lupus erythematosus, diabetes, thyroid adenoma, adenocarcinoma of the prostate, pancreatitis, infections

and Smithers (84) expanded this viewpoint. They suggested that many characteristics of such malignancies could result from the immunologic expression of a clone of foreign cells that had retained the capacity for antibody production. Such cells might produce a widespread systemic disease dominated by multiple immunologic abnormalities. The production of a varying number of autoantibodies directed against normal host constituents would characterize this state. Autoimmune hemolytic anemia, within this concept, is only one manifestation of the immunologic aberration (81). The entire clinical and laboratory pattern is similar to a graft-host disease syndrome.

Oliner and associates (86) and Stastny and associates (87) have investigated these problems through an experimental F_1 hybrid animal test system. Their data strongly support the theoretical concepts described above. These observations have led to the postulation of a mechanism of autoantibody formation in human diseases emphasizing the "lymphoproliferative" aspects of autoimmunization (88). The theoretical and clinical applications of this postulate are presented in Chapters 13 and 15 in the sections dealing with the concept of a foreign clone. The experimental studies involved in the graft-host or runt disease concept are summarized in Chapter 22.

Other relationships between autoimmune hemolytic anemia and reticuloendothelial neoplasia appear to be possible. Animal investigations indicate that neoplasia may follow rather than precede immunologic abnormalities. Studies of NZB mice by Bielschowsky and Bielschowsky (89), Holmes and Burnet (90), East and associates (91) and Mellors (92) indicate that malignancy may develop long after the occurrence of autoimmune hemolytic anemia. This malignancy may take the form of thymomas, plasmacytomas, the leukemias, undifferentiated lymphomas and reticulum cell sarcoma. The similarity of these neoplastic processes to those seen in our patients is striking. In addition, there is an increased susceptibility for malignant transformation after exposure to the carcinogen 2-aminofluorene (89).

The thymus gland has also shown a similar temporal relationship. Neonatal thymectomy may result in a wasting disease with an antiglobulin positive hemolytic anemia (93). Such animals are not competent immunologically. They have an increased resistance to virus induced lymphocytic leukemia, probably related to atrophy of lymphogenous tissue. However,

such immunologically incompetent animals also show an increased susceptibility for the development of granulocytic leukemia (94) and reticulum cell sarcoma (95).

Walford and Hildemann (96) employed coisogenic C_3H mice which differed only in a weak (H_1) histocompatibility antigen in splenic transplantation studies. After 1 year a high incidence of lymphomas was found in the absence of an overt runting syndrome. Schwartz and associates (97, 98) have recently expanded their observations of transplanted F_1 hybrid mice with immunologic abnormalities. They have similarly observed the development of malignancies, primarily reticulum cell sarcoma, after the initiation of runt disease and autoimmune hemolytic anemia.

Human Autoimmune Hemolytic Anemia Terminating in Reticuloendothelial Neoplasia

These experimental studies appear to have their spontaneous counterpart in human disease. Ben-Ishay and associates (99) described a patient with cold acting autoimmune hemolytic anemia associated with leukopenia and thrombocytopenia. This autoimmune state persisted for 18 years before terminating in an acute leukemic process. A similar patient was encountered in the present series.

Case 37. A 44-year-old white female developed fatigue, jaundice and anemia. Various hematinics gave no response and her hematocrit persisted at approximately 22 per cent. Multiple transfusions were utilized. Seven years later workup revealed a reticulocytosis of 5.8 per cent, jaundice and bone marrow erythrocytic hyperplasia. Splenectomy was carried out with a diagnosis of hemolytic anemia. Four years later Raynaud's phenomenon was diagnosed and cholecystectomy was carried out for cholelithiasis and jaundice. The hematocrit persisted at approximately 20 to 25 per cent with moderate reticulocytosis. Serologic studies revealed a potent cold hemagglutinin with complete agglutination at room temperature. Direct and indirect antiglobulin and bromelin tests were 4+. Attempts to elute the antibody at 37°C. consistently led to complete hemolysis. Physical examination was negative. Prednisone therapy was initiated and maintained at 15 to 20 mg. per day for the next 52 months. During this time the hematocrit approximated 25 per cent without transfusion therapy. Physical examination was normal except for intermittent purpura. The potent cold hemagglutinin and Raynaud's phenomenon persisted. Seventeen years after onset of hemolytic anemia the peripheral white blood count gradually rose to 50,000/mm.[3] and abnormal monocytes were found. Heterophile agglutinin studies were negative. Bone marrow aspiration revealed a typical pattern of acute monocytic leukemia; morphologic changes in the peripheral blood confirmed this observation. In spite of increasing prednisone therapy, severe anemia with reticulocytosis, a progressively enlarging liver, osteoporosis with multiple fractures, jaundice and gastric ulcers developed leading to death. Autopsy confirmed the leukemic state. Total course of hemolytic anemia was 215 months with the last 12 months complicated by an associated acute monocytic leukemia.

Bowdler and Glick (100) reported a case in which autoimmune hemolytic anemia underwent therapeutic remission following splenectomy. Three years after the onset of the autoimmune hemolytic process, lymphadenopathy developed and Hodgkin's disease was diagnosed. Becker (101) reported a patient with autoimmune hemolytic anemia who developed widespread cytomegalic disease and a terminal lymphoma. Miller (102) examined the association of various connective tissue types of autoimmune disease in patients with lymphomas. In 264 patients with malignant lymphomas, a 1.86 per cent incidence of an associated autoimmune disease was found. Five of 17 patients with this association had a history of a previously existing autoimmune disease followed by the subsequent development of a lymphoma.

Analysis of Present Series

The current report summarizes the data obtained from 114 examples of reticuloendothelial neoplasia associated with autoimmune hemolytic anemia. Table 48 indicates the temporal relationship of onset of the two conditions. It is apparent that the time of onset of autoimmune hemolytic anemia and reticuloendothelial neoplasia is variable. A simultaneous diagnosis of both conditions could be made in 36 cases or 31.6 per cent of the series. Reticuloendothelial neoplasia preceded the onset of autoimmune hemo-

TABLE 48. *The temporal relationship between onset of reticuloendothelial neoplasia and autoimmune hemolytic anemia in 113 patients*

Type of Neoplasia	Total Patients	Onset of Neoplasia in Reference to Autoimmune Hemolytic Anemia		
		Before	Simultaneous	After
Chronic lymphocytic leukemia	48	31	17	0
Acute lymphocytic leukemia	10	7	3	0
Acute monocytic leukemia	12	5	5	2
Granulocytic leukemia (acute and chronic)	7	4	3	0
Hodgkin's disease	13	10	3	0
Lymphosarcoma	7	6	1	0
Reticulum cell sarcoma	4	3	0	1
Giant follicular lymphoma	1	1	0	0
Plasma cell myeloma	9*	3	4	2*
Thymoma	3*	0	0	3*
Total	114	70	36	8
Per cent of 114 cases		61.4	31.6	7

* One patient had both plasma cell myeloma and thymoma.

lytic anemia in 70 cases or 61.4 per cent of the series. In eight instances (seven patients), autoimmune hemolytic anemia initially occurred and was subsequently followed by reticuloendothelial neoplasia.

This latter group of patients with autoimmune hemolytic anemia terminating in neoplasia of the reticuloendothelium was examined in detail. The protocols of four of these patients have already been presented as Cases 6, 20, 36 and 37. The following three cases complete this group.

Case 38. A 55-year-old white female developed fatigue and fever and received Achromycin therapy. Anemia was present 2 months later with a 0.0 per cent reticulocyte count and a WBC of 4,500/mm.[3]. Physical examination revealed the spleen palpated 2.5 cm. below the costal margin. Bone marrow aspiration demonstrated an aplastic process which was confirmed by bone marrow biopsy. The hematocrit dropped to 15 per cent with 0.3 per cent reticulocytes. An attempt to transfuse the patient demonstrated positive direct and indirect antiglobulin tests. Prednisone therapy lead to a reticulocytosis of 5.9 per cent, and the hematocrit rose to 35 per cent in 3 months. The WBC returned to normal. The spleen reached a size of 5 cm. below the costal margin before becoming non-palpable. Maintenance prednisone therapy varying from 2.5 mg. to 15 mg. daily was given over the next 79 months. During this time neither hepatosplenomegaly nor lymphadenopathy was present and the hematocrit ranged from 24 to 36 per cent. The antiglobulin and bromelin tests initially became negative but returned to positive for the last 2 years of the patient's clinical course. She suddenly developed severe bone pain, and over the next month multiple pathologic fractures developed. An abdominal mass became palpable. Biopsy of bone lesions revealed a classic pathologic picture of reticulum cell sarcoma. Death occurred with increasing osteolytic lesions and bone pain. Total course of hemolytic anemia was 87 months with a terminal reticulum cell sarcoma for 4 months.

Case 39. A 65-year-old-female was found to have anemia, reticulocytosis and leukopenia. Past history revealed poliomyelitis with bladder paresis at age 17, carcinoma of the cervix treated with radiation at age 37 and biologically false positive serologic reactions first noted at age 63. Her symptoms and laboratory abnormalities persisted and the patient was seen in consultation 15 months after the onset of anemia. Physical examination was negative. The hematocrit was 24 per cent with a 15.6 per cent reticulocyte count; thrombocytes and WBC counts were depressed. Nucleated erythrocytes and spherocytes were seen in the peripheral blood. Biologically false positive serologic reactions were found and multiple LE cell preparations were negative. The bone marrow was moderately hypocellular and erythrocytic hyperplasia was demonstrated. The urine had 1+ albumin, and *Escherichia coli* and *Streptococcus faecalis* infections were diagnosed. Multiple antiglobulin tests were performed and found to be positive on three occasions and negative on four. Donath-Landsteiner and Ham tests were negative. Prednisone therapy was given, resulting in a rise in the hematocrit to 31 per cent and a reticulocytosis of 25 per cent. Prednisone was reduced. Fever and hematuria developed and a hemolytic crisis occurred. The hematocrit dropped to 22 per cent, the reticulocyte count was 36.2 per cent and indirect bilirubin rose to 14 mg. per cent. Repeat bone marrow revealed only marked erythrocytic hyperplasia with megaloblastic changes. The patient developed axillary adenopathy and rapid deterioration with fever was apparent. Lymphohematogenous tuberculosis

was diagnosed with acid fast organisms growing from sputum, bone marrow and blood cultures. The liver and spleen were not enlarged. Repeat bone marrow examination was again carried out and sheets of blast cells were now found. Four additional consultants agreed independently with the diagnosis of acute monocytic leukemia, in spite of the presence of lymphohematogenous tuberculosis. Vincristine therapy was initiated. Extensive skin bleeding and multiple infarcts occurred. The patient died 20 months after the onset of autoimmune hemolytic anemia and 9 days after the diagnosis of acute monocytic leukemia.

Case 40. An 80-year-old white male consulted his own physician for abdominal pain, a 40-pound weight loss and anemia. No diagnosis was made. Over the next 4 years the anemia persisted, two bone marrow examinations revealed erythrocytic hyperplasia and megaloblastic changes, and jaundice developed on at least three occasions. Thirty-five transfusions were given with frequent reactions noted. The hematocrit approximated 18 per cent with a reticulocytosis ranging from 13 to 46 per cent. The WBC and thrombocyte counts were normal. Bilirubin was 4.4/4.2 mg. per cent and total protein, A/G ratio and urinalysis were normal. Free hemoglobin was demonstrated in the serum on two occasions. Several direct antiglobulin tests were negative. Four years after the onset of hemolytic anemia the patient was seen for hematologic consultation. Physical examination was negative. The hematocrit was 14 per cent with a 4.6 per cent reticulocyte count, bilirubin of 0.6/2.5 mg. per cent and A/G ratio of 3.9/5.6 gm. per cent. Electrophoresis revealed a gamma spike typical of plasma cell myeloma. There was 2+ proteinuria and Bence-Jones protein was demonstrated. A bone survey was negative. Bone marrow aspiration revealed plasma cell myeloma and marked erythrocytic hyperplasia with megaloblastic changes. A Schilling test was normal. The direct antiglobulin test was positive. Subsequent direct antiglobulin tests were positive on six occasions and negative on six other occasions. The isoantibodies anti-K and anti-Le[a] were found in the serum. The patient was treated with cyclophosphamide without response. Prednisone, 60 mg. a day, was given and caused a progressive rise of the hematocrit to 40 per cent with a sustained reticulocytosis. The patient's course was complicated by repeated pneumonia and fluid retention. Repeated episodes of jaundice occurred with a decrease in prednisone therapy. Marked bone pain developed and osteoporosis was seen on x-ray. Death

TABLE 49. *Statistical data obtained from seven patients (four females, three males) with autoimmune hemolytic anemia (AHA) terminating in reticuloendothelial neoplasia (REN) (all patients had died at time of analysis)*

Test Procedures	Total	Statistical Data		
		Range	Mean	Median
Clinical data				
Age (years)	7	44–80	63	65
Duration of AHA before REN (months)	7	10–203	61	34
Survival from onset of AHA (months)	7	20–215	75	58
Survival from onset of REN (months)	7	0.3–41	15	9
Laboratory data				
Initial hematocrit (%)	7	8–25	19.6	19
Lowest hematocrit (%)	7	8–22	17	18
Initial reticulocytes (%)	7	0–46	9.1	4.5
Therapeutic reticulocytes (%)	7	0–36.2	12.1	8.5
Initial WBC (10^3/mm.^{3})	7	2.7–9.7	5.2	3.8
Initial thrombocytes (10^3/mm.^{3})	6	3.3–225	166	200

		Increased	Decreased	Normal
Bone marrow aspiration				
Total cellularity	7	3	2	2
Erythrocyte precursors	7	4	2	1
Leukocytes	7	0	1	6
Megakaryocytes	7	0	1	6
Megaloblasts	7	4	0	3
Plasma cells	7	2	0	5

		Weakness	Dizziness	Fever	Bleeding
Presenting symptoms					
Abnormal	7	7	6	3	4

		Spleen	Liver	Lymph nodes	Jaundice
Presenting Signs					
Abnormal	7	3	2	3	4

occurred 58 months after the onset of hemolytic anemia and 10 months after diagnosis of plasma cell myeloma.

Tables 49 to 51 summarize the statistical, laboratory and clinical data obtained in these seven patients. The clinical histories have been presented in some detail as it is impossible to group them into any specific clinical pattern. Only two common characteristics are present. All cases had autoimmune hemolytic anemia associated with neoplasia of the reticuloendothelium. In addition, all cases were characterized by the initial onset of autoimmune hemolytic ane-

mia followed by the subsequent development of the neoplastic process.

No particular predisposition on the basis of sex was noted with three males and four females involved. The median age of this patient group was 65 years. Autoimmune hemolytic anemia developed prior to neoplasia of the reticuloendothelium in a range extending from 10 to 203 months. A median of 34 and a mean of 61 months of preexisting autoimmune hemolytic anemia were found. The lengths of time, with the possible exception of one case of thymoma, make it unlikely that an undiagnosed underlying

TABLE 50. *Type of subsequent reticuloendothelial neoplasm and other clinical syndromes present in seven patients with autoimmune hemolytic anemia*

Case	Neoplasia	Other Clinical Syndromes
20	Thymoma	Weed killer sensitivity; erythrocytic aplasia
6	Thymoma	Pernicious anemia, thyroid adenoma, diabetes, systemic lupus erythematosus, positive serology, adenocarcinoma of the prostate, infections, pancreatitis
36	Thymoma, plasma cell myeloma	Thyroid adenoma, diabetes, cystitis, positive serology
40	Plasma cell myeloma	Repeated pneumonia
38	Reticulum cell sarcoma	Aplastic bone marrow
37	Acute monocytic leukemia	Raynaud's phenomenon
39	Acute monocytic leukemia	Adenocarcinoma of the cervix, poliomyelitis, biologically false positive serology, pyelonephritis, lymphohematogenous tuberculosis

TABLE 51. *Additional laboratory data obtained from seven patients with autoimmune hemolytic anemia terminating in reticuloendothelial neoplasia*

Case	Urine	Bilirubin, Direct/Indirect	Albumin/ Globulin	Serum Electrophoresis	LE Cells	Serology for Syphilis	Antibody Identification	Cr51 Half-life Survival Time
		mg. %	*gm. %*					*days*
20	Normal		3.4/3.2	Broad alpha-2 globulin		0	Panhemmag-glutinin	
6	Diabetes, cystitis	0.2/0.4	4.4/2.4 3.5/4.1	Broad gamma, 24.2% of protein	+	+		
36	Diabetes, cystitis	?/1.6	4.1/1.6		0	+	Panhemag-glutinin	
40	Bence-Jones protein	4.4/4.2	4.3/2.1 3.9/5.6	Gamma myeloma spike	0	0	Panhemag-glutinin	14
38	Normal				0	0	Panhemag-glutinin	12
37	Proteinuria	Icterus index, 35	4.4/2.0	Broad gamma, 20% of protein		0	Cold acting panhemag-glutinin	18 (postsplenectomy)
39	Proteinuria, cystitis	0.7/1.4	2.9/3.2	Normal	0	+		20

neoplasia existed concomitant with hemolytic anemia. In general, chronic ailments were present. The median duration of disease in the seven patients was 58 months with a mean of 75 months. The eventual development of reticuloendothelial neoplasia was generally disastrous. Five of the seven patients who died did so within a year of developing such neoplasia. A median of 9 and a mean of 15 months' duration was seen.

The associated neoplasia was malignant in five cases and benign in three cases. The three benign tumors were thymomas and these may have been of epithelial origin. One patient developed both a benign and a malignant abnormality of the reticuloendothelium. In addition to the three thymomas, acute monocytic leukemia was present in two cases, plasma cell myeloma in two cases and reticulum cell sarcoma in one patient. Nothing in the presenting symptoms, signs, hematologic data or serologic studies during the state of autoimmune hemolytic anemia was of significance in predicting the eventual development of neoplasia.

In two patients (Cases 37 and 40) the clinical course was characterized by a relatively simple association of hemolytic anemia and neoplasia. In two other patients (Cases 38 and 20) the hemolytic anemia was unusual in that one patient had an aplastic bone marrow and the other had pure erythrocytic aplasia following exposure to a toxic substance. This latter patient who developed a thymoma appeared similar to a patient reported by Ross and associates (73). In the remaining three cases complex clinical pictures were present. The simultaneous development of Addisonian pernicious anemia, positive antiglobulin tests and positive LE cells in a patient with a thyroid adenoma, diabetes and positive serologic tests for syphilis were noted in Case 6. This patient subsequently developed recurrent infections, adenocarcinoma of the prostate, interstitial pancreatitis and a thymoma. The association of hemolytic anemia, thymoma, plasmacytoma, thyroid adenoma, positive serologic tests for syphilis, diabetes and cystitis was seen in Case 36. An additional patient, Case 39, had a history of carcinoma of the cervix treated with x-ray and radium, longstanding chronic pyelonephritis secondary to an atopic bladder after poliomyelitis, and a biologically false positive serology. Her hemolytic anemia terminated in an acute fulminating disease with lymphohematogenous tuberculosis and a bone marrow typical of acute monocytic leukemia.

Etiologic Considerations

The temporal variations described above must be considered in any discussion of etiology. Many investigators have suggested various mechanisms which might relate neoplasia of the reticuloendothelium to autoimmune hemolytic anemia. Five major postulates have been offered:

(a) The relationship between autoimmune hemolytic anemia and reticuloendothelial neoplasia is purely fortuitous and no etiologic significance is present. This suggestion may be discarded. The combination of these two pathologic states occur with such regularity (25 per cent of cases of chronic lymphocytic leukemia) that some explanation appears to be necessary.

(b) Malignant cells may contain foreign antigens with a structural similarity to erythrocyte antigens. The antibody produced could then cross react with erythrocytes leading to autoimmune hemolytic anemia. Levine and associates (103), Stefanini and associates (104) and Kissmeyer-Nielsen and associates (105) have all suggested such a sequence. This explanation appears unlikely. No experimental proof has been offered and instances of a preceding autoimmune hemolytic anemia are not explained by this postulate.

(c) Neoplastic cells of the reticuloendothelium may retain their ability to produce antibodies but lose the ability to recognize self constituents. A situation analogous to experimental runt disease will result, and widespread immunologic abnormalities, including autoimmune hemolytic anemia, may occur. The concepts of Greene (82, 83), Kaplan and Smithers (84) and Dameshek and Schwartz (38, 88) are important in this respect. This postulate leaves unsolved three problems. (1) It does not explain the occurrence of autoimmune hemolytic anemia preceding the onset of reticuloendothelial neoplasia. (2) Why may neoplasia exist for years before autoimmune hemolytic anemia develops? (3) If neoplastic cells are immunologically foreign, why are they not rejected through the usual immune homeostatic mechanism? Although this hypothesis appears as a powerful theoretical tool, it does not appear adequate to explain all instances of autoimmune hemolytic anemia.

(d) Autoimmune hemolytic anemia leads to the production of reticuloendothelial neoplasia. Ben-Ishay and associates (99), in describing a case of pancytopenia and autoimmune hemolytic anemia which terminated after 18 years in acute leukemia, have suggested such a role. These investigators felt that the preceding immunologic disorder conditioned the tissues to develop the neoplastic state. Animal studies involving the NZB mice (89–92), neonatal thymectomized mice (93) and transplanted F_1

hybrids (97, 98) all support such a relationship. Metcalf (106) has demonstrated that repeated antigenic stimulation may result in reticuloendothelial neoplasia. A possible mechanism would involve the longstanding, rapid proliferation of immunocompetent cells, which must be present in chronic autoimmune hemolytic anemia. The development of thymic germinal centers and of lymph node, spleen and liver reticuloendothelial hyperplasia would appear as the morphologic counterpart of this activity. The rapid turnover and growth of such cells may increase the risk of and vulnerability to somatic mutation and eventual neoplasia. As a general explanation for the association of autoimmune hemolytic anemia and reticuloendothelial neoplasia, however, this seems inadequate. The great majority of such associations are characterized by a preexisting malignancy, rather than by a prior autoimmune hemolytic state.

(e) Autoimmune hemolytic anemia results from "a functional instability of globulin production by the lymphocyte." Bowdler and Glick (100) have suggested that an early stage of lymphoma is present and that the involved cells are responsible for autoantibody production. The lymphoma is conceived of as existing in an early phase prior to the development of histologically recognizable lesions. This postulate represents a modification of the runt disease suggestion, with the same basic problems. In addition, the long periods of autoimmune hemolytic anemia which may exist before neoplasia becomes apparent make this suggestion unlikely.

None of the five postulated mechanisms appears to be satisfactory as a general explanation for *all* instances of an associated autoimmune hemolytic anemia and reticuloendothelial neoplasia. The therapeutic response and disease activity of the two states are frequently dissociated in the same patient. The temporal variations in onset are also great. It commonly appears as if the two disease processes exist independently in one individual. In view of this, another mechanism may be postulated.

It is unlikely that either autoimmune hemolytic anemia or reticuloendothelial neoplasia are directly involved in the crea-

tion of the other state, except in isolated instances. Rather, it may be hypothesized that both conditions result from the same fundamental abnormality (81). A more general applicable theory may be constructed by blending the concepts of graft-host disease and a genetic abnormality.

It is proposed that some individuals have a basic defect in their immune apparatus which limits their ability to initate normal immune responses. There is some evidence in the autoimmune hemolytic anemias that this aberration may be genetically mediated (107–109). These individuals are poor antibody producers. The deficiency would prevent the establishment of an efficient immune homeostatic mechanism. Abnormal cells produced in vivo, which normally are recognized as foreign and destroyed, may be permitted to survive because of the malfunction of the immune apparatus. Either permanent somatic mutations or virus modifications could be involved in the creation of such foreign host cells. The reticuloendothelial system would be particularly vulnerable to the creation of such cells because their growth and turnover rate is of the highest magnitude. The survival and replication of such modified immunocompetent cells could result in autoimmune hemolytic anemia through a graft-host disease mechanism. A permanent somatic mutation will result in malignancy. Virus modifications can lead to either malignancy or autoimmune hemolytic anemia without malignancy. One cell clone may create both of these abnormalities, e.g., a malignant immunocompetent cell clone producing multiple autoantibodies. This is probably unusual, if it occurs at all. It is more likely that multiple modified cells are produced and persist throughout the natural history of the disease. This concept is supported by the observation that warm acting erythrocyte autoantibodies are generally of both kappa and lambda type L chains in the same individual (60, 61). In addition, serum electrophoretic patterns in autoimmune hemolytic anemia frequently show a polyclonal gamma abnormality.

This postulate suggests that autoimmune hemolytic anemia and reticuloendothelial neoplasia both result from the same abnormality, but that neither state induces the other. Miller (102) has similarly considered this view. The concept of a vulnerable immunodeficient individual has certain advantages. Many confusing clinical and laboratory observations are clarified by this hypothesis. These include: (a) Reticuloendothelial neoplasia and autoimmune hemolytic anemia may occur simultaneously or in random order. In addition, either disease state can occur independently. The number, types and sequences of involvement of immunocompetent cells would determine the clinical pattern. (b) Autoimmune hemolytic anemia and reticuloendothelial neoplasia may exist in the same patient and may clinically appear dissociated. (c) Both autoimmune hemolytic anemia and neoplasia of the reticuloendothelium have a high rate of association with other malignancies (see Chapter 10). The growth rate of the involved tissues is frequently less than that of the reticuloendothelium. Therefore, malignancy of such areas will be less common than that seen with the reticuloendothelium. (d) The familial predisposition demonstrated in the NZB mice and now frequently described in the human being (107–109) can be explained by this concept. The sibling data previously described (Cases 3 to 5) suggest that the predisposition does not result in an isolated defect of erythrocyte homeostasis. Rather a more fundamental abnormality allowing both autoimmune hemolytic anemia and the other associated diseases to develop must be postulated. The high incidence of other autoimmune diseases in family members of patients with idiopathic autoimmune hemolytic anemia strongly supports this argument (109). This hypothesis is compatible both with a genetic defect or vertical transmission of a virus in an immunodeficient population. (e) Evidence that autoimmune hemolytic anemia is one part of a diffuse, immunologic, systemic disease is compatible with this postulate. An immunodeficient state would explain complex clinical patterns with association of lesions such as thymoma, various malignancies, pernicious anemia, biologically false positive serologic tests, positive LE cell preparations, thyroid adeno-

mas, ulcerative colitis, etc. (f) The perplexing relationship between agammaglobulinemia, hypogammaglobulinemia (seen in approximately one-third of patients with chronic lymphocytic leukemia (110)), the lymphomas, leukemias and thymomas (77) becomes understandable with this postulate. The tendency of patients with agammaglobulinemia to develop lymphomas (111, 112), leukemias (112) and rheumatoid arthritis (113, 114) would also strongly support this concept. (g) Patients with reticuloendothelial neoplasia have restricted humoral antibody and delayed hypersensitivity responses. A pathophysiologic contradiction is apparent in such patients. Their clinical picture may be dominated by a blend of abnormal increased and decreased immunologic activity. This observation is understandable if an individual is immunodeficient and develops autoimmunization.

Experimental support for this hypothesis is fragmentary but highly suggestive. Thymectomized animals have been shown to be immunologically incompetent. In addition, they may develop a wasting disease with autoimmune hemolytic anemia and amyloidosis (115). Miller (116) has shown that genetically modified host cells, which would be eliminated in a normal animal, may survive in animals with a defective immune apparatus. The possible etiologic role of viruses in autoimmune hemolytic anemia and reticuloendothelial neoplasia has assumed great importance. Such infections are common in the presence of inadequate immune homeostasis. Miller and associates (117) have suggested that vertical transmission of viruses simulating a genetic predisposition may be involved in the creation of such syndromes. This concept is supported by studies involving NZB mice. Mellors and Huang (118) demonstrated virus particles in NZB neoplastic cells. Employing cell free extracts, they successfully transmitted the immunologic and neoplastic abnormality of the NZB mice to Swiss mice (119).

The most elegant and exhaustive review of "immunologic deficiency diseases" has been presented by Good and associates (120). The above postulate incorporates many of their concepts. The clinical reports of Thompson and Johnson (121), Colomb

and associates (122), Hoffbrand (123),
Mathews (124), and Anderson and Vye
(125) illustrate human syndromes best explained by this hypothesis. Further studies
on the relationship of autoimmune hemolytic anemia and reticuloendothelial neoplasia are indicated. Clarification of this
association would offer an experimental tool
of great potential in the study of neoplasia
and autoimmunity.

BIBLIOGRAPHY

1. Pappenheim, A.: Bemerkungen über Leukanämie in Anschull an vorstehende Mit-
   telung von Hans Hirschfeld. Folia Haemat.
   (Leipzig) **3**: 339, 1906.
2. Hirschfeld, H.: Ueber Leukänamie. Folia Haemat. (Leipzig) **3**: 332, 1906.
3. Brill, N. E.: Chronic hemolytic icterus complicated by a myeloid leukemia. Med. Clin.
   N. Amer. **8**: 153, 1924.
4. Paschkis, K.: Über atypische hämolytische
   Anämien. Z. Klin. Med. **105**: 301, 1927.
5. Holler, G., and Paschkis, K.: Zur Klinik
   der splenomegalen Lymphogranulomatose.
   Wien. Arch. Inn. Med. **14**: 149, 1927.
6. Davidson, L. S. P.: Macrocytic haemolytic
   anaemia. Quart. J. Med. **1**: 543, 1932.
7. Watson, C. J.: Hemolytic jaundice and macrocytic hemolytic anemia. Ann. Intern. Med.
   12: 1782, 1939.
8. Davis, L. J.: Symptomatic haemolytic anaemia. Edinburgh Med. J. **51**: 70, 1944.
9. Marchal, G., Mahoudeau, D., Leloc', K., and
   Brun, C.: L'activité érythrophagique dans
   les formes anémiques de la lymphogranulomatose maligne. Bull. Soc. Med. Hop. Paris
   57: 15, 1941.
10. Singer, K.: Über das hämolytisch-anämische
    Syndrom als klinische Erscheinungsform
    des Lymphogranuloms. Med. Klin. **32**: 179,
    1936.
11. Marchal, G.: L'anemié de la maladie de
    Hodgkin. Rev. Hemat. (Paris) **2**: 479, 1947.
12. Paraf, A., and Dausset, J.: Les ictères hémo-
    lytiques au cours des affections malignes
    (leucémies, granulomatose maligne, can-
    cers). Sem. Hop. Paris **28**: 290, 1952.
13. Singer, K., and Dameshek, W.: Symptomatic
    hemolytic anemia. Ann. Intern. Med. **15**:
    544, 1941.
14. Jensen, K. B.: Anaemia in Hodgkin's disease
    and chronic lymphatic leukaemia. Danish
    Med. Bull. **4**: 150, 1957.
15. Waggener, R. E., Pratt, P. T., and Hunt,
    H. B.: Erythrocyte survival in leukemia,
    Hodgkin's disease and malignant lymphoma
    as determined by radiochromate. Amer. J.
    Roentgen. **79**: 1045, 1958.
16. Giannopoulos, P. P., and Bergsagel, D. E.:
    The mechanism of the anemia associated
    with Hodgkin's disease. Blood **14**: 856, 1959.

17. Veeger, W., Woldring, M. G., van Rood, J. J.,
    Eernisse, J. G., Leeksma, C. H. W., Verloop,
    M. C., and Nieweg, H. O.: The value of
    the determination of the site of red cell
    sequestration in hemolytic anemia as a pre-
    diction test for splenectomy. Acta Med.
    Scand. **171**: 507, 1962.
18. Cline, M. J., and Berlin, N. I.: Anemia in
    Hodgkin's disease. Cancer **16**: 526, 1963.
19. Gall, E. A., and Mallory, T. B.: Malignant
    lymphoma; clinico-pathologic survey of 618
    cases. Amer. J. Path. **18**: 381, 1942.
20. Goia, I.: Le sang dans la lymphogranuloma-
    tose maligne. Sang **7**: 354, 1933.
21. Wasserman, L. R., Stats, D., Schwartz, L., and
    Fudenberg, H.: Symptomatic and hemo-
    pathic hemolytic anemia. Amer. J. Med.
    18: 961, 1955.
22. Matthias, J.: Haemolytic anaemia in leu-
    kaemia and lymphoma: incidence, prognos-
    tic significance and effect of treatment. Pre-
    sented at the Tenth International Congress
    of the International Society of Hematology,
    Stockholm, 1964.
23. Gruelund, S.: A case of lymphogranulomatosis
    (Hodgkin) with hemolytic anemia. Acta
    Med. Scand. **129**: 361, 1947.
24. Brown, R. J. K., and Meynell, M. J.: Haemo-
    lytic anaemias associated with Hodgkin's dis-
    ease. Lancet **2**: 835, 1949.
25. Trinick, R. H.: Lymphocytes and intravascu-
    lar haemolysis. Lancet **1**: 225, 1949.
26. Von Sulzer, H. J.: Hämolytische Anämie
    durch Autoantikörper bei Lymphogranulo-
    matosis Hodgkin. Schweiz. Med. Wschr.
    82: 1103, 1952.
27. Rundles, R. W., and Barton, W. B.: Triethyl-
    ene melamine in the treatment of neoplastic
    disease. Blood **7**: 483, 1952.
28. Hennemann, G.: Beobachtung über das
    gleichzeitige Auftreten von Lymphogranulo-
    matose und hämolytischer Anämie. Medi-
    zinische **27**: 914, 1953.
29. Grobbelaar, B. G.: Haemolytic anaemia and
    erythrocyte sensitization in the malignant
    reticuloses. S. Afr. Med. J. **32**: 271, 1958.
30. Kyle, R. A., Kiely, J. M., and Stickney, J. M.:
    Acquired hemolytic anemia in chronic
    lymphocytic leukemia and the lymphomas.
    Survival and response to therapy in twenty-
    seven cases. Arch. Intern. Med. (Chicago)
    104: 61, 1959.
31. Dausset, J., and Colombani, J.: The serology
    and the prognosis of 128 cases of autoim-
    mune hemolytic anemia. Blood **14**: 1280,
    1959.
32. Crosby, W. H., and Rappaport, H.: Autoim-
    mune hemolytic anemia. I. Analysis of
    hematologic observations with particular
    reference to their prognostic value. A survey
    of 57 cases. Blood **12**: 42, 1957.
33. Bousser, J., Leconte des Floris, R., Christol, D.,
    and Rousère, J.: Les anémies hémolytiques
    à autoanticorps symptomatiques de lym-

phomes malins (étude de 16 cas personnels). Sem. Hop. Paris **37**: 2537, 1961.

34. Videbaek, A.: Autoimmune haemolytic anaemia in some malignant systemic diseases. Acta Med. Scand. **171**: 463, 1962.
35. Eisner, E., Ley, A. B., and Mayer, K.: Coombs'-positive hemolytic anemia in Hodgkin's disease. Ann. Intern. Med. **66**: 258, 1967.
36. Scott, J. L.: The effect of nitrogen mustard and maintenance chlorambucil in the treatment of advanced Hodgkin's disease. Cancer Chemother. Rep. **27**: 27, 1963.
37. Ranløv, P., and Videbaek, A.: Cyclic haemolytic anaemia synchronous with Pel-Ebstein fever in a case of Hodgkin's disease. Acta Med. Scand. **174**: 583, 1963.
38. Dameshek, W., and Schwartz, R. S.: Leukemia and autoimmunization. Some possible relationships. Blood **14**: 1151, 1959.
39. Introzzi, A. S., Quirno, N., and Pavlovsky, A.: Anemia hemolitica adquirida. Linfosarcomatosis. Resultado de la esplenectomia. Bol. Trab. Acad. Argent. Cir. **27**: 638, 1943.
40. Stats, D., Rosenthal, N., and Wasserman, L. R.: Hemolytic anemia associated with malignant diseases. Amer. J. Clin. Path. **17**: 585, 1947.
41. Aubert, A., and Brendemoen, O. J.: Acquired hemolytic anaemia and lymphoblastoma. Scand. J. Clin. Lab. Invest. **1**: 95, 1949.
42. Dustin, P., and Drochmans, P.: Ictère hémolytique acquis et prolifération néoplasique: deux cas. Acta Clin. Belg. **7**: 483, 1952.
43. Fisher, J. H., Welch, C. S., and Dameshek, W.: Splenectomy in leukemia and leukosarcoma. New Eng. J. Med. **246**: 477, 1952.
44. Rosenthal, M. C., Pisciotta, A. V., Komninos, Z. D., Goldenberg, H., and Dameshek, W.: The autoimmune hemolytic anemia of malignant lymphocytic disease. Blood **10**: 197, 1955.
45. Rosenberg, S. A., Diamond, H. D., Jaslowitz, B., and Carver, L. F.: Lymphosarcoma: a review of 1269 cases. Medicine (Balt.) **40**: 31, 1961.
46. Bigley, R. H., Koler, R. D., Pirofsky, B., and Osgood, E. E.: A comparison of chronic leukemic lymphocytic leukemia, chronic subleukemic lymphocytic leukemia and lymphocytic sarcoma. Cancer Chemother. Rep. **16**: 231, 1962.
47. Scott, R. B., and Robb-Smith, A. H. T.: Histiocytic medullary reticulosis. Lancet **2**: 194, 1939.
48. Krah, E.: Inkomplette Kälte-autoantikörper. Klin. Wschr. **29**: 674, 1951.
49. Sievers, K., and Harwerth, H. G.: Zur Therapie symptomatischer hämolytischer Anämien. Acta Haemat. (Basel) **9**: 208, 1953.
50. Giraud, G., Cazal, P., Latour, H., Lévy, A., and Puech, P.: Hémoglobinuries paroxystiques par autoanticorps froids au cours

d'une lymphosarcomatose. Montpellier Med. **48**: 462, 1955.
51. Widmann, H.: Akute subleukämische Plasmozytose auf der Basis eines Reticulosarkoms mit erworbener hämolytischer Anämie. Deutsch. Med. Wschr. **82**: 1298, 1957.
52. Boulet, P., Mirouze, J., Barjon, P., Jaffiol, C., and Robinet, J.: Etude d'une dysprotéinémie avec épisodes successifs splénique, ganglionnaire et hémolytique. Bull. Soc. Med. Hop. Paris **76**: 826, 1960.
53. Dacie, J. V.: *The Haemolytic Anaemias, Part III*, Ed. 2. Grune & Stratton, Inc., New York, 1967.
54. Evans, T. S., and Doan, C. A.: Hemolytic crises of acquired hypersplenism in the course of giant follicle lymphoma. In *Proceedings of the Third International Congress of the International Society of Hematology*. William Heineman, Ltd., London, 1951.
55. Kistner, S., and Norberg, S.: The simultaneous occurrence of two different myeloma proteins. Scand. J. Clin. Lab. Invest. **17**: 321, 1964.
56. Bachmann, R.: Simultaneous occurrence of two immunologically different M-components in serum. Acta Med. Scand. **177**: 593, 1965.
57. Costea, N., Yakulis, V. J., Libnoch, J. A., Pilz, C. G., and Heller, P.: Two myeloma globulins (IgG and IgA) in one subject and one cell line. Amer. J. Med. **42**: 630, 1967.
58. Harboe, M., Van Furth, R., Schubothe, H., Lind, G., and Evans, R. S.: Exclusive occurrence of kappa chains in isolated cold haemagglutinins. Scand. J. Haemat. **2**: 259, 1965.
59. Schubothe, H.: The cold hemagglutinin disease. Seminars Hemat. **3**: 27, 1966.
60. Leddy, J. P., and Bakemier, R. F.: Structural aspects of human erythrocyte auto-antibodies. I. L chain types and electrophoretic dispersion. J. Exp. Med. **121**: 1, 1965.
61. Eyster, M. E., Nachman, R. L., Christenson, W. N., and Engle, R. L.: Structural characteristics of red cell autoantibodies. J. Immun. **96**: 107, 1966.
62. Cline, M. J., and Berlin, N. I.: Studies of the anemia of multiple myeloma. Amer. J. Med. **33**: 510, 1962.
63. Forster, G., and Moeschlin, S.: Extramedulläres, leukämisches Plasmazytom mit Dysproteinämie und erworbener hämolytischer Anämie. Schweiz. Med. Wschr. **84**: 1106, 1954.
64. Cassell, M., and Chaplin, H.: Studies on anti-eluate sera. II. Comparison of a conventional antiglobulin serum with three anti-eluate sera in the study of 70 patients with acquired hemolytic anemia. Vox Sang. **5**: 43, 1960.
65. Massei, G., and Pallone, E.: Due osservasioni di anemia emolitica acquisata immunologica

in corso di plasmacitomatosi. Minerva Med. **48**: 2730, 1957.

66. Pirofsky, B.: Serologic and clinical findings in autoimmune hemolytic anemia. Series Haemat. **9**: 47, 1965.

67. Hennemann, H. H., Falck, I., and Gillert, K. E.: Hämolytisches Syndrom mit positivem Coombs-test bei einer Lymphadenose und einem Plasmozytom. Z. Ges. Inn. Med. **8**: 321, 1953.

68. Bohrod, M. G., and Bottcher, E. J.: Multiple myeloma, hemolytic anemia, and protein phagocytosis. Arch. Path. (Chicago) **76**: 700, 1963.

69. Wright, C. S., Dodd, M. C., Bouroncle, B. A., Doan, C. A., and Zollinger, R. M.: Studies of hemagglutinins in hereditary spherocytosis and in acquired hemolytic anemia. J. Lab. Clin. Med. **37**: 165, 1951.

70. Frenger, W., Ringelmann, R., and Scheifferth, F.: Hämolytisches Syndrome bei blastomatösen Erkrankungen des lymphoretikulären Systems. Med. Welt. **31**: 1552, 1961.

71. Yamada, A.: Investigations on clinical observations of autoimmune hemolytic anemia and characteristics of the warm autoantibody obtained from patients red cells. Acta Haemat. Jap. **27**: 19, 1964.

72. Osgood, E. E.: The survival time of patients with plasmocytic myeloma. Cancer Chemother. Rep. **9**: 1, 1960.

73. Ross, J. F., Finch, S. C., Street, R. W., and Strieder, J. W.: The simultaneous occurrence of benign thymoma and refractory anemia. Blood **9**: 935, 1954.

74. Janbon, M. M., Bertrand, L., and Bonnet, H.: Sarcome du thymus avec anémie hémolytique par autoanticorps. Montpellier Med. **49**: 161, 1956.

75. Halperin, I. C., Minogue, W. F., and Komninos, Z. D.: Autoimmune hemolytic anemia and myasthenia gravis associated with thymoma. New Eng. J. Med. **275**: 663, 1966.

76. Jacox, R. F., Mongan, E. S., Hanshaw, J. B., and Leddy, J. P.: Hypogammaglobulinemia with thymoma and probable pulmonary infection with cytomegalovirus. New Eng. J. Med. **271**: 1091, 1964.

77. Mongan, E. S., Kern, W. A., and Terry, R.: Hypogammaglobulinemia with thymoma, hemolytic anemia, and disseminated infection with cytomegalovirus. Ann. Intern. Med. **65**: 548, 1966.

78. Wilmers, M. J., and Russell, P. A.: Autoimmune hemolytic anemia in an infant treated by thymectomy. Lancet **2**: 915, 1963.

79. Richmond, J., Woodruff, M. F. A., Cumming, R. A., and Donald, K. W.: A case of idiopathic thrombocytopenia and autoimmune hemolytic anemia. Lancet **2**: 125, 1963.

80. Aisenberg, A. C.: Studies on delayed hyper-

sensitivity in Hodgkin's disease. J. Clin. Invest. **41**: 1964, 1962.

81. Pirofsky, B.: Autoimmune hemolytic anemia and neoplasia of the reticuloendothelium. With a hypothesis concerning etiologic relationships. Ann. Intern. Med. **68**: 109, 1968.

82. Greene, H. N.: An immunological concept of cancer: a preliminary report. Brit. Med. J. **2**: 1374, 1954.

83. Greene, H. N., Wakefield, J., and Littlewood, G.: The nature of cancer anaemia and its bearing on the immunological theory of cancer. Brit. Med. J. **2**: 779, 1957.

84. Kaplan, H. S., and Smithers, D. W.: Autoimmunity in man and homologous disease in mice in relation to the malignant lymphomas. Lancet **2**: 638, 1959.

85. Ahrengot, V.: De serologiske forhold hos en patient med immunologtisk haemolyisk anaemi og en antistofholdig abdominalcyste. Nord. Med. **50**: 1570, 1953.

86. Oliner, H., Schwartz, R. S., and Dameshek, W.: Studies in experimental autoimmune disorders. I. Clinical and laboratory features of autoimmunization (runt disease) in the mouse. Blood **17**: 20, 1961.

87. Stastny, P., Stembridge, V. A., Vischer, T. L., and Ziff, M.: Homologous disease, a model for autoimmune disease. Ann. N. Y. Acad. Sci. **124**: 158, 1965.

88. Dameshek, W.: Theories of autoimmunity. In *Conceptual Advances in Immunology and Oncology*. Hoeber Medical Division, Harper & Row, Publishers, New York, 1963.

89. Bielschowsky, M., and Bielschowsky, F.: Reaction of the reticular tissue of mice with autoimmune haemolytic anaemia to 2-amino-fluorene. Nature (London) **194**: 692, 1962.

90. Holmes, M. C., and Burnet, F. M.: The natural history of autoimmune disease in NZB mice. A comparison with the pattern of human autoimmune manifestations. Ann. Intern. Med. **59**: 265, 1963.

91. East, J., deSousa, M. A. B., and Parott, D. M. V.: Immunopathology of New Zealand black (NZB) mice. Transplantation **3**: 711, 1965.

92. Mellors, R. C.: Autoimmune disease in NZB-B1 mice. II. Autoimmunity and malignant lymphoma. Blood **27**: 435, 1966.

93. Good, R. A., Peterson, R. D. H., Martinez, C., Sutherland, D. E. R., Kellum, M. J., and Finstad, J.: The thymus in immunobiology: with special reference to autoimmune disease. Ann. N. Y. Acad. Sci. **124**: 73, 1965.

94. Kuni, A., and Furth, J.: Inhibition of lymphoma induction in virus-infected rats by thymectomy. An affinity of the lymphoma virus for myeloid cells. Cancer Res. **24**: 493, 1964.

95. Metcalf, D., Wiadrowski, M., and Bradley,

R.: Analysis of the role of the thymus in leukemia development using thymectomy and thymus grafts. In *Murine Leukemia,* edited by M. A. Rich and J. B. Maloney. National Cancer Institute, U. S. Government Printing Office, Washington, D. C., 1966.

96. Walford, R. L., and Hildemann, W. H.: Life span and lymphoma-incidence of mice injected at birth with spleen cells across a weak histocompatibility locus. Amer. J. Path. 47: 713, 1965.

97. Schwartz, R. S., and Beldotti, L.: Malignant lymphomas following allogenic disease: transition from an immunological to a neoplastic disorder. Science 149: 1511, 1965.

98. Armstrong, M. Y., Andre-Schwartz, J., and Schwartz, R. S.: Immunological homeostasis and leukemia: an experimental model in the mouse. In *Perspectives in Leukemia.* Grune & Stratton, Inc., New York, 1968.

99. Ben-Ishay, D., Freund, M., and Groen, J. J.: A case of autoimmune hemolytic anemia with circulating cold agglutinins presenting for many years as "hypersplenism" and terminating in leukemia. Blood 22: 100, 1963.

100. Bowdler, A. J., and Glick, I. W.: Autoimmune hemolytic anemia as the herald state of Hodgkin's disease. Ann. Intern. Med. 65: 761, 1966.

101. Becker, F. P.: Autoimmune hemolytic anemia with terminal lymphoma and cytomegalic inclusion disease. New York J. Med. 64: 1211, 1964.

102. Miller, D. G.: The association of immune disease and malignant lymphoma. Ann. Intern. Med. 66: 507, 1967.

103. Levine, P., Bobbit, O. B., Waller, R. K., and Kuchmichel, A.: Isoimmunization by a new blood factor in tumor cells. Proc. Soc. Exp. Biol. Med. 77: 403, 1951.

104. Stefanini, M., Magalini, S. I., and Patterson, J. H.: The relation of neoplastic tissue antigens to "autoimmune" hematologic syndromes (abstract). Clin. Res. Proc. 4: 82, 1956.

105. Kissmeyer-Nielsen, F., Bichel, J., and Bjerre Hanson, P.: Specific autoantibodies in immunohaemolytic anaemia. Acta Haemat. (Basel) 15: 189, 1956.

106. Metcalf, D.: Induction of reticular tumours in mice by repeated antigenic stimulation. Acta Un. Int. Cancr. 19: 657, 1963.

107. Fialkow, P. J., Fudenberg, H., and Epstein, W. V.: "Acquired" antibody hemolytic anemia and familial aberrations in gamma globulins. Amer. J. Med. 36: 188, 1964.

108. Cordova, M. S., Baéz-Villaseñor, J., Mendez, J. J., and Compos, E.: Acquired hemolytic anemia with positive antiglobulin (Coombs' test) in mother and daughter. Arch. Intern. Med. (Chicago) 117: 692, 1966.

109. Pirofsky, B.: Hereditary aspects of autoimmune hemolytic anemia; a retrospective analysis. Vox. Sang. 14: 334, 1968.

110. Pisciotta, A. V., Jermain, L. F., and Hinz, J. E.: Chronic lymphocytic leukemia, hypogammaglobulinemia and autoimmune hemolytic anemia—an experiment of nature. Blood 15: 748, 1960.

111. Fudenberg, H., and Solomon, A.: "Acquired agammaglobulinemia" with autoimmune hemolytic disease: graft-versus-host reaction? Vox Sang. 6: 68, 1961.

112. Page, A. R., Hansen, A. E., and Good, R. A.: Occurrence of leukemia and lymphoma in patients with agammaglobulinemia. Blood 21: 197, 1963.

113. Fudenberg, H., German, J. L., and Kunkel, H. G.: The occurrence of rheumatoid factor and other abnormalities in families of patients with agammaglobulinemia. Arthritis Rheum. 5: 565, 1962.

114. Good, R. A., and Rotstein, J.: Rheumatoid arthritis and agammaglobulinemia. Bull. Rheum. Dis. 10: 203, 1960.

115. Kellum, M. J., Sutherland, D. E., Eckert, E., Peterson, R. D. A., and Good, R. A.: Wasting disease, Coombs-positivity, and amyloidosis in rabbits subjected to central lymphoid tissue extirpation and irradiation. Int. Arch. Allerg. 27: 6, 1965.

116. Miller, J. F. A. P.: Influence of thymectomy on tumor induction by polyoma virus in C57 B1 mice. Proc. Soc. Exp. Biol. Med. 116: 323, 1964.

117. Miller, J. F. A. P., Osoba. D., and Dukor, P.: A humoral thymus mechanism responsible for immunologic maturation. Ann. N. Y. Acad. Sci. 124: 95, 1965.

118. Mellors, R. C., and Huang, C. Y.: Immunopathology of NZB/B1 mice. V. Virus-like (filterable) agent separable from lymphoma cells and identifiable by electron microscopy. J. Exp. Med. 124: 1031, 1966.

119. Mellors, R. C., and Huang, C. Y.: Immunopathology of NZB/B1 mice. VI. Virus separable from spleen and pathogenic for Swiss mice. J. Exp. Med. 126: 53, 1967.

120. Good, R. A., Kelly, W. D., Rotstein, J., and Varco, R. L.: Immunological deficiency diseases, agammaglobulinemia, hypogammaglobulinemia, Hodgkin's disease and sarcoidosis. Progr. Allerg. 6: 187, 1962.

121. Thompson, E. N., and Johnson, R. S.: A case of primary idiopathic hypogammaglobulinemia associated with haemolytic anaemia. Postgrad. Med. 38: 292, 1962.

122. Colomb, D., Croizat, P., Morel, P., Creyssel, R., Jouvenceaux, A., and Desmonceaux, H.: Reticulolymphoblasts sarcomatosis with acquired hemolytic anemia caused by cold antibodies and cryoglobulinemia having complicated a paraffinoma after 50 years development. Lyon Med. 94: 635, 1962.

123. Hoffbrand, B. I.: Haemolytic anaemia in Hodgkin's disease associated with immunoglobulin deficiencies. Brit. J. Cancer 18: 98, 1964.

124. Mathews, R. J.: Idiopathic autoimmune hemolytic anemia and idiopathic thrombocytopenic purpura associated with diffuse hypergammaglobulinemia, amyloidosis, hypoalbuminemia and plasmacytosis. Amer. J. Med. 39: 972, 1965.

125. Anderson, E. T., and Vye, M. V.: Dysproteinemia of the myeloma type associated with a thymoma. Ann. Intern. Med. 66: 141, 1967.

Chapter 7

Infectious Disease and Autoimmune Hemolytic Anemia

Historical Review

The ability of infectious agents to cause erythrocyte damage and lysis assumed importance early in the study of hemolytic anemia. In 1898 Hayem (1) became aware of this relationship and termed acquired hemolytic anemia "ictère infectieux chronique splénomégalique." In 1902 Macintosh and Cleland (2) described a patient suffering from fever, splenomegaly, profound anemia and infectious disease. Widal and associates (3) in 1907 stressed the hemolytic role of malaria, streptococci, staphylococci, tuberculosis, the clostridia organisms and ancylostomiasis. In 1910 Gaucher and Giroux (4) and de Beurmann and associates (5) related the development of hemolytic anemia to syphilis. Tileston (6) expanded these observations and specifically implicated the secondary stage of syphilis.

Lederer (7, 8) and Brill (9) described a form of hemolytic anemia characterized by an explosive onset, severe clinical course and rapid recovery apparently related to transfusion therapy. Fever was prominent and an infectious etiology was considered. The sudden onset of hemolytic anemia in the presence of infection was striking, and Lederer termed this syndrome "acute hemolytic (infectious) anemia." Brill described the process as "acute febrile anemia." For many years Lederer-Brill anemia was a well recognized entity. The relation to infectious disease was confirmed by many observers (10). An acute onset and rapid recovery appeared as characteristic features of the disease.

It gradually became apparent that acquired hemolytic anemia might appear in association with another pathologic state. Watson (11) termed this secondary hemolytic anemia, and Singer and Dameshek (12) called it symptomatic hemolytic anemia. Infectious disease was emphasized as a pertinent pathologic state. Singer and Dameshek (12) reported the development of acute hemolytic anemia in a patient suffering from a type 17 pneumococcal infection. Spontaneous disappearance of hemolytic anemia resulted upon resolution of the pneumonia.

Dameshek and Schwartz (13, 14) suggested an immunologic pathogenesis in some cases of acquired hemolytic anemia. Infectious agents were considered to initiate hemolytic anemia through a different mechanism. Kracke (15) in discussing the pathogenesis of hemolytic anemia stated, "there is evidence that certain infectious diseases such as malaria, syphilis, tuberculosis, Hodgkin's and various liver diseases may be causative." Davis (16) in 1943 established separate categories of bacterial infections and hemolysins as etiologic agents in the production of acquired hemolytic anemia. The problem of accurately separating immunologic from infectious etiologies is apparent and still with us.

The distinction between the etiologic role of infectious agents and autoimmune mechanisms has been accepted and fortified through the years. Various parasites such as *Plasmodium falciparum* (17, 18), Toxoplasma (19–21) and Leishmania

(22–24) have been shown to induce hemolytic anemia. Bacteria such as *Bartonella bacilliformis* (25), *Bartonella muris* (26) and *Clostridium welchii* (27–30) also may lead to severe hemolytic states. Salmonella (31–34), cholera (35), streptococcal (36–39), enterococcal (39), staphylococcal (39, 40) and pneumococcal (12, 39, 41) infections have all been reported in hemolytic syndromes. Hemolytic anemia has been associated with the virus infections of pneumonia (42, 43), influenza (44–46), hepatitis (47), herpes infections (48, 49), cytomegalic disease (50), Coxsackie infections (51, 52), Newcastle disease (48), measles (53) and varicella (54).

A survey of the literature relating infectious agents to hemolytic anemia clearly indicates that different mechanisms are involved. At least two broad pathogenic categories are present. Hemolytic anemia may occur through direct action of the infecting agent or its products on the erythrocyte, with subsequent damage and lysis of cells. In addition, infectious agents may initiate a sequence of events leading to the host production of humoral antibodies which damage host erythrocytes. This chapter is limited to reviewing the latter mechanism. The theoretical pathways through which such a state may arise are discussed in Chapter 14. Although the clinical syndromes described below are called "autoimmune," many if not all actually result from immunologic but not autoimmune mechanisms. As such, they may be more accurately described as antiglobulin positive hemolytic anemia.

Incidence of Autoimmune Hemolytic Anemia Etiologically Related to Infectious Disease

There is a tendency to ignore the relationship between infectious disease and hemolytic anemia characterized by positive antiglobulin tests. Several reasons exist for this attitude. Infectious processes are common and an association with autoimmune hemolytic anemia is relatively uncommon. Accordingly, many investigators consider a relationship unproven. Autoimmune hemolytic anemia in such circumstances is considered to be idiopathic. The

association of an infectious process with hemolytic anemia frequently occurs in the infant or child. The separation of adult and pediatric hematologic problems prevents many investigators from studying such patients. Hemolytic anemia induced by infection is frequently explosive, with rapid and complete recovery. Hematologic consultation may not be obtained and serologic studies may not be done. The immunologic character of the hemolytic state may therefore not be documented. It is also well known that infectious agents and their products may directly affect the erythrocyte, leading to hemolysis. This pathogenesis is frequently assumed, with the result of limiting clinical studies and foregoing serologic investigations.

We are in a curious situation with certain infectious processes and hemolytic anemia. Certain infections such as virus pneumonia and infectious mononucleosis immediately suggest an immunologic process when hemolytic anemia occurs. Other infectious states complicated by hemolysis are totally ignored as to possible immunologic mechanisms.

Dacie (53) encountered 23 patients with an infectious history in his series of 175 cases of autoimmune hemolytic anemia. Twelve were examples of the warm acting type. An etiologic relationship of the hemolytic state to the infection was not assumed in these cases, although significance was ascribed to the cases having an associated virus pneumonia. Dausset and Colombani (45) similarly appear reluctant to ascribe etiologic significance to infectious processes in autoimmune hemolytic anemia. One hundred and twenty-eight patients were studied in their series. Five patients with cold acting erythrocyte autoantibodies had an associated influenza infection or virus pneumonia; these were unchallenged. Ninety-three patients were classified as having idiopathic autoimmune hemolytic anemia and an infectious disease was noted in nine.

Other investigators have been more impressed with the association of autoimmune hemolytic anemia and infectious disease. Horowitz and associates (55) noted "Lederer's anemia" accompanying urinary tract infections. Githens and Hathaway (56) similarly observed the association of auto-immune hemolytic anemia with urinary tract infections. Giesy and associates (57) recorded positive antiglobulin tests in patients with urinary tract obstruction. Wasikowa and Wilkomerska-Kajetanowicz (58) reported four patients with hemolytic anemia of an infectious etiology. Beretta (59) related the development of autoimmune hemolytic anemia to chronic focal tonsillitis in five patients.

There is little doubt that infectious processes may be associated with hemolytic anemia and/or positive antiglobulin tests. Excellent theoretical model systems exist to explain this relationship. Immunologic mechanisms apparently have a role in the development of these states. Whether these are autoimmune or immunologic but not autoimmune will have to be determined in the future. The type of infectious agent, its incidence and the clinical pattern it presents are still obscure. The present series of patients with autoimmune hemolytic anemia has been analyzed in an attempt to resolve some of these problems.

Analysis of Present Series

Two hundred and thirty-four patients with warm acting autoimmune hemolytic anemia have been studied. Forty-four cases were considered as idiopathic forms and 190 as symptomatic types associated with a significant pathologic state. Infectious disease occupied an important segment of the secondary or symptomatic varieties. This series does not include cold acting varieties of autoimmune hemolytic anemia. Accordingly, virus pneumonia with cold acting erythrocyte autoantibodies does not contribute to the following statistical data. Twenty-four patients were studied who had an unequivocal relationship between an infectious process and warm acting autoimmune hemolytic anemia. They represent an incidence of 10.3 per cent of the total series and 12.6 per cent of secondary varieties.

These figures may be compared to calculations made from Dacie's series (53). Twelve cases were studied, representing an incidence of 9.3 per cent of patients with warm acting autoimmune hemolytic anemia and 30.0 per cent of secondary varie-

ties. In the series of Dausset and Colombani (45), there were 106 examples of warm acting autoimmune hemolytic anemia. Nine cases with an infectious disease association were seen and classified as idiopathic. This constituted 8.5 per cent of the total series. Accordingly, these three large series are in remarkable agreement as to the incidence of associated infectious disease in warm acting autoimmune hemolytic anemia.

The relationship of infectious disease to the development of autoimmune hemolytic anemia is even more extensive than that described above. In addition to the 24 patients with an unequivocal association in the current series, 51 other patients had a significant infectious disease history. In most cases another pathologic state was also present and appeared to be related to autoimmune hemolytic anemia. It therefore was not possible to implicate directly the infectious process in the production of the hemolytic state. In other cases the infectious process occurred either before or after the development of hemolytic anemia. A time sequence was present which made it possible but not unequivocal for a relationship to exist. Significant infectious disease therefore occurred in close temporal proximity to the development of warm acting autoimmune hemolytic anemia in 75 patients, an incidence of 32.1 per cent of the entire series.

It should be emphasized that the above data do not summarize the total infectious disease exposure of our patients with autoimmune hemolytic anemia. Rather, the 24 and 51 patient groups were selected on the basis of an unequivocal or possible etiologic relationship to autoimmune hemolytic anemia. An extremely high incidence was noted when the entire series of patients was analyzed for infectious disease occurring during the course of their ailment. Only a small percentage of patients studied were free of complicating infectious disease.

Etiologic Implications in the Association of Infectious Disease and Autoimmune Hemolytic Anemia

It is extremely difficult to evaluate the role of infectious disease in autoimmune hemolytic anemia. This applies particularly to the patient group with a possible but not unequivocal relationship. A fortuitous or nonetiologic status must be considered. The current series is heavily weighted with secondary varieties of autoimmune hemolytic anemia. As a general rule these patients were extremely ill. The frequent occurrence of infectious disease in a population of such debilitated individuals is not unexpected and may not have etiologic significance. In addition, a large number of patients with neoplastic processes of the reticuloendothelium are included in this series. It is well known that such patients have a peculiar predilection for developing infectious disease. Complicating infectious disease must be anticipated when it is realized that these patients were also extensively treated with corticosteroids, immunosuppressive agents and marrow depressing drugs. The occurrence of infectious processes may therefore not be related to the development of autoimmune hemolytic anemia.

This skeptical view is healthy but it may be totally erroneous. In the previous chapter the premise is developed that autoimmune hemolytic anemia may be a manifestation of a defective immune apparatus. Patients in such cases would be immunodeficient and unable to marshal a normal immune response (60). In such conditions infectious disease may have an important although not etiologic relationship to autoimmune hemolytic anemia. Autoimmune hemolytic anemia, reticuloendothelial neoplasia and infectious disease could result from the same abnormality of the immune apparatus. They may arise at different times in the natural history of the disease and they have different prognostic significance.

There is no reason to assume that infectious disease is related to the development of hemolytic anemia in only one manner. Many different organisms are involved, and the clinical and laboratory observations are variable. It is probable that several entirely different pathophysiologic mechanisms are activated. The five possibilities described below offer the clinician a wide range of mechanisms to consider in dealing with this problem. Only three involve immunologic pathways.

(a) Infectious agents may directly affect the erythrocyte. The action of malaria parasites in damaging the erythrocyte is prototypical of this group. It is interesting that the exact etiology of blackwater fever is not clearly understood. Zuckerman (17) has reviewed this entire subject and has even suggested that autoimmunity may be present.

(b) Products released from the infectious agent may damage the erythrocyte. Hemolytic anemia in the presence of *Clostridium welchii* is typical of this mechanism. The toxin of this organism functions as a lecithinase leading to severe hemolysis (61).

(c) Infectious agents or their products may initiate antibody production in a host and the resulting antibody may damage host erythrocytes. An antiglobulin positive type of hemolytic anemia develops. The formation of cross reacting antibodies, hapten formation, denaturation of the erythrocyte surface, innocent bystander states and the adsorption of immune complexes are all possible pathways for such an immune but not autoimmune pathogenesis.

(d) Infectious agents may induce autoimmune hemolytic anemia by creating a "foreign" immunocompetent cell, as was suggested in the case of infectious mononucleosis (62), or through mechanisms not as yet elucidated.

(e) Infectious disease may occur as the result of a basic defect of the immune apparatus in an immunodeficient individual. This defect may also be responsible for the development of autoimmune hemolytic anemia and reticuloendothelial neoplasia (60).

This wide diversity of possible modes of action of infectious disease can create complex clinical relationships. This may explain in part the difficulty in relating autoimmune hemolytic anemia to infectious processes. The clinical patterns encountered in the current series with the various infectious agents associated with autoimmune hemolytic anemia are presented below.

Virus Infections

Virus infections are clinically related to autoimmune hemolytic anemia in two major situations. Exacerbation of the hemolytic state may follow the development of relatively minor virus infections. In addition, a virus infection may be related to the development of autoimmune hemolytic anemia in a cause and effect relationship. These two clinical sequences have been noted by several investigators and are emphasized in the reports of Kölbl (63), Neimann and associates (64), Kissmeyer-Nielsen (65), Wuilleret (66) and Dionigi (67). It is striking how frequently children are involved in this phenomenon.

Six patients in the current series had virus infections with an unequivocal cause and effect relationship to hemolysis. Fifteen additional patients had a possible etiologic relationship. The types of virus infections and numbers of patients involved are summarized in Table 52. Several distinctive characteristics were noted in patients developing warm acting autoimmune hemolytic anemia related to a virus infection. No predisposition on the basis of sex is apparent; three males and three females were involved. The age distribution differed from that of the total series as well as from that of the idiopathic forms of autoimmune hemolytic anemia. The young were particularly prone to develop this association. The age of these patients at the onset of autoimmune hemolytic anemia ranged from 5 weeks to 23 years. The median age was 14 and the mean was 12 years.

Fever was characteristic and was present in all six patients. The onset of autoimmune hemolytic anemia was frequently explosive. A normal, healthy child would suddenly become acutely ill with severe hemolysis. Jaundice was present in five of the six patients. Reticuloendothelial hyperplasia was noted in all. Hepatosplenomegaly and lymphadenopathy were present in two, and isolated hepatosplenomegaly was present in two others. An enlarged liver was found in one patient and lymphadenopathy was discovered in another patient. Although the characteristic onset of autoimmune hemolytic anemia suggested a severe disease, complete recovery was the rule. Four of the six patients recovered swiftly and completely; followup has not revealed any evidence of

TABLE 52. *Virus infections with an unequivocal or possible etiologic relationship to autoimmune hemolytic anemia (21 patients seen among 234 cases of warm acting autoimmune hemolytic anemia)*

Virus Infection	Total Patients	Etiologic Relation to Autoimmune Hemolytic Anemia	
		Unequivocal	Possible
Infectious mononucleosis	3	3	0
Measles	1	1	0
Cytomegalic inclusion disease	1	1	0
Herpes zoster	8	1	7
Herpes simplex	1	0	1
Virus pneumonia	3	0	3
Virus upper respiratory infection	2	0	2
Infectious hepatitis	2	0	2
Total	21	6	15

residual disease. One patient died (Case 1). The underlying virus infection, cytomegalic virus disease, was the cause of death with autoimmune hemolytic anemia well controlled. One patient has had persisting autoimmune hemolytic anemia with relapses and exacerbations. Her course, however, has been complicated by continual virus infection (Case 44). Hemolytic anemia in this patient group persisted for a duration ranging from 1 week to 7 months. The longest duration appeared in the patient with the chronic infectious state. In the remaining five patients the duration of hemolytic disease was less than 2 months.

Specific Virus Associated Syndromes

Infectious Mononucleosis

Acute hemolytic anemia developing in association with infectious mononucleosis is a particularly inappropriate syndrome for children to develop. It is frequently heard of but infrequently seen. Dameshek (42) in 1943 reported the first patient with this combined disease. Although a number of reports are now available, the combination is relatively rare. This may be appreciated when the prevalence of infectious mononucleosis is considered. Dacie (53) has encounted only one case in 14 years of study in this field. Green and Goldenberg (68) in 1960 could document only 21 cases in the literature.

At least three forms of hemolytic anemia may occur with infectious mononucleosis when classification is dependent on serologic criteria. In one type erythrocyte autoantibodies have not been demonstrated (69–75). In a second form, positive antiglobulin reactions suggesting warm acting erythrocyte autoantibodies have been associated with infectious mononucleosis (68, 76–86). Berté (87) specifically described an autohemolysin active at room temperature in the face of negative tests for cold agglutinins. In a third type, cold agglutinins have been documented in the association of infectious mononucleosis and autoimmune hemolytic anemia (42, 71, 72, 75, 88–90). The observation of Rosenfield and associates (91) that sera of uncomplicated cases of infectious mononucleosis may contain cold hemagglutinins with a specificity of anti-i has clarified this latter group. This observation has been repeatedly confirmed (92–95) and implicated in a hemolytic state. The role of anti-i autoantibodies is discussed more extensively in Chapter 20.

Clinical Patterns

Autoimmune hemolytic anemia associated with infectious mononucleosis can present a variable clinical course. The usual pattern is that of a severe but transient illness, with spontaneous recovery in a few weeks. Hemolytic anemia may occur simultaneously with or during the course of infectious mononucleosis. Splenomegaly and lymphadenopathy have generally been present. Weakness, fever and jaundice are common. Thrombocytopenia may occur in this disease leading to an Evans' syndrome (85). Hemoglobinuria has been encountered by several observers (42, 68, 70, 80, 88). Although spontaneous recovery is the rule, it is not inevitable. Corticosteroid therapy and splenectomy have been employed in severe or chronic hemolytic episodes. It is interesting to note that Thurm and Bassen (72) and also Wasserman and

associates (82) have seen hemolytic anemia and infectious mononucleosis in patients with thalassemia. Splenectomy had to be performed to control the hemolytic syndrome in both patients.

In the present series three cases of infectious mononucleosis were associated with warm acting erythrocyte autoantibodies. Two males and one female were involved. The ages of the patients were 15, 18 and 23 years, respectively. Spontaneous recovery without specific therapy developed in all. Positive direct antiglobulin tests and warm acting erythrocyte autoantibodies were found in all three cases. The following protocol illustrates an extremely mild syndrome.

Case 41. A 23-year-old white medical student was investigated because of malaise, anorexia, jaundice, fever and dark urine. Physical examination revealed a pharyngeal exudate and 2+ cervical lymph nodes. The spleen was palpated 2 cm. below the costal margin and the liver, which was not tender, was palpated at the costal margin. The hematocrit 10 months before had been 46 per cent. It was now found to be 41.5 per cent with a reticulocyte count of 1.7 per cent. The peripheral blood smear was diagnostic for infectious mononucleosis. Heterophile agglutinin studies were positive at a titer of 1792 in unabsorbed tests and at 224 with absorption procedures. Alkaline phosphatase, transaminase and Bromsulphalein values were abnormally elevated. Cephalin flocculation was 4+. Bilirubin was 5.8/0.2 mg. per cent. The direct antiglobulin test was 1+ and the bromelin test was negative. No specific therapy other than bedrest was employed. The patient improved, with disappearance of symptoms, jaundice and adenopathy in 2 weeks. The antiglobulin test returned to negative. Followup 1 year later revealed that the patient's condition was entirely normal.

The above patient presented with infectious mononucleosis, jaundice and hepatitis. The antiglobulin test was unexpectedly found to be positive. There was no clinical evidence for hemolytic anemia. Spontaneous recovery occurred with disappearance of the positive antiglobulin test. The benign clinical course of infectious mononucleosis and positive antiglobulin tests illustrated in this patient are not typical of the combined syndrome. The following protocol demonstrates the severity which can be seen.

Case 42. An 18-year-old white male was first examined because of fever and a sore throat. Two weeks later fever was more extreme and jaundice was noted. Both the liver and spleen were palpated 3 cm. below the coastal margin. Cervical nodes of 1+ were found. The hematocrit was 17 per cent with a 5 per cent reticulocyte count. The white blood cell count (WBC) was 20,000/mm.³ with atypical lymphocytes, nucleated erythrocytes and spherocytes. Total bilirubin was 0.54/7.14 mg. per cent. Increased free hemoglobin was found in the plasma. Liver chemistries were normal. Bone marrow aspiration revealed erythrocytic hyperplasia. Heterophile agglutinin titers of 1800 were initially obtained and rose to 2560. Direct antiglobulin and bromelin tests were strongly positive. A cold agglutinin with a titer of 16 was found in the serum. Six transfusions were given over the next 6 days. The hematocrit stayed at 18 per cent during this time, and then gradually rose to 25 per cent 3 weeks after the onset of disease. One week later the hematocrit was 36 per cent. In 1 month it reached 41.5 per cent and the patient was completely asymptomatic. The heterophile agglutinin titer was 0 and antiglobulin tests were negative. Followup examination 31 months later demonstrated a normal patient with negative serologic studies.

In this patient severe autoimmune hemolytic anemia was superimposed on a relatively mild case of infectious mononucleosis. The onset of hemolytic anemia was explosive, and hemolysis was rapid and extensive. Although no specific therapy was employed other than transfusions the hemolytic syndrome abruptly terminated after 1 week, and spontaneous recovery occurred. Remission has now persisted without relapse for about 3 years.

Measles

The association of warm acting autoimmune hemolytic anemia with measles does not appear to have been previously reported. Dacie (53) described a child who developed a potent Donath-Landsteiner antibody and paroxysmal cold hemoglobinuria following measles. A positive direct antiglobulin test was found at the onset of he-

molytic anemia. This reverted to negative as the child recovered. The Donath-Landsteiner antibody persisted for a longer period of time. Dacie (53) also mentions a 6-year-old child who developed an ultimately fatal case of autoimmune hemolytic anemia following measles. A warm acting erythrocyte autoantibody was present but the etiologic relationship to the virus was unclear. A relationship of measles to autoantibody production is suggested by Ottaviani and associates (96). They described thrombocytopenia and platelet autoantibodies developing during measles.

In the current series, one patient was seen whose case clearly demonstrated that warm acting autoimmune hemolytic anemia may result from exposure to the measles virus.

Case 43. A healthy 2-year-old female child was vaccinated with a live measles preparation. One week later fever was noted. Four days later chills and diarrhea developed. The next day pallor was present with jaundice and dark urine. The temperature was 101°F., the liver was 2 cm. below the coastal margin and the spleen not felt. The hematocrit was 22 per cent, the WBC was 7,300/mm.³ and spherocytes were found in the peripheral blood. Hemoglobinuria was demonstrated. Two days later the hematocrit had dropped to 12 per cent, the reticulocyte count was 1.3 per cent, the WBC was 34,500/mm.³, the bilirubin was 1.2/1.2 mg. per cent and free serum hemoglobin was 98 mg. per cent. Hemoglobinuria persisted. Bone marrow aspiration revealed erythrocytic hyperplasia. Direct antiglobulin and bromelin tests were positive. Dexamethasone, 4 mg., was given intravenously and oral prednisone, 40 mg. per day, was started. The spleen was palpable and remained so for 2 days; the liver was 4 cm. below the costal margin. The hematocrit dropped to 10.8 per cent and the WBC reached 135,000/mm.³ Five days after the start of corticosteroids the reticulocyte count reached 37 per cent and the hematocrit started to rise. Over the next week the hematocrit rose to 31 per cent. The WBC decreased to 12,000/mm.³ and hemoglobinuria disappeared. Two weeks after the onset of hemolytic anemia, the antiglobulin and bromelin tests reverted to normal. The liver and spleen were no longer palpable and prednisone therapy was gradually tapered off. Five weeks later all hematologic values were normal. Two weeks later prednisone was discontinued. A followup examination 8 months after the onset of disease was negative, with normal hematologic and serologic studies.

There is little doubt that administration of a live measles virus preparation precipitated acute hemolytic anemia of a warm acting erythrocyte autoantibody type. A severe hemolytic process with hemoglobinuria developed. A dramatic therapeutic response occurred concomitant with corticosteroid therapy. Followup examination suggests that only a transient disease state was present, and there is no evidence of either relapse or an underlying precipitating disease.

The initiation of autoimmune hemolytic anemia by introducing viruses through vaccination is not unique. Kölbl (63) has recorded a similar case following smallpox vaccination, and Dameshek and Schwartz (97) have reported a case following poliomyelitis vaccination.

Cytomegalic Virus Disease

The association of cytomegalic virus disease and autoimmune hemolytic anemia was reported in 1964 in separate publications by Zuelzer and associates (98), Becker and Eddy (99), and Pirofsky (100). Zuelzer and associates (50) have carried out the most significant investigation in this area. Their studies are reviewed in detail in Chapter 14. Evidence is presented that cytomegalic virus is a frequent accompaniment of autoimmune hemolytic anemia in childhood. Zuelzer feels that the hemolytic state best correlates with, and is etiologically related to, activity of the cytomegalic virus. He rejects an autoimmune etiology and notes little relationship between erythrocyte autoantibody activity, as determined by antiglobulin testing, and hemolytic anemia. The exact relationship between autoantibody formation and cytomegalic virus is obscure.

Since these original publications, other workers have encountered the association of cytomegalic virus and autoimmune hemolytic anemia. Mongan and associates (101) reported a patient with a thymoma, hypogammaglobulinemia, autoimmune hemolytic anemia and cytomegalic

virus disease. It is interesting to note that the case reported by Becker and Eddy (99) terminated with development of a lymphoma. Wong and Warner (102) have noted cytomegalic inclusion disease in 14 adults. Four patients had reticuloendothelial neoplasia; a thymoma was noted in one of these. Three patients had ulcerative colitis, which may also have autoimmune significance (see Chapter 9). A review of the literature indicates that, of the 41 adults previously reported as having cytomegalic virus disease, 15 had reticuloendothelial neoplasia and four had other autoimmune states. A possibility exists that patients liable to develop this syndrome have an impaired immune apparatus (60). Thymoma, hypogammaglobulinemia, lymphomas, autoimmune hemolytic anemia and a spreading cytomegalic virus disease may all be manifestations of the inability to marshal a normal immune response. Further clinical and investigational studies in this area are needed.

In the current series cytomegalic virus disease and autoimmune hemolytic anemia were seen in one patient (Case 1). This infant was ill at birth. A warm acting type of autoimmune hemolytic anemia was apparent at 5 weeks of age. Death occurred at 7 weeks of age from cytomegalic virus disease. The objection that cytomegalic virus with a ubiquitous distribution represents superinfection in a debilitated patient with autoimmune hemolytic anemia does not appear valid in the case of this patient. Cytomegalic disease dominated the clinical picture, antedated the autoimmune hemolytic anemia and led to the patient's death.

Herpes Zoster

Although varicella (54) and herpes simplex (48, 49) have been reported in association with autoimmune hemolytic anemia, no such relationship with herpes zoster has been suggested. In the current series eight patients developed herpes zoster in a time sequence significant in relation to the development of autoimmune hemolytic anemia. However, seven of these patients had an accompanying malignancy of the reticuloendothelium (three patients had chronic lymphocytic leukemia, two had Hodgkin's disease, and one each had acute monocytic leukemia and plasma cell myeloma). These patients have not been included as either unequivocally or possibly related to the development of autoimmune hemolytic anemia. One patient developed herpes zoster in a close relationship to autoimmune hemolytic anemia. Her clinical course is extremely complex, and infectious diseases other than herpes zoster were present. Accordingly, the author will not object if the reader rejects the proposed association.

Case 44. A female child was born with a widespread infectious disease diagnosed as systemic moniliasis. She had repeated bouts of pneumonia and she developed bronchiectasis as an infant. At age 6, diabetes was diagnosed and lobectomy was performed. Extensive amphotericin therapy was given. Repeated attacks of systemic moniliasis and bacterial infections occurred. Amphotericin therapy was repeated at ages 8, 10 and 11. At age 12½, extensive herpes zoster developed. Her physical examination was negative and hematocrit 40 per cent. Four weeks later abdominal pain was noted, and the liver was palpated 2 cm. below the costal margin. One week later she returned with a suppurative otitis media, and her spleen was palpated 2 cm. below the costal margin. The hematocrit had dropped to 23 per cent. Nucleated erythrocytes and spherocytes were found in the peripheral smear. The liver and spleen rapidly enlarged to 6 and 4 cm. respectively, below the costal margins. Jaundice and fever developed. A nose and throat culture grew pneumococci and coagulase positive staphylococci. The hematocrit was 18.8 per cent, the reticulocyte count was 42 per cent and the bilirubin was 1.2/1.6 mg. per cent. Bone marrow aspiration revealed erythrocytic hyperplasia with megaloblastic changes. A Cr^{51} half-life survival of 3.6 days with splenic sequestration was found. Heterophile agglutinin and lupus erythematosus (LE) studies were negative. Direct and indirect antiglobulin and bromelin studies were strongly positive and elution demonstrated a panhemagglutinin. No therapy except oral amphotericin was given in view of her severe diabetes. One month later the hematocrit was 15 per cent with a 30 per cent reticulocyte count and the bilirubin was 1.0/2.5 mg. per cent. The hematocrit dropped to 12.5 per cent, and intravenous hydrocortisone and oral prednisone were started. Two units of blood were transfused with moderately severe

reactions. The hematocrit gradually rose. Prednisone was rapidly decreased, down to 2.5 mg. daily, in five weeks. This dose was continued for 1 additional month, during which time the hematocrit remained at 40 per cent. Her clinical course was complicated by a beta-streptococci abscess of her arm and jaw. Six weeks after discontinuation of prednisone the hematocrit had dropped to 28 per cent with a 19 per cent reticulocyte count. The spleen and liver were both palpable and a *Streptococcus faecalis* cystitis was present. When the hematocrit dropped to 19 per cent, prednisone therapy was again employed, and it was followed by a therapeutic remission. Her hematocrit rose to 38 per cent and prednisone therapy was maintained at 5 mg. daily. Followup is continuing. The antiglobulin and bromelin tests have remained consistent positive.

This complex patient was born with systemic moniliasis and developed juvenile diabetes and multiple infections. A herpes zoster infection occurred and was followed by severe warm acting autoimmune hemolytic anemia. Two remissions have been induced with corticosteroid therapy. Multiple infections have continued to complicate the patient's clinical course. The temporal relationship of herpes zoster to the development of autoimmune hemolytic anemia is striking. However, this patient has so many infectious disease problems, as well as juvenile diabetes, that a specific etiologic relationship is problematical.

Other Virus Diseases Associated with Autoimmune Hemolytic Anemia

Other viruses have been implicated in an etiologic relationship with warm acting autoimmune hemolytic anemia. Although no unequivocal examples of these were seen in the current series, excellent reports are available in the literature. The occurrence of a warm acting type of autoimmune hemolytic anemia during Influenza A infection has been reported by Beickert and Spróssig (103) and d'Oelsnitz and associates (104). In both examples cold agglutinins were absent and the antiglobulin test was positive. In the case reported by Beickert and Spróssig, polyarteritis and thrombocytopenic purpura were also present. Hemolytic anemia characterized by cold hemagglutinins during Influenza A and B infections has also been reported and is described in Chapter 11. A possible mechanism for this action has been described by Springer and Ansell (105). They noted that influenza virus led to erythrocyte agglutination and destroyed the M, N, Lu^a and Lu^b antigens.

Betke and associates (51) and Vivell (52) reported the association of Coxsackie A virus infections in children having autoimmune hemolytic anemia. The virus was isolated from the stools and blood, neutralizing convalescing antibodies were demonstrated and the antiglobulin test was positive.

Borbolla and Barquetchediak (54) reported a complex case of a 6-year-old child who developed autoimmune hemolytic anemia during convalescence from varicella. The antiglobulin test, the Kahn test and heterophile agglutinins were positive.

Moolten and Clark (106, 107), and Moolten and associates (48) have etiologically related Newcastle disease virus, herpes simplex and other viruses in human hemolytic anemia characterized by autohemagglutination. These studies have not been confirmed. The pertinent reports are discussed in Chapter 14. The possible etiologic relationship of such viruses to autoimmune hemolytic anemia still must be clarified. Todd and O'Donohue (49) have reported herpes simplex stomatitis in a child who developed autoimmune hemolytic anemia. The autoantibody had anti-hr″(e) specificity. The simultaneous occurrence of herpes simplex and autoimmune hemolytic anemia was seen in one patient of the current series (Case 21). This individual had chronic lymphocytic leukemia, positive antiglobulin tests with minimal evidence of hemolysis and a preexisting herpes simplex stomatitis for over 2 years. This condition responded poorly to continual gamma-globulin therapy.

In addition to the cases mentioned above, six patients in the current series had virus infections which possibly suggested a relationship to a warm acting variety of autoimmune hemolytic anemia. The time sequence of virus infection was suggestive but not diagnostic of an etiologic relationship.

Three patients had primary atypical virus pneumonia. One patient (Case 9) developed an upper respiratory virus infection 1 month after virus pneumonia. This in turn was followed by idiopathic thrombocytopenic purpura. Autoimmune hemolytic anemia occurred shortly thereafter. A second patient developed severe anemia with a hematocrit of 21.5 per cent during convalescence from virus pneumonia. Anemia has persisted for over 72 months. This patient has been classified as having an idiopathic form of autoimmune hemolytic anemia. Positive antiglobulin tests were not obtained until 14 months after the onset of disease. Case 19 developed virus pneumonia followed by viral myocarditis and aplastic anemia. Approximately 5 years later Hodgkin's disease occurred and terminated in autoimmune hemolytic anemia.

Additional virus infections which were encountered but not considered to be unequivocally related to autoimmune hemolytic anemia include two cases of upper respiratory infections and two cases of acute hepatitis. The latter group is discussed in detail in Chapter 9.

Bacterial Infections

There is little doubt that bacterial as well as viral infections may have a close relationship to hemolysis and positive antiglobulin tests. In some instances the relationship is undoubtedly fortuitous. In other cases a cause and effect state cannot be denied. The possibility that the basic disease process reflects an abnormality of the immune apparatus must be considered. In such states infectious disease and autoimmune hemolytic anemia may both result from the same pathologic process. Separation of these possible relationships is difficult.

Analysis of the frequency of bacterial infections complicating autoimmune hemolytic anemia is inadequate to deal with this problem. In the current series, 234 patients were reviewed from this aspect. It was rare to observe a patient in whom the clinical course had not been obscured at some time by the development of an infectious process. In the following discussion a deliberate attempt has been made to minimize this association in order to emphasize more firmly the unequivocal relationships that exist. Such an unequivocal status has been accepted when the relative time sequence in the development of bacterial infection and autoimmune hemolytic anemia was striking. In addition, the absence of other significant pathologic states reinforced the interpretation of an unequivocal relationship. When the time relationship was striking but other significant pathologic states were present, a possible relationship has been considered.

The early literature supplies excellent evidence that bacterial infections can induce acute hemolytic syndromes. Reports are available indicating this sequence for *C. welchii* (27–30), *Bartonella bacilliformis* (25) and *B. muris* (26), syphilis (4–6), tuberculosis (108–110), cholera (35), salmonella (31, 34, 111), streptococci (36–39), enterococci (39), staphylococci (39, 40), pneumococci (12, 39, 41), *Escherichia coli* (55) and typhoid fever (32, 33, 112, 113). In some cases hemolysis results from the direct action of the invading organism or its products. In other cases, positive antiglobulin tests have been observed. It is therefore important to examine a large number of cases of warm acting autoimmune hemolytic anemia for the frequency of such bacterial associations. The theoretical mechanisms that may result in an antiglobulin positive type of hemolytic anemia with infection are presented in Chapter 14.

Incidence of Etiologically Significant Bacterial Infections

Bacterial infections which appeared in an unequivocal etiologic relationship to autoimmune hemolytic anemia were seen in 18 patients of our current series, an incidence of 7.6 per cent. Significant bacterial disease was discovered in a close temporal sequence to the onset of autoimmune hemolytic anemia in an additional 36 patients. An etiologic relationship was not unequivocal in these cases. There was either another significant pathologic state or a clinical

course which could not be interpreted in a cause and effect manner. Table 53 summarizes the data concerning the site of infection, the number of patients involved, identification of the organisms when known and the unequivocal or possible etiologic relationship.

Clinical Patterns

The 18 patients with an unequivocal etiologic relationship presented a clinical pattern with similarities and dissimilarities from the pattern seen with virus infections. Different populations of patients were involved in the two groups of infections. With virus infections there was no predisposition on the basis of sex. In contrast, a high incidence of males was en-

TABLE 53. *Site and type of bacterial infections with an unequivocal or possible etiologic relationship to autoimmune hemolytic anemia (55 patients involved in a series of 234)**

Type of Infection	Total Patients	Etiologic Relationship to Autoimmune Hemolytic Anemia	
		Unequivocal	Possible
Urinary tract infection	24	5	19
E. coli		1	
S. faecalis		1	
Pseudomonas		1	
Unknown		2	
Pneumonia	13	4	9
K. pneumoniae		1	
Beta-streptococci		1	
Alpha-streptococci		1	
Mixed type		1	
Tuberculosis	6	4	2
Acute cholecystitis†	3	3	0
Meningitis	2	1	1
Staphylococcus epidermis		1	
Staphylococcus pyodermia	1	1	0
Septicemia	3	1	2
Pseudomonas†		1	
Thrombophlebitis	3	0	3
Total	55	19	36

* Specific organisms, when known, refer to the unequivocal group.

† Both states were simultaneously present in the same patient.

TABLE 54. *Statistical data obtained from 24 patients (eight females, 16 males) with an infectious disease unequivocally associated with autoimmune hemolytic anemia*

Clinical Data	Type of Infectious Disease	
	Virus	Bacterial
No. of patients	6	18
Sex (no./%)		
Female	3/50	5/28
Male	3/50	13/72
Age		
Range	5 wk.–23 yr.	5 mo.–87 yr.
Mean (years)	12	52
Median (years)	14	55
Survival (no./%)		
Living	5/83	14/77
Dead	1/17	4/23
Dead of disease	1/17	3/17
Complete recovery	4/67	15/83
Duration of followup of living cases (months)		
Range	7–97	2–90
Mean	36	25
Median	19	16

countered with bacterial infections. The predisposition for the young, as seen with virus infections, was not found. Patients with bacterial infections presented an age range from 5 weeks to 87 years, with a median age of 55 years. Only three of the 18 were not adults.

The clinical picture of the bacterial infection group resembled that seen with associated viral disease. The onset of disease was often abrupt although not necessarily explosive. It was not unusual, however, to discover positive antiglobulin reactions in patients with chronic disease in whom hemolytic anemia was not suspected. The major similarity between virus associated and bacterial associated autoimmune hemolytic anemia was an excellent prognosis. Recovery from autoimmune hemolytic anemia appeared to be complete and possibly permanent in 15 of the 18 patients with associated bacterial infections. The three patients who died had active hemolytic anemia for 1 week in two cases and for 8 months in the third. The remaining 15 patients have not had recurrences of autoim-

mune hemolytic anemia in followups ranging from 2 to 90 months. Long survivals without relapse were characteristic. One patient in this group died postoperatively for an unrelated abnormality. Table 54 summarizes the statistical data obtained for the patients with both viral and bacterial disease unequivocally related to autoimmune hemolytic anemia.

Special Syndromes Seen with Associated Bacterial Infections

The large number of clinical patterns and the limited number of patients in each category prevent generalization. Accordingly, case histories are employed in order to present the variable as well as typical aspects seen in each type of infectious association.

Urinary Tract Infections

Horowitz and associates (55), Githens and Hathaway (56) and Giesy and associates (57) have all been impressed with the association of urinary tract infections and autoimmune hemolytic anemia. In the current series, 24 patients were found to have an associated urinary tract infection in a close temporal relationship to the onset of autoimmune hemolytic anemia. Nine of these infectious states were diagnosed as cystitis. Five cases presented an unequivocal relationship between the infection and the development of positive antiglobulin tests. One female patient had cystitis, and four male patients had prostatitis with urinary retention and cystitis. Variable clinical patterns were seen.

Case 45. A 39-year-old white female was investigated by her physician because of fatigue and low grade anemia. During the next 3 months anemia became more marked in spite of oral iron therapy. The hematocrit reached 20 per cent, and 13 ml. of intramuscular iron were given. The stools were free of blood and reticulocytosis was not documented. She was seen in hematologic consultation 1 month later. Physical examination revealed the liver 4 cm. below the costal margin as the only abnormality. The hematocrit was 14 per cent with a 0.1 per cent reticulocyte count. Marked hypochromia of erythrocytes was seen. Thrombocytes were elevated to 750,000/mm.^{3} and the WBC was normal. Bone marrow examination indicated a hypercellular pattern with erythrocytic hyperplasia. The protein bound iodine was 6.4 μg. per cent. A Schilling test was normal. The serum iron was 205 μg. per cent with an iron binding capacity of 46 μg. per cent. Antiglobulin and bromelin tests were negative. Upper and lower gastrointestinal series x-rays were normal. Three blood transfusions were given and a 1-month trial of pyridoxine was employed. The hematocrit progressively dropped from its transfused level. Six weeks later the hematocrit was 24 per cent and the reticulocyte count was 2.1 per cent. Urinalysis revealed 2+ albuminuria, pus cells and many bacteria. The direct antiglobulin test was positive and the bromelin test was negative. Oral sulfa therapy was given. The hematocrit dropped to 21 per cent over the next 3 weeks and then started to rise. Seven weeks after the start of oral sulfa therapy the hematocrit reached 36 per cent and urinalysis was normal. Sulfa therapy was continued 1 additional week. Two months later the hematocrit was 41 per cent with normal urine and serologic studies.

In the above patient severe hypochromic anemia did not respond to oral or parenteral iron or to pyridoxine therapy. No evidence of hypothyroidism or blood loss was found. Hemolytic anemia was unsuspected except for the presence of bone marrow erythrocytic hyperplasia. The development of a positive direct antiglobulin test and laboratory evidence of cystitis suggested a relationship. Oral sulfa therapy was employed without hematinics or corticosteroids. A gradual but progressive return to normal hematologic status occurred. Followup examination 7 months after the onset of anemia has not revealed either relapse or the presence of other underlying pathologic states that could be responsible for the hematologic problem.

Four additional examples of urinary tract infections etiologically related to positive antiglobulin tests were studied. Similar clinical courses were found in all four patients. Anemia was not present and an autoimmune or hemolytic state was not suspected. Urinary obstruction secondary to prostatic hypertrophy and infection were common to all. The offending organisms were identified in three patients. These included a combination of *E. coli* and Pseudomonas in one patient, *Streptococcus faecalis* in a second and Pseudomonas in a third. This last patient also developed pseudomonas septicemia. The antiglobulin positive state was discovered during routine blood cross matching procedures performed prior to surgery. Relief of obstruction and correction of the infection postoperatively frequently led to a rapid disappearance of the positive antiglobulin test. Followup investigations have not suggested any other associated pathologic state which could be responsible for the positive antiglobulin test.

Case 46. An 87-year-old white male entered the urologic service with urinary retention secondary to benign prostatic hypertrophy. Congestive heart failure was the only pertinent observation obtained by history and physical examination. Laboratory studies, including an extensive but routine hematologic examination, were all within normal limits. Urinary cultures revealed *E. coli* and Pseudomonas. Routine blood cross matches performed prior to surgery revealed incompatibilities both of the major and minor types. Serologic investigation demonstrated positive direct and indirect antiglobulin and bromelin tests. A panhemagglutinin was identified. Perineal prostatectomy was performed. Pathologic examination showed stromal and glandular hyperplasia of the prostate with acute and chronic prostatitis and focal abscess formation. Surgery was complicated by a blood loss of 1500 ml. In the absence of compatible blood, albumin and 0.2 per cent sodium chloride were infused. The hematocrit dropped to 24.5 per cent 24 hours postoperatively and hypotension occurred. Cross matching was again carried out and this time was found compatible. Repeat serologic studies revealed negative direct and indirect antiglobulin and bromelin tests. Four units of blood were transfused without difficulty, with supplementary parenteral hydrocortisone. Eight days after prostatectomy, direct and indirect antiglobulin and bromelin tests were still negative. Evaluations 3 and 8 months postoperatively did not suggest a hemolytic state. All serologic studies were negative.

This protocol is typical of the patients who entered with prostatitis, urinary retention and infection. A hemolytic state was not clinically suspected. Positive serologic findings were noted as an incidental observation during preoperative preparation. Surgery and antibiotic therapy led to disappearance of the positive antiglobulin test in a variable but generally short period of time. The benign hematologic state of these patients should not be interpreted as an inactive process or "false positive" antiglobulin reaction. The potency of the autoantibody and its potential danger are illustrated in the next case.

Case 47. A 78-year-old male entered the urologic service with prostatism, urinary obstruction and cystitis. History and physical examination were negative except for the urologic condition. Laboratory studies, including routine hematologic examinations, were normal. *Streptococcus faecalis* was obtained on urine culture. Routine blood cross matching prior to surgery was interpreted as normal. Transurethral resection of a 45-gm. prostate was carried out. Pathologic examination revealed benign stromal and grandular hypertrophy of the prostate. Bleeding during surgery was extremely difficult to control, and 6 units of blood were transfused. Following transfusion, hemoglobinuria, hemoglobinema and jaundice were noted. Bleeding continued and required repeated transurethral fulguration and suprapubic ligation of the bladder neck. Renal shutdown and multiple cardiovascular problems occurred during the next 3 days, resulting in death.

A serologic investigation was performed. The preoperative blood sample of the patient revealed positive direct and indirect antiglobulin and bromelin tests. A circulating autoantibody was found in the serum. Accordingly, the six transfusions administered during surgery were incompatible. On the 3rd day after the operation, just prior to death, the antiglobulin and bromelin reactions still remained positive. Autopsy did not reveal any cause of the positive antiglobulin reaction.

In this case inaccurate cross match studies failed to demonstrate the presence of an erythrocyte autoantibody in a patient not suspected of having a hemolytic state. Rapid transfusion of incompatible blood was employed during surgery. Extensive hemolysis and renal shutdown followed, with death in 3 days.

The disappearance of positive serologic tests after surgical correction of benign prostatic hypertrophy, as noted in Case 46, was seen in another case, and in two additional patients with renal carcinoma. These cases have been reported in detail by Giesy and associates (57). It must not be assumed, however, that removal of either abnormal prostatic or renal tissue specifically eliminates the source of autoantibody producing cells. In another patient, prostatic hypertrophy and urinary retention with positive serologic tests were complicated by pseudomonas septicemia. Acute cholecystitis occurred during treatment. Cholecystectomy was performed and antibiotics were given. The positive serologic tests reverted to normal in 4 days. Three weeks later prostatectomy was carried out without difficulty. Accordingly, bacterial infection appeared to be the common feature in these patients.

Urinary tract infections in the remaining 19 patients developed in a time relationship to the onset of autoimmune hemolytic anemia which suggested an etiologic role. The presence of other significant pathologic states has relegated these infections to the category of a possible but not unequivocal relationship. In addition, many other patients had a history of previous urinary tract infections or subsequently developed such infections during their illness. In Chapter 3 the large number of abnormalities relating to the urinary tract is summarized for the entire series of 234 patients.

Bacterial Pneumonia

The association of bacterial pneumonia and autoimmune hemolytic anemia has been reported by several investigators. Singer and Dameshek (12) noted this association with pneumococcal pneumonia, and Stratton (40) noted it with staphylococcal pneumonia. In both cases the hemolytic disease disappeared with correction of the infectious process.

Bacterial pneumonia occurred in a close temporal relationship to the onset of autoimmune hemolytic anemia in 13 patients of the current series. In four, a cause and effect relationship of infection to autoimmune hemolytic anemia was apparent. No specific clinical pattern was obvious in these four cases. One child and three adults were involved. Different organisms were implicated in each case. These included *Klebsiella pneumoniae*, beta-hemolytic streptococci, alpha-streptococci and mixed organisms. In the nine patients with a possible but not unequivocal relationship, staphylococci and *E. coli* infections were common.

Autoimmune hemolytic anemia related to bacterial pneumonia differed clinically from that seen with urinary tract infections. Anemia was generally obvious and a hemolytic state was easily documented. Correction of the infectious state generally resulted in correction of hemolytic anemia.

Case 48. A 2-year-old white child was investigated because of a high temperature. Pneumonia and empyema were diagnosed. Beta-hemolytic streptococci were cultured as the causative agent. Physical examination was normal, aside from the pulmonary abnormalities. The hematocrit was 30 per cent and the WBC was 51,000/mm.[3] Surgical drainage and antibiotics were employed. The hematocrit remained unchanged and the WBC decreased. Twenty days later an elevated temperature and abdominal pain developed. Acute appendicitis with a perforated abscess was diagnosed. The hematocrit was 30 per cent and the WBC was 7,800/mm.[3] Blood cross match revealed incompatible reactions and serologic studies indicated strong positive direct and indirect antiglobulin and bromelin tests. The hematocrit dropped to 17 per cent, the WBC rose to 25,000/mm.[3] and thrombocytes were normal. The reticulocyte count was 1.1 per cent. Occasional plasma cells were seen in the peripheral blood. The bone marrow was hypercellular with erythrocytic and granulocytic hyperplasia. Extensive antibiotic therapy was given. In 2 months the patient was asymptomatic. The hematocrit was 34 per cent and the reticulocyte count was 0.7 per cent. The WBC remained elevated at 18,300/mm.[3] and erythrocyte serologic tests were still positive. Two years later the patient was reexamined with cerebellar ataxia and acute pharyngitis and tonsillitis. The examination was otherwise normal. The hematocrit was 35 per cent and all serologic studies were negative.

In the above case a child with a severe infection had persisting anemia associated with erythrocytic hyperplasia and positive antiglobulin and bromelin tests. Correction of the infectious disease led to a gradual elevation of the hematocrit and disappearance of positive erythrocyte serologic tests. The clinical course was prolonged. It did not resemble the abrupt onset and recovery seen in children with a viral disease and

autoimmune hemolytic anemia. Persistence of the hematologic disease is possibly related to persistence of the infectious process. A more explosive nature is illustrated in the following case.

Case 49. A 51-year-old white male alcoholic presented a long history of repeated pneumonia, emphysema, herpes zoster and possible cirrhosis. He entered the hospital with fever, chills and hemoptysis. Pneumonia was diagnosed and *Klebsiella pneumoniae* was isolated from the sputum. The hematocrit was 41 per cent and the WBC was 1,120/mm.[3] Large doses of intramuscular penicillin were given over the next 2 weeks without a therapeutic effect. Cephalothin therapy was then employed. Six days later the hematocrit had dropped to 20 per cent. An attempt to transfuse the patient revealed incompatibilities, and positive direct antiglobulin tests were obtained. The liver was palpated 4 cm. and the spleen 3 cm. below the costal margin. Toxic granulation of leukocytes was seen and bone marrow aspiration revealed granulocytic hyperplasia with a shift to the left. The albumin-globulin (A/G) ratio was 2.6/4.6 gm. per cent. The indirect bilirubin was elevated to 1.2 mg. per cent. Four units of blood were transfused. One week later the hemolytic process was still apparent and pneumonia was unchanged; antiglobulin tests continued positive. Cephalothin was stopped and kanamycin was given. The pneumonia improved and sputum cultures no longer grew out *Klebsiella pneumoniae*. The hematocrit gradually rose. Two weeks later *Pseudomonas* was found in the sputum, and erythromycin was added to the therapy with continual improvement. Eleven days later the antiglobulin test became negative. Followup 1 year later revealed no evidence of a hemolytic state.

In this example extensive *Klebsiella pneumoniae* was complicated by a severe hemolytic process and positive antiglobulin tests. The process was initiated soon after the start of cephalothin therapy. It is possible that a "false positive" antiglobulin test secondary to cephalothin was present. However, the severe hemolytic anemia makes it unlikely that a drug induced reaction was the only explanation. Correction of the infectious process eventually was reflected in correction of the hemolytic state. Disappearance of the positive antiglobulin test correlated with this improvement.

Case 50. A 45-year-old white female entered the hospital with cough, fatigue, a temperature of 104°F. and x-ray evidence of bilateral pneumonia. Sputum cultures revealed mixed organisms, with alpha-streptococci predominating. Her son had made an uncomplicated recovery from a similar pneumonia 1 month previously. The hematocrit was 32 per cent and the WBC was 15,000/mm.³ Physical examination was negative except for pneumonia. Chloramphenicol therapy was given. One week later the hematocrit was 24 per cent with a 12 per cent reticulocyte count. Mild jaundice was noted. Direct antiglobulin and bromelin tests were strongly positive. Otitis media and a nasal ulcer were noted. Prednisone therapy, 60 mg. per day, was started. Twelve days later the hematocrit reached 30 per cent with a 1.4 per cent reticulocyte count. The pneumonia was markedly improved. The hematocrit progressively improved as prednisone was decreased and finally discontinued 3 months after initiation of therapy. Antiglobulin tests reverted to normal 2½ months after first being found positive. Followup 90 months later revealed no hematologic or serologic abnormalities and no other disease state.

In the above case corticosteroid therapy was employed with an excellent therapeutic response. However, the infectious disease simultaneously improved. It is problematical whether corticosteroid therapy initiated hematologic remission or whether this response would have occurred spontaneously with the disappearance of pneumonia.

In the patients with autoimmune hemolytic anemia and bacterial pneumonia, the clinical pattern was dominated by the infectious process. The severity of the combined disease correlated with the severity of the pneumonic state. Hemolytic anemia generally appeared as merely a troublesome complication. It differed, therefore, from the pattern noted with virus diseases associated with autoimmune hemolytic anemia. In such patients hemolytic anemia frequently dominated the clinical manifestations of the combined disease.

Tuberculosis

The association of tuberculosis and hemolytic anemia has frequently been recognized in the earlier literature. Tuberculosis of the spleen complicated by hemolytic anemia is a well documented syndrome. The reports of Griffin (108), Thompson (114), Engelbreth-Holm (109), Howells (110) and Guszich (115) have emphasized this association. The elegant studies of Boyden (116, 117) have delineated the pathways through which products of the tuberculous organism may induce an antiglobulin positive type of hemolytic anemia (see Chapter 14).

It is surprising that reports of autoimmune hemolytic anemia associated with tuberculosis are so uncommon, in view of this past experience. This combined syndrome apparently has been forgotten by many clinicians. The simultaneous occurrence of the two states generally leads to confusion.

In the current series six patients had active tuberculosis concomitant with autoimmune hemolytic anemia. In four of these patients an unequivocal relationship existed. In the two remaining cases pathologic states were present which distorted an etiologic relationship. One patient had Addisonian pernicious anemia, autoimmune hemolytic anemia and bilateral apical tuberculosis; acid fast organisms were found in the sputum (Case 81). A second patient had hemolytic anemia for 20 months, chronic pyelonephritis, a biologically false positive serology and a history of radiation treatment following carcinoma of the cervix. The patient died with widespread lymphohematogenous miliary tuberculosis and acute monocytic leukemia (Case 39).

In four patients an unequivocal relationship of autoimmune hemolytic anemia to tuberculosis was found. The infection was active in all and generally severe. One patient died with miliary tuberculosis, one had caseous pneumonia, one had a large open cavity and a fourth patient had previous miliary tuberculosis with active pulmonary tuberculosis and acid fast organisms in the sputum.

Case 51. A 62-year-old Negro male was diagnosed as having active pulmonary tuberculosis with positive sputum cultures. Streptomycin and isoniazid (INH) therapy was given with good results. Two years later the sputum was again found to contain acid fast organisms in multiple cultures. Extensive drug therapy was given with persistence of positive cultures. Ten months later a large open cavity was demonstrated. The hematocrit was 44 per cent. The liver, spleen and lymph nodes were not enlarged. Pulmonary lobectomy was decided upon. Routine preoperative blood cross matches revealed positive direct antiglobulin and bromelin tests. Elution identified a panhemagglutinin. Laboratory investigation demonstrated an hematocrit of 38 per cent, a reticulocyte count of 1.5 per cent, negative serologic tests for syphilis, a normal bone marrow, an A/G ratio of 4.8/2.8 gm. per cent and serum bilirubin of 0.7/0.8 mg. per cent. Lobectomy was performed and 3 units of blood were transfused without difficulty. Prednisone, 60 mg. per day, was given. This was rapidly decreased and finally discontinued 2 weeks later. The hematocrit progressively dropped to 34 per cent 1 month postoperatively, and then started to climb. Sputum cultures became negative and streptomycin and INH therapy was continued. Followup 19 months later demonstrated a hematocrit of 40 per cent, negative antiglobulin tests and positive direct and indirect bromelin tests. Elution revealed a panhemagglutinin which could be demonstrated in the antiglobulin procedure. No other disease state was apparent.

Case 52. A 56-year-old white male was investigated because of fatigue, weakness, productive cough, night sweats and a progressive weight loss of 40 pounds in 6 months. The liver was felt 4 cm. below the costal margin, but the spleen and lymph nodes were not palpated. Bilateral pleural effusions were found. Extensive bilateral caseous pneumonia was demonstrated with sputum cultures positive for tuberculosis. Urine cultures and cultures of the pleural effusion were negative. The hematocrit was 42 per cent and serologic tests for syphilis were negative. Streptomycin, INH and para-amino-salicylic acid therapy was given. After 5 months the sputum cultures were still positive and caseous pneumonia persisted. Thoracoplasty was decided upon. The hematocrit ranged from 38 to 42 per cent. Routine blood cross match studies were incompatible. Serologic investigation revealed positive direct antiglobulin and bromelin tests. Surgery was carried out and transfusions were given without difficulty. The sputum cultures became negative and persisted as negative for 27 months. During this time the hematocrit ranged from 44 to 50 per cent. Unfortunately no further antiglobulin or bromelin tests were performed. Twenty-seven months postoperatively a sputum culture was positive for acid fast organisms and normal hematologic

values were found. No other disease process was apparent. The patient was then lost to followup.

The above two patients presented similar clinical patterns. Active severe pulmonary tuberculosis was present. No evidence of other organ involvement was obtained. Antituberculous drug therapy was not successful. Nothing in the clinical course or routine hematologic studies suggested either hemolytic anemia and/or erythrocyte autoantibodies. Routine blood cross matches performed as a presurgical procedure uncovered the positive antiglobulin state. Surgery was performed and transfusions were given without difficulty. In the one case in which adequate followup was obtained, erythrocyte autoantibodies could be demonstrated 19 months later, although sputum cultures were then negative. In both cases the positive antiglobulin and bromelin tests were troublesome for the clinician. However, this did not influence the course of disease or therapy. The similarity of this sequence to that encountered in many patients with urinary tract infections is striking.

Not all examples of positive antiglobulin tests complicating active tuberculosis have a benign prognosis. The following two cases illustrate severe clinical courses.

Case 53. A 55-year-old white male developed miliary tuberculosis and was treated with streptomycin. One year later renal and testicular tuberculosis necessitated a nephrectomy. His course over the next 12 years was complicated by a fistula in ano and polyneuropathy. Periodic routine hematologic studies were negative. The patient eventually developed weakness, pallor, fever and jaundice. Hepatosplenomegaly and lymphadenopathy were not found. Several months prior to this episode the hematocrit was 43 per cent. It was now found to be 18 per cent with a 26 per cent reticulocyte count. Nucleated erythrocytes and spherocytes were seen in the peripheral blood and the WBC was 19,000/mm.^{3} Total bilirubin was 0.8/1.6 mg. per cent and the A/G ratio 3.5/3.0 gm. per cent. A broad gamma peak was found on electrophoresis which contained 34 per cent of the total protein. Six LE cell preparations were negative, as were serologic tests for syphilis. Bone marrow aspiration revealed erythrocytic hyperplasia with megaloblastic changes. Direct and indirect antiglobulin and bromelin tests were strongly positive; cold agglutinins and cryoglobulins were not found. Three blood transfusions were given with some febrile reactions. Prednisone therapy was initiated when the hematocrit reached 16.6 per cent and the reticulocyte count was 33 per cent. Four days later the hematocrit had risen and reached normal values in 7 weeks. Prednisone was decreased but maintained at 10 mg. daily. INH therapy was given. Active pulmonary tuberculosis with positive sputum cultures became apparent 5 months after the onset of hemolytic anemia and the start of prednisone therapy. The antiglobulin test had then reverted to normal. Sputum cultures became normal with antituberculous drug therapy. Prednisone was discontinued 5 months later. Followup 34 months after the onset of hemolytic anemia revealed an hematocrit of 48.5 per cent, 34 per cent eosinophiles and negative sputum cultures. No other disease process was apparent.

Case 54. A 57-year-old Negro male was first investigated because of chronic bronchitis and tender inguinal adenopathy. Physical examination, bronchograms, serologic tests for syphilis and hematologic values were normal. Over the next 2 years generalized adenopathy developed without hepatosplenomegaly. Acute migratory polyarthritis occurred, and polyarteritis and rheumatoid arthritis were considered but could not be diagnosed. Over the next 7 years undiagnosed intermittent acute arthritis occurred. Progressive pulmonary difficulties thought to be emphysema developed. A peptic ulcer was documented and subtotal gastrectomy was performed. Workup at this time revealed a hematocrit of 39 per cent, an A/G ratio of 3.1/5.1 gm. per cent and normal serologic tests for syphilis, bilirubin and urinalysis. Inguinal adenopathy of 2+ and a liver palpated at the costal margin were noted. Eighteen months later the patient entered with fatigue, jaundice and marked weight loss. The liver was 5 cm. below the costal margin and the spleen was palpated 2 cm. below the costal margin. Tender inguinal nodes of 3+ were found. The hematocrit was 24 per cent with a 2.2 per cent reticulocyte count. The A/G ratio was 2.4/6.2 gm. per cent and bilirubin was 6.5/1.1 gm. per cent. Serum electrophoresis revealed a broad gamma band encompassing 73 per cent of the total protein. Urinalysis demonstrated traces of protein, microscopic hematuria and pus cells. Bone marrow aspiration was normal except for an increased number of normal plasma cells. Direct antiglobulin and bromelin tests were strongly positive. Five units of blood were transfused but the hematocrit continued

to drop. Coma developed as jaundice deepened. The bilirubin reached 23.6/4.8 mg. per cent and the patient died in liver failure. Autopsy revealed pyelonephritis, postnecrotic cirrhosis and extensive, active miliary tuberculosis specifically involving the liver, spleen and lymph nodes.

These two patients had clinical courses which contrast strongly with those of the two previous cases of tuberculosis. Not only were positive antiglobulin tests obtained, but marked hemolytic anemia also developed. Both patients had extensive tuberculosis activity, with the miliary form noted in both. In Case 53, pulmonary tuberculosis might have been quiescent and positive sputum cultures may have been precipitated by corticosteroid therapy. In Case 54, the tuberculosis diagnosis was not apparent until autopsy; corticosteroids had not been given. It might be argued that postnecrotic cirrhosis or pyelonephritis was the basic pathologic state associated with autoimmune hemolytic anemia in this latter case. Although this cannot be refuted, the past history and autopsy indicate that miliary tuberculosis was the major pathologic abnormality. Necropsy revealed extensive miliary tuberculous lesions of the liver, spleen and lymph nodes.

Several other patients with autoimmune hemolytic anemia presented either an old tuberculous history or x-ray evidence of inactive tuberculosis. Neither an unequivocal nor possible relationship of such tuberculosis to autoimmune hemolytic anemia has been suggested. Active tuberculosis would appear to be a necessary postulate in the assumption of an etiologic relationship to positive antiglobulin tests and/or autoimmune hemolytic anemia. Fisher (118), however, found evidence of old tuberculosis in five of 11 random cases of acquired hemolytic anemia.

Acute Cholecystitis

Autoimmune hemolytic anemia was diagnosed in an etiologic relationship to acute cholecystitis in three patients. One patient had prostatic hypertrophy, urinary retention, pseudomonas cystitis and septicemia. Hemolytic anemia was not clinically apparent, although antiglobulin and bromelin tests were positive. Surgical correction of concomitant acute cholecystitis led to the reversal of positive antiglobulin and brome-lin tests in 4 days. In a second case acute cholecystitis developed in a patient with questionable rheumatoid arthritis and a nonfunctioning kidney. A persisting pseu-domonas urinary tract infection was also present. The patient had a reversed A/G ratio, a polyclonal broad gamma band on serum electrophoresis (41 per cent of total protein) and a normal bone marrow with benign plasma cell hyperplasia. Hepato-splenomegaly, 1+ axillary adenopathy and a palpable gall bladder were found. Anemia, leukopenia and positive antiglobulin tests were demonstrated. A chronic course re-sulted. Death occurred 15 months later af-ter a hysterectomy was performed. An undiagnosed systemic disease was probably present in this patient.

Case 55. A 50-year-old white female had a thyroidectomy performed for hyperthyroidism. Replacement thyroid therapy was given and maintained. Rheumatoid arthritis with mild activity had been present for several years. Five years later epigastric pain, nausea and vomiting developed. Over the next 2 months jaundice oc-curred. The liver, spleen and lymph nodes were not palpated, but the gall bladder was felt by some observers. The hematocrit of 44 per cent progressively dropped to 35 per cent. The re-ticulocyte count, WBC, serologic tests for syph-ilis, thymol turbidity, transaminase and A/G ratio were all normal. The bilirubin was 2.4/0.4 mg. per cent with elevated serum alkaline phos-phatase. Cholecystectomy was planned. Preop-erative workup revealed incompatible blood cross matches. Positive direct antiglobulin and bromelin tests were found. Elution identified a panhemagglutinin. In addition, the serum con-tained anti-Le^a and anti-P$_1$. Cholecystectomy was performed and a chronically infected gall bladder with stones was removed. Transfusions were not given. The hematocrit dropped to 32 per cent 2 weeks postoperatively, and intramus-cular iron was employed as the only therapy. The hematocrit rose progressively and appeared normal 5 weeks after surgery. The antiglobulin test became negative. Followup 6 months later revealed normal hematologic values.

The above protocol again illustrates a chronic infectious process which did not sug-gest the presence of either hemolytic anemia

or erythrocyte autoantibodies. Correction of the infectious process led to disappear-ance of the anemic state and to negative conversion of the positive antiglobulin test. Serologic investigation was initiated only because of incompatible blood cross matches performed preoperatively.

Meningitis

Two examples of bacterial meningitis in association with anemia and positive anti-globulin tests were seen in the current series. In one, a 6-month-old child developed *Haemophilus influenzae* meningitis. After recovery, bronchitis and otitis media devel-oped. A persistent low grade anemia became apparent. Hematologic workup 7 months after the development of meningitis re-vealed normal physical findings, a hemato-crit of 20.5 per cent, a reticulocyte count of 4.8 per cent and marked hypochromia of erythrocytes. Positive direct antiglobulin tests with negative bromelin tests were ob-tained. Iron therapy led to a rapid return toward normal of the hematocrit and disap-pearance of positive antiglobulin tests. The possibility that positive serologic tests were related to iron deficiency rather than to bac-terial meningitis must be considered. In sup-port of an infectious etiology is the observa-tion of Hagberg (119) that the erythrocytes of a child with *H. influenzae* meningitis had a shortened erythrocyte survival time. This hemolysis, however, may reflect the type of treatment rather than a direct effect of the microorganism (120).

In the second patient a much clearer re-lationship could be established.

Case 56. A male child was born with a menin-gomyelocele, congenital hydrocephalus and Ar-nold-Chiari malformations. A right-sided Halter valve was inserted. At age 18 months the patient was hospitalized with a fever of 105°F., otitis media and meningitis. Both the spleen and liver were palpated 5 cm. below the costal margin, and lymph nodes were palpated along the shunt. His previous hematocrit of 42 per cent (3 months earlier) had dropped to 22 per cent with a 1.2 per cent reticulocyte count. The WBC was 27,800/mm.^{3}, and thrombocytes, bilirubin and bone marrow examinations were normal. The erythrocytes appeared hypochromic and micro-cytic, but serum iron was elevated at 154 μg.

per cent. Protein of 3+ was found in the urine. Direct antiglobulin tests were positive on four occasions, with two negative bromelin tests. The Halter valve was removed and cultures demonstrated *Staphylococcus epidermidis*. Extensive antibiotic therapy was given. The hematocrit rose to 25 per cent with a 4.2 per cent reticulocyte count over the next 12 days. Oral iron therapy was started. The antiglobulin test became negative 1 week later. On followup examination 7 months later the hematocrit was 32 per cent. Hepatosplenomegaly and lymphadenopathy were then absent. The patient is alive 37 months after meningitis without any evidence of another disease process.

A clear association of *Staphylococcus epidermidis* meningitis, anemia and positive antiglobulin tests was seen in this patient. A hypochromic erythrocytic blood picture was found despite adequate serum iron. A similar observation was made in many of the patients having an associated bacterial infection and autoimmune hemolytic anemia. Correction of the infectious process led to improvement of anemia and negative conversion of positive antiglobulin tests.

Other Bacterial Infections

An extensive variety of infectious disease was encountered in an etiologic relationship to autoimmune hemolytic anemia. One patient had a continuous staphylococcal pyoderma, chronic anemia and consistently positive antiglobulin tests. This patient was an alcoholic, was infested with lice and had early Laennec's cirrhosis. The bone marrow revealed benign plasmacytosis. There was persistent eosinophilia in the peripheral blood. Death occurred 8 months after the onset of the hemolytic disease.

Pseudomonas septicemia occurred in one patient simultaneously with the development of positive antiglobulin tests. This patient has previously been mentioned as having urinary retention with pseudomonas cystitis and acute cholecystitis. The exact etiologic relationship to autoimmunization is not clear. Kissmeyer-Nielsen (65) has reported the development of hemolytic anemia in a patient with streptococcal septicemia. Septicemia was unfortunately common in patients of the current series with autoimmune hemolytic anemia. This complication

was found in 12 additional cases. In only two instances was a relationship to autoimmune hemolytic anemia considered possible. In nine of these cases an underlying neoplasia of the reticuloendothelium was present (four plasma cell myeloma, two Hodgkin's disease, two chronic lymphocytic leukemia, one acute lymphocytic leukemia). The remaining cases included two patients with scleroderma and one patient with a myeloproliferative syndrome. The responsible bacterial agents were staphylococci in four cases, *E. coli* in three cases, and pneumococci in three cases. In two patients the organism was not identified.

Thrombophlebitis has been noted to have a relationship to autoimmune hemolytic anemia by several investigators (121). Dacie (53) has also mentioned multiple embolization as a postoperative complication and cause of death. Both of these conditions were encountered in our patient population, although no specific cause and effect relationship between infected embolization, thromboses and autoimmune hemolytic anemia could be determined. Superficial vein thrombophlebitis was seen in five patients. This complication frequently was persistent, difficult to eradicate and likely to recur. Multiple pulmonary embolization was also seen in five patients. This generally occurred as a terminal event. One patient had idiopathic thrombocytosis with thrombocyte counts consistently over one million. Cases 22 and 29 describe the clinical course of two patients with embolization and autoimmune hemolytic anemia and Case 57 describes an example of complicating thrombophlebitis. Chronic lymphocytic leukemia, chronic granulocytic leukemia and an aspergillosis infection, respectively, were present in these three patients.

Several infectious states not seen in the current series have been reported by various investigators to be associated with autoimmune hemolytic anemia. Nussbaum and Dameshek (122) noted hemolytic anemia and thrombocytopenia in a patient with a meningococcal infection. Dacie (53) mentions a case of meningococcal septicemia complicated by a microangiopathic type of hemolytic anemia. This state possibly results from small blood vessel damage secondary to meningococcal endotoxin. Bedarida and associates (37) have emphasized a relationship between streptococcal focal infections and autoimmune hemolytic anemia. Beretta (59) has noted a similar relationship of focal tonsillitis to a hemolytic state. *Salmonella typhi* has been implicated by many investigators in a hemolytic state characterized by positive antiglobulin tests. The reports of Shaw (123), Gordon Smith (124), McFadzean and Choa (32), Ruggieri (33) and Retief and Hofmeyer (113) should be consulted. Grobbelaar (112) found positive antiglobulin tests in 30 of 100 blood samples obtained from patients suspected of having typhoid fever. Other Salmonella organisms have been similarly associated with autoimmune hemolytic anemia. *Salmonella dublin* (111), *Salmonella aertrycke* (53) and a Salmonella infection associated with polyarthritis (34) have all been reported.

Yeast and Fungus Infections

Moniliasis

Moniliasis was commonly encountered in the current series. This is not unexpected in a group of patients with severe illness. The use of corticosteroid therapy, immunosuppressive drugs and marrow depressing chemotherapy magnifies this problem. In addition, the large number of cases with neoplasia of the reticuloendothelium supplies a population likely to develop monilia infections. Although monilia infections were frequently encountered, they were of major clinical significance in only seven cases. In none of these patients could an unequivocal or possible relationship to autoimmune hemolytic anemia be determined. One patient (Case 42) was born with systemic moniliasis, developed juvenile diabetes and had multiple infectious problems. Autoimmune hemolytic anemia occurred soon after a severe herpes zoster infection. Both moniliasis and autoimmune hemolytic anemia have persisted in a chronic stage. The remaining six patients all had neoplasia of the reticuloendothelium and received extensive chemotherapy. Visceral moniliasis was present in four of these patients. The relatively insidious development of moniliasis made it impossible to determine an accurate relationship to the onset of autoimmune hemolytic anemia.

Fungus Infections

Only one case of a fungus infection associated with autoimmune hemolytic anemia was seen in the current series.

Case 57. A 45-year-old white male developed fatigue, fever, hematuria and purpura. Physical examination was negative. The hematocrit was 33 per cent, the reticulocyte count was 1.2 per cent, the WBC was 3,800/mm.^{3} and the thrombocyte count was 12,000/mm.^{3} The bone marrow appeared somewhat hypocellular, with decreased megakaryocytes and erythrocytic hyperplasia. Prednisone therapy was given with a continuation of bleeding and persistent thrombocytopenia. One month later a pulmonary lesion was noted and sputum and bronchoscopy cultures revealed *Aspergillus fumigatus*. Amphotericin therapy was initiated. In spite of this the fungal pneumonia progressed over the next month. Pursfucin was started, with gradual improvement of the pneumonic process during the next 2 months. Thrombocytopenia and bleeding persisted. Six months after the onset of disease the hematocrit had dropped to 19 per cent in spite of 14 units of blood administered in the last 3 months. The reticulocyte count was 3.6 per cent, a spleen tip was palpated by one observer and the direct antiglobulin test was weakly positive. Over the next 8 months the direct antiglobulin test was positive on three occasions and negative on seven occasions. Direct bromelin tests were all negative. Elution was unsuccessful. The patient's course was complicated by thrombophlebitis. Without specific therapy the hematocrit attained levels of 35 per cent with reticulocyte counts as high as 6.8 per cent. Thrombocyte counts reached 64,000/mm.^{3} and the WBC reached 11,000/mm.^{3} Recurrence of aspergillosis pneumonia occurred 9 months after the onset of disease. This again responded to Pursfucin therapy. Over the next year the patient continued to have recurrent episodes of purpura, thrombocytopenia and anemia with hematocrits ranging from 23 to 35 per cent. Leukopenia was not a problem. Death occurred 23 months after the onset of disease with thrombocytopenia, bleeding and infection.

The above patient has been classified as having an Evans' syndrome type of idiopathic autoimmune hemolytic anemia. It is difficult to determine exactly what relationship, if any, exists between the aspergillosis infection and the autoimmune process. Thrombocytopenia occurred 1 month prior to demonstration of fungal pneumonitis. However, fever and the bone marrow findings were not typical of idiopathic thrombocytopenic purpura. It is probable that aspergillosis was already present. An alternative explanation must be considered. Corticosteroid therapy may have activated the fungus infection and aided in establishing its chronic course. As such, the infection may be unrelated to the primary disease state.

Parasitic Infestations

In the current series of patients with autoimmune hemolytic anemia, parasitic infestation was neither encountered nor searched for. This is not surprising as our geographic area is remarkably free from such infections. In view of the association of other infectious diseases with autoimmune hemolytic anemia, however, it appeared to be important to study such a possible relationship. Dr. Robert L. Cella of the Permanente Medical Group, Oakland, California, recently encountered a case of *Strongyloides stercoralis* infection associated with positive antiglobulin tests. The following case is presented through his courtesy.

Case 58. A 29-year-old Philippino was diagnosed as having a peptic ulcer. He had recurrent abdominal distress. The patient revisited the Philippines at age 47 and upon return to Oakland developed diarrhea. At age 51 melena occurred and a weight loss of 5 pounds was noted. He entered the hospital complaining of weakness and dizziness. Physical examination was normal. The hematocrit was 21 per cent, the reticulocyte count was 7.8 per cent and the WBC and thrombocytes were normal. The erythrocytes appeared hypochromic and a 17 per cent eosinophilia was found. Urinalysis, creatinine, A/G ratio, Bromsulphalein, serum glutamic oxalacetic transaminase, LE cell preparations, latex fixation and antinuclear antibodies were all normal. The initial bilirubin was 0.2/0.6 mg. per cent and this rose to 0.1/1.1 mg. per cent. The Venereal Disease Research

Laboratory (VDRL) test for syphilis was weakly reactive and the Kolmer test was nonreactive. The direct antiglobulin test was 4+ and indirect tests were negative. Repeat direct antiglobulin tests were consistently positive with erythrocytes obtained from the bottom and top of centrifuged specimens. The patient's stools were strongly guaiac positive and large numbers of larvae of *Strongyloides stercoralis* were found. X-ray studies did not reveal any abnormalities of the upper or lower gastrointestinal tract. The hematocrit dropped to 18 per cent and 4 units of blood were transfused without difficulties. Thiabendazole (Mintezol) therapy was initiated. After the first course of therapy *Strongyloides stercoralis* larvae were absent in casual stool specimens, but were found in concentrated preparations. A second course of thiabendazole converted subsequent stool specimens to normal. The VDRL test became nonreactive, but direct antiglobulin tests persisted as 2+. The patient's hematocrit progressively rose and ranged at 44 per cent. Eosinophilia has disappeared. Follow-up is continuing 22 months since the first demonstration of the parasite. Positive antiglobulin tests and normal hematologic values are present.

The above case clearly demonstrates the presence of positive antiglobulin tests associated with severe parasitic infestation of the gastrointestinal tract. Because of the blood loss it is difficult to determine whether hemolytic anemia also occurred. Eradication of the parasitic infection resulted in symptomatic improvement, cessation of gastrointestinal bleeding and correction of the anemic state. A weakly reactive VDRL test was converted to a nonreactive state. The antiglobulin test, however, has remained positive although less strong. Followup 22 months after onset has not revealed any underlying pathologic state which could be related to the development of a positive antiglobulin test. Dr. Cella suggests that the patient has an abnormal circulating erythrocyte autoantibody, unrelated to parasitic infestation, creating persisting positive antiglobulin tests. The strong antiglobulin reactions encountered during active parasitic infection could result from an increased production of all types of globulin. Although this explanation of a fortuitous occurrence is possible, other suggestions may be made. Products released from the parasite may initiate an antiglobulin positive immunohemolytic anemia. Such products may also cross react with human erythrocyte antigens, leading to a termination of tolerance and true autoimmunization. As such, mechanisms similar to those theorized in Chapter 14 for other infectious agents may have been involved in this case.

Summary of Autoimmune Hemolytic Anemia Related to Infectious Disease

The reader who has struggled through the large number of case histories presented in this chapter must be complimented for his tenacity. He has undoubtedly been left with an impression of a confusing spectrum of heterogeneous clinical states somewhat tenuously related by positive antiglobulin tests. The author must confess to a similar feeling of confusion. These data require several interpretations in order to clarify the status of autoimmune hemolytic anemia complicated by infectious disease.

1. Infectious disease immediately preceding or occurring during the course of autoimmune hemolytic anemia is common. In some instances the onset of infection and the clinical course of the patient leave little doubt that an unequivocal cause and effect etiologic relation exists. In other cases a possible etiologic role may be present. In most instances no direct relationship can be documented with our current testing procedures.

2. The clinical course of patients with infectious disease and positive antiglobulin tests is highly variable. Several characteristic patterns were observed. An infectious disease may lead to the explosive onset of autoimmune hemolytic anemia. A severe clinical course with rapid and complete recovery may follow. This sequence simulates what has been described as Lederer-Brill's anemia and generally involves a virus infection in the young. Bacterial infections may also occur in a manner to suggest an unequivocal relationship of infection, hemolytic anemia and positive antiglobulin tests. The onset of the hemolytic state is generally more gradual and convalescence is more prolonged than is the case with virus disease. There is some evidence, which is only suggestive at this time, that yeast, fungi and parasitic worms may be involved in a similar relationship.

3. In contrast to patients presenting the triad of infection, hemolytic anemia and positive antiglobulin tests, another clinical relationship was observed. In this syndrome infectious disease occurs in a close temporal sequence with the development of positive antiglobulin tests. However, a hemolytic state is equivocal and anemia may not even be present. The author has reluctantly called these cases "autoimmune hemolytic anemia" although they may not be autoimmune, hemolytic or even anemic. The difficulty that the immunohematologist has in ignoring a positive antiglobulin test is apparent. In the current series patients with bacterial infections constituted the majority of such cases. Urinary tract infections and tuberculosis appeared prominent in this group. In many instances anemia was not documented and positive antiglobulin tests were discovered only during preoperative blood cross matches. Positive antiglobulin tests frequently reverted to negative after surgical correction of abnormalities which predisposed to persistence of the infectious state. In several instances when anemia was present, a hypochromic, microcytic pattern was found, suggesting iron deficiency. Serum iron values generally were normal or elevated, and anemia was corrected as the infection was eliminated. Iron therapy was generally given to such patients, and it is accordingly difficult to evaluate the relationship of the antiglobulin test to the anemic state. The deficiency of a retrospective analysis immediately becomes apparent in this area. Critical testing of erythrocyte survival time was not performed and the presence of hemolysis is problematical.

4. A large variety of different infectious agents was encountered in the cases reported in the current series. Even with the same agent, e.g., infectious mononucleosis or tuberculosis, wide variations in the clinical course were apparent. Heterogeneity in the clinical state appeared as the summation of a large number of infectious agents and their individual capability of inducing var-

iable degrees of hemolytic anemia. None of the infectious agents presented a specific clinical pattern predisposing to the development of autoimmune hemolytic anemia.

5. Patients with a significant complicating infection constitute an important etiologic subgroup of all cases of autoimmune hemolytic anemia. However, autoimmune hemolytic anemia complicating infection is still rare. This may be appreciated when compared to the frequency of infection due to the same organisms described above in any large general hospital. The investigator must ask why antiglobulin tests are positive in some cases and not in others.

6. The clinical and laboratory heterogeneity seen strongly suggests that different pathophysiologic mechanisms are involved. At least four major relationships may be postulated. In some cases the relationship is fortuitous. In others the normal erythrocyte is probably not the target for the immunologic event. Innocent bystander states, the adsorption of immune complexes and complement, cross reacting antibodies and modification of autologous erythrocyte antigens can occur and result in an antiglobulin positive hemolytic anemia. The similarity is striking between the type of organisms encountered in our patients and those theoretically predictable as involving the erythrocyte in an immune but not autoimmune relationship (see Chapter 14). A third relationship may be truly autoimmune with a possible termination of tolerance occurring secondary to infectious organisms. In other cases an aberrant immune apparatus may lead to both infectious disease and autoimmune states in an immunodeficient individual.

7. The combination of the above listed variables (a large number of different infectious agents, the variability of such agents, different pathophysiologic mechanisms through which such agents may induce an antiglobulin positive state) creates clinical heterogeneity. Clinical observations are currently the only available tool to study this phenomenon. New laboratory diagnostic methods for analyzing this relationship are desperately needed. Future studies should clarify the various connections between infectious disease and autoimmune hemolytic anemia.

BIBLIOGRAPHY

1. Hayem, G.: Sur une variété particulière d'ictère chronique. Ictère infectieux chronique splénomégalique. Presse Med. **6**: 121, 1898.
2. Macintosh, A. H., and Cleland, J. B.: A case of rapidly increasing anaemia with irregular pyrexia and death. Aust. Med. Gaz. **21**: 422, 1902.
3. Widal, F., Abrami, P., and Brulé, M.: Pluralité d'origine des ictères hémolytiques: recherches cliniques et experimentales. Bull. Soc. Hop. Paris **24**: 1354, 1907.
4. Gaucher, and Giroux, Ann. Mal. Vener. **251**: 1910. Quoted by Tileston, W.: Medicine (Balt.) **1**: 355, 1922.
5. de Beurmann, Bith, and Cain, Bull. Soc. Med. Hos. Paris **30**: 636, 1910. Quoted by Tileston, W.: Medicine (Balt.) **1**: 355, 1922.
6. Tileston, W.: Hemolytic jaundice. Medicine (Balt.) **1**: 355, 1922.
7. Lederer, M.: A form of acute hemolytic anemia probably of infectious origin. Amer. J. Med. Sci. **170**: 500, 1925.
8. Lederer, M.: Three additional cases of acute hemolytic (infectious) anemia. Amer. J. Med. Sci. **179**: 228, 1930.
9. Brill, I. C.: Acute febrile anemia—a new disease. Arch. Intern. Med. (Chicago) **37**: 244, 1926.
10. Giordano, A. S., and Blum, L. L.: Acute hemolytic anemia (Lederer's type). Amer. J. Med. Sci. **194**: 311, 1937.
11. Watson, C. J.: Hemolytic jaundice and macrocytic hemolytic anemia: certain observations in a series of 35 cases. Ann. Intern. Med. **12**: 1782, 1939.
12. Singer, K., and Dameshek, W.: Symptomatic hemolytic anemia. Ann. Intern. Med. **15**: 544, 1941.
13. Dameshek, W., and Schwartz, S. O.: The presence of hemolysins in acute hemolytic anemia; preliminary note. New Eng. J. Med. **218**: 75, 1938.
14. Dameshek, W., and Schwartz, S. O.: Acute hemolytic anemia (acquired hemolytic icterus, acute type). Medicine (Balt.) **19**: 231, 1940.
15. Kracke, R. R.: *Diseases of the Blood and Atlas of Hematology.* J. B. Lippincott Company, Philadelphia, 1941.
16. Davis, L. J.: Haemolytic anaemias. Edinburgh Med. J. **50**: 589, 1943.
17. Zuckerman, A.: Autoimmunization and other types of indirect damage to host cells as factors in certain protozoan diseases. Exp. Parasit. **15**: 138, 1964.
18. Adner, M. M., Altstatt, L. B., and Conrad, M. E.: Coombs-positive hemolytic disease in malaria. Ann. Intern. Med. **68**: 33, 1968.

19. Zuelzer, W. W.: Infantile toxoplasmosis, with a report of three new cases, including two in which the patients were identical twins. Arch. Path. (Chicago) **38**: 1, 1944.

20. Bain, A. D., Bowie, J. H., Flint, W. F., Beverley, J. K. A., and Beattie, C. P.: Congenital toxoplasmosis simulating hemolytic disease of the newborn. J. Obstet. Gynaec. Brit. Emp. **63**: 826, 1956.

21. Nelson, L. G., and Hodgman, J. E.: Congenital toxoplasmosis with hemolytic anemia. Calif. Med. **105**: 454, 1966.

22. Burchenal, J. H., Bowers, R. F., and Haedicke, T. A.: Visceral leishmaniasis complicated by severe anemia: improvement following splenectomy. Amer. J. Trop. Med. **27**: 699, 1947.

23. Rachmilewitz, M., DeVries, A., and Gurevitch, G.: Further observations on the anaemia in kala-azar. Acta Haemat. (Basel) **7**: 179, 1952.

24. Martins, J. M., Alencar, J. E., and de Magalhães, V. B.: The anemia of kala-azar. Rev. Inst. Med. Trop. S. Paulo **7**: 47, 1965.

25. Ricketts, W. E.: *Bartonella bacilliformis* anemia (Oroya fever). A study of 30 cases. Blood **3**: 1025, 1948.

26. Weinman, D.: Infectious anemias due to Bartonella and related red cell parasites. Bull. N. Y. Acad. Med. **22**: 647, 1946.

27. Bull, C. G., and Pritchett, J. W.: Toxin and antitoxin of and protective inoculation against *Bacillus welchii*. J. Exp. Med. **26**: 117, 1917.

28. Draper, G., and Barach, A.: Studies on experimental anemias: effects on rabbits of infection of hemolytic toxin of Welch bacillus. J. Clin. Invest. **4**: 507, 1927.

29. Isham, R. L., and Finch, S. G.: Postabortal *Clostridium welchii* with massive hemolysis: report of a case. New Eng. J. Med. **254**: 317, 1956.

30. Bennet, J. M., and Healey, P. J. M.: Spherocytic hemolytic anemia and acute cholecystitis caused by *Clostridium welchii*. New Eng. J. Med. **268**: 1070, 1963.

31. Davis, L. J.: Symptomatic haemolytic anaemia. Edinburgh Med. J. **51**: 70, 1944.

32. McFadzean, A. J. S., and Choa, G. H.: Haemolytic anaemia in typhoid fever. Brit. Med. J. **2**: 360, 1953.

33. Ruggieri, P. A.: Hemolytic anemia in typhoid fever. Delaware Med. J. **33**: 77, 1961.

34. McCormick, J. S., and Micks, R. H.: Anaemia of haemolytic type and polyarthritis caused by Salmonella infection. Irish J. Med. Sci. **429**: 421, 1961.

35. De, S. N., Sengupta, K. P., and Chanda, N. N.: Intravascular hemolysis in cholera. Lancet **1**: 807, 1954.

36. Kissmeyer-Nielsen, F.: A case of autoimmune haemolytic anaemia with a very remarkable course. Vox Sang. **2**: 88, 1957.

37. Bedarida, G., Bernasconi, C., and Pollini, G.: On the relations between streptococcal focal infections and auto-immune hemolytic anemia (study on 4 cases). Haematologica **46**: 1085, 1961.

38. Fuà, C.: Anemia emolitica acuta, successiva ad infezione streptococcica, guarita con splenectomia. Minerva Med. **52**: 323, 1961.

39. Gasser, C.: *Die hämolytischer Syndrome in Kindersalter.* Georg Thieme Verlag KG., Stuttgart, 1951.

40. Stratton, F.: Erythrocyte anti-bodies and autoimmunity. Lancet **2**: 626, 1963.

41. Shumway, C. N.: Spherocytic hemolytic anemia associated with acute pneumococcal infection in rabbits. J. Lab. Clin. Med. **51**: 240, 1958.

42. Dameshek, W.: Cold hemagglutinins in acute hemolytic reactions in association with sulfonamide medication and infection. J. A. M. A. **123**: 77, 1943.

43. Finland, M., and Barnes, M. W.: Cold agglutinins. Arch. Intern. Med. (Chicago) **101**: 462, 1958.

44. Laroche, C., Milliez, P., Dreyfus, B., Dausset, J., and Leprat, J.: Ictère hémolytique aigu post-grippal. Bull. Soc. Med. Hop. Paris **67**: 779, 1951.

45. Dausset, J., and Colombani, J.: The serology and the prognosis of 128 cases of autoimmune hemolytic anemia. Blood **14**: 1280, 1959.

46. Puxeddu, A., Colonna, A., Nenci, G. G., et al.: Su di un raro caso di anemia emolitica autoimmune da virus influenzale B. Haematologica **50**: 1073, 1965.

47. Hennemann, H., Möller, H., and Gillert, K. E.: Nach Hepatitis Epidemica erworbener hämolytischer Ikterus mit positivem Coombs Test. Klin. Wschr. **30**: 809, 1952.

48. Moolten, S. E., Clark, E., Glasser, M. F., Katz, E., and Mitler, B. S.: Blood stream invasion by Newcastle disease virus associated with hemolytic anemia and encephalopathy. Report of three cases. Amer. J. Med. **14**: 294, 1953.

49. Todd, R. M., and O'Donohoe, W. V.: Acute acquired haemolytic anaemia associated with herpes simplex infection. Arch. Dis. Child. **33**: 524, 1958.

50. Zuelzer, W. W., Stulberg, C. S., Page, R. H., Teruya, J., and Brough, A. J.: The etiology and pathogenesis of acquired hemolytic anemia. Transfusion **6**: 438, 1966.

51. Betke, K., Richarz, H., Schubothe, H., and Vivell, O.: Beobachtungen zu Krankheitsbild Pathogenese und Ätiologie der akuten erworbenen hämolytischen Anämie (Lederer-Anämie). Klin. Wschr. **31**: 373, 1953.

52. Vivell, O.: Ergebnisse virologischer Studien bei Fällen von akuter häemolytischer Anämie (Lederer-Brill). Mschr. Kinderheilk. **102**: 113, 1954.

53. Dacie, J. V.: *The Haemolytic Anaemias, Part II*, Ed. 2. Grune & Stratton, Inc., New York, 1962.
54. Borbolla, L., and Barquetchediak, A.: Anemia hemolítica de etiología viral (revisión de la literatura). Presentación de un caso en la convalescencia de una varicela con Coombs positivo. Rev. Cubana Pediat. **25**: 557, 1953.
55. Horowitz, H. I., Javid, J., and Spaet, T. H.: Lederer's anemia accompanying urinary tract infections. Amer. J. Dis. Child. **99**: 757, 1960.
56. Githens, J. H., and Hathaway, W. E.: Autoimmune hemolytic anemia and the syndrome of hemolytic anemia, thrombocytopenia and nephropathy. Pediat. Clin. N. Amer. **9**: 619, 1962.
57. Giesy, J. D., Pirofsky, B., and Hodges, C. V.: Positive antiglobulin reactions complicating urological surgery. J. Urol. **95**: 809, 1966.
58. Wasikowa, R., and Wilkomerska-Kajetanowicz, J.: Four cases of acquired hemolytic anemia of infectious etiology with different clinical courses. Pediat. Pol. **36**: 969, 1961.
59. Beretta, L.: Rapporti tra anemia emolitica autoimmune e tonsillite cronica focale. Considerazioni su cinque casi clinici. Arch. Ital. Otol. **75**: 78, 1964.
60. Pirofsky, B.: Autoimmune hemolytic anemia and neoplasia of the reticuloendothelium. With a hypothesis concerning etiologic relationships. Ann. Intern. Med. **68**: 109, 1968.
61. MacFarlane, R. G., Oakley, C. C., and Anderson, C. G.: Haemolysis and production of opalescence in serum and lecitho-vitillin by alpha toxin of *Clostridium welchii*. J. Path. Bact. **52**: 99, 1941.
62. Dameshek, W.: Theories of antibody production. In *Conceptual Advances in Immunology and Oncology*. Hoeber Medical Division, Harper & Row, Publishers, New York, 1963.
63. Kölbl, H.: Klinik und Therapie der akuten erworbenen hämolytischen Anämien im Kindesalter. Ostdeutsch. Z. Kinderheilk. **11**: 27, 1955.
64. Neimann, N., Michon, P., Pierson, M., and Lascombes, G.: L'anémie hémolytique acquise par auto-anticorps chez le nourrisson. Arch. Franc. Pediat. **13**: 247, 1956.
65. Kissmeyer-Nielsen, F.: Specific auto-antibodies in immunohaemolytic anaemia. With a note on the pathogenesis of autoimmunization. In *P. H. Anderson, Papers in Dedication of his Sixtieth Birthday*. Einar Munksgaard, Forlag, Copenhagen, 1957.
66. Wuilleret, B.: L'anémie hémolytique acquise par autoanticorps de l'enfant C. P. étudiée à la lumière des tests immunohémolytiques érythrocytaires. Helv. Paediat. Acta **13**: 140, 1958.
67. Dionigi, R.: Sindromi emolitiche in corso di affezioni virali. Riv. Pat. Clin. **15**: 657, 1961.
68. Green, N., and Goldenberg, H.: Acute hemolytic anemia and hemoglobinuria complicating infectious mononucleosis. Arch. Intern. Med. (Chicago) **105**: 108, 1960.
69. Wilson, S. J., Ward, C. E., and Gray, L. W.: Infectious lymphadenosis (mononucleosis) and hemolytic anemia in a Negro; recovery following splenectomy. Blood **4**: 189, 1949.
70. Appleman, D. H., and Morrison, M. M.: Concomitant infectious mononucleosis and hemolytic anemia. Blood **4**: 186, 1949.
71. Punt, K., and Verloop, M. C.: Een Geval van acute haemolytische Anaemie bij Mononucleosis infectiosa. Nederl. T. Geneesk. **99**: 3128, 1955.
72. Thurm, R. H., and Bassen, F.: Infectious mononucleosis and acute hemolytic anemia; report of two cases and review of the literature. Blood **10**: 841, 1955.
73. Evans, R. S., and Weiser, R. S.: The serology of auto-immune hemolytic disease: observations on forty-one patients. Arch. Intern. Med. (Chicago) **100**: 371, 1957.
74. Bean, R. H. D.: Haemolytic anaemia complicating infectious mononucleosis, with report of a case. Med. J. Aust. **1**: 386, 1957.
75. DiPiero, G., and Arcangeli, A.: Anemia emolitica acquisata con auto-anticorpi incompleti a freddo in corso di mononucleosi infettiva. Haematologica **43**: 91, 1958.
76. Sawitsky, A., Papps, J. P., and Wiener, L. M.: The demonstration of antibody in acute hemolytic anemia complicating infectious mononucleosis. Amer. J. Med. **8**: 260, 1950.
77. Huntington, P. W.: Hemolytic anemia in infectious mononucleosis. A case report. Delaware Med. J. **23**: 165, 1951.
78. Samuels, M. L.: Hemolytic anemia complicating infectious mononucleosis. Report of three cases. U. S. Armed Forces Med. J. **4**: 1778, 1953.
79. Hall, B. D., and Archer, F. C.: Acute hemolytic anemia associated with infectious mononucleosis. New Eng. J. Med. **249**: 973, 1953.
80. Crosby, W. H., and Rappaport, H.: Reticulocytopenia in autoimmune hemolytic anemia. Blood **11**: 929, 1956.
81. Fordham, C. C.: Acute hemolytic anemia complicating infectious mononucleosis. U. S. Armed Forces Med. J. **7**: 98, 1956.
82. Wasserman, L. R., Stats, D., Schwartz, L., and Fudenberg, H.: Symptomatic and hemopathic hemolytic anemia. Amer. J. Med. **18**: 961, 1955.
83. Hortemo, T.: Hemolytisk anemi ved mononucleosis infectiosa. Nord. Med. **59**: 468, 1958.
84. Perrier, C. V., and Rousso, C.: Un cas de mononucléose infectieuse avec anémie hé-

molytique et test de Coombs positif. Schweiz. Med. Wschr. **89**: 766, 1959.

85. Smith, D. S., Abell, J. D., and Cast, I. P.: Auto-immune haemolytic anaemia and thrombocytopenia complicating infectious mononucleosis. Brit. Med. J. **1**: 1210, 1963.

86. Fekete, A. M., and Kerpelman, E. J.: Acute hemolytic anemia complicating infectious mononucleosis. J. A. M. A. **194**: 1326, 1965.

87. Berté, S. J.: Acute hemolytic anemia in infectious mononucleosis. New York Med. J. **51**: 781, 1951.

88. Ellis, L. B., Wollenman, O. J., and Stetson, R. P.: Autohemagglutinins and hemolysins with hemoglobinuria and acute hemolytic anemia in an illness resembling infectious mononucleosis. Blood **3**: 419, 1948.

89. Mermann, A. C.: Acute hemolytic anemia with infectious mononucleosis. U. S. Armed Forces Med. J. **3**: 1551, 1952.

90. Kostinas, J. E., and Cantow, E. F.: Studies on infectious mononucleosis. II. Autohemolysis. Amer. J. Med. Sci. **252**: 296, 1966.

91. Rosenfield, R. E., Schmidt, P. J., Calvo, R. C., and McGinniss, M. H.: Anti-i, a frequent cold agglutinin in infectious mononucleosis. Vox Sang. **10**: 631, 1965.

92. Jenkins, W. J., Koster, H. G., Marsh, W. L., and Carter, R. L.: Infectious mononucleosis: an unsuspected source of anti-i. Brit. J. Haemat. **11**: 480, 1965.

93. Calvo, R., Stein, W., Kochwa, S., and Rosenfield, R. E.: Acute hemolytic anemia due to anti-i: frequent cold agglutinins in infectious mononucleosis. J. Clin. Invest. **44**: 1033, 1965.

94. Wollheim, F. A., and Williams, R. C.: Studies on the macroglobulins of human serum. 1. Polyclonal immunoglobulin class M (IgM) increase in infectious mononucleosis. New Eng. J. Med. **274**: 61, 1966.

95. Troxel, D. B., Innella, F., and Cohen, R. J.: Infectious mononucleosis complicated by hemolytic anemia due to anti-i. Amer. J. Clin. Path. **46**: 625, 1966.

96. Ottaviani, P., Mandelli, F., and Deriu, L.: Porpora trombocitopenica acuta da autoanticorpi in corso di rosolia. Policlinico (Prat.) **71**: 1250, 1964.

97. Dameshek, W., and Schwartz, R.: Hemolytic mechanisms. Ann. N. Y. Acad. Sci. **77**: 589, 1959.

98. Zuelzer, W. W., Stulberg, C. S., and Page, R. H.: Demonstration of recurrent cytomegalic inclusion virus disease in the etiology and mechanism of autoimmune hemolytic anemia. Blood **24**: 841, 1964.

99. Becker, F. P., and Eddy, J. R.: Auto-immune hemolytic anemia with terminal lymphomas and cytomegalic inclusion disease. New York J. Med. **64**: 1211, 1964.

100. Pirofsky, B.: Serologic and clinical findings in autoimmune hemolytic anemia. Series Haem. **9**: 47, 1965.

101. Mongan, E. S., Kern, W. A., and Terry, R.: Hypogammaglobulinemia with thymoma, hemolytic anemia, and disseminated infection with cytomegalovirus. Ann. Intern. Med. **65**: 548, 1966.

102. Wong, T. W., and Warner, N. E.: Cytomegalic inclusion disease in adults. Arch. Path. (Chicago) **74**: 403, 1962.

103. Beickert, A., and Sprössig, M.: Immunhämotologische und virologisch-serologische Beobachtungen bei erworbener hämolytischer Anämie im Verlaufe einer "asiatischen" Grippe. Klin. Wschr. **37**: 146, 1959.

104. d'Oelsnitz, M., Vincent, L., and Lippmann, C.: Ictère hémolytique et hémoglobinurie d'origine grippale. Arch. Franc. Pediat. **16**: 391, 1959.

105. Springer, G. F., and Ansell, N. J.: Inactivation of human erythrocyte agglutinogens M and N by influenza viruses and receptor-destroying enzyme. Proc. Nat. Acad. Sci. U. S. A. **44**: 182, 1958.

106. Moolten, S. E., and Clark, E.: Viremia in acute hemolytic anemia and in autohemagglutination. Arch. Intern. Med. (Chicago) **89**: 270, 1952.

107. Moolten, S. E., and Clark, E.: The red blood cell as a vehicle of virus transport. II. Role of blood-borne viruses in autohemagglutination and in hemolytic anemia. Trans. N. Y. Acad. Sci. **14**: 235, 1952.

108. Griffin, H. Z.: Tuberculosis of the spleen. Med. Clin. N. Amer. **3**: 765, 1919.

109. Engelbreth-Holm, J.: Study of tuberculous splenomegaly and splenogenic controlling of cell emission from bone marrow. Amer. J. Med. Sci. **195**: 32, 1938.

110. Howells, L.: Tuberculous splenomegaly. Brit. J. Tuberc. **33**: 178, 1939.

111. Davidson, L. S. P., and Fullerton, H. W.: Some rare types of macrocytic anaemia. Quart. J. Med. **7**: 43, 1938.

112. Grobbelaar, B. G.: Auto-sensitization of red blood cells in various diseases with particular reference to the pathogenesis of haemolytic anaemia. (thesis). University of Witwatersrand, 1958.

113. Retief, F. P., and Hofmeyer, N. G.: Acute haemolytic anaemia as a complication of typhoid fever. S. Afr. Med. J. **39**: 96, 1965.

114. Thompson, W. P.: Hemolytic jaundice. Its diagnosis, behavior and treatment: a review of forty-five cases. J. A. M. A. **107**: 1776, 1936.

115. Guszich, A.: Hämolytische Krisen verusachende "isolierte" Milztuberculose. Beitr. Klin. Chir. **195**: 372, 1957.

116. Boyden, S. V.: Fixation of bacterial products by erythrocytes *in vivo* and by leucocytes. Nature (London) **171**: 402, 1953.

117. Boyden, S. V., and Andersen, M. E.: Agglutination of normal erythrocytes in mixtures of antibody and antigen, and haemolysis in the presence of complement. Brit. J. Exp. Path. **36**: 162, 1955.

118. Fisher, J. A.: The cryptogenic acquired haemolytic anaemias. Quart. J. Med. **16**: 245, 1947.

119. Hagberg, B.: Hyperhemolysis following septic conditions in children (a preliminary report). Acta Soc. Med. Upsal. **56**: 273, 1951–1952.

120. Margolis, J.: Haemolytic anaemia in *Haemophilus influenzae* meningitis treated with specific rabbit serum. Med. J. Aust. **1**: 912, 1955.

121. Young, L. E., Miller, G., and Christian, R. M.: Clinical and laboratory observations on autoimmune hemolytic disease. Ann. Intern. Med. **35**: 507, 1951.

122. Nussbaum, M., and Dameshek, W.: Transient hemolytic and thrombocytopenic episode (? acute transient thrombohemolytic thrombocytopenic purpura), with probable meningococcemia. Report of a case. New Eng. J. Med. **256**: 448, 1957.

123. Shaw, A. B.: Haemoglobinuria in typhoid fever. Report of two cases. Lancet **2**: 813, 1951.

124. Gordon Smith, C. E.: Haemoglobinuria in typhoid fever treated with Chloramphenicol. Lancet **2**: 1020, 1951.

Chapter 8

Collagen Diseases, Diseases of Hypersensitivity and Autoimmune Hemolytic Anemia

Historical Concepts

At the turn of the century it became apparent that immunologic processes could lead to systemic disease. Anaphylaxis and serum sickness appeared as the prototype of immunologically mediated clinical syndromes (1). The possibility was considered that similar immunologic mechanisms might be involved etiologically in various idiopathic systemic human diseases. Evidence gradually accumulated that disease processes characterized by angiitis involved anaphylactic hypersensitivity. These syndromes differed from classical anaphylaxis and serum sickness because it was not possible to demonstrate foreign antigens responsible for hypersensitivity.

Klinge (2) in 1933 utilized the concepts of allergy and hypersensitivity to derive the pathogenesis of various rheumatoid diseases. He emphasized that fibrinoid degeneration of collagen was present in rheumatism. This resembled hypersensitivity responses in rabbits exposed to foreign proteins. Rich (3), on the basis of pathologic similarities, conceived of anaphylactic hypersensitivity as a pathologic mechanism leading to several related but distinct clinical diseases. These included polyarteritis nodosa, rheumatic fever, systemic lupus erythematosus and rheumatoid arthritis. Rich and Gregory (4) offered experimental support for this concept. They demonstrated that repeated and protracted anaphylactic

episodes of the serum sickness type in rabbits led to blood vessel changes. These closely resembled changes found in rheumatic fever and systemic lupus erythematosus. In addition, they emphasized the similarity of clinical and laboratory characteristics seen in serum sickness and lupus erythematosus. These included fever, skin lesions, purpura, arthritis, necrotizing inflammatory arterial lesions, focal collagen degeneration, focal necrosis of lymph nodes and spleen, myocarditis, valvulitis, inflammation of serous membranes and pneumonitis. Dixon (5, 6) performed similar studies involving the continual production of immune complexes in rabbits. These studies demonstrated the development of chronic glomerulonephritis. The fibrinoid depositions about the nephrotic tubules were shown to consist of foreign antigen and antibodies produced by the host rabbit.

In 1941 Banks (7) pointed out that a common pathologic background existed in various human diseases of unknown etiology. Fibrinoid degeneration of collagen appeared as a fundamental lesion in rheumatic fever, rheumatoid arthritis, lupus erythematosus, polyarteritis nodosa, dermatomyocitis and scleroderma. Banks suggested that a common etiology might be involved. Klemperer and associates (8) in 1942 also recognized the involvement of collagen tissues as a common pathologic abnormality in these diseases. They introduced the term "diffuse collagen disease" as a pathologic and anatomic concept suggesting that various diseases have as their primary abnormality marked damage to collagen tissue. This terminology was employed only to emphasize morphologic similarities (9). However, the term "collagen disease" was quickly accepted and considered to indicate a common etiology. Baehr and Pollack (10) objected to this concept and pointed out that collagen damage could only occur in three basic ways. These included degeneration, fibrosis and cellular reaction. Fibrinoid degeneration of collagen can appear as the end stage of any of these three processes. Although a common morphologic abnormality was present, as in scleroderma and lupus erythematosus, the clinical pictures varied so widely that an etiologic relationship was unlikely. The same rationale was applied to the morphologic changes of serum sickness, rheumatoid arthritis, rheumatic fever, polyarteritis nodosa and thromboangiitis obliterans.

The relationship of immunologic events to collagen disease was purely speculative. The lack of a demonstrable foreign antigen prevented any generalized immunologic approach to this problem. The concept of autoimmunity burst with a spectacular effect upon this background of theoretical and anatomic data. The possibility that a host constituent might be the antigen required for the hypersensitivity hypothesis offered a framework upon which these pathologically related diseases could be investigated. The involvement of a variety of different host antigens, either individually or in various combinations, could be hypothesized. With this concept the dissimilarities of clinical patterns in the same disease and among the different syndromes became understandable. Dameshek (11) elegantly expanded this view in considering the hematologic manifestions of such diseases.

The Association of Collagen Disease and Autoimmune Hemolytic Anemia

Several of the postulated etiologies of autioimmune hemolytic anemia consider erythrocyte autoantibody formation as only one part of a more generalized disease (12). Complex multisystem involvement may occur. Collagen diseases may be considered to result from a similar aberration, with the clinical variations reflecting the number and type of host antigens concerned. These two postulates would strongly suggest a relationship between the two states. A high rate of association might be anticipated. The following chapter is devoted to a review of this relationship. Both collagen disease and other hypersensitivity reactions are considered.

In the current series of patients with autoimmune hemolytic anemia, 35 examples of either collagen or hypersensitivity diseases were studied. In several instances more than one pathologic state of this type was present in the same patient. Only 30 patients are therefore included in this group. This represents an incidence of 12.8 per cent in patients with autoimmune hemolytic anemia. In some patients a collagen disease was suspected but could not be diagnosed. In other instances an additional pathologic state was present and considered more likely to be related to the development of autoimmune hemolytic anemia. On this basis only 17 patients, or 7.3 per cent of the series, were diagnosed as having an unequivocal relationship between autoimmune hemolytic anemia and hypersensitivity or collagen diseases. The remaining 18 syndromes are considered as exhibiting a possible relationship. The number of patients and variety of associated diseases are summarized in Table 55. The individual syndromes are discussed below.

Systemic Lupus Erythematosus

Historical and Pathophysiologic Review

Kaposi (13) in 1872 originally described lupus erythematosus. Osler in 1895 (14) emphasized the significance of systemic manisfestations of this disease. In 1935 Baehr and associates (15) documented the clinical and pathologic findings in 23 patients and established the modern era of study. The clinical picture they presented was limited to what we now consider the acute type. Clinical descriptions have since been expanded to include subacute and

TABLE 55. *The number and variety of collagen and hypersensitivity diseases associated in an unequivocal or possible etiologic state with autoimmune hemolytic anemia (30 patients studied with 35 disease states)*

Associated Disease	No.	Relationship of Associated Diseases to Autoimmune Hemolytic Anemia		
		Unequivocal	Possible	Other significant diagnoses in possible groups
Lupus erythematosus	16	10		
Systemic type	10	10		
Possible systemic type	5	0	5	5 Idiopathic hemolytic anemia
Discoid type	1	0	1	Idiopathic hemolytic anemia
Rheumatoid arthritis	5	3	2	1 Idiopathic; 1 infectious
Scleroderma	3	2	1	Lupus erythematosus
Rheumatic fever	3	0	3	2 Idiopathic; 1 pernicious anemia
Recurrent polyarthritis	2	0	2	2 Idiopathic hemolytic anemia
Polyarteritis nodosa	1	1	0	
Serum sickness	1	1	0	
Erythema nodosa	1	0	1	Idiopathic hemolytic anemia
Erythema multiforma	1	0	1	Chronic lymphocytic leukemia
Sjögren's syndrome	1	0	1	Scleroderma
Porphyria cutanea tarda	1	0	1	Lupus erythematosus
Total	35	17	18	

chronic varieties of systemic lupus erythematosus (16, 17). However, the pathologic observations made by these investigators are still pertinent. There was evidence of pleuritis and/or pericarditis in 17 patients and verrucous endocarditis in 13. A variety of different vascular lesions were found. These included simple dilation of capillary beds, endothelial proliferation in capillaries, arterioles and venules, and degeneration or necrosis of vessel walls with adjacent thromboses and hemorrhage. "Wire loop" hyaline thickening lesions of glomerular tufts were frequently seen.

In 1948 Hargraves and associates (18) described a characteristic cell in the bone marrow of patients with lupus erythematosus. This cell, which appeared to be a neutrophilic granulocyte which had phagocytized nuclear material, was termed the lupus erythematosus (LE) cell. This observation supplied a diagnostic tool of surprising sensitivity. Its presence permitted the discovery and diagnosis of many cases which otherwise would have remained obscure.

Haserick and associates (19, 20) demonstrated that the LE cell phenomenon was dependent on the action of a gamma-G immunoglobulin. This suggested that an immunologic mechanism might be involved. Miescher (21) expanded this approach and considered the reacting globulin (LE factor) to be an autoantibody directed against the cell nucleus. Evidence rapidly accumulated that autoantibodies directed against cell nuclei, deoxyribonucleic acid and deoxyribonucleic acid-histone complexes were common in systemic lupus erythematosus (22). The antibody nature of such substances has been demonstrated by precipitation, complement fixation, immunofluorescence, specific adsorption, tanned red cell hemagglutination, latex particle agglutination, passive cutaneous anaphylaxis and delayed cutaneous hypersensitivity. Such observations suggested that autoimmunization played a prominent role in systemic lupus erythematosus. The immunologic literature has been summarized by MacKay and Burnet (23). The association of hypergammaglobulinemia, biologically false positive serologic reactions, lowered serum complement, antilysosome substances, antithrombin agents, antimuscle antibodies, leukopenia, thrombocytopenia and autoimmune hemolytic anemia all support the premise that a widespread systemic autoimmune process is involved. (24, 25). Although humoral autoantibodies have been shown to be capable of initiating damage to cellular elements of the blood, the potential danger of such substances reacting with the vascular endothelium is less clear. Fabius (26) and Piomelli and associates (27) failed to demonstrate circulating autoantibodies with the capacity to damage the vascular network or to result in angiitis.

Many observers have documented the occurrence of systemic lupus erythematosus in several family members. Pirofsky and Shearn (28) in 1953 suggested that a "familial predisposition" for systemic lupus erythematosus existed. They emphasized the necessity of investigating examples of rheumatic fever and glomerulonephritis in family members of patients with lupus erythematosus. Leonhardt (29) has exhaustively reviewed the familial evidence in a brilliant monograph. Holman and Deicher (30), Pollack and associates (31) and Ansell and associates (32) reported that antinuclear factors may be found in the sera of relatives of patients with systemic lupus erythematosus even though an active disease process cannot be documented. Leonhardt (29) conceived of an inheritable increased propensity to produce antibodies which might result in lupus erythematosus. Ziff (33) postulated that autoimmune phenomena might appear as the "consequence of the genetically transmitted failure of a mechanism normally present for the acquisition of immune tolerance to normal body constituents during embryonic life." Pollack and associates (31) suggested the presence of a hereditary derangement of immunologic homeostasis.

These studies have implicated an autoimmune etiology in systemic lupus erythematosus. Other collagen disease syndromes have been seen with similar clinical, pathologic and laboratory characteristics. This tends to support the concept of related etiologies. It is difficult to classify several disease states with similar pathophysiologic abnormalities and different but variable anatomic defects. The exact relationship of systemic lupus erythematosus to other collagen diseases is still to be determined. Autoimmune hemolytic anemia occurring in association with systemic lupus erythematosus supports the premise that autoimmunization is of fundamental importance in these diseases. The nature of this association is explored below.

Incidence of Autoimmune Hemolytic Anemia in Systemic Lupus Erythematosus

From 1950 to 1953 a number of reports documented the association of autoimmune hemolytic anemia and systemic lupus erythematosus. Positive antiglobulin tests and a hemolytic syndrome in patients with lupus erythematosus were commonly reported (16, 34–44). The studies of Pisciotta and associates (35) established the LE cell factor as distinct from the erythrocyte autoantibody.

Anemia is characteristic of systemic lupus erythematosus. Michael and associates (38) noted that only 16 of 111 cases initially were not anemic. Fifteen of these cases subsequently developed anemia. Jessar and associates (45) found anemia in 80 per cent of the 323 cases they summarized. Shearn and Pirofsky (16) described a normochromic, normocytic anemia in 33 of their 34 patients. Dubois (46) noted that 48 of his 62 patients had hemoglobin values below 11.0 gm. per cent. Harvey and associates (17) analyzed 138 cases and found anemia in 70 per cent on first examination. During the course of disease 78 per cent developed anemia.

Harvey and associates (17) felt that anemia in systemic lupus erythematosus resulted from retarded erythropoiesis rather than from hemolysis. They were able to document hemolytic anemia in only three of their 138 cases. No relationship between positive antiglobulin tests and clinical evidence of hemolytic anemia was apparent. Antiglobulin tests were performed in 34 patients with positive reactions in six. Only one patient had hemolytic anemia. Pisciotta and associates (35) noted the persistence of positive antiglobulin tests after cessation of hemolysis. Evans and associates (36) found positive antiglobulin tests without hemolytic anemia in four cases of lupus erythematosus. In contrast, Shearn and Pirofsky (16) obtained positive antiglobulin reactions in three of the four anemic cases they tested. Wasserman and associates (47) obtained positive antiglobulin reactions in 31 of 72 patients with lupus erythematosus. However, only six patients had hemolytic anemia. One of these cases had a negative antiglobulin test.

The dissociation of positive antiglobulin tests and hemolysis in systemic lupus erythematosus makes it difficult to derive accurate incidence figures for autoimmune hemolytic anemia. The data of Harvey and associates (17) suggest an incidence of hemolytic anemia of only 2.2 per cent, with positive antiglobulin tests in 17.6 per cent. Michael and associates (38) quote Rosenfield and Vogel as obtaining positive antiglobulin tests in 25 per cent of 25 cases of systemic lupus erythematosus. The patient population of Wasserman and associates (47), which may duplicate that reported by Rosenfield and Vogel, had a hemolytic anemia incidence of only 8.3 per cent. In contrast, positive antiglobulin tests were found in 43 per cent of the total series. Cowling and Thomas (48) observed autoimmune hemolytic anemia in 23 per cent of 39 cases of systemic lupus erythematosus. MacKay and Burnet (23) state that a typical warm antibody type of autoimmune hemolytic anemia, with positive direct antiglobulin tests, may occur in 25 per cent of cases of systemic lupus erythematosus. The source of their patient population is not stated but presumably it duplicates the cases of Cowling and Thomas (48) from the same institution. Videbaek (49) feels that 40 per cent of patients with systemic lupus erythematosus eventually develop autoimmune hemolytic anemia.

Incidence of Systemic Lupus Erythematosus in Autoimmune Hemolytic Anemia

The association of systemic lupus erythematosus and autoimmune hemolytic anemia has been noted in most studies of autoimmune hemolytic anemia. The incidence of such an association has varied greatly. Dausset and Colombani (50) reported only two cases of systemic lupus erythematosus in 128 patients, an incidence of 1.6 per cent. Dacie (51) found six examples in his 175 patients, an inci-

dence of 3.4 per cent. More recently, his series of 250 patients includes 15 patients with systemic lupus erythematosus, an incidence of 6 per cent (52). Dameshek and Komninos (53) found two patients with this association in 43 cases, an incidence of 4.6 per cent. Evans and Weiser (54) had three examples in a series of 41 patients, a 7.3 per cent incidence. Videbaek (49) found 10 cases of concomitant autoimmune hemolytic anemia and systemic lupus erythematosus in 41 patients with autoimmune hemolytic anemia, an incidence of 24.4 per cent.

It is striking that the lowest incidence of lupus erythematosus occurred in studies reporting many cases of idiopathic autoimmune hemolytic anemia. The series of Dausset and Colombani (50) contained 72.7 per cent of iodiopathic cases, and Dacie (51) found an incidence of 64.7 per cent (excluding paroxysmal cold hemoglobinuria cases). In contrast, Videbaek's series (49), showing a high incidence of associated systemic lupus erythematosus, was dominated by secondary varieties (88 per cent). Videbaek speculates that the high incidence of idiopathic autoimmune hemolytic anemia and the low incidence of associated systemic lupus erythematosus may be related. Lupus erythematosus may not be diagnosed because of insufficient diagnostic procedures or followup examinations. Such patients would have an erroneous diagnosis of idiopathic autoimmune hemolytic anemia.

In the current series lupus erythematosus was either diagnosed or strongly suspected in 16 patients. The difficulty of diagnosing lupus erythematosus in the absence of a positive LE cell test has been discussed in Chapter 3. In 10 patients a diagnosis of systemic lupus erythematosus was unequivocal. This represents a 4.3 per cent incidence of systemic lupus erythematosus in patients with autoimmune hemolytic anemia. One additional patient developed discoid lupus erythematosus 51 months after the onset of autoimmune hemolytic anemia, and her disease was classified as an idiopathic variety. Five additional patients had clinical pictures, supplemented in two cases by pertinent family histories, that strongly suggest systemic lupus erythematosus. A definitive diagnosis of systemic lupus erythematosus was not made, primarily because negative LE cell preparations were found. These cases have also been classified as idiopathic autoimmune hemolytic anemia. These 16 patients with either a definite or strong presumption of an associated lupus erythematosus syndrome constitute 6.8 per cent of the total number of patients with autoimmune hemolytic anemia.

There is little doubt that the hematologic patient population influences the comparative incidences of associated disease states in autoimmune hemolytic anemia. Our series more closely resembles those of Dacie (52), Dameshek and Komninos (53) and Evans and Weiser (54), than the extremes of either Dausset and Colombani (50) or Videbaek (49). In spite of this, there is little doubt that Videbaek's basic premise is accurate. Many cases of autoimmune hemolytic anemia classified as idiopathic undoubtedly represent undiagnosable systemic lupus erythematosus. Some will eventually develop clinical and laboratory manifestations permitting such a diagnosis. Others must remain as idiopathic until the diagnosis of lupus erythematosus is placed on a finer pathologic basis.

Age and Sex

Patients in the current series with the combined syndrome were predominantly female. Thirteen of the 16 patients, or 81.3 per cent, were women. This sex distribution is similar to that found in uncomplicated systemic lupus erythematosus. Jessar and associates (45), Dubois (46), Shearn and Pirofsky (16) and Harvey and associates (17) recorded a female incidence of 85, 89, 91 and 78 per cent, respectively, in systemic lupus erythematosus.

An age range from 2½ to 75 years was found in our group of patients having autoimmune hemolytic anemia associated with systemic lupus erythematosus. The medium age was 30 years, and a mean of 37.5 years was obtained. When compared with the entire group of patients having autoimmune hemolytic anemia, or with those of the idiopathic variety, a younger population appears to be involved. In spite of this, patients with systemic lupus erythematosus and an associated autoimmune hemolytic anemia appear to be older than individuals having uncomplicated systemic lupus erythematosus. Patients with systemic lupus erythematosus had mean ages of 27 and 29 years, respectively, in the series reported by Dubois (46) and Harvey and associates (17).

Duration of Disease

Accurate statistical data for duration of survival of patients with autoimmune hemolytic anemia and systemic lupus erythematosus could not be obtained in the current series. Eight patients are still living, five have died and three have been lost to followup. In spite of the inability to supply final statistical figures it is apparent that a chronic disease syndrome with long survivals is present. Patients who subsequently died survived through a range of 16 to 85 months, with a median survival of 62 months. Even longer survivals are noted in the living patients. This group has been followed through a range of 17 to 192 months. A median and mean approximating 7 years is present in this surviving group. Similar long survivals have been noted by Videbaek (49).

Onset of Autoimmune Hemolytic Anemia in Relation to Systemic Lupus Erythematosus

Autoimmune hemolytic anemia may occur either simultaneously with systemic lupus erythematosus, at any time during the course of the disease, or substantially prior to the time when a diagnosis of lupus erythematosus can be made. In the current group of 16 patients a simultaneous occurrence was noted in five patients, a preexisting systemic lupus erythematosus was present in six patients and autoimmune hemolytic anemia antedated lupus erythematosus in four patients. A time relationship could not be accurately determined in one case. Systemic lupus erythematosus preceded autoimmune hemolytic anemia by approximately 5 years in the six cases studied. Autoimmune hemolytic anemia existed for a mean of 34 months before the development of systemic lupus erythematosus in the four cases with this type of onset.

Dubois (55) in 1952 first pointed out that autoimmune hemolytic anemia may be the initial sign of systemic lupus erythematosus. He reported three cases in which autoimmune hemolytic anemia existed 6 months, 3 weeks and 2 weeks, respectively, before the diagnosis of systemic lupus erythematosus. The data are not impressive, and it is likely that our current clinical orientation would have resulted in the simultaneous diagnosis of lupus erythematosus and autoimmune hemolytic anemia. Videbaek (49) has presented more convincing data, which our patients appear to confirm. Ten patients with autoimmune hemolytic anemia and systemic lupus erythematosus were studied. In two cases simultaneous onsets were noted. In five, a preexisting systemic lupus erythematosus was present. In three patients autoimmune hemolytic anemia antedated diagnosable systemic lupus erythematosus. In this latter group autoimmune hemolytic anemia existed for 2, 3 and 6 years, respectively, before lupus erythematosus was diagnosed. In five patients lupus erythematosus was present for 2, 4½, 5, 6½ and 15 years, respectively, before autoimmune hemolytic anemia occurred.

Signs and Symptoms

All patients in the present series complained of weakness when first seen; this was frequently associated with lightheadedness or dizziness. Arthritis, arthralgia and fever were noted in approximately 50 per cent of the patients. Bleeding, which was apparently due to an associated thrombocytopenia, was present in three cases. Gastrointestinal complaints were noted in five patients and photosensitivity was noted in two.

Abnormalities discovered on physical examination were common. Enlargement of various reticuloendothelial organs was frequent. An enlarged liver was found in nine patients, splenomegaly was found in eight and lymphadenopathy was found in six. Jaundice was clinically apparent in six patients. Other physical findings appeared to be related to systemic lupus erythematosus. Five patients had skin lesions, two had alopecia, two had pericarditis, two had pleuritis and one patient had neuropathic and psychotic episodes.

Laboratory Studies

Anemia was present in all patients having autoimmune hemolytic anemia and systemic lupus erythematosus. Hematocrit values ranging from 11 to 35 per cent were found at the onset of hemolytic anemia. The lowest hematocrit values obtained during the course of disease did not differ substantially from those obtained on initial examination. All patients with this associated syndrome had positive antiglobulin reactions. The observation that positive antiglobulin tests do not correlate with a hemolytic syndrome in systemic lupus erythematosus was partially confirmed. Positive antiglobulin and bromelin tests were found during quiescent hematologic periods in the absence of hemolysis. This observation is not specific for systemic lupus erythematosus. With adequate followup examinations carried out for a sufficient length of time, hemolysis and overt hemolytic anemia could eventually be demonstrated in almost every case.

The tendency to regard positive antiglobulin tests as unrelated to hemolysis may partially be dependent on equating reticulocytosis with a hemolytic state. Only three of the 12 examined cases in this series had a significant elevation of the reticulocyte count on initial study. Normal mean and median reticulocyte values for the entire group were obtained. The initiation of corticosteroid therapy, however, resulted in an adequate response. In all patients reticulocytosis occurred, and a median value of 12.2 per cent and mean of 10 per cent were obtained.

In seven patients nucleated erythrocytes and in six patients spherocytes were found on the peripheral blood smear. The initial white blood counts (WBC) were normal in statistical terms. However, leukopenia was present in seven of the 13 initial examinations, and leukopenic values developed in nine of 12 cases with adequate followup. Thrombocyte values also appeared normal in statistical analysis. However, marked thrombocytopenia (under 10,000/mm.^{3}) was present with bleeding in three patients. Two of these patients were initially diagnosed as having an Evans' syndrome type of idiopathic autoimmune hemolytic anemia until the associated state of systemic lupus erythematosus developed (Case 2). These observations strongly suggest that any case of idiopathic autoimmune hemolytic anemia with thrombocytopenia and/or leukopenia should be carefully followed for the eventual development of systemic lupus erythematosus.

Bone marrow examinations were not particularly helpful in this series of patients. Erythrocytic hyperplasia occurred in only five instances, and megaloblastic changes occurred in only two cases. Two patients had marked depression of the erythrocytic series. One case appeared as erythrocytic aplasia and the other as aplastic anemia. Both have been carried as idiopathic forms and included in Chapter 4. Case 61 presents the protocol of one of these patients.

Urinary tract abnormalities were common in the present series. Marked proteinuria was found in six cases and hematuria in three. The blood urea nitrogen was elevated in five of the six patients tested. Bilirubin values, primarily in indirect testing, were abnormal in four of nine tested patients. The albumin-globulin (A/G) ratio was abnormal in four of eight cases. Abnormal electrophoretic studies consisting primarily of broad elevations of the gamma zone were seen in four of the five sera tested. Positive serologic tests for syphilis were found in four of eight tested patients. In three instances these appeared as biologically false positive reactions. In one case past exposure to syphilis existed and a gonorrhea infection was present. LE cell tests were positive in eight of the 12 cases tested. These statistical, clinical and laboratory values are summarized in Table 56.

Clinical Patterns

Systemic lupus erythematosus is a disease characterized by protean manifestations. Autoimmune hemolytic anemia may present a variable clinical pattern. The combination of autoimmune hemolytic anemia with systemic lupus erythematosus can be anticipated to give rise to complex disease states of great variability.

These two states may occur in close temporal proximity to each other or one may precede the other from short to extremely long intervals. Autoimmune hemolytic anemia has a variable influence on the clinical manifestations of systemic lupus erythematosus. In some instances the combined disease pattern may be dominated by autoimmune hemolytic anemia. In others, autoimmune hemolytic anemia presents as only an interesting laboratory manifestation in active lupus erythematosus.

Extremely long survivals of patients with the combined syndrome have been noted in this series and in that of Videbaek (49). This is surprising when the relatively poor prognosis of each separate state is considered. The following protocol illustrates the clinical course of one patient.

Case 59. A 39-year-old white female developed arthralgia and alopecia. One sister had rheumatoid arthritis. Systemic lupus erythematosus was diagnosed in the patient, and gold therapy was given. A relatively benign clinical state resulted. Seven years later splenomegaly was first noted. Over the next 2 years multiple arthralgias and migratory arthritis occurred. Chloroquine therapy was initiated. Fourteen years after the onset of diagnosable lupus erythematosus, anemia developed and hematologic consultation was carried out. Physical examination revealed a spleen 12 cm. below the costal margin and a liver palpated at the costal margin. Lymph nodes were not enlarged. The hematocrit was 32 per cent, the reticulocyte count was 0.7 per cent, the WBC was 1,300/mm.^{3} and thrombocytes were 89,000/mm.^{3} A previous bone marrow aspiration was reviewed and found normal. LE cells, serum electrophoresis and urinalysis were normal. Total serum bilirubin was elevated. Direct antiglobulin and bromelin tests were postive. Prednisone therapy was initiated, with symptomatic improvement and reduction of arthritis. Maintenance prednisone of 7.5 to 15 mg. daily was given. The hematocrit elevated slightly, the WBC rose to 4,100/mm.^{3} and thrombocytes reached 206,000/mm.^{3} Twenty-one months after the start of prednisone, a "butterfly" facial rash developed. The spleen could no longer be palpated. Direct antiglobulin and bromelin tests were still positive. The brome-

TABLE 56. *Statistical data obtained from 16 patients (13 females, three males) with autoimmune hemolytic anemia (AHA) and lupus erythematosus (LE)*

Test Procedures	Total	Statistical Data		
		Range	Mean	Median
Clinical data				
Age (years)	16	3–75	38	30
Duration of LE before AHA* (months)	6	4–163	61	53
Duration of AHA before LE* (months)	4	2–67	34	33
Survival with LE, dead (months)	5	16–85	55	62
Survival with LE, living (months)	8	17–192	87	82
Laboratory data				
Initial hematocrit (%)	14	11–35	23	22.5
Lowest hematocrit (%)	14	11–31	20.5	21
Initial reticulocytes (%)	12	0.2–6.3	2.2	1.4
Therapeutic reticulocytes (%)	9	3.2–19.0	10	12.2
Initial WBC (10^3/mm.^{3})	13	1.8–37	7.5	4.2
Initial thrombocytes (10^3/mm.^{3})	12	1.6–300	142	200

		Normal	Abnormal	
Other laboratory abnormalities				
Bilirubin	9	5	4	
Albumin-globulin ratio	8	4	4	
Serum electrophoresis	5	1	4	
Serologic tests for syphilis	8	4	4	
LE cell test	12	4	8	
Blood urea nitrogen	6	1	5	
Proteinuria	12	6	6	
Hematuria	12	9	3	

		Increased	Decreased	Normal
Bone marrow aspiration				
Total cellularity	12	2	1	9
Erythrocyte precursors	12	5	2	5
Leukocytes	12	2	1	9
Megakaryocytes	12	3	2	8
Megaloblasts	12	2	0	10

		Weakness	Dizziness	Fever	Arthritis	Weight loss
Presenting symptoms Abnormal	14	14	7	3	8	5

		Spleen	Liver	Lymph nodes	Jaundice
Presenting signs Abnormal	14	8	9	6	5

* Five patients had simultaneous diagnosis of LE and AHA. The relationship was not determined in one patient.

lin technique revealed a panhemagglutinin in the serum. On the last followup examination the hematocrit was 33 per cent with normal WBC and thrombocyte counts. The total duration of lupus erythematosus is 192 months. Autoimmune hemolytic anemia has been diagnosed for 29 months, with the patient still living.

This patient had a clinical pattern suggestive of discoid lupus erythematosus progressing into systemic manifestations. A chronic state occurred, and 163 months after the onset of lupus erythematosus, splenomegaly, positive antiglobulin tests, elevated bilirubin and mild anemia were demonstrated. Prednisone induced and has maintained a remission. Throughout the long clinical course an extremely mild disease has been present. The onset of autoimmune hemolytic anemia did not change the benign clinical pattern.

Not all patients are as fortunate as the one described above. Severe and fulminating patterns may be seen.

Case 60. A 19-year-old white female was found to have positive serologic tests for syphilis. Two years later a biologically false positive reaction was proved when negative treponemal immobilization reactions were found. The patient was asymptomatic for 9 additional years. At age 30 leukopenia, anemia and positive LE cells were documented, resulting in a diagnosis of systemic lupus erythematosus. Chloroquine therapy and prednisone, 20 mg. daily, were started. Three months later carcinoma of the cervix was found and radiation was employed. Five months later the hematocrit was 23 per cent and positive direct antiglobulin tests were discovered. Hematologic studies were carried out. Arthralgia and Raynaud's phenomenon were present. The liver was 4 cm. and the spleen was 2 cm. below the costal margin. The hematocrit after transfusion was 32 per cent with a 1.7 per cent reticulocyte count. The WBC was 4,100/mm.³, thrombocytes were 106,000/mm.³, bilirubin was 0.15/0.10 mg. per cent and the A/G ratio was 3.3/3.4 gm. per cent. Electrophoresis revealed a broad gamma band containing 48 per cent of the total protein. Bone marrow examination was normal. The urine revealed proteinuria and hematuria. The Cr⁵¹ half-life (T/2) survival time was 14 days. Repeated LE cell preparations were then negative and Kline, Kolmer and Veneral Disease Research Laboratory tests were positive. A negative Kolmer-Reiter test was found. Direct and indirect antiglobulin and bromelin tests were positive. A low titer cold hemagglutinin and a warm acting panhemagglutinin were demonstrated in the serum. Radiation therapy of 5,050 r was given for spreading carcinoma of the cervix. The hematocrit rapidly dropped to 15 per cent with a 3 per cent reticulocyte count. Generalized urticaria developed. Prednisone therapy was increased to 60 mg. daily with a 13.4 per cent reticulocyte count. The hematocrit reached 36 per cent. Multiple rectal fistulae developed, followed by peritonitis. Death occurred 16 months after the simultaneous diagnosis of systemic lupus erythematosus and autoimmune hemolytic anemia.

The onset of disease in the above patient was heralded by a biologically false positive serologic reaction which developed more than 11 years before evidence of systemic lupus erythematosus was found. The role of biologically false positive serologic reactions as initial evidence of systemic lupus erythematosus has been emphasized by Haserick and Long (56). These workers noted positive serologic tests for periods as long as 7 years before systemic disease could be diagnosed. The development of systemic lupus erythematosus in the above patient was associated with autoimmune hemolytic anemia. This combination led to rapid death when combined with multiple infections and a spreading carcinoma.

Autoimmune hemolytic anemia may antedate clinical evidence of systemic lupus erythematosus. In such patients the clinical picture is dominated by a hemolytic state. Case 2 illustrates such a patient in whom hemolytic anemia preceded diagnosable systemic lupus erythematosus for a long period of time.

One patient (Case 4) in the current series had a family history of associated autoimmune hemolytic anemia. The two additionally involved siblings did not have diagnosable systemic lupus erythematosus. One sister had an Evans' syndrome type of idiopathic autoimmune hemolytic anemia, and a second sister had plasma cell myeloma associated with the autoimmune hemolytic state (Cases 3 and 5).

Five patients in the present series had probable systemic lupus erythematosus in association with autoimmune hemolytic anemia. Negative LE cell preparations prevented a definitive diagnosis. The following protocol illustrates one example.

Case 61. A 53-year-old white female developed generalized arthralgia and severe fatigue. Symptomatic therapy, including small doses of corticosteriods, was ineffective. Her hematocrit was 34 per cent. Four months later syncope developed. Physical examination was negative except for pallor. The hematocrit was found to be 14 per cent with a 0.0 per cent reticulocyte count. Bone marrow aspiration demonstrated erythrocytic aplasia with an increased number of granulocytes and megakaryocytes; LE cells were not found. An attempt to cross match the patient for transfusions revealed incompatible reactions. The direct and indirect antiglobulin and bromelin tests were postitive and a panhemagglutinin was identified in the serum. Prednisone therapy was initiated and followed by reticulocytosis. In 2 months the hematocrit reached 35 per cent and prednisone was maintained at 2.5 mg. daily. The patient remained asymptomatic except for arthralgia. Two years later the antiglobulin tests reverted to negative. She stayed in hematologic remission except for one episode when her hematocrit transiently dropped to 24 per cent and positive antiglobulin tests were found. At this time carcinoma of the colon was found and resected. Maintenance prednisone, 2.5 mg. daily, has been continued. A negative antiglobulin test and an hematocrit of 39 per cent was found at last followup 78 months after the onset of hemolytic disease.

The family history of this patient revealed one sister with systemic lupus erythematosus, a second sister with rheumatoid arthritis and a third sister with chronic granulocytic leukemia. Four grandnieces have "nephrosis of unknown etiology" and one grandneice has idiopathic thrombocytopenic purpura with 4+ proteinuria.

This patient has been classified as having idiopathic autoimmune hemolytic anemia. Positive LE cell tests would have led to the diagnosis of systemic lupus erythematosus. The remaining four patients in whom a definitive diagnosis of systemic lupus erythematosus has not been made have similarly suggestive clinical patterns.

Many of the patients discussed in this section had complex clinical disease. Two of these cases have been previously described. Case 7 presented with pernicious anemia and subsequently developed multiple infections, a thymoma, interstitial pancreatitis and an adenocarcinoma of the prostate. A nodular thyroid and diabetes were present prior to the development of positive LE cells and antiglobulin tests. Case 8 had porphyria cutanea tarda, an Evans' syndrome, lung abscess, scleroderma and liver disease in association with positive LE cell and antiglobulin tests. It is difficult to avoid the conclusion that such patients have a defect of their immune apparatus resulting in the development of widespread systemic immunologic disease.

Discoid Lupus Erythematosus

One patient in the current series had idiopathic autoimmune hemolytic anemia and subsequently developed discoid lupus erythematosus. There is general agreement that discoid and systemic lupus erythematosus are manifestations of the same process (16, 17). Accordingly, autoimmune hemolytic anemia may be related to the discoid lupus state.

Case 62. A 30-year-old white female developed a virus infection. She had a prior history of sensitivity to sulfa drugs. Therapy with chloramphenicol was started. Four months later severe menorrhagia developed and the hematocrit dropped to 21 per cent. Intramuscular iron therapy and two transfusions were given. The hematocrit rapidly dropped to 21 per cent and petechiae were noted. Physical examination was negative. The WBC was 2,000/mm.³, thrombocytes were 70,000/mm.³ and the reticulocyte count was 0.2 per cent. The bone marrow was markedly hypocellular, and a diagnosis of aplastic anemia was made. Leukopenia and reticulocytopenia persisted and the thrombocyte count dropped to 2,000/mm.³ LE cell preparations, serology and urinalysis were normal. The bilirubin was 0.3/0.9 mg. per cent and the A/G ratio was 3.7/4.12 gm. per cent. A broad gamma band containing 27.1 per cent of the total protein was found. Direct antiglobulin tests were positive. Prednisone therapy was given. A rapid elevation of the hematocrit to 44 per cent occurred. Leukopenia disappeared in 2 weeks, but thrombocytopenia persisted for 3 years before values returned to normal. Antiglobulin and bromelin tests became negative in 3 weeks and remained so. Prednisone therapy was discontinued after 7 months. The patient remained asymptomatic. Fifty-one months after the onset of aplasia and hemolysis she noted photosensitivity. Skin lesions developed over her face and neck. Skin biopsy was compatible with discoid lupus erythematosus. Her hematologic values were all negative. Followup is continuing 97 months after the onset of autoimmune hemolytic anemia. Discoid lupus erythematosus without systemic manifestations has been present for 46 months.

This patient was included in the group of idiopathic autoimmune hemolytic anemias. The relationship to lupus erythematosus is still problematical. Careful followup is needed to determine whether a pattern of systemic lupus erythematosus will eventually develop.

Other Collagen Diseases and Autoimmune Hemolytic Anemia

The premise that collagen diseases and autoimmune hemolytic anemia may be frequently associated is supported by the evidence in the case of systemic lupus erythematosus. Little support for this relationship, however, is found when other collagen diseases are examined. Rheumatoid arthritis, rheumatic fever and scleroderma are common diseases. Even uncommon syndromes such as polyarteritis nodosa and dermatomyositis are more frequently being recognized because of a high degree of clinical alertness. In spite of the prevalence of collagen diseases, their association with autoimmune hemolytic anemia is rare. This suggests that either nonimmunologic mechanisms are concerned in their pathogenesis or else entirely different immunologic pathways are involved in the disease complex. The relationship of autoimmune hemolytic anemia to these syndromes is summarized below.

Rheumatoid Arthritis

Autoimmune hemolytic anemia developing in patients with rheumatoid arthritis is uncommon. Evans and Weiser (54) mention one such patient in their series of 41 cases of autoimmune hemolytic anemia. Dacie (51) encountered three such patients in his series of 175 cases of autoimmune hemolytic anemia. In two patients cold acting autoantibodies were present and one had a warm acting erythrocyte autoantibody. Dacie states that the association of rheumatoid arthritis with autoimmune hemolytic anemia usually leads to the eventual discovery of systemic lupus erythematosus. Our experience confirms this.

A patient seen in conjunction with a rheumatologist illustrates the problem of classification in such cases. The patient had rheumatoid arthritis for 5 years and developed joint deformities and crippling. Severe anemia resulted and was characterized by jaundice, reticulocytosis and positive antiglobulin tests. A therapeutic response to corticosteroids occurred. LE cell preparations were repeatedly positive. This author diagnosed autoimmune hemolytic anemia and systemic lupus erythematosus. The rheumatologist classified the case as rheumatoid arthritis and autoimmune hemolytic anemia with false positive LE cell tests. The author employed the LE cell test as diagnostic. The rheumatologist emphasized the clinical pattern of deforming joint changes to diagnose rheumatoid arthritis. Currently there is no diagnostic procedure to clarify this dilemma. Either systemic lupus erythematosus and rheumatoid arthritis will be consolidated as manifestations of the same disease process or else accurate differential procedures must be developed to separate these as specific entities. Hejmans and associates (57) have pointed out the serologic overlap between these states.

In the current series five patients with rheumatoid arthritis developed autoimmune hemolytic anemia in a time sequence suggesting a relationship. Other patients with rheumatoid arthritis were seen in the present series and are not included in this group. In such patients the arthritis appeared to be unrelated to autoimmune hemolytic anemia. In several instances other associated pathologic states were considered to be significant.

Two of the five patients had only a possible relationship. One had concomitant acute cholecystitis and a pseudomonas infection (Case 55). She has been categorized in the infectious group. A second patient developed rheumatoid arthritis 16 months after the onset of autoimmune hemolytic anemia and her case was classified as idiopathic autoimmune hemolytic anemia. This diagnosis may be challenged and changed in the future.

A relatively uniform pattern was noted in the association of autoimmune hemolytic anemia and rheumatoid arthritis. All five patients are women. Their ages range from 45 to 76 years, with a mean of 58 years. Longstanding arthritis was characteristic of this group. One patient died after 76 months of rheumatoid arthritis activity. The four living patients have had rheumatoid arthritis for 15, 112, 122 and 225 months, respectively. Duration of survival after the onset of autoimmune hemolytic anemia is also long. The one dead patient had autoimmune hemolytic anemia for 15 months. One patient has been lost to followup after 6 months of autoimmune hemolytic anemia. The remaining three living patients have survived 15, 72 and 128 months, respectively, since the onset of autoimmune hemolytic anemia. In one patient rheumatoid arthritis and autoimmune hemolytic anemia were simultaneously diagnosed. In another case the hemolytic process antedated rheumatoid arthritis by 16 months. In the remaining three patients rheumatoid arthritis was present 48, 61 and 219 months, respectively, before the development of autoimmune hemolytic anemia.

All patients had weakness at the onset of their disease. Two patients also had fever. Splenomegaly was noted in three patients, hepatomegaly was found in two and lymphadenopathy was found in one. Other abnormal states were common. Two patients entered in congestive heart failure. Acute and chronic cholecystitis were found in two other patients. Pseudomonas pyelonephritis, pneumonia, a thyroid nodule and carcinoma of the cervix were each found in individual patients. These observations are summarized in Table 57.

Clinical Patterns

A remarkably similar clinical course was present in all patients. The appearance was that of a chronic disease compatible with long survivals.

Case 63. A 44-year-old white female developed carcinoma of the cervix which was treated by total hysterectomy. The next year rheumatoid arthritis was diagnosed. Over the next 2 years LE cell preparations were normal. Prednisone, 15 to 20 mg. daily, gave symptomatic relief. When prednisone therapy was discontinued an anemia unresponsive to hematinics was noted. At prednisone doses over 15 mg. daily, normal hematocrits were present. Hematologic workup was carried out 4 years after the onset of rheumatoid arthritis. Definite rheumatoid joint deformities were present. Inguinal adenopathy was documented without hepatosplenomegaly. The hematocrit was 31 per cent, the reticulocyte count was 3 per cent, the WBC was 4,000/mm.^{3} and thrombocytes were 200,000/mm.^{3} Total bilirubin was normal, as were LE cell preparations and serologic tests for syphilis. The bone marrow revealed erythrocytic hyperplasia. Direct antiglobulin tests were negative and bromelin test 1+. Elution demonstrated a panhemagglutinin erythrocyte autoantibody documented only by enzyme techniques. A Cr^{51} T/2 time of 12 days was obtained; no splenic sequestration could be demonstrated. Prednisone, 20 mg., induced hematologic improvement. Over the next 3 years repeated attempts to discontinue prednisone inevitably resulted in a recurrence of anemia. Reduction was finally accomplished and the hematocrit has been maintained at 36 per cent without prednisone for the last 41 months. Direct antiglobulin and bromelin tests are negative, but bromelin procedures still demonstrate a panhemagglutinin in the patient's serum. Rheumatoid arthritis has progressed, leaving the patient as a crippled semi-invalid. Followup is continuing 127 months after the onset of rheumatoid arthritis and 72 months after the diagnosis of autoimmune hemolytic anemia.

Several interesting aspects of this case deserve emphasis. The clinical pattern was dominated by rheumatoid arthritis. The anemic state was primarily a laboratory curiosity. There is little doubt that hemolytic anemia was concurrently present. Anemia, reticulocytosis, erythrocytic hyperplasia and a shortened erythrocyte survival time were demonstrated. Serologically the antiglobulin test has been consistently negative. Equally consistent have been positive bromelin tests. Successful elution of a panhemagglutinin supports the premise that erythrocyte autoantibodies are present. Note should be made of the chronic nature of the ailment, compatible with the ex-

TABLE 57. *Statistical data obtained from five patients, all females, with rheumatoid arthritis (RA) and autoimmune hemolytic anemia (AHA)*

Test Procedures	Total	Statistical Data		
		Range	Mean	Median
Clinical data				
Age (years)	5	45–76	58	51
Duration of RA before AHA* (months)	3	48–219	109	61
Duration of RA, living (months)	4	15–225	110	112
Duration of AHA, living (months)	3	15–128	72	72
Laboratory data				
Initial hematocrit (%)	5	15–35	25.2	27
Lowest hematocrit (%)	5	15–31	24.3	27
Initial reticulocytes (%)	3	0.3–12.1	4.9	2.4
Therapeutic reticulocytes (%)	2	3–13.4		
Initial WBC (10^3/mm.^{3})	5	2.5–6.2	3.9	3.7
Initial thrombocytes (10^3/mm.^{3})	3	200	200	200
Serologic test for syphilis	5	Positive in one patient		

	Total	Increased	Decreased	Normal
Bone marrow aspiration				
Total cellularity	4	0	0	4
Erythrocyte precursors	4	3	0	1
Leukocytes	4	0	0	4
Megakaryocytes	4	0	0	4
Megaloblasts	4	0	0	4

	Total	Weakness	Dizziness	Fever	Arthritis	Weight loss
Presenting symptoms						
Abnormal	5	5	1	2	5	1

	Total	Spleen	Liver	Lymph nodes	Jaundice
Presenting signs					
Abnormal	5	3	2	1	2

* One patient had simultaneous onset of RA and AHA. One patient had AHA 16 months before RA.

pected natural history of rheumatoid arthritis.

Case 64. A 46-year-old white female was found to have anemia unresponsive to various hematinics. A family history of pernicious anemia in two close relatives was obtained. One year later jaundice was noted and the spleen was palpated at the costal margin. The patient was referred for hematologic evaluation. The hematocrit was 21 per cent, the reticulocyte count was 12.1 per cent, and the WBC was 3,700/mm.^{3} Positive Kolmer, Kahn and Kline tests for syphilis were obtained. LE cell preparations were

negative. The bone marrow revealed erythrocytic hyperplasia and a Cr^{51} T/2 of 3.2 days was found. Direct antiglobulin and bromelin tests were positive. Prednisone, 60 mg. a day, was given with a rapid elevation of the hematocrit to 36 per cent. Prednisone was gradually decreased, and at levels of 25 mg. a day, migratory arthritis became apparent. Six months after the start of prednisone this therapy was discontinued. The hematocrit rapidly dropped to 22 per cent and the reticulocyte count rose to 13.4 per cent. Arthritis was very severe. Prednisone was again administered and a hematologic and arthritic remission occurred. Scarlet fever developed 1 year later without apparent sequelae. Thirteen months later, deep thromboses of the right femoral vein occurred. Maintenance prednisone therapy of 15 mg. daily was continued. Since then the patient's course has been complicated by a peptic ulcer and staphylococcal pneumonia. Arthritis has continued with deformities of the fingers and a limitation of activity. The antiglobulin test became negative with prednisone therapy. This remained negative for 46 months and then became positive. Bromelin tests have remained consistently positive. Followup is continuing 128 months since the onset of anemia and 112 months after rheumatoid arthritis was diagnosed.

The above patient differs from the case previously presented. Her clinical course was dominated by anemia. Rheumatoid arthritis appeared only as an annoying additional disease. However, the patient has been on continual corticosteroid therapy for 114 months, and the severity of rheumatoid arthritis cannot be truly evaluated. The case history has been presented in detail to illustrate the difficulties in classification of such combined diseases. There is no doubt that autoimmune hemolytic anemia and rheumatoid arthritis are present. Is the association simply fortuitous? Is autoimmune hemolytic anemia of an idiopathic type? What is the etiologic relationship of rheumatoid arthritis to the immunohemolytic state? Does this patient possibly have systemic lupus erythematosus? The author has classified the case as idiopathic autoimmune hemolytic anemia, and a possible relationship to rheumatoid arthritis is considered. The absence of positive LE cell tests has prevented a diagnosis of systemic lupus erythematosus. It is quite apparent that the interrelationships between these various syndromes must still be clarified.

Scleroderma

Scleroderma is generally not complicated by anemia. Wasserman and associates (47) did not document a hemolytic process in 25 cases. When anemia develops, it is generally mild and of either a hypochromic microcytic (58) or normochromic normocytic type (59). In 1955 Fudenberg and Wintrobe (60) reported the first example of autoimmune hemolytic anemia associated with scleroderma. Their patient had both cold and warm acting erythrocyte autoantibodies. Therapeutic remission followed corticosteroid therapy. The cessation of hemolysis correlated with reduced titer levels of the warm acting autoantibody. The association of autoimmune hemolytic anemia and scleroderma has since been infrequently noted by other observers. Baloch (61) reported seven patients with scleroderma and cold hemagglutinins.

In the current series three patients with scleroderma had an associated autoimmune hemolytic anemia. All three were females and their ages at the time of onset of disease ranged from 21 to 50 years. Two patients have died, one after a 9-month course and one after 24 years of illness. The one surviving patient has been ill for 65 months. Marked variations in clinical patterns were observed. Complex mixtures of scleroderma intermingled with other collagen disease patterns, as well as relatively simple courses, were seen.

Case 65. A 43-year-old female was discovered to have carcinoma of the cervix. This was treated with radiation. She was well for the next 7 years. At that time diffuse muscle pains were noted. Over the next 4 months all joints became involved and appeared red, hot and tender. Severe thirst was present. Choking, dyspnea and dysphagia developed and became progressively more severe. A weight loss of 65 pounds occurred over a 1-year period of time. When first examined her lips were tight, muscles were atrophic and fingertips were tender and red. The thyroid was diffusely enlarged, and the spleen was palpated 5 cm. and liver 10 cm. below the costal margins. The hematocrit was 40.3 per cent, the reticulocyte count was 1.8 per cent and the WBC and thrombocytes were normal. Urinalysis revealed proteinuria and microscopic hematuria. The A/G ratio was 2.9/7.6 gm. per cent and electrophoresis revealed a broad polyclonal gamma elevation. Tests for syphilis and LE cell preparations were negative. The latex test for rheumatoid arthritis was positive. Liver damage was apparent with abnormal transaminase, thymol turbidity and cephalin flocculation studies. The direct antiglobulin test was positive. Corticosteroid therapy was initiated. The patient progressively deteriorated with liver failure, marked dysphagia and two episodes of pneumonia. Congestive heart failure with pericarditis developed. Scleroderma of the kidney became apparent. Urinary infections and a beta-streptococcal septicemia developed. The antiglobulin and bromelin tests remained consistently positive, although the hematocrit never dropped below 36.5 per cent. Mild thrombocytosis was noted and nucleated erythrocytes were found in the peripheral blood. 6-Mercaptopurine therapy was given. Death occurred 1 week later. Total course of scleroderma was 9 months, with positive antiglobulin tests obtained during the last 5 months of her illness.

This patient presented progressive systemic disease characterized by skin, muscle, joint, heart, pericardial, liver and kidney involvement. It is not known whether the thyroid was similarly involved in scleroderma or whether an unrelated thyroiditis was present. Positive antiglobulin and bromelin tests were obtained throughout the greater part of the patient's course. However, anemia never developed and hemolysis was not apparent. Autoimmune hemolytic anemia, accordingly, was simply an interesting laboratory observation.

The remaining two patients had more complex clinical patterns. One patient (Case 7) had photosensitivity, porphyria cutanea tarda, scleroderma, an Evans' syndrome, positive LE cell preparations, liver disease (lupoid hepatitis?) and a lung abscess. Positive antiglobulin tests and a mild reticulocytosis were present but anemia never assumed clinical significance. This patient has been classified in the systemic lupus erythematosus group. A complex clinical pattern was also seen in the third patient with scleroderma.

Case 66. A 21-year-old white female developed Raynaud's disease. Deposition of calcium became apparent and calcinosis circumscripta was diagnosed. Over the next 15 years progressive edema of the lower extremities occurred. Vein stripping was carried out. At age 41 progressive ascites and pulmonary edema developed. Laparotomy for an acute abdomen was performed. Hepatosplenomegaly was discovered and a biopsy diagnosis of portal cirrhosis was made. Several gastrointestinal hemorrhages developed and transfusions were given. Transfusion reactions were occasionally noted. Parotid

gland swelling developed and biopsy was diagnosed as Sjögren's disease. Over the next few months jaundice became apparent. The liver was palpated 6 cm. and the spleen 3 cm. below the costal margin. A diagnosis of scleroderma was made and prednisone therapy started. Repeated gastrointestinal hemorrhages occurred. A positive direct antiglobulin test was found 2 days after transfusion and anti-K was eluted from the erythrocytes. Anti-K was found in her serum and the patient was typed as K (−). A splenorenal shunt with splenectomy was performed. The patient did well for 2 years until gastrointestinal bleeding recurred. Prednisone was again given with marked clinical improvement. Another massive gastrointestinal hemorrhage developed. At this time strongly positive direct and indirect antiglobulin and bromelin tests were obtained. Elution revealed a panhemagglutinin. She received 9 units of K (−) washed erythrocytes without difficulties. Total bilirubin ranged from 4.4/5.4 mg. per cent to 13.2/15.4 mg. per cent. The A/G ratio was 3.0/3.0 gm. per cent and serum electrophoresis revealed a broad polyclonal gamma band. Multiple LE cell preparations and serologic tests for syphilis were negative. Direct and indirect antiglobulin tests remained strongly positive. A portal-caval shunt was performed and 10 units of washed K (−) erythrocytes were transfused without reactions. A postoperative wound infection occurred and staphylococcal septicemia with death followed. Autopsy confirmed the presence of scleroderma. Her total course since the start of Raynaud's disease was 24 years. Scleroderma was apparent for 48 months, and positive antiglobulin tests were found the last 5 months of her disease.

Although there are marked differences in the clinical patterns of these three patients, certain similarities are apparent. Positive antiglobulin and bromelin tests were found late in the course of disease in all three. In addition, hemolytic anemia either could not be diagnosed or hemolysis was only minimal. Autoimmune hemolytic anemia appeared as a curious laboratory observation or complication of transfusion therapy, rather than as an important part of the clinical disease. A "pure," uncomplicated sclerodermatous process was not present in any of the three patients. An interrelationship with other collagen diseases was apparent in all. One patient had suggestive evidence of acute rheumatoid arthritis and thyroiditis. Another patient had porphyria cutanea tarda, Evans' syndrome, systemic lupus erythematosus and possibly lupoid hepatitis. The last patient had Raynaud's disease, calcinosis circumscripta and Sjögren's syndrome with scleroderma. The relationship of scleroderma to lupus erythematosus has been noted by Beigelman and associates (58), Talbott and Ferrandis (63), Bardawil and associates (64) and Kampmeier (65). Positive LE cell tests of doubtful significance in cases of scleroderma have also been reported by Longhi (66) and Piper and Helwig (67). Hypothyroidism associated with scleroderma has been noted by Miller and associates (68) and Hashimoto's thyroiditis by MacKay and Burnet (23).

Rheumatic Fever

A history or physical evidence of previous rheumatic fever was commonly obtained in the 234 patients of this series with autoimmune hemolytic anemia. Active rheumatic fever, however, was not encountered concurrently with autoimmune hemolytic anemia. In only three instances did rheumatic fever attain clinical significance. In two, progressive cardiac decompensation from rheumatic valvular disease was present. In the third, rheumatic fever was followed by prophylactic sulfa ingestion for 7 years until hypothyroidism developed. Nine years later arthritis and idiopathic autoimmune hemolytic anemia became apparent. In none of these patients was there an unequivocal etiologic relationship of rheumatic fever to autoimmune hemolytic anemia.

Rheumatic fever is a relatively common disease. In addition, many studies suggest either a hypersensitivity or autoimmune pathogenesis. It is therefore surprising that an association with autoimmune hemolytic anemia has not been described. This lack of relationship was confirmed by the current series. The report of Evans and Weiser (54) is one of the few noting such an association. Of their 41 cases of autoimmune hemolytic anemia, rheumatic valvular disease and acute rheumatic fever were each noted in one case. Giraud and associates

(69) reported one child who developed autoimmune hemolytic anemia 1 year after the onset of acute polyarthritis and chorea.

On a theoretical basis the lack of association of autoimmune hemolytic anemia with rheumatic fever is not unexpected. There is little to indicate a widespread immunologic defect. A lymphoproliferative aspect of rheumatic fever has not been noted. Rather, the hypersensitivity postulate is dependent on an anaphylactic reaction involving sensitized vascular tissue and streptococcal antigens. The hypothesis of Kaplan (70) requires a cross reacting antibody. This antibody is stimulated by streptococcal antigens and reacts with subsarcolemma and intermyelofibrilla sarcoplasm. With current etiologic concepts, involvement of the erythrocyte is not anticipated. The development of a clone of "foreign" immunocompetent cells is not assumed and termination of tolerance is not suggested.

Recurrent Arthritis of Unknown Etiology

Two patients with recurrent polyarthritis of unknown etiology were seen in the present series of patients with autoimmune hemolytic anemia. The association of arthritis with autoimmune hemolytic anemia was not sufficiently striking to warrant the assumption of an etiologic relationship. One male patient developed acute arthritis at age 45. Recurrent episodes of polyarthritis occurred. Sixteen years later Butazolidin was started for the arthritic condition. Two months later he developed an aplastic bone marrow and idiopathic autoimmune hemolytic anemia. The second patient also has been classified as an idiopathic form (Case 13). During her 17 years of disease she has developed recurrent polyarthritis, colitis, erythema nodosa and thyroiditis. In addition, one sibling developed a Stevens-Johnson syndrome. McCormick and Micks (71) have reported the association of hemolytic anemia and polyarthritis in the presence of salmonella infection.

Polyarteritis Nodosa

Polyarteritis nodosa is one of the more uncommon collagen diseases. The association of hemolytic anemia with polyarteritis nodosa is rare. Dacie (52) suggests that the anemia of polyarteritis nodosa is probably of a microangiopathic type (72, 73) rather than autoimmune. Lovshin (74) in 1942 described four cases of polyarteritis nodosa associated with acquired hemolytic anemia. Dameshek and Rosenthal (75) in 1951 mentioned four additional cases of probable autoimmune etiology. A positive antiglobulin test was noted in one patient. Other studies of autoimmune hemolytic anemia have not encountered this association. Wasserman and associates (47) specifically mention seven cases of polyarteritis nodosa without a hemolytic complication. In the current series only one patient presented this combination of diseases.

Case 67. An 18-year-old white male was investigated because of fever, edema and rectal bleeding. Examination revealed petechiae, hepatosplenomegaly, anemia and microscopic hematuria. A history of plastic solvent inhalation was obtained. Investigative studies led to a diagnosis of ulcerative colitis and infectious hepatitis. Transfusions were given and resulted in delayed febrile reactions. In 4 months complete recovery with disappearance of hepatosplenomegaly was noted. The patient returned 2 years later with an identical clinical pattern of hepatosplenomegaly, skin lesions, colitis and microscopic hematuria. Anemia was present with a hemoglobin value of 5 gm. per cent. Skin biopsy was nondiagnostic but calf muscle biopsy revealed polyarteritis nodosa. Spontaneous remission occurred without specific therapy over the next 2 months. Three months later the patient was again seen with pallor, headaches, anorexia and a weight loss of 11 pounds. The spleen was palpated 3 cm. and the liver 5 cm. below the costal margins. An erythematous rash resembling those seen in Henoch-Schönlein disease was seen over the feet and ankles. Some petechiae were noted. A febrile course with temperatures to 106°F. resulted. The hematocrit was 16 per cent with a 1.1 per cent reticulocyte count. The WBC was 24,800/mm.^{3} and thrombocytes were over 300,000/mm.^{3} Bone marrow aspiration revealed generalized hyperplasia. Serologic tests for syphilis and five LE cell preparations were negative. Febrile agglutinins, purified protein derivative and bentonite flocculation tests were all negative. The urinalysis was now normal. Bilirubin was 1.2/0.0 mg. per cent and the A/G ratio was 2.6/3.9 gm. per cent. Serum electro-

phoresis revealed a broad polyclonal gamma elevation containing 46 per cent of the total protein. Alkaline phosphatase, Bromsulphalein, transaminase, and thymol turbidity studies were all abnormal. Direct antiglobulin studies were positive on four occasions. The patient was treated with penicillin and streptomycin. Two transfusions were given and were followed by severe delayed febrile reactions. Intramuscular iron was started and discontinued after sensitivity reactions were noted. The reticulocyte count rose to 6.2 per cent and the hematocrit spontaneously reached 33 per cent. The patient was then lost to followup.

This complex patient with polyarteritis nodosa diagnosed by biopsy had, in addition, ulcerative colitis, hepatitis, a rash suggestive of Henoch-Schönlein's syndrome, hematuria and autoimmune hemolytic anemia. The blending of various immunologically mediated diseases is reminiscent of the patterns seen in lupus erythematosus and scleroderma.

Sjögren's Disease

Parotitis was related to systemic lupus erythematosus in 1952 by Shearn and Pirofsky (16). Morgan and Castleman (76, 77) more definitely implicated Sjögren's disease and Mikuliez's syndrome to lupus erythematosus and collagen diseases. Jones (78) in 1958 suggested that Sjögren's disease may result from an autoimmune aberration. This concept was supported by obtaining positive precipitant reactions between sera from patients with Sjögren's disease and lacrimal gland tissue. Positive LE cell preparations in Sjögren's disease have been noted by Shipton (79), Heaton (80) and Bloch and associates (81). Bunim (62, 82) and Bloch and associates (81) have also demonstrated the presence of rheumatoid factor and circulating autoantibodies directed against cell nuclei, cell cytoplasm, denatured gamma-globulin and thyroglobulin.

These serologic studies suggesting an aberrant immune apparatus are supported by clinical observations. A frequent association of Sjögren's disease with other autoimmune syndromes has been noted. Jones (78) emphasized the relationship of this disease to rheumatoid arthritis and Hashimoto's disease. Heaton (80) suggested that Sjögren's disease, Mikuliez's syndrome and Felty's syndrome may all be manifestations of lupus erythematosus. Shearn (83, 84) reported the association of Sjögren's disease and scleroderma and emphasized the interrelationship of connective tissue disease. The association of disseminated lupus erythematosus and Sjögren's disease has been reported by Morgan (77) and Bain (85). The systemic nature of this disease and its blending into other immunologically mediated syndromes have been clearly demonstrated (81, 82, 84, 86).

Autoimmune hemolytic anemia is not generally considered to be a complication of Sjögren's disease. Gordon and Shanbrom (87) reported one example of this association. Their patient was found to have positive antiglobulin tests which subsequently disappeared after corticosteroid therapy. Anemia and a hemolytic syndrome were not apparent when positive antiglobulin tests were found.

In the current series Sjögren's syndrome was present in one patient (Case 66). She presented with Raynaud's disease, calcinosis circumscripta and scleroderma. Direct and indirect antiglobulin tests were positive. The presence of a hemolytic state was difficult to document because of continual gastrointestinal tract bleeding secondary to portal hypertension.

Dermatomyositis

Dermatomyositis may appear as an acute, subacute or chronic disease localized to the skin and muscles. Polymyositis may be a variant of the same condition. Systemic manifestations are uncommon. Pathologically, the skin is infiltrated by lymphocytes which may appear diffuse or localized in well defined perivascular foci. Such lymphorrhages may simulate germinal centers. Muscular damage may be extensive and consists of edema, degeneration and fragmentation of muscle fibers with replacement by dense collagen tissue.

Positive LE cell preparations may sometimes be found. A peculiar predilection to develop malignancies has been noted in patients with dermatomyositis. These malig-

nancies generally involve the gastrointestinal tract, but lymphomas and sarcomas have also been described.

Autoimmune hemolytic anemia is unusual, in spite of the lymphoproliferative aspect of this disease and the predilection for malignant growth. Wasserman and associates (47) did not encounter a hemolytic syndrome in 14 cases of dermatomyositis. The association of autoimmune hemolytic anemia and dermatomyositis was not seen in our current series of 234 patients. Only two reports have been noted in the literature. Jones and Tillman (88) documented one case of dermatomyositis complicated by the presence of a warm acting serum panhemagglutinin. An ovarian cyst was discovered and surgical removal of a pseudomucinous cystadenoma corrected the hemolytic anemia. The serum panhemagglutinin, however, could still be demonstrated 3 months after surgery. Activity of dermatomyositis did not appear to be clinically related to the presence or correction of the hemolytic state. Unger (89) has also reported an example of hemolytic anemia with positive antiglobulin tests in a patient with uncomplicated dermatomyositis.

Hypersensitivity Reactions

Several patients in the current series presented with disease states generally considered to be hypersensitive in etiology. It frequently was difficult to relate such states to autoimmune hemolytic anemia.

Drug Dependent Anaphylaxis

The relationship of various drugs to hemolytic anemia and positive serologic studies is discussed in detail in Chapter 10. Such cases are probably examples of antiglobulin positive hemolytic anemia and generally do not have systemic manifestations. However, one patient was studied with a clinical pattern suggesting anaphylaxis or serum sickness following drug exposure. Transient autoimmune hemolytic anemia was seen as part of this syndrome.

Case 68. A 27-year-old white male was investigated because of weakness and arthralgias. Pyuria was discovered and oral sulfa therapy was initiated. Facial edema and a fever to 104°F.

developed. Sulfa therapy was discontinued and intramuscular penicillin was started. The fever promptly disappeared. The patient became acutely ill and developed generalized anasarca and back and bone pain. The WBC rose to 108,000/mm.³ with an eosinophilia of 88 per cent. The hematocrit dropped to 32 per cent. Direct antiglobulin and bromelin tests were positive. All therapy was discontinued and gradual symptomatic improvement occurred. In 10 days the hematocrit reached 41 per cent and the WBC had dropped to 9,000/mm.³ An 18 per cent eosinophilia persisted. Pruritus remained as his only complaint and physical examination was negative. Followup examination 10 months later revealed an hematocrit of 45 per cent and a WBC of 6,900/mm.³, without eosinophilia. Negative antiglobulin tests were obtained.

An acute drug reaction occurred in this patient and was associated with a transient episode of autoimmune hemolytic anemia. Either sulfa or penicillin may have initiated the acute hypersensitivity state which resembled serum sickness. The reaction was most probably due to penicillin sensitivity. The similarity of this reaction to that reported by Walsh and Zimmerman (90) for penicillin hypersensitivity and positive LE cell preparations is striking. It also bears some relationship to variations of the hydralazine syndrome which may activate autoimmune processes such as systemic lupus erythematosus. This subject has been extensively reviewed by Alarcón-Segovia and associates (91). The relationship between such drug reactions and autoimmune hemolytic anemia is obscure. The above patient has been classified as having an idiopathic variety of autoimmune hemolytic anemia.

Other Hypersensitivity Reactions

Other syndromes suggesting a hypersensitivity reaction were encountered. One patient with chronic lymphocytic leukemia and autoimmune hemolytic anemia developed erythema multiforme. This patient was hypersensitive to insect products and a mosquito bite generally required vigorous corticosteroid therapy and possibly hospitalization. No particular clinical relationship of the hemolytic state to such hypersensitivity reactions were noted.

Christen and Jaccottet (92) have described a similar patient in whom a bee sting precipitated relapse of autoimmune hemolytic anemia. Copps (93) has reported a patient who developed erythema multiforme and primary atypical pneumonia with hemolytic anemia.

An additional patient (Case 13) has been classified as having an idiopathic variety of autoimmune hemolytic anemia. She suffered from idiopathic migratory polyarthritis, colitis, thyroiditis and erythema nodosa. Hemolytic anemia had been present for many years and required splenectomy. Positive antiglobulin tests were not obtained, however, until erythema nodosa developed.

Summary

The frequent association of lupus erythematosus and autoimmune hemolytic anemia supports the postulate that a multisystem immunologic abnormality is present in such syndromes. However, the current series does not particularly suggest a similar relationship between autoimmune hemolytic anemia and other collagen diseases, or diseases with a hypersensitivity etiology. The three patients with scleroderma and the one patient with polyarteritis nodosa who developed autoimmune hemolytic anemia demonstrate that such combinations do occur. However, the autoimmune hemolytic state frequently appeared as a laboratory curiosity, and hemolysis and/or anemia were minimal or absent. The blending of the various clinical states into complex disease syndromes makes definitive classification difficult.

A clinical review of the various syndromes suggest that difficulties in diagnosis are related to shaky and nonspecific pathologic criteria. This frequently prevents an accurate statement of the interrelationship between various collagen diseases. Specific diagnostic procedures to separate these entities accurately must be established. The converse must also be considered. It is possible that we are dealing with a single disease process which may manifest in various clinical and pathologic patterns. An aberrant immune apparatus may represent the common pathophysiologic abnormality. Only by clarifying this problem can a meaningful interpretation be made of the role of associated autoimmune hemolytic anemia in connective tissue disease.

BIBLIOGRAPHY

1. von Pirquet, C., and Schick, B.: *Die serum Krankheit,* 1905. English translation: *Serum Sickness,* The Williams & Wilkins Company, Baltimore, 1952.
2. Klinge, F.: Der Rheumatismus: Pathologisch-anatomische und experimentell-pathologische Tatsachen un ihre aus Wertung für das ärtzliche Rheumaproblem. Ergebn. Allg. Path. **27**: 1, 1933.
3. Rich, A. R.: Hypersensitivity in disease. Harvey Lect. **42**: 106, 1946–1947.
4. Rich, A. R., and Gregory, J. E.: Experimental anaphylactic lesions of the coronary arteries of the "sclerotic type," commonly associated with rheumatic fever and disseminated lupus erythematosus. Bull. Hopkins Hosp. **81**: 312, 1947.
5. Dixon, F. J.: The role of antigen-antibody complexes in disease. Harvey Lect. **58**: 21, 1963.
6. Dixon, F. J.: Experimental serum sickness. In *Immunological Diseases,* edited by M. Samter. Little, Brown and Company, Boston, 1965.
7. Banks, B. M.: Is there a common denominator in scleroderma, dermatomyositis, disseminated lupus erythematosus, the Libman-Sacks syndrome and polyarteritis nodosa? New Eng. J. Med. **225**: 433, 1941.
8. Klemperer, P., Pollack, A. P., and Baehr, G.: Diffuse collagen disease. Acute disseminated lupus erythematosus and diffuse scleroderma. J. A. M. A. **119**: 331, 1942.
9. Klemperer, P.: The concept of collagen diseases. Amer. J. Path. **26**: 505, 1950.
10. Baehr, G., and Pollack, A. D.: Disseminated lupus erythematosus and diffuse scleroderma. J. A. M. A. **134**: 1169, 1947.
11. Dameshek, W.: Hemolytic anemia. Amer. J. Med. **18**: 315, 1955.
12. Pirofsky, B.: Autoimmune hemolytic anemia and neoplasia of the reticuloendothelium. With a hypothesis concerning etiologic relationships. Ann. Intern. Med. **68**: 109, 1968.
13. Kaposi, M. K.: Neue Beiträge zur Kenntnis des Lupus erythematosus. Arch. Derm. Syph. (Berlin) **4**: 36, 1872.
14. Osler, W.: On the visceral complications of erythema exudativum multiforme. Amer. J. Med. Sci. **110**: 629, 1895.
15. Baehr, G., Klemperer, P., and Schifrin, A.: A diffuse disease of the peripheral circulation (usually associated with lupus erythematosus and endocarditis). Trans. Ass. Amer. Physicians **50**: 139, 1935.
16. Shearn, M. A., and Pirofsky, B.: Disseminated lupus erythematosus. Arch. Intern. Med. (Chicago) **90**: 790, 1952.
17. Harvey, A. M., Shulman, L. E., Tumulty, P. A., Conley, C. L., and Schoenrich, E. H.: Systemic lupus erythematosus: review of the literature and clinical analysis of 138 cases. Medicine (Balt.) **33**: 291, 1954.
18. Hargraves, M. M., Richmond, H., and Morton, R.: Presentation of two bone marrow elements: the "tart" cell and the "L.E." cell. Proc. Mayo Clin. **23**: 25, 1948.
19. Haserick, J. R., Lewis, L. A., and Bortz, D. W.: Blood factor in acute disseminated lupus erythematosus: I. Determination of gamma globulin as specific plasma fraction. Amer. J. Med. Sci. **219**: 660, 1950.
20. Haserick, J. R., and Lewis, L. A.: Blood factor in acute disseminated lupus erythematosus: II. Induction of specific antibodies against L.E. factor. Blood **5**: 718, 1950.
21. Miescher, P.: The antigenic constituents of the neutrophilic leukocyte with special reference to the L. E. phenomenon. Vox Sang. **2**: 145, 1957.
22. Kunkel, H. G., Holman, H. R., and Deicher, H. R. G.: Multiple "autoantibodies" to cell constituents in systemic lupus erythematosus. In *Cellular Aspects of Immunity,* edited by G. E. B. Wolstenholme and M. O'Connor. Little, Brown and Company, Boston, 1959.
23. MacKay, I. R., and Burnet, F. M.: *Autoimmune Diseases.* Charles C Thomas, Publisher, Springfield, Ill., 1963.
24. Holman, H. R.: Systemic lupus erythematosus. In *Immunological Diseases,* edited by M. Samter. Little, Brown and Company, Boston, 1965.
25. Kunkel, H. G., and Tan, E. M.: Autoantibodies and disease. Advances Immun. **4**: 351, 1964.
26. Fabius, A. J. M.: Failure to demonstrate precipitating antibodies against vessel extracts in patients with vascular disorders. Vox Sang. **4**: 247, 1959.
27. Piomelli, S., Stefanini, M., and Mele, R. H.: Antigenicity of human vascular endothelium: lack of relationship to the pathogenesis of vasculitis. J. Lab. Clin. Med. **54**: 241, 1959.
28. Pirofsky, B., and Shearn, M. A.: The familial occurrences of disseminated lupus erythematosus. New York J. Med. **53**: 3022, 1953.
29. Leonhardt, T.: Family studies in systemic lupus erythematosus. Acta Med. Scand. **176**: (suppl.): 416, 1964.
30. Holman, H. R., and Deicher, H. R.: The appearance of hypergammaglobulinemia, positive serologic reactions for rheumatoid arthritis and complement fixation reactions with tissue constituents in the sera of relatives of patients with systemic lupus erythematosus. Arthritis Rheum. **3**: 244, 1960.
31. Pollack, V. E., Mandema, E., and Kark, R. M.: Antinuclear factors in the serum of relatives of patients with systemic lupus erythematosus. Lancet **2**: 1061, 1961.

32. Ansell, B. M., Johnson, G. D., and Weir, D. M.: Antinuclear factors and systemic lupus erythematosus. Lancet 2: 606, 1961.
33. Ziff, M.: Genetics, hypersensitivity, and the connective tissue diseases. Amer. J. Med. 30: 1, 1961.
34. Berman, L., Axelrod, A. R., Goodman, H. L., and McCloughry, R. I.: So-called "lupus erythematosus inclusion phenomenon" of bone marrow and blood. Amer. J. Clin. Path. 20: 403, 1950.
35. Pisciotta, A. V., Giliberti, J. J., Greenwalt, T. J., and Engstrom, W. W.: Acute hemolytic anemia in disseminated lupus erythematosus. Treatment with Cortisone; report of case. Amer. J. Clin. Path. 21: 1139, 1951.
36. Evans, R. S., Takahashi, K., Duane, R. T., Paine, R., and Liu, C.: Primary thrombocytopenic purpura and acquired hemolytic anemia; evidence for a common etiology. Arch. Intern. Med. (Chicago) 87: 48, 1951.
37. Marshall, J., Zoutendyk, A., and Gear, J.: Serum autoantibodies in diseases of the skin. S. Afr. Med. J. 25: 764, 1951.
38. Michael, S. R., Vural, I. L., Bassen, F. A., and Schaefer, L.: Hematologic aspects of disseminated (systemic) lupus erythematosus. Blood 6: 1059, 1951.
39. Zoutendyk, A., and Gear, J. H. S.: Lupus erythematosus—an auto-antibody disease? Brit. Med. J. 2: 1175, 1950.
40. Wiener, A. S.: Autoantibody formation and disease. Brit. Med. J. 2: 163, 1950.
41. Conley, C. L.: Disorders of the blood in disseminated lupus erythematosus. Amer. J. Med. 13: 1, 1952.
42. Kuhns, W. J., and Bauerlein, T. C.: Exchange transfusion in hemolytic anemia complicating disseminated lupus erythematosus. Arch. Intern. Med. (Chicago) 92: 284, 1953.
43. Gold, S. C., and Gowing, N. F.: Systemic lupus erythematosus. A clinical and pathological study. Quart. J. Med. 22: 457, 1953.
44. Baike, A. G.: The direct Coombs test in disseminated lupus erythematosus. Glasgow Med. J. 34: 10, 1953.
45. Jessar, R. A., Lamont-Havers, W., and Ragan, C.: Natural history of lupus erythematosus disseminatus. Ann. Intern. Med. 38: 717, 1953.
46. Dubois, E. L.: The effect of the L.E. cell test on the clinical picture of systemic lupus erythematosus. Ann. Intern. Med. 38: 1265, 1953.
47. Wasserman, L. R., Stats, D., Schwartz, L., and Fudenberg, H.: Symptomatic and hemopathic hemolytic anemia. Amer. J. Med. 18: 961, 1955.
48. Cowling, D. C., and Thomas, I. D.: The significance of the L. E. cell test. Med J. Aust. 1: 905, 1957.
49. Videbaek, A.: Auto-immune haemolytic anaemia in systemic lupus erythematosus. Acta Med. Scand. 171: 187, 1962.
50. Dausset, J., and Colombani, J.: The serology and the prognosis of 128 cases of autoimmune hemolytic anemia. Blood 14: 1280, 1959.
51. Dacie, J. V.: The Haemolytic Anaemias, Part II, Ed. 2. Grune & Stratton, Inc., New York, 1962.
52. Dacie, J. V.: The Haemolytic Anaemias, Part III, Ed. 2. Grune & Stratton, Inc., New York, 1967.
53. Dameshek, W., and Komninos, Z. D.: The present status of treatment of auto-immune hemolytic anemia with ACTH and Cortisone. Blood 11: 648, 1956.
54. Evans, R. S., and Weiser, R. S.: The serology of autoimmune hemolytic disease. Observations on forty-one patients. Arch. Intern. Med. (Chicago) 100: 371, 1957.
55. Dubois, E. L.: Acquired hemolytic anemia as the presenting syndrome of lupus erythematosus disseminatus. Amer. J. Med. 12: 197, 1952.
56. Haserick, J. R., and Long, R.: Systemic lupus erythematosus preceded by false positive serologic tests for syphilis: presentation of five cases. Ann. Intern. Med. 37, 559, 1952.
57. Hejmans, W., Doniach, D., Roitt, I. M., and Holborow, E. J.: Serological overlap between lupus erythematosus, rheumatoid arthritis and thyroid auto-immune disease. Brit. Med. J. 2: 909, 1961.
58. Beigelman, P. M., Goldner, F., and Bayles, T. B.: Progressive systemic sclerosis (scleroderma). New Eng. J. Med. 249: 45, 1953.
59. Orabona, M. L., Albano, O.: Progressive systemic sclerosis (or visceral scleroderma). Acta Med. Scand. 160: (suppl.): 333, 1958.
60. Fudenberg, H., and Wintrobe, M. M.: Symptomatic hemolytic anemia: report of a case with scleroderma. Ann. Intern. Med. 43: 201, 1955.
61. Baloch, G. M. K.: Pathogénie de la sclérodermie et de l'acrosclérose, et leur association avec le phénomène de Raynaud. Pakistan J. Health 2: 116, 1952 (in Presse Med. 1: 889, 1953).
62. Bunim, J. J.: A broader spectrum of Sjögren's syndrome and its pathogenetic implications. Ann. Rheum. Dis. 20: 1, 1961.
63. Talbott, J. H., and Ferrandis, R. M.: Collagen Diseases. Grune & Stratton, Inc., New York, 1956.
64. Bardawil, W. A., Toy, B. L., Galins, N., and Bayles, T. B.: Disseminated lupus erythematosus, scleroderma, and dermatomyositis as manifestations of sensitization to DNA-protein. I. An immunohistochemical approach. Amer. J. Path. 34: 607, 1958.
65. Kampmeier, R. H.: Collagen diseases—unanswered questions on pathogenesis and etiology. Arch. Intern. Med. (Chicago) 106: 753, 1960.
66. Longhi, A.: Contributo allo studio della

malattia sclerodermica; osservazioni cliniche. Arch. Ital. Derm. Sif. **27**: 469, 1955.

67. Piper, W. N., and Helwig, E. B.: Progressive systemic sclerosis. Visceral manifestations in generalized scleroderma. Arch. Derm. (Chicago) **72**: 535, 1955.

68. Miller, R. D., Keating, F. R., and Winkelmann, R. K.: Progressive systemic sclerosis. Acrosclerosis with extensive visceral involvement: report of case. Proc. Mayo Clin. **34**: 58, 1959.

69. Giraud, G., Cazal, P., Latour, H., Lévy, A., Puech, P., and Roujon, J.: Anémie hémolytique par auto-anticorps au cours du rhumatisme articulaire aigu. Montpellier Med. **48**: 468, 1955.

70. Kaplan, M. H.: Autoantibodies to heart and rheumatic fever: the induction of autoimmunity to heart by streptococcal antigen cross-reactive with heart. Ann. N. Y. Acad. Sci. **124**: 904, 1965.

71. McCormick, J. S., and Micks, R. H.: Anaemia of haemolytic type and polyarthritis caused by Salmonella infection. Irish J. Med. Sci. **429**: 421, 1961.

72. Brain, M. C., Dacie, J. V., and Hourihane, D. O'B.: Microangiopathic haemolytic anaemia: the possible role of vascular lesions in pathogenesis. Brit. J. Haemat. **8**: 358, 1962.

73. Brain, M. C., and Hourihane, D. O'B.: Microangiopathic haemolytic anaemia: the occurrence of haemolysis in experimentally produced vascular disease. Brit. J. Haemat. **13**: 135, 1967.

74. Lovshin, L. L.: Periarteritis nodosa: association of acquired hemolytic anemia. Cleveland Clin. Quart. **19**: 28, 1942.

75. Dameshek, W., and Rosenthal, M. C.: Treatment of acquired hemolytic anemia with note on relationship of periarteritis nodosa to hemolytic anemia. Med. Clin. N. Amer. **35**: 1423, 1951.

76. Morgan, W. S., and Castleman, B.: A clinicopathologic study of Mikuliez's disease. Amer. J. Path. **29**: 471, 1953.

77. Morgan, W. S.: The probable systemic nature of Mikuliez's disease and its relation to Sjögren's syndrome. New Eng. J. Med. **251**: 5, 1954.

78. Jones, B. R.: Lacrimal and salivary precipitating antibodies in Sjögren's syndrome. Lancet **2**: 773, 1958.

79. Shipton, E.: A contribution to the study of collagen disease and the L.E. phenomenon. Med. J. Aust. **1**: 911, 1957.

80. Heaton, J. M.: Sjögren's syndrome and systemic lupus erythematosus. Brit. Med. J. **1**: 466, 1959.

81. Bloch, K. J., Buchanan, W. W., Wohl, M. J., and Bunim, J. J.: Sjögren's syndrome: a clinical, pathological, and serological study of sixty-two cases. Medicine (Balt.), **44**: 187, 1965.

82. Bunim, J. J.: Clinical, pathologic and serologic studies in Sjögren's syndrome. Ann. Intern. Med. **61**: 509, 1964.

83. Shearn, M. A.: Sjögren's syndrome in association with scleroderma. Ann. Intern. Med. **52**: 1352, 1960.

84. Shearn, M. A.: The Sjögren-Mikuliez syndrome—its relationship to connective tissue disorders. Calif. Med. **95**: 159, 1961.

85. Bain, G. O.: The pathology of Mikuliez-Sjögren disease in relation to disseminated lupus erythematosus. A review of the autopsy findings and presentation of a case. Canad. Med. Ass. J. **82**: 143, 1960.

86. Bloch, K. J., and Bunim, J. J.: Sjögren's syndrome and its relation to connective tissue diseases. J. Chronic Dis. **16**: 915, 1963.

87. Gordon, M. E., and Shanbrom, E.: The systemic manifestations of Sjögren's syndrome: report of glandular function with histologic, bacterial and viral studies. Ann. Intern. Med. **48**: 1342, 1958.

88. Jones, E., and Tillman, C.: Case of hemolytic anemia relieved by removal of ovarian tumor. J. A. M. A. **128**: 1225, 1945.

89. Unger, L. J.: The effect of ACTH in acquired hemolytic anemia. Amer. J. Clin. Path. **21**: 456, 1951.

90. Walsh, J. R., and Zimmerman, H. J.: The demonstration of the "L.E." phenomenon in patients with penicillin hypersensitivity. Blood **8**: 65, 1953.

91. Alarcón-Segovia, D., Wakim, K. G., Worthington, J. W., and Ward, L. E.: Clinical and experimental studies of the hydralazine syndrome and its relationship to systemic lupus erythematosus. Medicine (Balt.) **46**: 1, 1967.

92. Christen, J. P., and Jaccottet, M.: Anémie hémolytique immunologique par auto-anticorps. 1° partie: clinique. Helv. Paediat. Acta **13**: 131, 1958.

93. Copps, S. C.: Primary atypical pneumonia with hemolytic anemia and erythema multiforme. Clin. Pediat. **3**: 491, 1964.

Chapter 9

The Gastrointestinal Tract and Autoimmune Hemolytic Anemia

Historical Review

Immunologic concepts have been employed in gastrointestinal pathology for many years. The gastrointestinal tract is continually exposed to foreign antigenic substances. Many workers therefore considered that allergic or hypersensitivity mechanisms probably play an important etiologic role in gastrointestinal disease. Emphasis was initially placed on hypersensitivity reactions mediated by exogenous antigens.

In recent years the role of autologous antigens has concerned investigators. The concept of autoimmunization supplied a valuable theoretical tool for such investigations. All parts of the gastrointestinal tract have been involved in speculative approaches employing an autoimmune pathogenesis. Cirrhosis, hepatitis, ulcerative colitis, regional enteritis, malabsorption syndromes, pancreatitis, atrophic gastritis and Addisonian pernicious anemia are some of the prominent syndromes mentioned.

Historically, hemolytic anemia and gastrointestinal disease have been closely associated. Early studies were confused by an intertwining of liver disease, jaundice and hemolytic anemia. This confusion was eventually clarified by demonstrating that jaundice could result from an increased rate of erythrocyte destruction and the release of hemoglobin products (1, 2). In the studies that followed, gastrointestinal abnormalities were occasionally noted as related to erythrocyte injury and death. The early reports of Mouisset and associates (3), Eppinger (4), Mosse (5) and Chevalier and Tourkine (6) related chronic liver disease to hemolysis. By 1941 the relationship was sufficiently clear to permit Singer and Dameshek (7) to include chronic liver disease as a major category in symptomatic hemolytic anemia.

The association of hemolysis and the postulated immunologic mechanisms suggest that gastrointestinal tract disease may have a relationship to autoimmune hemolytic anemia. Chapter 9 is designed to investigate this association. The cases of autoimmune hemolytic anemia in the current series have been reviewed from the aspect of concomitant gastrointestinal disease. No attempt has been made to review the voluminous literature which relates autoimmune mechanisms to the gastrointestinal tract. Excellent surveys of this subject have been presented by Taylor (8), Cruickshank (9), Glynn and Holborow (10) and Tomasi (11).

Analysis of Present Series

In the current series 29 patients developed gastrointestinal disease in a close temporal relationship to autoimmune hemolytic anemia. In 16 the relationship was sufficiently striking to warrant the assumption of a cause and effect status. In the remaining 13 cases the time relationship was tenuous or an additional pathologic state was considered to be more significant. In such examples only a possible relationship is suggested. Accordingly, significant gastrointestinal disease was present in 12.4 per cent of patients with autoimmune hemolytic anemia. An unequivocal relationship was present in 6.8 per cent of the total series. The specific diseases and their unequivocal or possible etiologic relationship to autoimmune hemolytic anemia are summarized in Table 58.

These 29 cases do not represent the total number of gastrointestinal problems presented by our patients with autoimmune hemolytic anemia. Patients with cholecystitis, for example, have been included in Chapter 7 summarizing infectious disease. Malignancies of the gastrointestinal tract are discussed in Chapter 10. Other cases have been excluded when the time sequence or clinical course was not suggestive of a significant association. Several exceptions have been made purely at the author's discretion. Patients were included if associated pathologic states suggested multiple system defects. For example, three patients with scleroderma and one with polyarteritis nodosa had prominent gastrointestinal tract disease and are included in the analysis.

The clinical courses exhibited by patients in these categories varied greatly. Accordingly, no attempt has been made to analyze subjects as if a homogeneous group were involved. Rather, each syndrome is individually analyzed and the similarities and dissimilarities are emphasized in separate discussions.

Liver Disease

The liver is anatomically and physiologically well designed for involvement in immunologic events. The portal blood system assures exposure to antigenic materials absorbed through the gastrointestinal tract. In addition, a sinusoidal circulation and many phagocytic cells create a favorable environment for initiation of immunologic responses. The splenic venous blood passes through the liver circulation. Accordingly, the antibody producing capacity of the spleen is delivered almost totally to the

TABLE 58. *Number and variety of gastrointestinal diseases found in 234 cases of autoimmune hemolytic anemia (AHA) (29 patients had an unequivocal or possible significant association of the two states)*

Type of Disease	No.	Type of Association with Autoimmune Hemolytic Anemia	
		Unequivocal	Possible
Hepatic disease	14	6	8
Laennec's cirrhosis	5	4	1
Scleroderma	3	0	3
Postnecrotic cirrhosis	2	0	2
Biliary cirrhosis	1	1	0
Banti's syndrome	1	1	0
Infectious hepatitis	1	0	1
Toxic hepatitis	1	0	1
Folic acid deficiency	2	2	0
Malabsorption syndrome	2	1	1
Ulcerative colitis	5	3	2
Addisonian pernicious anemia	5	4	1
Pancreatitis	1	0	1
Total	29	16	13

liver. A favorable cellular distribution is also present. Although lymphocytes are not normally found in large numbers in the liver, lymphocytes and plasma cells may infiltrate the portal areas to a striking degree in various disease states. The Kupffer cells may also play a significant immunologic role. In addition to their phagocytic function they apparently possess the ability to produce immunoglobulins. Although the amount produced is normally insignificant, Cohen and associates (12) have demonstrated conspicuous gamma-globulin formation in infectious hepatitis and chronic postnecrotic hepatitis. The responsible cell is a reticuloendothelial structure possibly transitional to plasma cells (13). The major morphologic characteristics of the liver in relationship to immunologic phenomena have been summarized by Glynn and Holborow (10).

Pathologic changes in the liver resulting from immunologic reactivity have been investigated by Steiner and associates (14). They employed a test system based on the reaction of a heteroimmune serum with the liver. Observations were made of the following phenomena as part of the immunologic event: (a) edema of the perisinusoidal space, (b) vacuolar degeneration of parenchymal cells, (c) plasma cell infiltration, (d) necrosis of parenchymal cells (a varied distribution was found with a frequent midzonal or peripheral lobular localization), (e) rare fibrosis due to small areas of necrosis, and (f) vascular lesions similar to those seen after hyperimmunization with foreign proteins.

Historical Review

The study of liver disease has been complicated by insufficient knowledge of the pertinent pathophysiologic mechanisms. The classic division of hepatic cirrhosis into a Laennec's and a postnecrotic type has done little to clarify the problem. Current immunologic approaches may offer some aid in this problem.

Hughes (15) in 1933 and Gear (16) in 1946 suggested that the initial hepatic lesion in cirrhosis could result from immune or even autoimmune mechanisms. The possibility was considered that such lesions could even be self-perpetuating. In the early 1950's Waldenström (17), Kunkel and associates (18) and Saint and associates (19) described a group of patients with a form of cirrhosis which differed from the classical Laennec's type. Females were frequently involved and an alcoholic history often was not obtained. Most patients were young, and the onset of disease frequently resembled acute viral hepatitis. MacKay and associates (20, 21) gave the term active chronic hepatitis to this syndrome and listed the following criteria as characteristic (22): (a) persistent activity for at least 6 months, usually with relapsing or continuing jaundice, (b) high levels of serum transaminase, (c) elevated serum gamma-globulin values, (d) a "piecemeal" hepa-

tocellular necrosis found on biopsy characterized by regeneration, diffuse lymphoid infiltration and fibrosis progressing to cirrhosis, (e) the presence of various autoantibodies, and (f) therapeutic benefit of immunosuppressive therapy and corticosteroids, particularly in the early stage of disease.

Joske and King (23) and MacKay and associates (24) reported that some patients with chronic active hepatitis have positive lupus erythematosus (LE) cell preparations and varying clinical manifestations of systemic lupus erythematosus. This group has been separated and classified as "lupoid hepatitis." Chronic active hepatitis may result from continual activity of virus hepatitis. An alternate explanation has been championed by MacKay and associates (24). The process is viewed as a self-perpetuating autoimmune disease. The presence of lupoid hepatitis, hypergammaglobulinemia, lymphocyte infiltration and various serologic reactions suggesting autoantibodies forms the basis for this immunologic pathogenesis.

Morphologic Changes

The morphologic counterpart of the suggested autoimmune state has been documented by Popper and associates (25). Necrosis of single hepatocytes on the periphery of the lobule appears to be characteristic. Destruction of the limiting plate of the parenchyma follows and is associated with an inflammatory reaction and proliferation of bile ductules. The lesion has been termed peripheral piecemeal necrosis and is characterized by the presence of many gamma-globulin producing cells. This lesion appears relatively early in viral hepatitis, as well as in drug induced hepatic injuries. It is absent in alcoholic hepatitis and in diffuse alcoholic septal and portal cirrhosis. However, it is well developed in the postnecrotic cirrhosis of alcoholics. The lesion is conspicuous in chronic active hepatitis and in lupoid hepatitis. It is absent in the early precirrhotic stage of primary biliary cirrhosis, when macroglobulin producing cells may be found. Piecemeal necrosis occurs in later stages of primary biliary cirrhosis where it acts to transform an incomplete septal or posthepatic type into cirrhosis. Popper and associates (25) feel that the histologic features of piecemeal necrosis are compatible with immune reactivity.

Autoantibodies in Liver Disease

The presence of circulating antibodies against hepatic antigens has been reported by many investigators (15, 16, 26–35) employing a variety of different serologic techniques. The significance of such observations is questionable. A specific antigen has not been identified, the sera of patients with nonhepatic disease frequently give similar reactions and the presumed hepatic autoantibodies have a high degree of reactivity with other tissues and their extracts. These observations do not satisfy the criteria outlined in Chapter 13 for the existence of autoantibodies. Accordingly, in various forms of chronic liver disease, nonspecific substances are found which possess the ability to react with the diseased liver. Popper and associates (25) summarized these studies by stating that "no evidence has been so far obtained that circulating antibodies as such initiate liver injury in the sense of an autoimmune process." They do not rule out the direct action of mesenchymal cells upon hepatocytes as the basis of autoimmunity. It is suggested that the best immunologic system may involve the action of immune complexes in accentuating and possibly perpetuating liver injury.

MacKay and associates (22) feel that an autoimmune mechanism is etiologically involved in active chronic hepatitis and lupoid hepatitis. They obtained positive LE cells (lupoid hepatitis) in 26 of 69 cases of active chronic hepatitis. Weir and associates (36) found antinuclear globulins in four of nine cases of postinfectious hepatitis and in one of four cases of portal cirrhosis. Calabresi and Greenberg (37) obtained positive antinuclear tests in 10 of 32 patients with various types of liver disease. Seven of the positive reactions were in patients with nutritional cirrhosis. Bouchier (38) analyzed the sera of 116 patients with various forms of liver disease for rheumatoid factor, antinuclear

factor, antithyroglobulin and LE cells. Rheumatoid factors (53 per cent), and antinuclear factor (42 per cent) and LE cells (16 per cent) were found in a substantial number of cases resembling active chronic hepatitis. Gajdusek (30) found anticytoplasmic reactivity in the sera of patients with active chronic hepatitis. This reaction was not specific for hepatic antigens. However, MacKay and Larkin (39) found that this immune complement fixation test was positive in 21 per cent of patients with active chronic hepatitis and in 40 per cent of patients with lupoid hepatitis. Hackett and Beech (40) found transient positive reactions in the same test system employing the sera of subjects undergoing routine prophylactic immunization. Reactions were found with adrenal, kidney, thyroid, liver and lung tissue. The significance of this nonspecific reaction is obscure. Unpublished studies in our laboratory employed a similar test system with heart antigens. The sera of patients undergoing open heart surgery were analyzed for the development of complement fixing ability. Over 100 cases were tested and all developed positive reactions. The time relationship postoperatively was such as to preclude immunologic significance. No correlation with the postcardiotomy syndrome or the febrile-lymphocyte splenomegaly syndrome was observed.

Limited attempts have been made to determine a specific hepatic antigen in such complement fixation testing. Asherson (41) felt that the reaction is associated with mitochondrial and cytoplasmic protein rather than with nuclear antigens. Deicher and associates (42) studied patients with primary biliary cirrhosis. They found both microsomal and mitochondrial antigens.

The relationship of autoimmunity to liver disease is unclear. Immunologic mechanisms appear to be involved, at least in the end stages, in a variety of different hepatic diseases. Whether such reactions are autoimmune must still be determined. The primary or secondary role of autoantibodies in initiating damage or reflecting progressive tissue injury is still to be clarified. In addition the potentially damaging action of such immune reactions, even when occurring in a secondary stage, must be considered and correlated with clinical events.

Hemolytic Anemia and Liver Disease

Hepatic disease is frequently accompanied by anemia. A hemolytic pathogenesis is not uncommon (3–6, 43–46). Watson (46) described hemolytic anemia complicating cirrhosis in more than 20 per cent of a large series. More recent studies have confirmed the presence of hemolysis in cirrhosis (47–50). Zieve (51) and Zieve and Hill (52) have suggested that hemolytic anemia may develop through two mechanisms. Cirrhosis may be associated with "hypersplenism." Hyperlipemia may also induce a hemolytic state by the release of lipase into the blood and the creation of lysolecithin. Sheehy and Berman (53) emphasized hemolysis superimposed on acute and chronic blood loss as an explanation for anemia. The bone marrow appeared to be unable to compensate adequately for these factors. Similar observations have been made by Boivin and associates (54). Pitcher and Williams (55) documented a hemolytic state in infectious hepatitis and obstructive jaundice. A reduction of the erythrocyte survival time is almost universally observed in a variety of liver diseases, with cirrhosis prominently involved (54–58). A similar hemolytic state has been described by Sjovall and Wallgren (59) in hepatolenticular degeneration. There is excellent evidence that hemolysis results from the release of copper, which in turn creates an enzootic jaundice (60).

Autoimmune Hemolytic Anemia and Liver Disease

Erythrocyte autoantibodies are not demonstrated in the majority of patients with liver disease and hemolytic anemia. However, a substantial number of cases with positive antiglobulin tests suggesting an autoimmune pathogenesis have been reported. Hyman and Southworth (47) found positive tests in six of 11 patients with chronic liver disease. Hennemann and associates (61) and Hennemann (62) also noted this relationship in infectious hepa-

titis. Heller and associates (63) reported the occurrence of positive antiglobulin and LE cell tests in a patient with chronic liver disease. Arrau and Matte (64) found warm acting erythrocyte autoantibodies in two of 18 patients with cirrhosis. Bakx and associates (65) noted a positive antiglobulin test and cold hemagglutinins in an infant with infectious hepatitis. Wasserman and associates (66) reported a case of infectious hepatitis and hemolytic anemia with an extremely high titer warm hemolysin. The autoantibody disappeared spontaneously with resolution of the hepatitis. Dausset and Marchal (67) demonstrated a hemagglutinin active against trypsinized erythrocytes in the serum of a patient with cirrhosis. This was distinct from an antibody directed against hepatic antigens. Bornemann and Michel (68) studied 40 patients with infectious hepatitis. Twelve patients had hemolytic anemia, and a positive antiglobulin test was obtained in one. Ruggieri and Bolognesi (69) investigated four patients with hemolytic anemia. Positive antiglobulin tests were found in two. A third patient had potent cold hemagglutinins.

Beickert and Siering (70) reported the development of pancytopenia 6 weeks after the onset of infectious hepatitis. Positive direct and indirect antiglobulin tests were found. A similar complication has been reported by Kivel (71). Kölle (72) also noted the development of hemolytic anemia after infectious hepatitis. His patient developed both warm and cold acting erythrocyte autoantibodies. Easton and associates (73) studied a patient with cirrhosis and hemolytic anemia. Strong positive anti-nongamma and weak positive anti-gamma antiglobulin reactions were obtained.

MacKay and associates (22) did not encounter positive antiglobulin reactions in patients with uncomplicated active chronic hepatitis. However, 12 per cent of patients with lupoid hepatitis had positive antiglobulin tests. Similar observations were previously made by Hutchings and Wigley (74).

The incidence of autoimmune hemolytic anemia complicating liver disease is difficult to ascertain. Fodor and Tănăsescu (75) reported hemolytic anemia in 2 per cent of 1200 patients with infectious hepatitis. A hemolytic component was present in 10 per cent of patients with chronic hepatitis. Positive antiglobulin tests were found in 28 of their subjects. In Dacie's series (76) of 250 cases of autoimmune hemolytic anemia, liver disease was present in two patients. One example each of chronic hepatitis and of portal cirrhosis were encountered.

Fourteen patients had significant liver disease in the current series of 234 examples of autoimmune hemolytic anemia. In six an unequivocal relationship to autoimmune hemolytic anemia was postulated. In eight cases a possible relationship existed. Seven varieties of liver disease are included in these two groups.

Alcoholic Cirrhosis

Five patients with Laennec's cirrhosis and positive antiglobulin tests were seen in the current series. In four patients a significant relationship existed between these two states. One subject had persistent pyoderma and recurrent infections. He has been included in the infectious disease category.

Three males and two females had this combination of diseases. All five were alcoholics and three were derelicts. Their ages ranged from 50 to 67 years with a median of 64 years. In all five patients Laennec's cirrhosis was diagnosed at approximately the same time as was hemolytic anemia. Four of the five patients have died. The duration of survival since the onset of the hemolytic state ranged from 2 weeks to 10 months, with a median of 7 months. This suggests that hemolytic anemia appeared in the end stage of disease. Two patients died in progressive liver failure, one with pulmonary insufficiency, and one postoperatively after resection of a colon carcinoma. The remaining patient has survived 12 months since the diagnosis of hemolytic anemia.

Weakness was a universal complaint, and abdominal swelling, confusion, depression and dizziness were also noted. The liver was enlarged in all five patients, and splenomegaly, lymphadenopathy and jaundice were noted in each of two subjects. Melena was absent and gastrointestinal bleeding was not demonstrated in the five cases.

The clinical and laboratory studies are summarized in Table 59. Anemia was moderately severe. Reticulocytosis was not prominent, although bone marrow erythrocytic hyperplasia was found in three patients. A megaloblastic bone marrow was present in one patient. Benign bone marrow plasmacytosis was seen in a second subject. Macrocytes were found in three peripheral blood specimens. Abnormal serum electrophoretic patterns characterized by a broad polyclonal gamma elevation were found in four cases tested.

Clinical Patterns

A similar clinical pattern was seen in the five patients, except for variations reflecting the underlying liver disease. Anemia, although severe, was a relatively insignificant part of a clinical syndrome dominated by liver disease.

Case 69. A 48-year-old white female was hospitalized with a fractured pubis incurred after a fall during excessive consumption of alcohol. Sixteen months later she was again hospitalized with ascites. A diagnosis of Laennec's cirrhosis was made. The patient was icteric with dry, hyperkeratotic skin. Marked ascites was present. The hematocrit was 29.5 per cent, the reticulocyte count was 2.1 per cent and the total bilirubin was elevated. A normal albumin-globulin (A/G) ratio was found. Bone marrow aspiration revealed megaloblastic changes. Both direct and indirect antiglobulin and bromelin tests were weakly positive. Elution obtained an erythrocyte autoantibody, but it was too weak to permit accurate identification. There was no free acid in the patient's stomach secretions. She was treated with Aldactone and hydrochlorothiazide. The hematocrit rose to 34 per cent. The liver was felt 4 cm. below the costal margin. Oral folic acid, 15 mg. daily, was given without a reticulocyte response. Progressive ascites continued. In spite of Mercuhydrin, Aldactone, Hykinone, chlorothiazide, potassium and brewer's yeast, progressive liver failure developed. Death occurred 6 months after positive antiglobulin tests were first obtained.

In the above subject the positive anti-

TABLE 59. *Statistical data obtained from five patients (two females, three males) with Laennec's cirrhosis and autoimmune hemolytic anemia*

Test Procedures	Total	Statistical Data		
		Range	Mean	Median
Clinical data				
Age (years)	5	50–67	62	64
Survival, dead (months)	4	0.5–10	6	7
Laboratory data				
Initial hematocrit (%)	5	22–29.5	24.9	24
Lowest hematocrit (%)	5	19–29.5	23.7	24
Initial reticulocytes (%)	5	0.2–7.5	2.36	1.5
Initial WBC (10^3/mm.^{3})	5	3.4–21.5	11.2	10.5
Initial thrombocytes (10^3/mm.^{3})	4	125–300	188	165
		Normal	Abnormal	
Other laboratory studies				
Total bilirubin	5	4	1	
A/G ratio	4	1	3	
Serum electrophoresis	4	0	4	
Serologic tests for syphilis	5	5	0	
		Increased	Decreased	Normal
Bone marrow aspiration				
Total cellularity	5	1	0	4
Erythrocyte precursors	5	3	0	2
Leukocytes	5	0	0	5
Megakaryocytes	5	0	0	5
Megaloblasts	5	1	0	4
Plasma cells	5	1	0	4
		Weakness	Dizzy	Fever	Bleeding
Presenting symptoms					
Abnormal	5	5	1	1	0
		Spleen	Liver	Lymph nodes	Jaundice
Presenting signs					
Abnormal	5	2	5	2	2

globulin and bromelin tests appeared as an interesting laboratory observation. There was little to suggest a hemolytic anemic state. Megaloblastic changes in the bone marrow were ascribed to the nutritional status and to folic acid deficiency. However, a reticulocyte response did not follow either oral or parenteral folic acid therapy. The clinical course was dominated by progressive liver failure which resulted in death.

Anemia apparently did not contribute to the patient's downhill course, and transfusions were not required.

Three other patients had similar clinical patterns. Relatively weak antiglobulin and bromelin tests were found in association with moderately severe anemia. Evidence for hemolysis was generally lacking. Progressive liver disease dominated the clinical course. One patient entered with severe anemia, hepatosplenomegaly and positive antiglobulin and bromelin tests. A therapeutic response did not occur with hematinics or prednisone. The chromium[51] half-life (T/2) time was normal and splenic sequestration was not present. A mass in the colon was found and laparotomy revealed a carcinoma of the colon. Portal hypertension was diagnosed at surgery and liver biopsy demonstrated Laennec's cirrhosis with congestive splenomegaly. Death occurred postoperatively with peritonitis.

The lack of relationship of positive antiglobulin tests to a hemolytic state is not unique in Laennec's cirrhosis. A similar lack of relationship was seen in other forms of liver disease. Feizi and Woodgate (77) mention two patients with juvenile cirrhosis (active chronic hepatitis) in whom positive direct antiglobulin tests also occurred in the absence of overt hemolytic anemia.

Postnecrotic Cirrhosis

Two examples of postnecrotic cirrhosis associated with autoimmune hemolytic anemia were seen in the current series. Widespread miliary tuberculosis involving the liver, spleen and lymph nodes was present in one case (Case 54). The patient died in liver failure with postnecrotic cirrhosis. A second patient had a complex clinical course which terminated in death. Autopsy revealed the presence of postnecrotic cirrhosis.

Case 70. A 10-year-old white female with polyarthritis was diagnosed as having rheumatic fever. Prophylactic oral sulfa therapy was given for 7 years. During the course of therapy, hypothyroidism was documented and thyroid therapy was employed. Drug reactions to sulfa and penicillin were encountered during this time. At age 19 arthralgia, fever and jaundice developed after severe sunburn. The spleen was palpated 6 cm. and the liver 4 cm. below the costal margins. A rash possibly related to penicillin administration was noted. The hematocrit was 27 per cent, total bilirubin was 2.5/3.5 mg. per cent and LE cell preparations were negative. The white blood cell count (WBC) was 2,000/mm.[3] and thrombocytes were normal. Bone marrow aspiration revealed erythrocytic hyperplasia. In spite of negative antiglobulin tests a diagnosis of autoimmune hemolytic anemia was made. Prednisone therapy induced a moderate rise in the hematocrit. Diabetes became apparent with such therapy. An attempt to withdraw prednisone led to enlargement of the spleen and a return of jaundice. Over the next 7 years the patient received intermittent prednisone therapy. The hematocrit ranged from 26 to 30 per cent. Repeat LE cell preparations and antiglobulin tests were negative. A Cr[51] T/2 time of 9 days, without splenic sequestration, was obtained 30 months after the onset of the hemolytic state. Splenectomy was elected 7 years after the onset of anemia. The spleen was palpated 10 cm. and the liver 4 cm. below the costal margins. The hematocrit was 33 per cent with a 1.0 per cent reticulocyte count. The WBC was 2,400/mm.[3] and thrombocytes were 27,000/mm.[3] A small stomach syndrome was extremely painful. Antiglobulin tests were still negative but the direct bromelin test was weakly positive. Elution was unsuccessful. The patient died after splenectomy with extensive bleeding. The spleen was found to be markedly fibrosed. An unsuspected finding was distortion of the liver and cirrhosis. Pathologic examination revealed postnecrotic cirrhosis.

This patient has been classified as having idiopathic autoimmune hemolytic anemia. The history of rheumatic fever, photosensitivity, hypothyroidism, diabetes, leukopenia, thrombocytopenia, sensitivity to penicillin and sulfa and persistent hemolytic anemia suggests a multisystem disease. Autopsy revealed a fibrotic spleen and severe postnecrotic cirrhosis. There is little doubt that positive LE cell preparations would have led to a diagnosis of lupoid hepatitis.

Autoimmune hemolytic anemia as a part of lupoid hepatitis was not encountered in the present series. This probably reflects the infrequency of this diagnosis at our institution.

Biliary Cirrhosis

The association of autoimmune hemolytic anemia with biliary cirrhosis has not been previously reported. One patient presented this combined syndrome in the present series.

Case 71. A 37-year-old white female developed edema, pruritus and hepatomegaly. Laparotomy and biopsy revealed biliary cirrhosis. Corticosteroid therapy was employed. Severe diabetes developed and required insulin. Persistent jaundice was noted at this time. Vaginal bleeding, epistaxis and xanthomata involving her hands, face and chest developed over the next 2 years. Increasing jaundice and edema, as well as a bleeding tendency, led to the therapeutic use of anabolic agents and cholestyramine. The liver further enlarged to 8 cm. below the costal margin. Fifty-eight months after the onset of her disease, dental extraction was followed by prolonged oral bleeding, hematuria and bacteremia. The liver was still 8 cm. below the costal margin, the spleen was not felt and cervical adenopathy was present. The hematocrit was 33.5 per cent, the reticulocyte count was 1.0 per cent, the WBC was 3,300/mm.^{3}, thrombocytes were 150,000/mm.^{3} and the prothrombin and proconvertin test (P & P) was 52 per cent. Bone marrow aspiration appeared normal. Direct antiglobulin tests were positive, but the direct bromelin test was negative. Progressive edema and ascites developed and were unresponsive to therapy. The total bilirubin rose to over 40 mg. per cent and the P & P dropped to 26 per cent. Hallucinations and coma developed with subsequent death. Duration of biliary cirrhosis was 60 months, with positive antiglobulin tests noted 2 months prior to death.

The above clinical protocol is very similar to that described for Laennec's cirrhosis. A positive antiglobulin test was the only suggestion of autoimmune hemolytic anemia and this appeared as a laboratory curiosity. The patient's clinical course was dominated by progressive liver disease, and neither hemolysis nor anemia appeared to be of importance in management or therapy.

Banti's Syndrome

The anemia found in Banti's syndrome is generally considered to result from "hypersplenism." It has not previously been related to autoimmune hemolytic anemia. One patient with this combined disease was studied in the present series of patients.

Case 72. A male child was the product of an 8 month pregnancy and delivered by section. His mother suffered from toxemia and a yeast infection prior to delivery. Hyaline membrane disease was diagnosed soon after birth, and the child received Similac with iron. His clinical course was complicated by frequent upper respiratory infections and bronchopneumonia. At age 16 months ileus occurred. The spleen was palpated 5 cm. below the costal margin. The hematocrit was 23 per cent and the reticulocyte count was

1.0 per cent. Thrombocytes were depressed and nucleated erythrocytes were found in the peripheral blood. The patient was treated with intramuscular iron, and the hematocrit rose to 33 per cent and reticulocytes to 4.2 per cent. He was returned 11 months later with diarrhea. The spleen was now palpated 8 cm. below the costal margin and guaiac positive stools were found. The hematocrit was 20 per cent with a 4.3 per cent reticulocyte count. Hypochromic erythrocytes were seen and a 10 per cent eosinophilia was found. Bone marrow aspiration revealed erythrocytic hyperplasia. The direct antiglobulin test was positive and the bromelin test was negative. The P & P was 32 per cent. Total bilirubin was 0.3/0.5 mg. per cent, the A/G ratio was 3.3/3.1 gm. per cent, the Bromsulphalein test was 2 per cent, thymol turbidity was 10.2 and serum iron was 37 μg. per cent with a normal serum iron binding capacity. Serum electrophoresis demonstrated a broad polyclonal elevation of gammaglobulin. A diagnosis of Banti's syndrome with esophageal varices was made after diagnostic studies. Iron therapy was given with a progressive rise of the hematocrit to 34 per cent in 1 month. The antiglobulin tests were then negative. The patient is alive 22 months since the demonstration of splenomegaly.

An interesting family history is present in this patient. The mother had a cholecystectomy at age 22 for cholelithiasis. Two brothers have anemia of unknown etiology and both have lymphadenopathy.

Although severe anemia was present in this case, there is little evidence of hemolysis. Gastrointestinal bleeding, hypochromia and a reticulocyte response to iron therapy strongly suggest blood loss with iron deficiency as the cause of anemia. The positive antiglobulin test was an isolated laboratory observation that did not reflect a significant clinical state. The family history, however, indicates a possible genetic background of hematologic disease. This observation suggests that the antiglobulin test might have significance. A familial predisposition in autoimmune hemolytic anemia has been postulated (78). Hereditary spherocytosis is absent in this family, and a specific abnormality has not been documented.

Acute Infectious Hepatitis

Viral states such as atypical pneumonia and infectious mononucleosis are commonly associated with erythrocyte autoantibody formation. Chronic liver disease frequently manifests autoimmune phenomena. These two observations would suggest that infectious hepatitis would show a significant association with autoimmune hemolytic anemia. This does not appear to be the case, and the association of these two states is uncommon.

Hemolytic anemia is not generally considered to be a complication of infectious hepatitis. Jones and Minot (79) in 1923 noted that patients with infectious hepatitis frequently manifested a drop in hemoglobin as icterus improved. On the basis of quantitative studies of bile pigment, they felt that hemolysis was an important factor. Many investigators (61, 62, 65, 66, 68–72, 75, 80) have confirmed the association of hemolytic anemia and infectious hepatitis. Sanchez-Medal (81) reviewed 338 cases of infectious hepatitis for evidence of hemolytic anemia. Hemolysis could be clearly shown in two patients and was possibly present in seven additional cases. An incidence of associated hemolytic anemia of 0.6 to 2.7 per cent may accordingly be estimated. This compares favorably with the experience of Fodor and Tănăsescu (75) who noted a 2 per cent incidence in 1200 cases of infectious hepatitis. Conrad and associates (82) have reported anemia (hematocrit below 40 per cent) and slight reticulocytosis in 19 of 25 cases of infectious hepatitis. They suggest that a hemolytic phase is typical of this disease. The evidence is not particularly convincing. Jandl and associates (83) postulate that splenomegaly is responsible for the premature destruction of erythrocytes in infectious hepatitis. The development of aplastic anemia after infectious hepatitis also suggests that the virus may be directly related to bone marrow damage. Levy and associates (84) and Schwartz and associates (85) have reported this rare complication. Such virus induced bone marrow depression may magnify minor degrees of erythrocyte destruction, leading to overt anemia.

Positive antiglobulin reactions suggesting an autoimmune etiology for the hemolytic state complicating infectious hepatitis are rare. Such cases have been reported by Hennemann (61), Bakx and associates (65), Bornemann and Michel (68), Beickert and Siering (70), Kölle (72) and Fodor and Tănăsescu (75). A hemolytic factor was mentioned by Wasserman and associates (66). Negative antiglobulin tests have been found by Schmidt (86), Raffensperger (80) and Sanchez-Medal (81).

In the current series of patients with autoimmune hemolytic anemia a past history of jaundice and/or "liver infection" was common. This is not particularly striking in our geographic area with endemic infectious hepatitis. A relationship of infectious hepatitis to subsequent autoimmune hemolytic anemia was not apparent. In two patients homologous serum jaundice developed after transfusion therapy. Although severe clinical disease resulted, the hemolytic process did not intensify.

In two patients a possible relationship of hepatitis to positive antiglobulin tests was observed. One had infectious mononucleosis with hepatitis (Case 41). Anemia was minimal in this patient, and hemolysis was not documented. In a second patient ulcerative colitis, infectious hepatitis and plastic solvent inhalation were simultaneously present (Case 67). Polyarteritis nodosa was eventually diagnosed, and the relationship of hepatitis to concomitant autoimmune hemolytic anemia is questionable.

Toxic Hepatitis

One patient in the current series developed toxic hepatitis after autoimmune hemolytic anemia. A relationship between these two states is not obvious. Her protocol is presented below.

Case 73. A 38-year-old white female developed hepatitis and jaundice, and made an uneventful recovery. Fifteen years later she complained of chills, fever and weakness. Anemia was discovered and jaundice was noted. The hematocrit dropped to 20 per cent. Five blood transfusions were given. She was investigated 5 weeks later. The liver, spleen and lymph nodes were not palpated. The hematocrit was 22 per cent and the reticulocyte count was 15.5 per cent. Bone marrow aspiration revealed erythrocytic hyperplasia. Direct and indirect antiglobulin and bromelin tests were positive, and elution obtained a panhemagglutinin. Corticosteroid therapy was given with an excellent therapeutic response. Over the next 13 months gradual reduction and finally discontinuation of corticosteroids was accomplished. The antiglobulin and bromelin tests persisted as positive for 20 months. Followup 50 months after the onset of anemia demonstrated negative antiglobulin tests and normal hematologic values. Twelve months later the patient fractured her ankle. Surgical open reduction was done. Postoperatively she developed paralytic ileus and pneumonia. Hematologic values were still normal. Death occurred 1 week later. Autopsy revealed bronchopneumonia, ulcerative cystitis, interstitial nephritis and toxic hepatitis.

Hepatitis had occurred 15 years prior to autoimmune hemolytic anemia in this patient. It is difficult to relate these two states. The patient had an excellent therapeutic response of hemolysis to corticosteroid therapy. An asymptomatic clinical course followed. Five years after the development of autoimmune hemolytic anemia the patient died after surgery for a traumatic fracture. The autopsy indicated that "the hepatic cells universally revealed extensive cloudy swelling with an enlargement of the sinusoids. Accumulation of inflammatory cells is not observed." A diagnosis of toxic hepatitis was made. As with the prior hepatitis, it is difficult to relate the hepatic lesion to autoimmune hemolytic anemia. The patient has accordingly been classified as having idiopathic autoimmune hemolytic anemia.

Scleroderma

Three patients of the present series had scleroderma and autoimmune hemolytic anemia; all three also had liver involvement. Portal hypertension was severe and dominated the clinical course in two patients (Cases 65 and 66). In a third patient (Case 7) liver disease was associated with ascites and hypoalbuminemia. In all three patients multiple system involvement was apparent and liver disease appeared as only one part of a severe systemic immune abnormality. Positive antiglobulin tests in all three were present without convincing evidence of hemolysis. In this regard scleroderma with liver disease resembled many of the other cases of liver disease.

Folic Acid Deficiency

In 1953 Spray and Witts (87) reported that an excessive bone marrow output of erythrocytes may deplete folic acid. Jonsson and associates (88) confirmed this observation. Folic acid utilization was found to reflect an increased production and delivery of erythrocytes. The administration of a folic acid antagonist, pyrimethamine, created megaloblastic bone marrow changes in patients with a hemolytic syndrome more easily than it did in normal individuals.

A folic acid deficiency complicating acquired hemolytic anemia was also noted by Gruelund (89) and Baikie and Pirrie (90). Chanarin and associates (91) investigated a case of hemolytic anemia characterized by positive non-gamma antiglobulin tests, autoagglutination in albumin solutions and megaloblastic bone marrow. Plasma levels of vitamin B-12 were normal and folic acid was rapidly cleared. The patient was treated with both prednisone and vitamin B-12. Thirteen additional cases of hemolytic anemia were studied. An increased rate of plasma folic acid clearance was noted in all. Willoughby and associates (92) investigated a similar patient. A megaloblastic bone marrow and macrocytosis suggested the presence of pernicious anemia. However, there was free acid in the stomach and serum vitamin B-12 levels were normal. The direct antiglobulin test was positive and elution studies obtained an erythrocyte autoantibody. A Cr^{51} T/2 survival time of 7 days was obtained. Vitamin B-12 therapy led to a 25 per cent reticulocyte count and to partial conversion of the marrow toward normal. The hematocrit rose but did not reach normal values. Folic acid therapy resulted in a reticulocyte count of 15 per cent and in the disappearance of the megaloblastic marrow picture. The hematocrit again rose but still did not reach normal levels. Prednisone therapy led to a complete hematologic remission.

The above observations suggesting a relative folic acid deficiency in autoimmune hemolytic anemia were confirmed in the current series. However, this state did not appear to be rare. Megaloblastic changes in the bone marrow were apparent in 25 of the 162 specimens examined. This 15 per cent incidence of morphologic abnormalities suggests that more elegant biochemical tests would reveal a substantially higher incidence of folic acid deficiency in autoimmune hemolytic anemia.

An increased turnover rate of erythrocytes is not the only mechanism leading to folic acid deficiency associated with autoimmune hemolytic anemia. Folic acid or vitamin B-12 deficient states may be etiologically related to a secondary form of autoimmune hemolytic anemia. In addition, autoimmune hemolytic anemia may develop in patients with subclinical deficiencies of folic acid and vitamin B-12. The hemolytic state in such patients would magnify the deficiency and make clinically apparent the underlying disease. There is some evidence for these alternative suggestions. In seven of the 25 patients with a megaloblastic bone marrow, the diagnoses of folic acid deficiency (two cases) and Addisonian pernicious anemia (five cases) were made.

Autoimmune hemolytic anemia may induce a secondary folic acid deficiency. The current series indicates that the reverse relationship also exists. Two patients were seen with a primary folic acid deficiency, anemia and positive antiglobulin tests.

Case 74. A 56-year-old white male alcoholic was hospitalized because of weight loss, cough, epigastric pains, vomiting, diarrhea and dyspnea. He had consumed 1 quart of wine daily and had a satisfactory diet until 6 months prior to the development of the above symptoms. Physical examination revealed pallor, edema, malnutrition, dehydration and a smooth tongue. Jaundice was absent and the liver was palpated 4 cm. below the costal margin. His hematocrit was 17.5 per cent and the reticulocyte count was 0.8 per cent. Thrombocytes and leukocytes were normal. Peripheral blood erythrocytes appeared macrocytic. Bone marrow aspiration revealed erythrocytic hyperplasia with megaloblastic changes. The total bilirubin was 0.8/0.4 mg. per cent, the A/G ratio was 3.0/1.9 gm. per cent and the transaminase was slightly elevated. Thymol turbidity, cephalin flocculation and alkaline phosphatase studies were normal. The blood urea nitrogen (BUN) was 42 mg. per cent. Free acid was demonstrated in stomach secretions. The direct antiglobulin test was positive and the bromelin test was negative. Folic acid, 0.5 mg. intramuscularly (I.M.), was given daily. Five days later the reticulocyte count reached 11.4 per cent and the hematocrit started to rise. A peak reticulocyte count of 16.3 per cent was attained and the hematocrit 2 weeks after start of folic acid was 30 per cent. Trace positive direct antiglobulin and bromelin tests were still present. Oral folic acid was given, and the hematocrit reached 47 per cent with a 0.5 per cent reticulocyte count 11 weeks after the start of therapy. Corticosteroids were not given. The patient is still receiving oral folic acid and is in hematologic remission.

Case 75. A 32-year-old white male suffered repeated strokes leading to hemiplegia. Over the next 5 years slurring of speech, inability to swallow and progressive neurologic crippling occurred. He developed repeated attacks of pneumonia secondary to aspiration. During this 14-year course his hematocrit consistently remained over 40 per cent. At age 48 he was hospitalized in semicoma with marked emaciation. Malnutrition and dehydration were diagnosed in a neurologic cripple who could not swallow adequately. The liver, spleen and lymph nodes were not palpated. The hematocrit was 17 per cent with a 0.3 per cent reticulocyte count. Macrocytosis was present. A megaloblastic bone marrow with an increased number of normal plasma cells was found. The total bilirubin was 0.4/0.2 mg. per cent and the A/G ratio was 3.2/3.8 gm. per cent. Serum electrophoresis revealed a broad gammaglobulin polyclonal peak. The BUN was 16 mg. per cent and free acid was found in the stomach. Direct and indirect antiglobulin and bromelin tests were positive. A cold hemagglutinin with a 128 titer was documented. Folic acid, 0.5 mg. I.M. daily, was given. On the 5th day the reticulocyte count reached 10.6 per cent and the hematocrit was rising. A peak reticulocyte count of 13.7 per cent was attained on the 8th day of therapy. Oral folic acid, 5 mg. daily, was given and a permanent tracheostomy was installed. The hematocrit reached 24 per cent after 2½ weeks of therapy. The patient was sent to a nursing home on oral folic acid therapy. During this time the direct antiglobulin test was positive on seven occasions. The patient was returned to the hospital 9 months later in coma and moribund. Folic acid therapy had been inadvertently discontinued. The hemacrit was 7.5 per cent and the reticulocyte count was 0.4 per cent. Direct antiglobulin and bromelin tests were positive. Folic acid was given parenterally and the patient died the next day. Autopsy revealed cystic degeneration in the caudate nucleus and thalamus, atrophic gastritis, bronchopneumonia and a normal spleen.

These two patients illustrate a clinical pattern which differs from that previously reported in the association of autoimmune hemolytic anemia with folic acid deficiencies. In the cases reported previously, idiopathic autoimmune hemolytic anemia was complicated by a secondary form of folic acid deficiency. In the two patients described above the fundamental defect was a macrocytic anemia due to a lack of folic acid. Positive antiglobulin tests and erythrocyte autoantibodies were unexpected. There was no evidence of hemolysis. Therapy consisted exclusively of minute amounts of folic acid. Hematologic remission occurred without resort to corticosteroids or to immunosuppressive therapy. It is doubtful whether true autoimmune hemolytic anemia was present. The possibility must be considered that the positive antiglobulin tests reflected abnormal erythrocytes with modified antigens resulting from the lack of folic acid.

Malabsorption Syndromes

The folic acid deficiency states described above resulted from a limited intake of food. Gastrointestinal pathology creating malabsorption might lead to a similar state and to the association of positive antiglobulin tests. Two such cases were studied in the current series. In one patient (Case 89) anemia was associated with positive antiglobulin tests for over 5 years. A hypochromic microcytic picture was present. A duodenal ulcer, subtotal gastrectomy, marginal ulcer, vagotomy and occasional melena complicated the diagnosis. A malabsorption syndrome with steatorrhea had been present for a 4-year period. Eventually a hysterectomy was performed and multiple hydatid ovarian cysts were discovered and removed. Anemia has not recurred since. Any relationship of the malabsorption syndrome to the positive antiglobulin tests is accordingly problematical. The case of the second patient is presented below.

Case 76. A 44-year-old white male developed severe diarrhea and weight loss. He was treated with corticosteroids and Azulfidine without a therapeutic response. He was hospitalized and intestinal biopsy revealed nontropical sprue. A glutin free diet was initiated with moderate relief. Recurrence of bloody diarrhea soon developed. Prednisone, 60 mg. daily, was begun and induced a therapeutic remission. Prednisone was reduced to 60 mg. every other day. Fever and sweating developed. The hematocrit was 36 per cent and the reticulocyte count was 1.1 per cent. The WBC was 5,700/mm.^{3} and thrombocytes were 202,000/mm.^{3} Bone marrow aspiration was normal except for hypochromic changes. The direct antiglobulin test was positive and the bromelin test was negative. A liver biopsy was performed and was complicated by fainting and shock. The hematocrit dropped to 18 per cent and the clotting time was prolonged. Multiple transfusions were given. A laparotomy was carried out to repair a lacerated liver biopsy wound. Unclotted blood in the amount of 5300 ml. was found in the peritoneal cavity. The thrombocytes had dropped to 35,000/mm.^{3} and fibrinogen to 100 mg. per cent. In spite of 33 transfusions and 12 gm. of fibrinogen, the patient died in shock.

The above patient with severe nontropical sprue died from a hemorrhage following liver biopsy. Multiple abnormalities of the clotting mechanisms were discovered. The positive direct antiglobulin test had not been anticipated and evidence of a hemolytic state was lacking. There is little to suggest either that autoimmune hemolytic anemia was present or that it contributed to the clinical picture.

Ulcerative Colitis

On theoretical grounds, diseases of the intestines should predispose a patient to the development of associated autoimmune hemolytic anemia. The gastrointestinal tract contains antigens common to the erythrocyte. In secretors, the ABO blood group substances are found in salivary, gastric and bowel secretions. The immunologic complexity of such mucopolysaccharides has been emphasized by Glynn and Holborow (10). Immunologic differences exist between similar antigens found in different tissues (93, 94). In addition, Holborow and Loewi (95) have demonstrated that different parts of complex mucopolysaccharide molecules may induce humoral antibody formation and delayed hypersensitivity.

Accordingly, immunologic aberrations involving the bowel may concomitantly involve immunologic reactivity directed against erythrocytes.

Evidence has accumulated which suggests that the bowel may be involved in autoimmune disease states. Bernier and associates (96) have produced ileitis in guinea pigs through autoantibody activity. Holborow and associates (97) failed to produce autoantibodies in experimental homologous bowel systems, but they induced autoantibody formation in rabbits immunized with rat colon. Ulcerative colitis in particular appears to be related to autoimmune phenomena. In 1925 Andresen (98) suggested that ulcerative colitis might reflect an allergic or hypersensitivity reaction to various foods. The clinical picture of an explosive onset characterized by ulcerative inflammatory changes is suggestive of a hypersensitivity reaction. The association of this disease with liver problems (99–101), ocular disorders (102), arthritis (103), myocarditis (104), glomerulitis (105, 106), purpura (106), leukopenia (107), splenomegaly (108), pyoderma (109), erythema nodosa (109, 110), thyroiditis (111, 112), lupus erythematosus (113–115), Sjögren's disease (116), polyarteritis nodosa (117), scleroderma (118), rheumatoid arthritis (103, 119, 120), myasthenia gravis (113), and autoimmune hemolytic anemia (121) is suggestive of a diffuse immunologic abnormality. We have studied ulcerative colitis associated with renal amyloidosis, which also suggests an immune aberration. A high incidence of cytomegalic inclusion disease in adults with ulcerative colitis (122) further suggests an immunologic deficiency. Hypergammaglobulinemia is common in ulcerative colitis and may also reflect an immune aberration. The role of immunologic mechanisms in ulcerative colitis has been reviewed by Gray (123) and by Kraft and Kirsner (124).

Autoantibody Formation in Ulcerative Colitis

The sera of patients with ulcerative colitis have been shown to contain antibodies reacting with extracts from the colon of newborn children who died without feeding (125, 126). Pheno-water extracts of the colon were studied and the antigen separated in the watery layer. This antigen was able to coat erythrocytes. Such observations suggest a polysaccharide nature of the antigen. Klavins (127) demonstrated that serum gamma-globulin from patients with ulcerative colitis would bind to colonic mucosal cell cytoplasm. His study also suggested a polysaccharide antigen. The presence of antinuclear globulins in the sera of patients with ulcerative colitis was demonstrated by Calabresi and associates (128) using a fluorescent antiglobulin technique. Broberger and Perlman (126) reported antibodies in the sera of six of 13 patients with ulcerative colitis which reacted with the colonic mucosa of normal human blood group O adults. Asherson and Broberger (129) demonstrated autoimmune complement fixation antibody reactions with sera from patients with ulcerative colitis. In addition, the white cells (lymphocytes?) from the peripheral blood of ulcerative colitis patients having circulating antibodies exert an immunologically specific cytotoxic effect on fetal colon cells (130, 131). Perlman and associates (132) have shown that the hemagglutinating antibody is primarily an IgM immunoglobulin.

The significanse of such antibodies in the sera of patients with ulcerative colitis is still obscure. Farr (133) points out that such antibodies do not necessarily indicate an immunologically induced state. Von Kleist and Burtin (134) have demonstrated such antibodies in the sera of normal individuals and in that of patients with carcinoma of the colon. Fletcher (135) noted high serum complement levels in ulcerative colitis, in contrast to the low levels generally observed in autoimmune diseases.

Glynn and Holborow (10) feel that current evidence is insufficient to implicate ulcerative colitis as part of a generalized autoimmune disease. Fong and associates (136), on the other hand, suggest that ulcerative colitis may be an autoimmune disease characterized by an underlying genetic predisposition to develop aberrant immunologic responses.

Autoimmune Hemolytic Anemia and Ulcerative Colitis

Anemia is commonly observed in ulcerative colitis and was encountered in 81 per cent of the series studied by Beal and associates (137). They suggest that blood loss and iron deficiency are of primary etiologic importance. Although a hemolytic stage could not be excluded, it was felt to be of limited significance.

Autoimmune hemolytic anemia, as characterized by positive antiglobulin tests, is considered to be rare in ulcerative colitis. This is erroneous. Lorber and associates (138) in 1955 first called attention to the association of ulcerative colitis with autoimmune hemolytic anemia; four cases were reported. An additional 14 cases have since been recorded (76, 136, 137, 139–145). Bardana and Pirofsky (121) have summarized these cases and added seven of their own patients.

Not all patients with an associated ulcerative colitis and positive antiglobulin test have had evidence of a hemolytic state. Hemolysis was apparent in only one of the four patients of Lorber and associates (138). The patient of Fong and associates (136) had little clinical evidence of hemolysis; however, a shortened erythrocyte survival time greater than that anticipated from blood loss was found. Hemolysis could not be proved for the patient studied by Beal and associates (137). Only two of Keene's (139) three patients and two of Dacie's (76) three patients had overt hemolytic anemia.

Analysis of Present Series

In the current series ulcerative colitis with positive antiglobulin tests was observed in five patients. The statistical, clinical and laboratory observations are summarized in Table 60. Three males and two females were involved. The subjects were relatively young with a median age of 27. Three patients died after durations of ulcerative colitis of 232, 163 and 16 months, respectively. One patient is alive after 13 months of disease. One patient was living when lost to followup after 36 months of disease. Ulcerative colitis was present prior to the development of positive antiglobulin tests in all five patients. The duration of preexisting colitis ranged from 3 to 225 months, with a mean of 87 and a median of 35 months. Autoimmune hemolytic anemia generally appeared as an end stage complication. Death occurred in a range from 2 to 7 months after the onset of positive antiglobulin tests. The one case still living has had positive antiglobulin tests for 10 months. The patient lost to followup was studied for only 1 month after hemolytic anemia was diagnosed.

Moderate anemia was generally present. Reticulocytosis was uncommon at the onset of hemolytic anemia. The reticulocyte count usually elevated with therapy. Leukopenia and thrombocytopenia were not a problem. A reversed A/G ratio with elevated globulin was found in two of four cases examined. In these, broad polyclonal gamma elevations were demonstrated. Such peaks contained 46 and 62 per cent, respectively, of the total protein. Erythrocytic hyperplasia was found in two of three bone marrows examined

Weakness, fever, bloody diarrhea, anorexia, weight loss and abdominal distress were common. Arthritis was present in only one of these patients. Physical examination was not remarkable. Enlargement of the liver, spleen and lymph nodes was infrequent. Jaundice was found in one case and an enlarged thyroid was found in two patients.

Clinical Patterns

Several clinical patterns were observed. One patient had an uncomplicated course with a clear relationship between ulcerative colitis and autoimmune hemolytic anemia.

Case 77. A 20-year-old white male developed bloody diarrhea, nausea, vomiting, malaise and severe dehydration. The physical examination was normal. Sigmoidoscopy and x-ray studies were diagnostic of ulcerative colitis. Small doses of prednisone and Azulfidine were given without response. The patient's weight decreased 40 pounds. A previous hematocrit of 42 per cent dropped to 32 per cent in 3 weeks. The reticulocyte count elevated to 6.3 per cent. Leukocytes, thrombocytes, total bilirubin, A/G ratio

TABLE 60. *Statistical data obtained from five patients (two females, three males) with ulcerative colitis (UC) and autoimmune hemolytic anemia (AHA)*

Test Procedures	Number	Statistical Data		
		Range	Mean	Median
Clinical data				
Age (years)	5	18–58	28	27
Duration of UC before AHA (months)	5	3–225	87	35
Survival with UC, dead (months)	3	16–232	137	163
Survival with AHA, dead (months)	3	2–7	5	7
Laboratory data				
Initial hematocrit (%)	5	16.1–38	26.1	24
Lowest hematocrit (%)	5	16.1–31.5	24.5	24
Initial reticulocytes (%)	4	0.5–6.3	2.2	1.9
Therapeutic reticulocytes (%)	4	2.2–12.6	5.9	4.3
Initial WBC (10^3/mm.^{3})	5	2.1–24.8	12.4	11.8
Initial thrombocytes (10^3/mm.^{3})	4	74–300	232	275

		Weak	Fever	Weight loss	abdominal pain	Bloody diarrhea
Presenting symptoms Abnormal	5	5	4	5	5	5

		Spleen	Liver	Lymph nodes	Jaundice
Presenting signs Abnormal	5	1	2	1	1

Patients	Additional Disease States
Case 77	None
Text case (see p. 215)	Mycosis fungoides, Hodgkin's disease
Case 67	Hepatitis, plastic solvent inhalation, hematuria, polyarteritis nodosa, hypergammaglobulinemia, Henoch-Schönlein's purpura
Case 78	Nodular thyroid, hypothyroidism, hypergammaglobulinemia, carcinoma of cecum
Case 79	Multiple infections, nodular thyroid, ovarian cysts

and serum electrophoresis were normal. A Cr^{51} T/2 time of 24 days was found. Direct antiglobulin tests were positive on two occasions. Prednisone, 60 mg. per day, was started and 7 ml. of intramuscular iron were given. In 2 weeks the reticulocyte count reached 12.6 per cent and there was symptomatic improvement. The hematocrit slowly rose and 2½ months after therapy it reached 48.5 per cent. Prednisone, which had been gradually reduced, was discontinued. Followup 9 months later revealed a hematocrit of 47 per cent, negative serologic studies and an asymptomatic patient.

This case presents a clear association of ulcerative colitis, anemia and positive antiglobulin tests. It is more difficult to determine whether hemolysis is also present. Although a mild reduction of erythrocyte survival was documented, its significance is

obscure in the presence of possible gastrointestinal blood loss.

The simplicity of the clinical state exhibited by the above patient was unique
in the present series. Complex multisystem
disease was encountered in the remaining
four patients. One patient developed ulcerative colitis and mycosis fungoides at age
29. Both conditions were moderately active
for 17 years. Lymphadenopathy developed
at that time and Hodgkin's disease was
diagnosed by biopsy. Sixteen months later
severe anemia with positive antiglobulin
tests was found. Death occurred in 7 months
with progressive Hodgkin's disease and
mycosis fungoides. A second patient (Case
67) presented the association of ulcerative
colitis, hepatitis, hepatosplenomegaly, plastic solvent inhalation, hematuria, hypergammaglobulinemia, polyarteritis nodosa
and a rash suggesting Henoch-Schönlein's
disease. Positive direct antiglobulin tests
and severe anemia developed. The cases of
the remaining two patients with ulcerative
colitis and autoimmune hemolytic anemia
are briefly described below.

Case 78. A 27-year-old white pregnant female
developed bloody diarrhea. Ulcerative colitis was
diagnosed and colostomy was performed. The
patient did well for many years except for anemia which required iron therapy. At age 40,
fatigue and fever resulted in hospitalization and
investigation. Physical examination demonstrated a liver palpated 4 cm. below the costal
margin, a 9 × 9 cm. abdominal mass, melanosis
of the skin, fever to 103°F. and a diffusely
enlarged nodular thyroid. The hematocrit was
24 per cent with a reticulocyte count of 0.5 per
cent. LE cells, heterophile agglutinins, serologic
tests for syphilis and cold hemmagglutinins were
negative. Bone marrow aspiration revealed erythrocytic hyperplasia. The total bilirubin was
normal and protein bound iodine values of 0.3
and 0.9 μg. per cent were obtained. The A/G
ratio was 2.0/4.8 gm. per cent. Serum electrophoresis demonstrated that 62 per cent of the
protein existed as a polyclonal gamma peak.
Direct antiglobulin and bromelin tests were
positive. Laparotomy revealed a carcinoma of
the cecum with metastasis. The liver and spleen
were not involved in the malignant process.
Prednisone was given with a progressive rise of
the hematocrit. Five months after resection of
the primary carcinoma, rapid growth of meta-

static lesions became apparent. 5-Fluorouracil
was given with a transient response. Death occurred from the malignancy. The hematocrit was
well maintained at 37 per cent.

Case 79. A 58-year-old white female developed bloody diarrhea, anorexia, nausea and
vomiting. Hospitalization was carried out and
diagnostic studies revealed ulcerative colitis. The
patient was unsuccessfully treated with penicillin, streptomycin and Azulfidine. A therapeutic
response to prednisone occurred. She returned
to the hospital 1 year later with fulminating
ulcerative colitis. Blood transfusions were given
and a symptomatic remission was produced with
adrenocorticotrophic hormone. Three months
later she again returned acutely ill. Extensive
active ulcerative colitis was present. The liver,
spleen and lymph nodes could not be felt. The
hematocrit was 35 per cent and the A/G ratio
was 3.2/2.3 gm. per cent. A fever of 104°F.
developed and *Escherichia coli* cystitis was
found. Rapid weight loss and frequent bloody
stools were present. Prednisone, 60 mg. per day,
was given without halting the disease. Moniliasis became apparent. The hematocrit dropped to
24 per cent and blood cross matches revealed
an incompatibility. Direct antiglobulin and
bromelin tests were positive with negative indirect studies. Elution revealed an erythrocyte
autoantibody. Blood transfusions were given
and were followed by severe reactions and shock.
Colectomy was planned and then canceled when
E. coli pneumonia developed. Tracheostomy was
performed. A staphylococcal pneumonia with
extensive oral moniliasis developed. The patient expired after a total course of 16 months
of severe ulcerative colitis. Positive antiglobulin
tests had been present during the last 2 months
of disease. Autopsy revealed multinodular thyroid disease and bilateral ovarian cysts, as well
as ulcerative colitis and pneumonia.

Two dissimilar relationships between
ulcerative colitis and positive antiglobulin
tests are apparent in the present patient
group. In two cases positive antiglobulin
tests developed in the absence of ulcerative
colitis activity. In Cases 66, 77 and 79 the
onset of autoimmune hemolytic anemia correlated with activity of the bowel disease.

It is exceedingly difficult to determine
whether hemolysis developed in the five
cases presented above. Such a diagnosis is
tenuous in the presence of gastrointestinal
bleeding. Accordingly, the clinical significance of the observed positive antiglobulin

tests is obscure. A hemolytic state probably contributed to the anemic condition in all five patients. However, in only two patients was hemolysis clinically important in the combined disease syndrome.

Ulcerative Colitis as a Multiple System Immunologic Disease

The complex multisystem involvement noted in four of the five subjects represents the most striking clinical observation of this patient group. In addition to ulcerative colitis and autoimmune hemolytic anemia, mycosis fungoides and Hodgkin's disease were present in one case. A second patient had hepatitis, hematuria, polyarteritis nodosa, hypergammaglobulinemia and a rash suggesting Henoch-Schönlein's disease. A third patient presented a clinical pattern of ulcerative colitis, positive antiglobulin tests, marked hypergammaglobulinemia, carcinoma of the cecum and a nodular thyroid with severe hypothyroidism. The fourth patient in this group had fulminating ulcerative colitis, autoimmune hemolytic anemia, multinodular thyroid disease, ovarian cysts and extensive infections including *E. coli* cystitis and pneumonitis, staphylococcal pneumonia and moniliasis. This pattern of a widespread multisystem disease state may have etiologic significance.

Lorber and associates (138) suggested that the colon may have a haptenic relationship to erythrocytes. Autoantibody formation directed against the colon could therefore lead to autoimmune hemolytic anemia. In support of this concept these authors reported that bowel surgery was followed by diminution or reversal of the positive antiglobulin test. This postulate no longer appears tenable. Fong and associates (136) demonstrated that autoantibodies directed against the colon were distinct from the erythrocyte autoantibody. In addition, two of Keene's cases (139) developed autoimmune hemolytic anemia 11 and 14 years, respectively, after total colectomy. Balint and associates (142) suggested that erythrocyte autoantibodies may develop in response to altered erythrocytic materials absorbed through the diseased bowel. This appears unlikely. If such a pathogenesis were involved, we would anticipate the frequent occurrence of positive antiglobulin tests in ulcerative colitis. In addition, Keene's cases (139) and the patients in the present series illustrate the development of positive antiglobulin tests after years of quiescent ulcerative colitis. Fong and associates (136) suggest that an "underlying genetic predisposition to aberrant immunologic responses" exists in patients with ulcerative colitis, and that this condition may be one of the autoimmune diseases. Bardana and Pirofsky (121) have expanded this view, and they suggest that the multisystem involvement in ulcerative colitis reflects an immunodeficient state. Multiple autoantibody formation would be responsible for variable complex clinical syndromes and it would develop through a defect in immune homeostasis and a graft-host disease pathogenesis.

The current series of patients would support this view. Ulcerative colitis appears to have a similar relationship to the development of autoimmune hemolytic anemia as do the collagen diseases, reticuloendothelial neoplasia (146) and pernicious anemia (147). It may be postulated that such patients are unable to establish a normal immune homeostatic mechanism. This permits the persistence of modified clones of cells maintaining immunocompetence. Multiple autoantibody formation may then occur similar to experimental graft-host disease. A multisystem immunologic disease can result and include various states considered as distinct unrelated entities by anatomic criteria. A common immunologic aberration would be the etiologic factor responsible for this confusing spectrum of associated pathologic states.

Addisonian Pernicious Anemia

In recent years impressive evidence has accumulated indicating that autoimmune mechanisms may be involved in the pathogenesis of Addisonian pernicious anemia and atrophic gastritis. Two separate autoantibody-antigen systems have been well documented.

TABLE 61. *Similarities between gastric parietal cell and thyroid microsomal antigens which react with organ specific autoantibodies**

Test procedures:	Both react in complement fixation Both react in immunofluorescence Antigen localized to microsomal fraction
Antigen inactivated by:	Enzymes: papain, trypsin Detergents: deoxycholate, Lubrol, Triton X-100 Alcohols: ethanol, n-butanol Heating to 100°C.
Antigen not affected by:	Enzymes: phospholipase, lipase, amylase Ethylenediaminetetraacetic acid Alkali Detergent: Tween 20 Ultrasound

* Modified from Roitt and associates (155).

Autoantibodies in Pernicious Anemia

One set of autoantibodies is directed against gastric intrinsic factor (148, 149) and is located in the gamma-globulin fraction of serum obtained from patients with pernicious anemia. It migrates as a gamma-globulin and can be precipitated by rabbit anti-7S human globulin antiserum (150). The autoantibody does not appear to be related to the duration of pernicious anemia or to previous treatment with hog extracts. Its incidence has ranged from 30 to 58 per cent, depending on the immunologic and biologic techniques employed for demonstration. Garrido-Pinson and associates (151) have presented evidence that two types of antibodies directed against human intrinsic factor are present. One type functions as a "blocking" antibody and is unable to react with preformed intrinsic factor B-12 complexes. A second type appears as a "binding" antibody reacting with either intrinsic factor or with intrinsic factor B-12 complexes. In 19 sera obtained from patients with pernicious anemia, both types of antibodies were present in eight, the

blocking antibody exclusively in two and the binding antibody alone in one.

The second form of autoantibody found in the sera of patients with pernicious anemia is directed against gastric parietal cells (152, 153). Demonstration is accomplished by complement fixation or by immunofluorescence. The complement fixing antigen is localized to the microsomal fraction of the parietal cells (154). It is very similar to thyroid microsomal antigen as summarized in Table 61, modified from Roitt and associates (155). There is a wide range of species cross reactivity. Human pernicious anemia serum leads to positive immunofluorescent tests with monkey, dog, cat, rat and mouse gastric parietal cells (155). The antigen arises early in fetal life and has been demonstrated in a 13-week-old human fetus (155). The antigastric parietal cell autoantibody has been demonstrated in 96 per cent of patients with pernicious anemia under 60 years of age and in 82 per cent of older patients. In healthy controls, Roitt and associates (155) found positive immunofluorescent reactions in 2 per cent of patients under 20 years of age, in 6 to 8 per cent of normal subjects aged 30 to 60 and in 16 per cent of elderly females. The sera of patients with atrophic gastritis were also analyzed. Subjects without a megaloblastic bone marrow and without a family history of pernicious anemia were studied. Roitt and associates (155) found that 61 per cent of the female patients had antiparietal cell autoantibodies.

Family Studies in Addisonian Pernicious Anemia

This immunologic evidence for an autoimmune state in pernicious anemia has been supplemented by two additional observations. Callender and Denborough (156) and McIntyre and associates (157) have demonstrated a genetic predisposition in the development of pernicious anemia. One hundred and six first degree and 77 second degree relatives of 39 patients with pernicious anemia were studied by Doniach and associates (158). Parietal cell antibodies were found in 36 per cent of these relatives, as compared with a 6 per cent incidence in matched controls ($X_2 = 28.5 \, P < 0.01$). The highest incidence occurred in sisters, and daughters had autoantibodies more frequently than did sons.

A relationship between thyroid disease and pernicious anemia has also become apparent. A significant clinical association of these two conditions has been documented by Tudhope and Wilson (159) and Williams and Doniach (160). There is excellent evidence that thyroid disease may be related to autoimmune mechanisms which also appear to be genetically mediated (Chapter 10). A comparison of the biochemical characteristics of gastric and thyroid microsomal antigens reveals many similarities, although organ specificity is distinct (Table 61). Therefore, it is not surprising that a serologic overlap has been observed in patients with thyroid disease and chronic gastritis (155, 158, 161, 162). Irvine and associates (162) found antigastric parietal cell autoantibody in the sera of 76 per cent of patients with Addisonian pernicious anemia, in 31 per cent of patients with Hashimoto's disease or spontaneous hypothyroidism and in 24 per cent of patients with thyrotoxicosis. Roitt and associates (155) have reported antigastric parietal cell autoantibodies in 32 per cent of 394 cases of Hashimoto's goiter and primary myxedema. Antithyroid cytoplasmic autoantibodies were also found in 55 per cent of 189 cases of Addisonian pernicious anemia. In an extensive serologic study of family members, Doniach and associates (158) found antigastric parietal cell autoantibodies in 20 per cent of 269 relatives of patients with thyroiditis. In 113 relatives of patients with Addisonian pernicious anemia, 50 per cent were found to have antithyroid autoantibodies.

These studies strongly suggest that an autoimmune basis exists for Addisonian pernicious anemia. A genetic predisposition is apparent. A close relationship to an additional autoimmune state involving the thyroid gland also appears to be well documented. The possibility must be considered that an aberrant immune apparatus exists and leads to an immunologic disease characterized by multiple autoantibody formation (147). In this context the possible relationship of autoimmune hemolytic anemia to Addisonian pernicious anemia assumes importance.

Autoimmune Hemolytic Anemia in Addisonian Pernicious Anemia

A hemolytic element is characteristic in Addisonian pernicious anemia, and a shortened erythrocyte survival time and hyperbilirubinemia are frequently observed. The exact role played by erythrocyte autoantibodies in contributing to or initiating the hemolytic phenomenon is difficult to ascertain. It is pertinent to note, however, that not only the patient's own erythrocytes are prematurely destroyed in pernicious anemia. Normal transfused erythrocytes are also destroyed in a random fashion, suggesting an extrinsic lytic mechanism (163).

The association of Addisonian pernicious anemia and positive antiglobulin tests has been infrequently recognized in the past (147, 164–170). Forshaw and Harwood (169) report it as common. Twenty-one of 59 patients with vitamin B-12 or folic acid deficiency were found to have positive antiglobulin tests. Only 14 were identified as having pernicious anemia; four positive antiglobulin reactions were obtained in this group. Hennemann (164) and Weiner (165) noted this relationship but considered the weak antiglobulin reactions to be of no importance. Other authors have been more impressed with this association (147, 166–168, 170). Edlen (167) and Schwartz and Costea (170) emphasized that both conditions were immunologically mediated.

Analysis of Present Series

From 1958 through 1966, 234 cases of autoimmune hemolytic anemia were studied in our laboratory. During the same period of time 103 patients with Addisonian pernicious anemia were admitted to our hospitals. Antiglobulin and enzyme procedures were performed on ten subjects for possible autoimmune hemolytic anemia. Within this group five patients were discovered to have Addisonian pernicious anemia and positive antiglobulin tests. A close temporal relationship suggested a significant association between the two states. The statistical data obtained from these patients are summarized in Table 62. Table 63 summarizes the antiglobulin and bromelin tests performed at diagnosis and during hematologic remission.

Three males and two females had the combined syndrome of Addisonian pernicious anemia and autoimmune hemolytic anemia. As anticipated, an elderly population was involved, with a median age of 67 years. In four of the five patients, positive antiglobulin tests were obtained simultaneously with the initial diagnosis of pernicious anemia. In the remaining patient, pernicious anemia had been diagnosed 69 months earlier; the patient was in severe relapse when positive antiglobulin tests were obtained. Survival figures cannot be derived as only one patient in the series has

TABLE 62. *Statistical data obtained from five patients (two females, three males) with Addisonian pernicious anemia (PA) and autoimmune hemolytic anemia (AHA)*

Test Procedures	Total	Statistical Data		
		Range	Mean	Median
Clinical data				
Age (years)	5	50–77	66	67
Duration of PA, living (months)	4	11–84	48	48
Duration of AHA, living (months)	4	11–62	34	33
Laboratory data				
Initial hematocrit (%)	5	13–29	18.9	18
Lowest hematocrit (%)	5	12.5–20.5	16.8	18
Initial reticulocytes (%)	5	0.5–1.1	0.8	0.9
Therapeutic reticulocytes (%)	5	10.8–32	21.9	21.4
Initial WBC (10^3/mm.^{3})	5	2.6–9.5	4.5	3.7
Initial thrombocytes (10^3/mm.^{3})	4	45–200	161	200

		Normal		Abnormal	
Other laboratory studies					
Total bilirubin	5	1		4	
A/G ratio	4	2		2	
Serum electrophoresis	3	1		2	
Serologic tests for syphilis	5	3		2	
LE cell preparations	3	2		1	
Free stomach acid	5	0		5	
Atrophic gastritis, x-ray	5	2		3	
Schilling test	5	0		5	
Schilling test with intrinsic factor	4	4		0	

Bone marrow	5	Megaloblastic with erythrocytic hyperplasia			

		Weakness	Dizziness	Fever	Weight Loss	Angina
Presenting symptoms						
Abnormal	5	5	2	0	4	2

		Spleen	Liver	Lymph nodes	Jaundice	Smooth tongue
Presenting signs						
Abnormal	5	2	2	0	4	3

TABLE 63. *Results of antiglobulin and bromelin tests in five patients with Addisonian pernicious anemia (tests performed at time of diagnosis and after hematologic remission)*

Case No.	Initial Testing				Testing in Remission				Elution	
	Direct		Indirect		Direct		Indirect			
	Antiglobulin	Bromelin	Antiglobulin	Bromelin	Antiglobulin	Bromelin	Antiglobulin	Bromelin	Success	Identification
80	2+	Negative	Negative	Negative	Negative	Negative			+	Panhemagglutinin
81	2+	4+	1+	4+	Negative	4+	Negative	4+	+	Panhemagglutinin
82	3+	1+	Negative	1+	Negative	1+			−	
83	1+	Negative								
6	1+	2+			Negative	Negative				

died. It is quite apparent, however, that a chronic disease state is present. The mean and median duration of illness is approximately 4 years after the onset of pernicious anemia. A mean survival approximating 3 years after documentation of positive antiglobulin tests is also present.

The five patients in the current series had classical Addisonian pernicious anemia. Anemia, macrocytosis, a megaloblastic bone marrow, absent free acid in gastric secretions (after histamine stimulation) and abnormal Schilling tests corrected by intrinsic factor were documented in all. Radiologic evidence of atrophic gastritis was present in three patients. Jaundice, a smooth tongue and mild neurologic disturbances were common. Lymphadenopathy was not found, but minimal hepatosplenomegaly was present in two patients.

A profound anemia was encountered in all cases. A mean hematocrit of 16.8 per cent was found. In addition to macrocytosis, peripheral blood nucleated erythrocytes were seen in four patients and spherocytes in one. The initial reticulocyte count was uniformly normal at diagnosis, and initiation of therapy resulted in a marked reticulocytosis. Four of five patients were leukopenic with a WBC of less than 4,000/mm.[3] Thrombocytopenia was not a problem. An elevation of serum bilirubin was seen in four of the five cases and a reversed A/G ratio was found in two of the sera tested. Serum electrophoresis demonstrated a broad polyclonal elevation of gammaglobulin in two of three analyzed specimens. Positive serologic values for syphilis were obtained in two of the five patients. Positive LE cell preparations were found in one of three patients examined.

Positive direct antiglobulin tests were obtained in all five patients. The reactions appeared to be moderately strong. The direct bromelin test was positive in only three of the five. Indirect testing for unbound erythrocyte autoantibody was carried out in three patients. The antiglobulin test was positive in one and the bromelin test was positive in two. In the same three cases an attempt was made to elute the antibody. Elution was successful and a weak panhemagglutinin was demonstrated in two. After hematologic remission had been induced with vitamin B-12, direct serologic tests were performed in four patients. In all, the direct antiglobulin test had reverted to normal. In two, positive direct bromelin tests were still demonstrated.

Clinical Patterns

Two of the five patients studied had a relatively simple clinical picture.

Case 80. A 60-year-old male had pernicious

anemia diagnosed at another institution and did well with vitamin B-12 therapy. After 6 years he spontaneously discontinued vitamin B-12. The regularity of vitamin B-12 injections prior to this total cessation of therapy is questionable. He entered the hospital 7 months later with fatigue, pallor and edema. Smooth tongue was noted as the only abnormality on physical examination. The hematocrit was 13 per cent and the reticulocyte count was 0.8 per cent. Macrocytes and nucleated erythrocytes were found in the peripheral blood. The serum total bilirubin was 1.1/1.5 mg. per cent and the A/G ratio was 4.2/2.6 gm. per cent. Serologic tests for syphilis were negative. There was no free acid in the gastric secretions. A Schilling test was 0.8 per cent and this increased to 20 per cent when intrinsic factor was given. Bone marrow examination revealed erythrocytic hyperplasia with megaloblastic changes. Direct and indirect antiglobulin and bromelin tests were strongly positive and elution revealed an autoantibody functioning as an erythrocyte panhemagglutinin. Parenteral vitamin B-12 therapy was given, resulting in a 10.8 per cent reticulocyte count in 4 days. The hematocrit rapidly rose toward normal. Intramuscular vitamin B-12 was continued at 60 μg. monthly. Followup 6 months later demonstrated a hematocrit of 43 per cent and a reticulocyte count of 0.6 per cent. Direct and indirect antiglobulin tests were now negative but strong positive bromelin reactions were obtained. A panhemagglutinin erythrocyte autoantibody could still be demonstrated. Followup 6 months later indicated a continuing hematologic remission.

Case 81. A 77-year-old Mexican-Indian entered with weakness, emaciation, cough and jaundice. Physical examination demonstrated mild neurologic abnormalities. The hematocrit was 15 per cent with a 1.1 per cent reticulocyte count. Macrocytes were present in the peripheral blood and a megaloblastic bone marrow was noted. Bile was present in the urine. Serologic tests for syphilis were negative. Free acid could not be demonstrated in the gastric secretions. A Schilling test of 0.8 per cent was obtained. Direct antiglobulin tests were positive and bromelin tests were negative. Elution revealed a weak erythrocytic autoantibody which functioned as a panhemagglutinin. Parenteral vitamin B-12 therapy was given. A reticulocyte count of 30 per cent was reached by the 5th day and the hematocrit rapidly rose to 40 per cent in 3½ weeks. The antiglobulin tests reverted to negative after 5 weeks of vitamin B-12 therapy. The patient had worked in a tuber-

culosis hospital, and chest x-rays indicated active tuberculous lesions. Sputum cultures grew out acid fast organisms. He was treated with streptomycin and isoniazid. Administration of vitamin B-12, 50 μg. I.M. monthly, was continued. Followup 11 months after the onset of disease revealed normal hematologic values and negative antiglobulin tests.

Both patients had a similar clinical pattern characterized by Addisonian pernicious anemia and positive antiglobulin tests. However, documentation of autoimmune hemolytic anemia is difficult. Anemia and a hemolytic state were present. Such observations are characteristic in both autoimmune hemolytic anemia and uncomplicated pernicious anemia. The exact role played by erythrocyte autoantibodies in producing or contributing to hemolysis is difficult to ascertain. Although erythrocyte autoantibodies may be involved in the hemolytic process, the primary erythrocyte defect is clearly a lack of vitamin B-12. Correction of the hemolytic process and disappearance of positive antiglobulin tests followed adequate replacement therapy with vitamin B-12. There was no necessity of employing more vigorous therapies such as corticosteroids, immunosuppressive drugs or splenectomy.

Three patients presenting with Addisonian pernicious anemia and positive antiglobulin tests had an entirely different clinical picture. Extremely complex patterns were found with multiple disease associations. In addition to Addisonian pernicious anemia and positive antiglobulin tests, one patient (Case 6) had positive LE cell preparations, positive serologic tests for syphilis and hypergammaglobulinemia. He also developed diabetes, thyroid disease, multiple infections, adenocarcinoma of the prostate, a spindle cell thymoma and interstitial pancreatitis. The other two patients are presented below.

Case 82. A 67-year-old white female was seen for weakness, dyspnea and angina. She had known of anemia since age 30 and had received intermittent transfusions without a definitive diagnosis. Physical examination demonstrated jaundice and a spleen 4 cm. and liver 2 cm. below the costal margins. A diffusely nodular thyroid gland was found. The hematocrit was

19.5 per cent and the reticulocyte count was 0.5 per cent. Nucleated erythrocytes and macrocytes were seen in the peripheral blood. Bone marrow examination revealed erythrocytic hyperplasia with megaloblastic changes. No free acid was found in the stomach, and atrophic gastritis was demonstrated by x-ray. The Schilling test was 2.3 per cent and this elevated to 8 per cent with intrinsic factor. Urine analysis revealed glycosuria and diabetes was diagnosed. The serum total bilirubin was 0.8/0.6 mg. per cent and the A/G ratio was 3.8/3.2 gm. per cent. Serologic tests for syphilis and LE cell tests were negative. The direct antiglobulin and bromelin tests were positive but elution was unsuccessful. Administration of prednisone, 60 mg. daily, was begun. In 1 week the reticulocyte count had risen to 2 per cent but the hematocrit had not changed. Two weeks later hematologic remission had not occurred, and parenteral vitamin B-12 was given. In 8 days the reticulocyte count reached 32 per cent and the hematocrit 33.5 per cent. Prednisone was reduced and discontinued over a 1-month period while maintenance vitamin B-12, 60 μg. I.M., was given monthly. A normal hematocrit was obtained 3 weeks after the start of vitamin B-12 therapy. Followup 2 years later revealed normal hematologic values, the absence of a palpable liver and spleen and negative antiglobulin tests. The direct bromelin test was still positive.

Case 83. A 17-year-old white female developed rheumatic fever with mitral and aortic valve involvement. At age 18 thyrotoxicosis occurred and a thyroidectomy was performed. At age 35, diabetes was diagnosed. The patient did well except for mild cardiac decompensation until age 47 when anemia was first noted. The bone marrow was hypocellular and no diagnosis was made. Corticosteroids were given for a short time with improvement. Over the next 2 years she developed jaundice, a 20-pound weight loss and an enlarged liver. When she was first seen, emaciation, jaundice and pruritus were present. The liver was at the costal margin and aortic stenosis and mitral insufficiency and stenosis were found. The hematocrit was 29 per cent and the bone marrow exhibited erythrocytic hyperplasia. The serum bilirubin was 0.6/3.7 mg. per cent and the A/G ratio was 3.8/3.3 gm. per cent. Serologic test for syphilis (Kline, VDRL, and Kolmer) were weakly positive. The peripheral erythrocytes appeared hypochromic and microcytic. Blood loss or a hemolytic state was assumed, but a specific etiology was not found. Iron therapy was given. During the next 6 months progressive fatigue and jaundice devel-

oped. The spleen was felt at the costal margin and the liver was palpated 3 cm. below the costal margin. The hematocrit dropped to 20.5 per cent with a 0.9 per cent reticulocyte count. Macrocytes were seen in the peripheral blood and the bone marrow revealed mild megaloblastic changes. No free acid was present in the gastric secretions. A Schilling test was 0.0 per cent and after giving intrinsic factor it rose to 12.6 per cent. The direct antiglobulin test was positive and a negative direct bromelin test was found. The A/G ratio was now 3.2/3.9 gm. per cent and electrophoresis revealed a broad polyclonal elevation of gamma-globulin. Vitamin B-12 was given parenterally and in 5 days a reticulocyte count of 21.4 per cent was reached. In 3 weeks the hematocrit was at 36 per cent. Parenteral vitamin B-12 therapy has been continued. Followup 4 years later revealed the patient to be clinically well except for mild cardiac complaints.

In the five cases of the current series, the antiglobulin test was positive during hematologic relapse of pernicious anemia. Therapeutic responses confirmed a relationship. In three patients corticosteroids were not employed. An excellent therapeutic response, with eventual disappearance of positive antiglobulin tests, occurred with parenteral vitamin B-12 therapy alone. In one patient prednisone therapy for 3 weeks did not result in remission. Vitamin B-12 therapy led to a rapid reticulocytosis and hematologic and serologic remission. In the remaining patient prednisone and parenteral vitamin B-12 therapy were given simultaneously, followed by an excellent therapeutic response.

The relationship of erythrocyte autoantibody formation to Addisonian pernicious anemia requires explanation. Fortuitous and independent development of both states in the same patient is possible but appears unlikely in view of the data indicating a close clinical and laboratory correlation. The antiglobulin reaction may be considered as a "false positive" test resulting from unknown changes of the erythrocyte membrane and the adsorption of normal globulins. No experimental proof of this mechanism exists. The elution of erythrocyte autoantibodies with panhemagglutinating activity against normal erythrocytes would appear to rule this out. An antiglobulin positive immunohemolytic state may occur due to antibody formation initiated against modified autologous antigens of the abnormal erythrocytes found in pernicious anemia. This view may be extended to include a termination of tolerance resulting in autoimmune hemolytic anemia. No proof or disproof of these latter two mechanisms is available.

On clinical grounds these suggestions appear inadequate to explain satisfactorily the association of erythrocyte autoantibody formation with Addisonian pernicious anemia. Three of the five patients presented in the current report had complex clinical disease states characterized by multiple system involvement. The associated ailments fall within the category of presumed autoimmune diseases. In addition to Addisonian pernicious anemia and erythrocyte autoantibody formation these three patients had thyroid disease and diabetes. The autoimmune status of thyroid disease and its serologic and clinical relationship to pernicious anemia has been well documented (155, 158–162). Rousso and Cruchand (171) have reported that 14.8 per cent of their patients with pernicious anemia had overt diabetes and that an additional 31.5 per cent had latent diabetes. The genetic and possible autoimmune implications of diabetes have been summarized by Burch and associates (172). In addition to these associated diseases, hypergammaglobulinemia and positive serologic tests for syphilis were found in two of the three patients. Migratory polyarthritis, rheumatic heart disease, positive LE cell preparations, interstitial pancreatitis, recurrent infections, active tuberculosis, carcinoma of the prostate and a thymoma occurred in various combinations in the patients having associated Addisonian pernicious anemia and erythrocyte autoantibody formation. It would appear reasonable to relate erythrocyte autoantibody formation in some manner to the obviously aberrant immunologic status of this group (147).

Irvine and associates (162) have stated that "in Addisonian pernicious anemia, in certain forms of thyroid disease and in idiopathic adrenal insufficiency there is a genetically determined disorder of immunologic tolerance characterized by the production of a multiplicity of antibodies that are precise in their specificity for distinct components of individual tissues." Ziff (173), Leonhardt (174) and Fudenberg and associates (175, 176) have all suggested that a genetically mediated abnormality of the immune apparatus is involved in the development of autoimmune disease. Pirofsky (146) has postulated that autoimmune hemolytic anemia and neoplasia of the reticuloendothelium occur in association with each other because of an aberrant immune apparatus which leads to defective immune homeostasis. Family studies have indicated that this abnormality results in a familial predisposition for complex autoimmune syndromes (78).

The patient data presented above support these theoretical concepts. It is postulated that an aberrant immune apparatus prevents the establishment of a normal immune homeostatic mechanism. Genetically mediated functions may be involved. An immunologically incompetent patient is the result. Defective immune homeostasis prevents the efficient removal of immunocompetent cells which have been modified by virus action or somatic mutation. The survival and replication of such cells may occur over a long period of time unless malignancy results. The creation and persistence of such multiple clones would result in autoantibody production directed against various host tissue antigens. The clinical manifestation of this process would be a variable, complex, multisystem, immunologically mediated disease. In this regard it could resemble syndromes seen in experimental graft-host reactions and in immunologically incompetent animals and humans. The association of Addisonian pernicious anemia, erythrocyte autoantibody production, thyroid disease, diabetes, hypergammaglobulinemia, positive serologic tests for syphilis, positive LE cell formation, multiple infections, interstitial pancreatitis, rheumatic heart disease, malignant transformations and thymoma formation can best be explained by such immunologic mechanisms. The observations of

Rousso and Cruchand (171), Lee and associates (177) and Reaves (178) are similar. Multiple autoantibody formation and associated diseases of a presumed autoimmune etiology were encountered. The concept of an immunologically incompetent individual appears to be most compatible with such clinical experiences. This view has been specifically applied to pernicious anemia by Clark and associates (179), Conn and associates (180) and Pirofsky and Vaughn (147). Although this postulate must still be considered as unproven, it indicates a fruitful direction for additional experimental studies.

Summary of Gastrointestinal Diseases and Their Relationship to Autoimmune Hemolytic Anemia

The material presented above indicates that autoimmune hemolytic anemia and/or positive antiglobulin tests are not uncommonly found in association with gastrointestinal disease. Liver disorders, ulcerative colitis and pernicious anemia are prominent in this relationship.

The clinical and hematologic picture frequently differs from that generally found in idiopathic autoimmune hemolytic anemia. Although the hemolytic process is occasionally severe, the clinical pattern is more often dominated by the associated gastrointestinal disease. Anemia may be mild or even absent. Hemolysis frequently cannot be demonstrated. Corticosteroid therapy may be of little use and correction of the gastrointestinal abnormality may induce the disappearance of positive antiglobulin tests. The positive antiglobulin test can appear as only a laboratory curiosity complicating efficient blood transfusion therapy. In this regard the association of gastrointestinal disease and positive antiglobulin tests has similarities to the erythrocyte serologic relationship frequently encountered with collagen diseases and various infectious agents.

Overt clinical importance of positive antiglobulin tests is frequently absent in gastrointestinal disease. In spite of this it would be an error to discount such abnor-

malities as "false positive" reactions. They may have important etiologic significance. Many of the discussed gastrointestinal ailments are closely related to immunologic phenomena. A defect of the immune apparatus may be responsible for the occurrence of both the gastrointestinal disease and the positive antiglobulin test. Such syndromes may represent a multisystem immunologically mediated disease.

BIBLIOGRAPHY

1. Vanlair, C. F., and Masius, J. R.: De la microcythémia. Bull. Acad. Roy. Med. Belg. 5: 515, 1871.
2. Hayem, G.: Sur une variété particulière d'ictère chronique. Ictère infectieux chronique splénomégalique. Presse Med. 6: 121, 1898.
3. Mouisset, A., Chalier, J., and Nove-Josserand, L.: Contribution a l'étude des ictères hémolytiques. Lyon Med. 114: 141, 1910.
4. Eppinger, H.: Zur Pathologie der Milzfunktion. Berlin Klin. Wschr. 50: 1509, 1913.
5. Mosse, M.: Polyglobulie und Lebererkrankung. Z. Klin. Med. 79: 431, 1914.
6. Chevalier, P., and Tourkine, J.: Le grand syndrome hémolytique dans les affections hépatospléniques. Folia Haemat. (Frankfurt) 19: 244, 1915.
7. Singer, K., and Dameshek, W.: Symptomatic hemolytic anemia. Ann. Intern. Med. 15: 544, 1941.
8. Taylor, K. B.: Immune mechanisms in gastroenterology. In Recent Advances in Gastroenterology, edited by J. Badenoch and B. N. Brook. Little, Brown and Company, Boston, 1965.
9. Cruickshank, B.: In Clinical Aspects of Immunology, edited by P. G. H. Gell and R. R. A. Coombs. F. A. Davis Company, Philadelphia, 1963.
10. Glynn, L. E., and Holborow, E. J.: Autoimmunity and Disease. F. A. Davis Company, Philadelphia, 1965.
11. Tomasi, T. B.: Diseases of the liver. In Immunologic Diseases, edited by M. Samter, Chapter 78. Little, Brown and Company, Boston, 1965.
12. Cohen, S., Ohta, G., Singer, E. J., and Popper, H.: Immunocytochemical study of gamma-globulin in liver, in hepatitis and postnecrotic cirrhosis. J. Exp. Med. 111: 285, 1960.
13. Schaffner, F., Barka, T., and Popper, H.: Hepatic mesenchymal cell reaction in liver disease. Exp. Molec. Path. 2: 419, 1963.
14. Steiner, J. W., Carruthers, J. S., Baumal, R., and Kalifat, S. R.: Experimental immunologic liver injury and the concept of auto-

destruction. Canad. Med. Ass. J. **85**: 1369, 1425, 1961.

15. Hughes, T. P.: Precipitin reaction in yellow fever. J. Immun. **25**: 275, 1933.

16. Gear, J.: Autoantigens and autoantibodies in the pathogenesis of disease with special reference to black water fever. Trans. Roy. Soc. Trop. Med. Hyg. **39**: 301, 1946.

17. Waldenström, J.: Leber, Blutproteine und Nahrungseiweiss Stoffwechsel-krankheiten. In *Verhandlungen der Dentochen Gesellschaft für Verdauungs-und Stoffwechsel-Krankheiten* (XV Tagung Bad Kissingen). Johann Ambrosius, Leipzig, 1952.

18. Kunkel, H. G., Ahrens, E. H., Eisenmenger, W. J., Bongiovanni, A. M., and Slater, R. J.: Extreme hypergammaglobulinemia in young women with liver disease of unknown etiology. J. Clin. Invest. **30**: 654, 1951.

19. Saint, E. G., King, W. E., Joske, R. A., and Finckh, E. S.: The course of infectious hepatitis with special reference to prognosis and the chronic stage. Aust. Ann. Med. **2**: 113, 1953.

20. MacKay, I. R., and Wood, I. J.: Autoimmunity in liver disease. In *Progress in Liver Disease,* edited by H. Popper and F. Schaffner. Grune & Stratton, Inc., New York, 1961.

21. MacKay, I. R.: The problem of persisting destructive disease of the liver. Gastroenterology **40**: 617, 1961.

22. MacKay, I. R., Weiden, S., and Hasker, J.: Autoimmune hepatitis. Ann. N. Y. Acad. Sci. **124**: 767, 1965.

23. Joske, R. A., and King, W. E.: The "L.E. cell" phenomenon in active chronic viral hepatitis. Lancet **2**: 477, 1955.

24. MacKay, I. R., Taft, L. I., and Cowling, D. C.: Lupoid hepatitis. Lancet **2**: 1323, 1956.

25. Popper, H., Paronetto, F., and Schaffner, F.: Immune processes in the pathogenesis of liver disease. Ann. N. Y. Acad. Sci. **124**: 781, 1965.

26. Olitzki, L., and Bernkopf, H.: A precipitation test in infective hepatitis. J. Infect. Dis. **76**: 60, 1945.

27. Bjorneboe, M., and Krag, P.: Studies on a complement fixation in hepatitis with liver extract as antigen. Acta Path. Microbiol. Scand. **24**: 352, 1947.

28. Eaton, M. D., Murphy, W. D., and Hanford, V. L.: Heterogenetic antibodies in acute hepatitis. J. Exp. Med. **79**: 539, 1949.

29. Rissel, E., Steffen, C., and Wewalka, F.: Serum Faktoren mit Gewebsantikörpereigenschaften bei Lebererkrankungen. Wien. Klin. Wschr. **69**: 885, 1957.

30. Gajdusek, D. C.: "Autoimmune" reaction against human tissue antigens in certain acute and chronic diseases. I. Serologic investigations. Arch. Intern. Med. (Chicago) **101**: 9, 1958.

31. Itano, T.: Serologic studies on hepatitis. Ikayama Igakkai Zasshi **71**: 7743, 1959.

32. Weir, D. M.: A complement-fixation reaction with serum and tissue extracts after the injection of carbon tetrachloride into rats. Lancet **1**: 1147, 1961.

33. Asherson, G. L., and Dumonde, D. C.: Characterization of autoantibodies produced in the rabbit by the injection of rat liver. Brit. J. Exp. Path. **43**: 12, 1962.

34. Jiminez Diaz, C., Segovia, J. M., Jiminez Casado, M., Ortega, A., Aguirre, M., and Durantez, J.: The presence of auto-active substances (autoantibodies?) in hepatic cirrhosis. Rev. Clin. Esp. **84**: 162, 1962.

35. Gökcen, M., and Zinneman, H. H.: Liver "autoantibodies" in a case of drug-induced jaundice. Gastroenterology **44**: 69, 1963.

36. Weir, D. M., Holborow, E. J., and Johnson, G. D.: A clinical study of serum antinuclear factor. Brit. Med. J. **1**: 933, 1961.

37. Calabresi, P., and Greenberg, M.: Circulating antinuclear globulins in patients with chronic liver disease. J. Clin. Invest. **39**: 976, 1960.

38. Bouchier, I. A.: Serologic abnormalities in patients with liver disease. Brit. Med. J. **1**: 592, 1964.

39. MacKay, I. R., and Larkin, L.: The significance of the presence in human serum of complement fixing antibodies to human tissue antigens. Aust. Ann. Med. **7**: 251, 1958.

40. Hackett, E., and Beech, M.: Transient appearance of "autoimmune" antibodies during prophylactic immunization. J. Immun. **85**: 533, 1960.

41. Asherson, G.: Antibodies against nuclear and cytoplasmic cell constituents in systemic lupus erythematosus and other diseases. Brit. J. Exp. Path. **40**: 209, 1959.

42. Deicher, H., Holman, H. R., and Kunkel, H. G.: Anti-cytoplasmic factors in the sera of patients with systemic lupus erythematosus and certain other diseases. Arthritis Rheum. **3**: 1, 1960.

43. Fellinger, K., and Klima, R.: Lebercirrhose und Anämien. Z. Klin. Med. **126**: 547, 1933–1934.

44. Lovibond, J. L.: Macrocytic haemolytic anaemia. Lancet **2**: 1395, 1935.

45. Davidson, L. S. P., and Fullerton, H. W.: Some rare types of macrocytic anaemia. Quart. J. Med. **7**: 43, 1938.

46. Watson, C. J.: Hemolytic jaundice and macrocytic hemolytic anemia: certain observations in a series of 35 cases. Ann. Intern. Med. **12**: 1782, 1939.

47. Hyman, G. A., and Southworth, H.: Hemolytic anemia associated with liver disease. Amer. J. Med. Sci. **221**: 448, 1951.

48. Chaplin, H., and Mollison, P. L.: Red cell life-span in nephritis and in hepatic cirrhosis. Clin. Sci. **12**: 351, 1953.

49. Jones, P. N., Weinstein, I. M., Ettinger, R. H., and Capps, R. B.: Decreased red cell survival associated with liver disease. Use of radioactive sodium chromate in measurement of red cell survival. Arch. Intern. Med. (Chicago) **95**: 93, 1955.

50. Jandl, J. H.: The anemia of liver disease: observations on its mechanism. J. Clin. Invest. **34**: 390, 1955.

51. Zieve, L.: Jaundice, hyperlipemia and hemolytic anemia: a heretofore unrecognized syndrome associated with alcoholic fatty liver and cirrhosis. Ann. Intern. Med. **48**: 471, 1958.

52. Zieve, L., and Hill, E.: Two varieties of hemolytic anemia in cirrhosis. Southern Med. J. **54**: 1347, 1961.

53. Sheehy, T. W., and Berman, A.: The anemia of cirrhosis. J. Lab. Clin. Med. **56**: 72, 1960.

54. Boivin, P., Hartmann, L., and Fauvert, R.: L'anémie des cirrhoses. Fréquence et méchanisme. Nouv. Rev. Franc. Hemat. **1**: 3, 1961.

55. Pitcher, C. S., and Williams, R.: Reduced red cell survival in jaundice and its relation to abnormal glutathione metabolism. Clin. Sci. **24**: 239, 1963.

56. Katz, R., Velasco, M., Guzman, C., and Alessandri, H.: Red cell survival estimated by radioactive chromium in hepatobiliary disease. Gastroenterology **46**: 399, 1964.

57. Prato, V., Chiandussi, L., Mazza, U., Massaro, A. L., and Fiorina, L.: L'anemia nella cirrosi del fegato. II. I sintomi di aumentata distruzione eritrocitaria. Arch. Sci. Med. (Torino) **119**: 87, 1965.

58. Kimber, C., Deller, D. J., Ibbotson, R. N., and Lander, H.: The mechanism of anaemia in chronic liver disease. Quart. J. Med. **34**: 33, 1965.

59. Sjovall, E., and Wallgren, A.: Some aspects of hepato-lenticular degeneration and its pathogenesis. Acta Psychiat. Neurol. **9**: 435, 1934.

60. McIntyre, N., Clink, H. M., Levi, A. J., Cumings, J. N., and Sherlock, S.: Hemolytic anemia in Wilson's disease. New Eng. J. Med. **276**: 439, 1967.

61. Hennemann, H., Möller, H., and Gillert, K. E.: Nach Hepatitis epidemica erworbener hämolytischer Ikterus mit positivem Coombs-test. Klin. Wschr. **30**: 809, 1952.

62. Hennemann, H.: Hämolytische Syndrome bei Erkrankungen der Leber und Gallenblase. Z. Klin. Med. **154**: 68, 1956–1957.

63. Heller, P., Zimmerman, H. J., Rozengvaig, S., and Singer, K.: The LE cell phenomenon in chronic hepatic disease. New Eng. J. Med. **254**: 1160, 1956.

64. Arrau, C. M., and Matte, H. O.: Alteraciones hematologicas, immunologicas y de la hemostosis en la cirrosis hepatica. Rev. Med. Chile **81**: 251, 1953.

65. Bakx, C. J. A., van Loghem, J. J., and Klomp-

Magnée, W.: Acquired haemolytic anaemia in a newborn. Vox Sang. **3**: 79, 1953.

66. Wasserman, L. R., Stats, D., Schwartz, L., and Fudenberg, H.: Symptomatic and hemopathic hemolytic anemia. Amer. J. Med. **24**: 648, 1958.

67. Dausset, J., and Marchal, G.: Cirrhose hépatique avec une substance sérique antifoie. In *Immunopathology, First International Symposium,* edited by P. Grabar and P. Miescher, p. 113. Schwabe and Company, Basel, 1959.

68. Bornemann, K., and Michel, D.: Hepatitis epidemica und Hämolyse. Neigung. Aerztl. Wschr. **10**: 813, 1955.

69. Ruggieri, P., and Bolognesi, G.: Anemia emolitica acquisita autoimmune e cirrosi epatica. Policlinico (Prat.) **62**: 1605, 1955.

70. Beickert, A., and Siering, H.: Immunpancytopenie mit auftreten heterophiler Antikörper bei akuter Hepatitis epidemica kompliziert durch eine schwere Myocarditis. Acta Haemat. (Basel) **19**: 51, 1958.

71. Kivel, R. M.: Hematologic aspects of acute viral hepatitis. Amer. J. Dig. Dis. **6**: 1017, 1961.

72. Kölle, G.: Zur Problematik der symptomatischen hämolytischen Anämie bei epidemischer Hepatitis. Wschr. Kinderheilk. **108**: 281, 1960.

73. Easton, J. A., Priest, C. J., and Giles, C. M.: An antibody against stored blood associated with cirrhosis of the liver and false positive serologic tests for syphilis. J. Clin. Path. **18**: 460, 1956.

74. Hutchings, H. E., and Wigley, R. A. D.: Lupoid hepatitis. New Zeal. Med. J. **58**: 12, 1959.

75. Fodor, O., and Tănăsescu, R.: Anemiile hemolitce immunologice posthepatice. Med. Intern. (Bucur.) **14**: 1469, 1962.

76. Dacie, J. V.: *The Haemolytic Anaemias, Part III,* Ed. 2. Grune & Stratton, Inc., New York, 1967.

77. Feizi, T., and Woodgate, D.: The direct antiglobulin (Coombs') test in hypertensive patients. Vox Sang. **12**: 273, 1967.

78. Pirofsky, B.: Hereditary aspects of autoimmune hemolytic anemia; a retrospective analysis. Vox Sang. **14**: 334, 1968.

79. Jones, C. M., and Minot, G. R.: Infectious (catarrhal) jaundice. An attempt to establish a clinical entity. Boston Med. Surg. J. **189**: 531, 1923.

80. Raffensperger, E. C.: Acute acquired hemolytic anemia in association with acute viral hepatitis. Ann. Intern. Med. **48**: 1243, 1958.

81. Sanchez-Medal, L.: Personal communication.

82. Conrad, M. E., Schwartz, F. D., and Young, A. A.: Infectious hepatitis—a generalized disease. Amer. J. Med. **37**: 789, 1964.

83. Jandl, J. H., Jacob, H. S., and Daland, G. H.: Hypersplenism due to infection. A study

of 5 cases manifesting hemolytic anemia. New Eng. J. Med. **264:** 1063, 1961.

84. Levy, R. H., Sawitsky, A., Florman, A. L., and Rubin, E.: Fatal aplastic anemia after hepatitis. New Eng. J. Med. **273:** 1118, 1965.

85. Schwartz, E., Baehner, R. L., and Diamond, L. K.: Aplastic anemia following hepatitis. Pediatrics **37:** 681, 1966.

86. Schmidt, K. E. A.: Über den erworbenen hämolytischen Ikterus und die intermittierende Hyperbilirubinämie nach Hepatitis epidemica. Deutsch. Arch. Klin. Med. **200:** 38, 1952.

87. Spray, G. H., and Witts, L. J.: The utilization of folic acid in anaemia and leukemia. Clin. Sci. **12:** 385, 1953.

88. Jonsson, U., Roath, O. S., and Kirkpatrick, C. I. F.: Nutritional megaloblastic anemia associated with sickle cell states. Blood **14:** 535, 1959.

89. Gruelund, S.: Megaloblastic hemolytic anemia. Acta Med. Scand. **239** (suppl.): 101, 1950.

90. Baikie, A. G., and Pirrie, R.: Megaloblastic erythropoiesis in idiopathic acquired hemolytic anemia. Scot. Med. J. **1:** 330, 1956.

91. Chanarin, I., Dacie, J. V., and Mollin, D. L.: Folic acid deficiency in haemolytic anaemia. Brit. J. Haemat. **5:** 245, 1959.

92. Willoughby, M. L. N., Pearce, M. A., Sharp, A. A., and Shields, M. J.: Megaloblastic erythropoiesis in acquired hemolytic anemia. Blood **17:** 351, 1961.

93. Brown, P. C., and Holborow, E. J.: An antigenic difference between A antigens of human epithelial and endothelial tissue. Nature (London) **193:** 1190, 1962.

94. Loewi, G., and Holborow, E. J.: Failure to elicit a delayed hypersensitivity reaction against blood group substance from erythrocytes. Nature (London) **194:** 1288, 1962.

95. Holborow, E. J., and Loewi, G.: The immune response to blood group substances. Immunology **5:** 278, 1962.

96. Bernier, J. J., Terris, G., and Lambling, A.: Production of ileitis in guinea pigs by means of autoantibodies. Arch. Mal. Appar. Dig. **50:** 1259, 1961.

97. Holborow, E. J., Asherson, G. L., and Wigley, R.: Auto-antibody production in rabbits. VI. The production of auto-antibodies against rabbit gastric, ileal and colonic mucosa. Immunology **6:** 55, 1963.

98. Andresen, A. F. R.: Gastrointestinal manifestations of food allergy. Med. J. Rec. **122** (suppl.): 271, 1925.

99. Gray, N., MacKay, I. R., Taft, L. I., Weiden, S., and Wood, I. J.: Hepatitis, colitis, and lupus manifestations. Amer. J. Dig. Dis. **3:** 481, 1958.

100. Miofilis, S. P.: Pericholangitis and ulcerative colitis. I. Pathology, etiology and pathogenesis. Ann. Intern. Med. **63:** 1, 1965.

101. Wilcox, R. G., and Isselbacker, K. J.: Chronic

liver disease in young people. Clinical features and course in thirty-three patients. Amer. J. Med. **30:** 185, 1961.

102. Billson, F. A., DeDombal, F. T., Watkinson, G., and Goligher, J. C.: Ocular complications of ulcerative colitis. Gut **8:** 102, 1967.

103. McEwen, C., Lingg, C., Kirsner, J. B., and Spencer, J. A.: Arthritis accompanying ulcerative colitis. Amer. J. Med. **33:** 923, 1962.

104. Kirsner, J. B., Palmer, W. L., Spencer, J. A., Bicks, R. O., and Johnson, C. F.: Corticotropin and adrenal steroids in the management of ulcerative colitis. Observations in 240 patients. Ann. Intern. Med. **50:** 891, 1959.

105. Jensen, E. J., Baggenstoss, A. H., and Bargen, J. A.: Renal lesions associated with chronic ulcerative colitis. Amer. J. Med. Sci. **219:** 281, 1950.

106. Lagercrantz, R., Winberg, J., and Zetterström, R.: Extra-colonic manifestations in chronic ulcerative colitis. Acta Paediat. **47:** 675, 1958.

107. Levine, M. L., Miranda, M., Engle, R. L., and Almy, T. P.: Leukocyte response in nonspecific ulcerative colitis. Gastroenterology **38:** 971, 1960.

108. Bargen, J. A.: Complications and sequelae of chronic ulcerative colitis. Ann. Intern. Med **3:** 335, 1929.

109. Nugent, F. W., and Rudolph, N. E.: Extracolonic manifestations of chronic ulcerative colitis. Med. Clin. N. Amer. **50:** 529, 1966.

110. Foster, J. J., and Brick, I. B.: Erythema nodosum in ulcerative colitis. Gastroenterology **27:** 417, 1954.

111. White, R. G., Bass, B. H., and Williams, E.: Lymphadenoid goitre and the syndrome of systemic lupus erythematosus. Lancet **1:** 368, 1961.

112. MacKay, I. R., and Burnet, F. M.: *Autoimmune Diseases*. Charles C Thomas, Publisher, Springfield, Ill., 1963.

113. Alarcón-Segovia, D., Herskovic, T., Dearing, W. H., Bartholomew, L. G., Cain, J. C., and Shorter, R. G.: Lupus erythematosus cell phenomenon in patients with chronic ulcerative colitis. Gut **6:** 39, 1965.

114. Brown, C. H., Shirley, E. K., and Haserick, J. R.: Gastrointestinal manifestations of systemic lupus erythematosus. Gastroenterology **31:** 649, 1956.

115. Bartholomew, L. G., Cain, J. C., Baggenstoss, A. H., and Hagedorn, A. B.: Further observations on hepatitis and cirrhosis in young women with positive clot tests for lupus erythematosus. Gastroenterology **39:** 730, 1960.

116. Clinicopathologic Conference. Amer. J. Med. **37:** 578, 1964.

117. Wasserman, F., Krosnick, A., and Tumen, H.: Necrotizing angiitis associated with ulcerative colitis. Amer. J. Med. **17:** 736, 1954.

118. Bicks, R. O., Goldgraber, M. B., and Kirsner,

J. B.: Generalized scleroderma associated with chronic ulcerative colitis. Amer. J. Med. **24**: 447, 1958.

119. Sloan, W. P., Bargen, J. A., and Gage, R. P.: Life histories of patients with chronic ulcerative colitis: a review of 2000 cases. Gastroenterology **44**: 444, 1950.

120. Fernandez-Herliky, L.: The articular manifestations of chronic ulcerative colitis. An analysis of 55 cases. New Eng. J. Med. **261**: 259, 1959.

121. Bardana, E. J., and Pirofsky, B.: Autoimmune hemolytic anemia and ulcerative colitis; a multisystem immunodeficiency disease? (to be published).

122. Wong, T. W., and Warner, N. E.: Cytomegalic inclusion disease in adults. Arch. Path (Chicago) **74**: 403, 1962.

123. Gray, J. G.: Immunology and ulcerative colitis. Brit. J. Clin. Prac. **16**: 729, 1962.

124. Kraft, S. C., and Kirsner, J. B.: Present status of immunologic mechanisms in ulcerative colitis. Gastroenterology **51**: 788, 1966.

125. Broberger, O., and Perlmann, P.: Autoantibodies in human ulcerative colitis. J. Exp. Med. **110**: 657, 1959.

126. Broberger, O., and Perlmann, P.: Demonstration of epithelial antigen in colon by means of fluorescent antibodies from children with ulcerative colitis. J. Exp. Med. **115**: 13, 1962.

127. Klavins, J. V.: Cytoplasm of colonic mucosal cells as site of antigen in ulcerative colitis. J. A. M. A. **183**: 547, 1963.

128. Calabresi, P., Thayer, W. R., and Spiro, H. M.: Demonstration of circulating antinuclear globulins in ulcerative colitis. J. Clin. Invest. **40**: 2126, 1961.

129. Asherson, G., and Broberger, O.: The incidence of haemagglutinating and complement fixing antibodies. Brit. Med. J. **1**: 1429, 1961.

130. Perlmann, P., and Broberger, O.: The possible role of immune mechanisms in tissue damage in ulcerative colitis. In *Mechanisms of Cell and Tissue Damage Produced by Immune Reactions,* (Second International Symposium on Immunopathology), edited by P. Grabar and P. Miescher. schwabe and Company, Basel, 1962.

131. Broberger, O., and Perlmann, P.: In vitro studies of ulcerative colitis. I. Reactions of patient's serum with human fetal colon cells in tissue culture. J. Exp. Med. **117**: 705, 1963.

132. Perlmann, P., Hammarström, S., Lagercrantz, R., and Gustafsson, B. E.: Antigen from colon of germfree rats and antibodies in human ulcerative colitis. Ann. N. Y. Acad. Sci. **124**: 377, 1965.

133. Farr, R. S.: Some comments regarding the allergic state. The initiation of antibody synthesis. Arch. Environ. Health (Chicago) **6**: 92, 1963.

134. Von Kleist, S., and Burtin, P.: On the specificity of autoantibodies present in colon cancer patients. Immunology **10**: 507, 1966.

135. Fletcher, J.: Serum complement levels in active ulcerative colitis. Gut **6**: 172, 1965.

136. Fong, S., Fudenberg, H., and Perlmann, P.: Ulcerative colitis with anti-erythrocyte antibodies. Vox Sang. **8**: 668, 1963.

137. Beal, R. W., Skyring, A. P., McRae, J., and Firkin, B. G.: The anemia of ulcerative colitis. Gastroenterology **45**: 589, 1963.

138. Lorber, M., Schwartz, L. I., and Wasserman, L. R.: Association of antibody-coated red blood cells with ulcerative colitis; report on 4 cases. Amer. J. Med. **19**: 887, 1955.

139. Keene, W. R.: Uncommon abnormalities of blood associated with chronic ulcerative colitis. Med. Clin. N. Amer. **50**: 535, 1966.

140. Ormerod, T. P.: Observations on the incidence and cause of anemia in ulcerative colitis. Gut **8**: 107, 1967.

141. Weiner, W., and Nussey, A. M.: Rhesustyping in unsuspected acquired hemolytic anemia. Lancet **1**: 257, 1961.

142. Balint, J. A., Hammack, W. J., and Patton, T. B.: Autoimmune hemolytic anemia complicating ulcerative colitis. Gastroenterology **42**: 740, 1962.

143. Gastaldi, F., Regazzine, A., Chiappino, G., and Fodeli, S.: Ulcerative colitis and acquired autoimmune hemolytic anemia (description of a case). Riv. Emoter. Immunoemat. **10**: 193, 1963.

144. Molaro, G. L., and Barillari, B.: On a case of ulcerative colitis with autoimmune hemolytic anemia. Riv. Emoter. Immunoemat. **11**: 43, 1964.

145. Bohnen, R. F., Ultmann, J. E., Gorman, J. G., Farhangi, M., and Scudder, J.: The direct Coombs test: its clinical significance. Ann. Intern. Med. **68**: 19, 1968.

146. Pirofsky, B.: Autoimmune hemolytic anemia and neoplasia of the reticuloendothelium. With a hypothesis concerning etiologic relationships. Ann. Intern. Med. **68**: 109, 1968.

147. Pirofsky, B., and Vaughn, M.: Addisonian pernicious anemia with positive antiglobulin tests; a multiple antoimmune disease syndrome. Amer. J. Clin. Path. **50**: 459, 1968.

148. Taylor, K. B.: Inhibition of intrinsic factor by pernicious anemia sera. Lancet **2**: 106, 1959.

149. Ardeman, S., and Chanarin, I.: A method for the assay of human gastric intrinsic factor and for the detection and titration of antibodies against intrinsic factor. Lancet **2**: 1350, 1963.

150. Taylor, K. B., Roitt, I. M., Doniach, D., Couchman, K. G., and Shapland, C.: Autoimmune phenomenon in pernicious anemia. I. Gastric antibodies. Brit. Med. J. **2**: 1347, 1962.

151. Garrido-Pinson, G. C., Turner, M. D., Crook-

ston, J. H., Sarnloff, I. M., Miller, L., and Segal, H. L.: Studies of human intrinsic factor auto-antibodies. J. Immun. **97**: 897, 1966.

152. Markson, J. L., and Moore, J. M.: Autoimmunity in pernicious anemia and iron deficiency anemia. Lancet **2**: 1240, 1962.

153. MacKay, I. R.: Autoimmune serologic studies in chronic gastritis and pernicious anemia. Gut **5**: 23, 1964.

154. Baur, S., Roitt, I. M., and Doniach, D.: Characterization of the human gastric parietal cell autoantigen. Immunology **8**: 62, 1965.

155. Roitt, I. M., Doniach, D., and Shapland, C.: Autoimmunity in pernicious anemia and atrophic gastritis. Ann. N. Y. Acad. Sci. **124**: 644, 1965.

156. Callender, S. T., and Denborough, M. A.: A family study of pernicious anemia. Brit. J. Haemat. **3**: 88, 1957.

157. McIntyre, P. A., Hahn, R., Couley, C. L., and Glass, B.: Genetic factors in predisposition to pernicious anemia. Bull. Hopkins Hosp. **104**: 309, 1959.

158. Doniach, D., Roitt, I. M., and Taylor, K. B.: Autoimmunity in pernicious anemia and thyroiditis. A family study. Ann. N. Y. Acad. Sci. **124**: 605, 1965.

159. Tudhope, G. R., and Wilson, G. M.: Deficiency of vitamin B-12 in hypothyroidism. Lancet **1**: 703, 1962.

160. Williams, F. D., and Doniach, I.: The post mortem incidence of focal thyroiditis. J. Path. Bact. **83**: 255, 1962.

161. Irvine, W., Davies, S. H., Delamore, I. W., and Williams, A. W.: Immunological relationship between pernicious anemia and thyroid disease. Brit. Med. J. **2**: 454, 1962.

162. Irvine, W. J., Davies, S. H., Teitelbaum, S., Delamore, I. W., and Williams, A. W.: The clinical and pathological significance of gastric parietal cell antibody. Ann. N. Y. Acad. Sci. **124**: 657, 1965.

163. Hamilton, H. E., DeGowin, E. L., Sheets, R. F., Janney, D. C., and Ellis, J. A.: Accelerated destruction of normal adult erythrocytes in pernicious anemia; contribution of hemolysis to the oligocythemia. J. Clin. Invest. **33**: 191, 1954.

164. Hennemann, H. H.: Klinische und serologische Studien bei erworbenen häemolytischen Anämien. Folia Haemat. (Frankfurt) **73**: 236, 1956.

165. Weiner, W.: To be or not to be an antibody: the "agent" in autoimmune hemolytic anemia. Blood **14**: 1057, 1956.

166. Krylov, A. A., and Schevchenko, A.: A case of Addison-Bierner anemia with positive Coombs test. Klin. Med. (Moskva) **39**: 126, 1961.

167. Edlen, A.: Tva Fall av Anemia perniciosa med förvärvad hamolytisk Anemi. Svensk. Lakartidn. **60**: 1933, 1963.

168. Radochova, D., Chrobak, L., Smid, A., and Svenda, J.: Survival of erythrocytes labeled with Cr⁵¹ in pernicious anemia with a positive direct Coombs test. Vnitrni Lek. **9**: 37, 1965.

169. Forshaw, J., and Harwood, L.: The direct antiglobulin (Coombs) test in megaloblastic anemia. J. Clin. Path. **18**: 119, 1965.

170. Schwartz, R. S., and Costea, N.: Autoimmune hemolytic anemia: clinical correlations and biological implications. Seminars Hemat. **3**: 2, 1966.

171. Rousso, C., and Cruchand, A.: Pernicious anemia. I. Clinical study of 54 cases, with special reference to associated diabetes. Helv. Med. Acta **33**: 175, 1966.

172. Burch, P. R. J., Rowell, N. R., and Burwell, R. G.: Autoimmunity and chromosomal aberrations. Lancet **2**: 170, 1966.

173. Ziff, M.: Genetics, hypersensitivity and the connective tissue diseases. Amer. J. Med. **30**: 1, 1961.

174. Leonhardt, T.: Familial studies in systemic lupus erythematosus. Acta Med. Scand. **176** (suppl.): 416, 1964.

175. Fudenberg, H., German, J. L., and Kunkel, H.: The occurrence of rheumatoid factor and other abnormalities in families of patients with agammaglobulinemia. Arthritis Rheum. **5**: 565, 1962.

176. Fudenberg, H.: Immunologic deficiency, autoimmune disease, and lymphoma: observations, implications and speculations. Arthritis Rheum. **9**: 464, 1966.

177. Lee, F. I., Jenkins, G. C., Hughes, D. I. D., and Kazantzis, G.: Pernicious anaemia, myxoedema, and hypogammaglobulinaemia. A family study. Brit. Med. J. **1**: 598, 1964.

178. Reaves, L. E.: Altered immunological mechanisms in diseases of unknown cause. Report of myasthenia gravis, pernicious anemia, and myxedema occurring in the same patient. Geriatrics **20**: 707, 1965.

179. Clark, R., Tornyos, K., Herbert, V., and Twomey, J. J.: Studies on two patients with concomitant pernicious anemia and immunoglobulin deficiency. Ann. Intern. Med. **67**: 404, 1967.

180. Conn, H. O., Binder, H., and Burns, B.: Pernicious anemia and immunologic deficiency. Ann. Intern. Med. **68**: 603, 1968.

Chapter 10

Miscellaneous Diseases and Autoimmune Hemolytic Anemia

In previous chapters it has been possible to discuss secondary or symptomatic forms of autoimmune hemolytic anemia within an organ system classification. This approach is satisfying from the aspect of familiarity. However, it is extremely limiting when applied to immunologically mediated disease states. The nature of immune processes is such that they may not conform to rigid anatomic barriers. This problem is further magnified with the autoimmune hemolytic anemias. In such states, as many as 13 separate pathophysiologic mechanisms may be involved. A heterogeneity of clinically recognized syndromes may be anticipated in view of this etiologic diversity.

The obvious solution is to discuss autoimmune hemolytic anemia, and probably all autoimmune disease, on an etiologic basis. Unfortunately, this approach is not as yet possible. In many instances the etiology is speculative and the exact pathogenesis is unclear. Accordingly, this volume has employed the usual pathologic classifications even though they have proven clumsy and uninformative. It is therefore not surprising that a group of pathologically distinct entities exists in relationship to autoimmune hemolytic anemia and that these entities are still unclassified in specific organ systems.

The object of the current chapter is to present our clinical experience with such unclassified secondary forms of autoimmune hemolytic anemia. The pathologic states involved may not appear to be related to previously presented syndromes. In spite of this, clinical analysis frequently indicates a relationship. Similar pathophysiologic mechanisms may be involved, although anatomic boundaries vary greatly. Whenever possible such relationships are emphasized in order to clarify the heterogeneous clinical spectrum.

Diseases of the Thyroid Gland

The thyroid gland has played an important role in the study of autoimmunization. Experimentation in this area validated the concept that antibodies may be produced by a host and may have specificity for unmodified host cellular constituents.

As early as 1927 Hektoen and associates (1) demonstrated that thyroglobulin could be antigenic. Witebsky and associates (2) incorporated thyroglobulin with Freund's adjuvant. Immunization of animals with this mixture led to autoantibody formation directed against thyroglobulin. These studies were an important milestone in the experimental approach to autoimmunization. They established the fact that autoantibody formation could result from a break in immunologic quarantine. In addition, a disease process similar to human thyroiditis could be experimentally produced by this procedure (3). Of major importance was the application of rational immunologic procedures which removed autoimmunity from a theoretical possibility to a sound experimental and clinical context. The identification of a specific antigen against which autoantibodies were directed was firmly established as a necessary prerequisite for diagnosis of autoimmunization.

Thyroid Autoantibodies

Two antigenic substances derived from the thyroid gland have been identified as reacting with autoantibodies. Both of these substances are clinically important in diseases of the thyroid gland.

Antibodies specifically directed against thyroglobulin have been demonstrated by tanned erythrocyte hemagglutination (2, 4), by precipitation reactions in agar (5), by immunofluorescence (6), by complement fixation (7) and by passive cutaneous anaphylaxis (8). Employing the latter procedure, Ovary and associates (8) have shown that thyroid autoantibodies produced in man, rabbit and guinea pig are species specific. Thyroglobulin autoantibodies are frequently found in human thyroid disease. Hashimoto's disease, primary myxedema, thyrotoxicosis, noncolloid goiter and carcinoma of the thyroid are prominent in this group (9). In addition, various nonthyroid diseases are also characterized by the frequent occurrence of thyroglobulin autoantibodies. These include systemic lupus erythematosus (10), active chronic hepatitis (11), Addisonian pernicious anemia (12) and Down's disease (13), and in mothers of infants with Down's disease (14). Extensive surveys of the distribution of antithyroid autoantibodies have been compiled (15, 16).

A microsomal antigenic substance of the thyroid gland has also been documented in an autoimmune relationship (17). The characteristics of this antigen are summarized in Table 61. A marked similarity to gastric parietal cell microsomal antigen is apparent. Autoantibodies directed against thyroid microsomal antigens are demonstrated in complement fixation (18) and immunofluorescent procedures (19). Anderson and associates (20) reported that autoantibodies reacting with the thyroid microsomal antigen are distinct from antithyroglobulin autoantibodies.

Thyroid Disease and Thyroid Autoantibody Formation

Autoantibody production directed against thyroglobulin apparently results from a break of immunologic quarantine. Two separate pathways may be involved and have different etiologic significance for thyroid disease. A cause and effect relationship is possible with antithyroid autoantibodies initiating thyroid disease. An alternate possibility must also be considered. Thyroglobulin autoantibody production may be causally unrelated to the disease process. It may represent a secondary phenomenon reflecting release of thyroglobulin into the circulation because of thyroid disease. A combination of these two postulates offers the most potential. Thyroid disease can lead to release of intracellular thyroglobulin with subsequent formation of autoantibodies. Such autoantibodies may then function as cytotoxic agents causing further damage to thyroid cells. Additional thyroglobulin would be released through such cellular damage and would further stimulate antithyroglobulin autoantibody formation. A vicious cycle would result. The cytotoxic action of thyroglobulin autoantibodies has been well documented (21–25).

The concepts presented above are dependent on a simple relationship between thyroid disease and antithyroid autoantibody formation. This viewpoint no longer appears tenable. Recent studies suggest that antithyroid autoantibody formation may be only one indication of a widespread pathophysiologic abnormality.

Evidence has accumulated indicating a genetic basis for thyroid disease. The familial occurrence of myxedema and Hashimoto's disease has been well documented (26). Hall and associates (27) reported the development of antibodies to thyroglobulin in families of patients with Hashimoto's disease. The distribution suggested a dominant genetic characteristic. Irvine and associates (28) and Beierwaltes (29) have reported Hashimoto's disease occurring in identical twins.

Thyroid disease with autoantibody formation may occur as one component of a multisystem complex characterized by immunologically mediated abnormalities. Beare (30) noted that patients with Hashimoto's disease were particularly prone to develop other disease states. The striking relationship to pernicious anemia has been summarized in Chapter 9. The association has been reported of thyroiditis with systemic lupus erythematosus (31, 32), rheumatoid arthritis (33), chronic hepatitis (32), Paget's disease (34), Sjögren's disease (35), scleroderma with renal involvement (32) and Addison's disease (20).

Autoimmune hemolytic anemia resembles thyroid disease in its immunologic background, genetic predisposition and multisystem associations. Wasastjerna (36) in 1959 reported the combination of these two states in a single patient. It is therefore pertinent to examine the current series of 234 patients with autoimmune hemolytic anemia from the aspect of associated thyroid disease.

Analysis of Present Series

Twenty-four patients with autoimmune hemolytic anemia, or 10.3 per cent of the current series, had clinically demonstrable thyroid disease. The specific types of thyroid pathology encountered are summarized in Table 64. All 24 patients had unequivocal thyroid abnormalities. In addition, a substantial number of patients had or were receiving thyroid therapy without adequate studies documenting thyroid malfunction. Such cases are not included for analysis. The present study is entirely retrospective. This precludes the possibility of deriving an accurate incidence of antithyroid autoantibodies in patients with autoimmune hemolytic anemia. The unexpected high incidence of clinically detected thyroid disease suggests that such a serologic study may be rewarding.

A marked predilection for females was noted in the association of thyroid disease and autoimmune hemolytic anemia. Twenty-one of the 24 patients (87.5 per cent) were women. A middle-aged population was involved with a median age of 40

TABLE 64. *Number and variety of thyroid diseases seen in 234 patients with autoimmune hemolytic anemia (24 patients studied with 25 thyroid abnormalities)*

Thyroid Disease	No.
Thyroid adenoma*	9
Thyroiditis	4
Hyperthyroidism	4
Hypothyroidism*	4
Nontoxic goiter	4
TOTAL	25

* Both conditions in a single patient.

years at the onset of detectable thyroid disease.

At the time of analysis, 12 patients were living, 11 had died and one was lost to followup. A chronic disease state was apparent. The 11 patients who died had a mean duration of 119 months of thyroid disease. The chronicity of the process was even more apparent when living patients were analyzed. Thyroid disease had been present for a median of 144 and a mean of 195 months. The development of autoimmune hemolytic anemia did not change the chronic nature of the syndrome.

Thyroid disease was present prior to the onset of autoimmune hemolytic anemia in 14 patients. Extremely long periods of pre-existing thyroid disease were noted, with a mean value approaching 18 years. In seven patients thyroid disease and autoimmune hemolytic anemia were simultaneously discovered. In the remaining three patients autoimmune hemolytic anemia was first documented and thyroid disease subsequently became apparent. The hemolytic process antedated clinical evidence of thyroid disease by 4, 15 and 191 months, respectively. The statistical data obtained from this patient group are summarized in Table 65.

The mean and median hematocrit at the onset of autoimmune hemolytic anemia approximated 28 per cent. The lowest hematocrit values developing during clinical progression of the disease were more im-

TABLE 65. *Statistical data obtained from 24 patients (21 females, three males) with thyroid disease (TD) and autoimmune hemolytic anemia (AHA)*

Test Procedures	Total	Statistical Data		
		Range	Mean	Median
Clinical data				
Age (years)	24	13–79	42	40
Duration of TD before AHA* (months)	14	3–466	212	182
Duration of AHA before TD* (months)	3	4–191	70	15
Survival with TD, dead (months)	11	2–528	119	26
Survival with TD, living (months)	12	13–468	195	144
Survival with AHA, dead (months)	11	2–85	26	10
Survival with AHA, living (months)	12	7–204	50	33
Laboratory data				
Initial hematocrit (%)	24	18–40.3	27.6	28
Lowest hematocrit (%)	24	16–36.5	23.5	21
Initial reticulocytes (%)	21	0–27.8	3.4	1.0
Therapeutic reticulocytes (%)	12	0–32	12.9	13.4
Initial WBC† (10^3/mm.^{3})	20	3.2–20	6.5	6.1
Initial thrombocytes (10^3/mm.^{3})	19	25–536	190	200
		Increased	Decreased	Normal
Bone marrow aspiration				
Total cellularity	16	4	0	12
Erythrocyte precursors	16	11	1	4
Leukocytes	16	2	0	14
Megakaryocytes	16	0	0	16
Megaloblasts	16	5	0	11
		Normal	Abnormal	
Other laboratory abnormalities				
Total bilirubin	19	7	12	
A/G ratio	13	6	7	
Serum electrophoresis	9	4	5	
Cr^{51} T/2 time	4	0	4	
Serologic tests for syphilis	15	12	3	
LE cell test	11	10	1	
		Weakness	Dizziness	Fever
Presenting symptoms				
Abnormal	24	24	13	9

		Spleen	Liver	Lymph nodes	Jaundice
Presenting signs					
Abnormal	24	13	14	8	9

* Seven patients had simultaneous onset of TD and AHA.
† Excluding three patients with leukemia.

pressive, with a median of 21 per cent. Reticulocytosis at the time of diagnosis of autoimmune hemolytic anemia was not striking. After therapy, however, reticulocytosis was the rule. One patient did not attain a substantial therapeutic response. This patient had bone marrow erythrocytic aplasia, marked hemochromatosis and severe hypothyroidism. When patients with leukemia and lymphosarcoma were excluded from analysis, no particular pattern of leukocyte or thrombocyte abnormalities was noted. Morphologic evidence of a hemolytic state was commonly found in the peripheral blood. Nucleated erythrocytes were seen in 10 patients and spherocytes were seen in eight cases. Bone marrow examinations performed at the onset of autoimmune hemolytic anemia were available in 16 patients. The only consistent abnormality was erythrocytic hyperplasia in 11 subjects. Megaloblastic changes were found in five patients, two of whom had Addisonian pernicious anemia.

The presenting signs and symptoms of the 24 patients at the time of onset of autoimmune hemolytic anemia are summarized in Table 65. Weakness was universally noted. Hepatosplenomegaly was found in over 50 per cent of the cases. Jaundice was observed in 38 per cent of the series.

Positive serologic tests for syphilis were found in three of 15 tested individuals. In two, a biologically false positive reaction was documented. Lupus erythematosus (LE) cell testing was performed in 11 patients and positive reactions were obtained in one. Total serum bilirubin was frequently elevated, particularly in indirect testing. The albumin-globulin (A/G) ratio was abnormal in over 50 per cent of tests. In two, hypogammaglobulinemia was noted with globulin values of 0.2 and 0.6 gm. per cent, respectively. Hypergammaglobulinemia was demonstrated in five patients. Serum electrophoresis studies were abnormal in five of nine tested sera. A monoclonal gamma-globulin spike was found in one patient with an associated plasma cell myeloma. The remaining four sera exhibited broad polyclonal elevations of gamma-globulin. The erythrocyte survival time was determined in four patients. Cr^{51} half-life $(T/2)$ values of 2.2, 8, 9 and 14 days, respectively, were found.

Clinical Patterns

Variable clinical pictures were encountered in the 24 patients having autoimmune hemolytic anemia and thyroid disease. Three patients had an uncomplicated, simple relationship between hemolytic anemia and thyroid disease. There was little or no evidence of a multisystem distribution of disease.

Case 84. A 13-year-old white female complained of fatigue. Physical examination revealed an enlarged thyroid gland. Hypothyroidism was diagnosed and thyroid therapy was given. Three years later pallor and icterus were noted. Physical examination demonstrated a spleen palpated 2 cm. below the costal margin. The thyroid gland was grossly enlarged. The hematocrit was 26 per cent and the reticulocyte count was 19.4 per cent. The white blood cell count (WBC), thrombocyte count, osmotic fragility, LE cell preparations and urine analysis were all normal. Indirect serum bilirubin was elevated. Direct and indirect antiglobulin and bromelin tests were 4+ and elution revealed an erythrocyte autoantibody. Prednisone, 40 mg. daily, was given. The hematocrit rapidly rose and reached normal levels in 1 month. Prednisone was reduced and eventually discontinued 5½ months after the start of therapy. The spleen was no longer palpable. After discontinuation of prednisone, fever developed and the thyroid became diffusely tender and warm. A diagnosis of subacute thyroiditis was made. These complaints gradually disappeared. Followup examination 2 years after the onset of hemolytic anemia revealed normal hematologic values. Serologic tests 7 months later were negative with normal antiglobulin and bromelin tests.

Case 85. A 46-year-old white male had a past history of asthma and had received intermittent corticosteroid therapy. Abdominal distress led to hospitalization, at which time a peptic ulcer was found. In addition, a diffusely enlarged thyroid gland was discovered. A diagnosis of Hashimoto's disease was made. Mild anemia was noted. Thyroid therapy was given with improvement. One year later anorexia, weight loss and fatigue developed. Over the next 9 months anemia and fever occurred. A tender liver palpated 2 cm. below the costal margin was discovered. The thyroid gland was diffusely enlarged and painful.

The hematocrit was 34 per cent and bone marrow aspiration revealed erythrocytic hyperplasia. The protein bound iodine (PBI) was 4.9 μg. per cent. Serum electrophoresis and LE cell preparations were normal. The direct antiglobulin test was trace positive and the bromelin test was 4+ positive. Thyroid therapy was increased with marked clinical improvement. The thyroid gland was no longer palpable but the liver continued to be felt 3 cm. below the costal margin. The hematocrit dropped to 31 per cent. Over the next 5 months it progressively rose to 41 per cent. Followup examination 2 years later indicated a continuing hematologic remission and inactive thyroiditis. The direct and indirect antiglobulin test was negative. Direct and indirect bromelin tests were 4+ and panel studies revealed a panhemagglutinin.

Several similarities are apparent in the clinical course of these two patients. Thyroiditis antedated the onset of autoimmune hemolytic anemia in both. In addition, the hemolytic state was only moderately severe. Hematologic remission was induced with prednisone in one patient and by controlling thyroiditis with thyroid therapy in the second. A return of thyroiditis developed with a discontinuation of prednisone in the first case. In both patients autoimmune hemolytic anemia correlated with activity of thyroiditis. Remission of both conditions has been maintained for over 2 years. No additional disease processes have become apparent.

A similar correlation of hemolytic and thyroid disease activity was seen in a third patient with hyperthyroidism.

Case 86. A 12-year-old white female developed abnormal menses, and lipodystrophy was considered. One year later an enlarged thyroid gland was discovered and potassium iodide and thyroid therapy were given. The patient did well for 7 years. A 30-pound weight loss and anemia then became apparent. A diffusely enlarged thyroid gland with exophthalmos was seen. Scleral icterus was also apparent and the spleen was felt 2 cm. below the costal margin. Thyroid myopathy was present and thyrotoxicosis diagnosed. The PBI was 10.3 μg. per cent and the I[131] thyroid gland uptake was 92 per cent. The hematocrit was 21 per cent and the reticulocyte count was 27.8 per cent. Bone marrow aspiration revealed erythrocytic hyperplasia. Spherocytes were found in the peripheral blood. A Cr[51] T/2 time of 2.2 days was obtained and splenic sequestration was demonstrated. The total bilirubin was 0.5/2.1 mg. per cent. The A/G ratio and LE cell preparations were normal. Kolmer, Kahn and Kline serologic tests for syphilis were positive but a treponemal immobilization test was negative. Direct and indirect antiglobulin tests and a trypsin indirect test were positive. Elution revealed an erythrocyte autoantibody. Prednisone, 60 mg. per day, was given with a rise in the hematocrit in 10 days. Propylthiouracil was also administered, with a rapid decrease of the PBI and I[131] thyroid uptake. Prednisone was gradually reduced. An attempt to discontinue prednisone 1 year later led to a rapid drop of the hematocrit. Maintenance prednisone was given over the next 3 years. Pregnancy then developed and anemia was noted. Direct antiglobulin and bromelin tests were positive. Delivery occurred without difficulty. A second pregnancy followed and the spleen was then palpated 3 cm. below the costal margin. Although the hematocrit was well maintained, splenectomy was performed. Direct bromelin and antiglobulin tests were still positive. Serologic tests for syphilis had all reverted to normal. Two weeks after splenectomy, steroid therapy was discontinued. A normal delivery resulted. A third normal delivery followed 14 months later. Examination 52 months after splenectomy demonstrated an hematocrit of 40 per cent and negative antiglobulin and bromelin tests. A multinodular enlarged thyroid was present and hypothyroidism was apparent. The patient is still living. Total course of thyroid disease is 210 months. Autoimmune hemolytic anemia has been present for the last 83 months of her clinical course.

In this patient thyrotoxicosis occurred simultaneously with autoimmune hemolytic anemia. Both diseases were severe and excellent therapeutic responses followed corticosteroids and propylthiouracil therapy. Biologically false positive serologic reactions for syphilis were obtained during the height of the combined disease syndrome. After remission these tests were negative. Although the clinical protocol suggests a widespread systemic immunologic disease, no definitive pattern has developed.

The three patients presented above have been grouped together because of two clinical similarities. An obvious relationship existed between thyroid disease activity and autoimmune hemolytic anemia. In addition, the two processes were the only diagnosable diseases present.

The remaining 21 patients with thyroid disease and autoimmune hemolytic anemia did not demonstrate a clear relationship between the two disease states. Four cases

TABLE 66. *Idiopathic or symptomatic classification of autoimmune hemolytic anemia seen in 24 patients with thyroid disease (the underlying pathologic state resulting in symptomatic classification is presented)*

Type of Autoimmune Hemolytic Anemia	No.
Idiopathic type	4
Symptomatic to:	20
Thyroiditis	2
Hyperthyroidism	1
Chronic lymphocytic leukemia	3
Chronic granulocytic leukemia	2
Plasma cell myeloma	2
Pernicious anemia	2
Ulcerative colitis	2
Hodgkin's disease	1
Lymphosarcoma	1
Lupus erythematosus	1
Scleroderma	1
Rheumatoid arthritis	1
Drug sensitivity	1

were considered as examples of idiopathic autoimmune hemolytic anemia. Two of the patients (Cases 13 and 70) classified as idiopathic eventually developed complex clinical courses with thyroid abnormalities appearing as one part of a multisystem disease. A fortuitous association of thyroid disease was initially assumed. Seventeen patients had additional pathologic processes which suggested a secondary form of autoimmune hemolytic anemia. Table 66 lists the classification of these 24 patients.

In the 17 patients with a secondary form of autoimmune hemolytic anemia, one or more additional pathologic states were present in addition to thyroid disease. Cases 6, 21, 29, 31, 36, 65, 78, 79, 82, 83, 95 and 97 may be consulted as typical examples. Many and varied associated diseases were found in patients with autoimmune hemolytic anemia and thyroid disease. The types involved represent a cross section of immunologically related diseases. These included malignancy, collagen disease, pernicious anemia, ulcerative colitis, liver disease, erythema nodosa, drug sensitivity and thymoma. The frequency and types of associated diseases are summarized in Table 67.

TABLE 67. *Number and variety of additional disease states found in 24 patients with autoimmune hemolytic anemia (AHA) and thyroid pathology (TD)*

	Diseases Seen in Addition to TD and AHA		
Type	No.	Type	No.
Diabetes	5	Scleroderma	1
Chronic lymphocytic leukemia	3	Lupus erythematosus	1
Migratory polyarthritis	3	Rheumatoid arthritis	1
Pernicious anemia	3	Erythema nodosa	1
Chronic granulocytic leukemia	2	Febrile-lymphocytic syndrome	1
Ulcerative colitis	2	Hodgkin's disease	1
Rheumatic fever	2	Lymphosarcoma	1
Drug reactions	2	Carcinoma, uterus	1
Liver disease	2	Carcinoma, cervix	1
Ovarian cysts	2	Carcinoma, prostate	1
Thymoma	2	Carcinoma, colon	1
Plasma cell myeloma	2	Pancreatitis	1

Infectious, severe: 14 (septicemia in 6)

	No. of Significant Diseases in Addition to TD and AHA				
	None	One	Two	Three	Four or more
No. of patients	5	9	5	2	3

Such an analysis suggests that positive antiglobulin tests and thyroid disease are frequently associated in a multiple system disease complex. Only five of the 24 patients had a simple association between these two conditions. Nine patients had one additional significant disease. Five subjects had two additional significant pathologic conditions. Two patients had three additional abnormalities and three patients had at least four significant abnormalities in addition to thyroid disease and autoimmune hemolytic anemia. These observations are also summarized in Table 67.

These data must be tempered by allowance for the possibly fortuitous occurrence of thyroid disease. The inference of etiologic implications may not be justified. However, half of the patients are still alive and may develop even more complex syndromes. In addition, infection as an index of immunologic deficiency has not been considered to indicate a significant pathologic state. This may be unwarranted. Fourteen of these 24 patients had serious multiple infectious episodes involving bacteria, viruses and monilia. Septicemia occurred in six. It is possible that such infections are also a manifestation of a deranged immune apparatus.

One explanation for such a clinical pattern is that a basic aberration of the immune apparatus permits the development of multiple autoantibodies. The inability to establish normal immune homeostatic mechanisms may be involved. Such a postulate has already been suggested in order to relate autoimmune hemolytic anemia to reticuloendothelial neoplasia (37), collagen diseases, Addisonian pernicious anemia (38) and ulcerative colitis (39). The association of thyroid disease with these abnormalities and autoimmune hemolytic anemia supports this suggestion.

Malignancies Other than Reticuloendothelial Types

Anemia has been recognized as a common accompaniment of malignant disease. Multiple etiologies may be involved. These include acute and chronic blood loss, decreased erythrocyte production due to disturbances of protein synthesis, an inadequate intake, absorption or storage of hematinic factors such as iron, folic acid and vitamin B-12, and a decrease in production of erythropoietin. Toxic depression of the bone marrow secondary to concomitant infection, uremia or a "tumor toxin" may also play a role. A myelophthistic abnormality may develop as part of tumor metastases. Erythropoiesis may also be depressed as part of therapy employing ionizing radiation, metabolic analogs, alkylating agents or other antitumor substances.

Hemolysis in Malignancy

Hemolysis must also be added to this list of possible etiologies. Waugh (40) and Stats and associates (41) pointed out that hemolytic mechanisms may be activated in malignancy, particularly when the bone marrow is involved. Paraf and Dausset (42) and Wasserman and associates (43) have summarized the early clinical literature. Extensive studies of the erythrocyte life span have confirmed the presence of a mild to moderate degree of hemolysis in many malignant states (44–50). Relatively minor shortening of the erythrocyte life span almost always results in anemia. This is surprising. The bone marrow normally has the capacity to increase erythrocyte production 6- to 8-fold under anemic stress. This safety margin is apparently lost in the presence of malignancies. The bone marrow frequently cannot increase its erythrocyte production capacity 3-fold. Accordingly, the hemolytic anemia of malignancy becomes overt because of two factors, i.e., increased hemolysis and a decreased compensatory capacity of the bone marrow. Wasserman and associates (43) have termed this phenomenon "hemopathic hemolytic anemia."

Autoimmune Hemolytic Anemia in Malignancy

Green and associates have emphasized an immunologic etiology for the hemolysis seen in malignancy. They postulated that malignant cells may act as a foreign population which has retained the capacity to produce antibodies (51). In this fashion antibody formation may be initiated against host erythrocytes. This hypothesis was tested with a modification of the antiglobulin test. Three hundred and forty-three patients with various types of malignancy were studied (52). Positive reactions were reported in 39 per cent of cases. In 108 cases of far advanced carcinoma, 57 per cent were found to have positive antiglobulin reactions. Control patients without carcinoma had a 15 per cent incidence of positive antiglobulin reactions in this modified procedure. The positive reactions were characteristically of the nongamma variety. In spite of this, successful elution of an erythrocyte autoantibody was reported in eight of 15 cases. Positive indirect tests were obtained in 56 of 74 patients with positive modified direct antiglobulin tests.

This experience differs from that usually observed. Shen and Homburger (45) and Hyman (49) generally observed negative antiglobulin reactions with disseminated malignancies. A positive antiglobulin reaction was found in one case in Hyman's series (49) of 34 patients. The diagnosis is not stated in this case and a lymphoma may have been present. Occasional examples of weak positive antiglobulin reactions in malignancy have been reported by many investigators (48, 53–61). Dacie (61) has studied three patients with carcinomatosis and autoimmune hemolytic anemia.

Analysis of Present Series

In the current series of 234 patients with autoimmune hemolytic anemia, 20 patients were found to have a prior, concomitant or subsequent malignancy of a nonreticulo-endothelial type. In 19 patients carcinoma was present and in one patient a malignant melanoma was found.

It is extremely difficult to evaluate the significance of such malignant growths in relation to autoimmune hemolytic anemia. A relatively elderly age group of patients are seen with autoimmune hemolytic anemia. This population might be expected to develop unrelated malignancies on a fortuitous basis.

In the current series an unequivocal relationship of malignancy to autoimmune hemolytic anemia was observed in only four patients. In nine patients neoplasia of the reticuloendothelium was present in addition to a second malignant growth. In two cases an idiopathic form of autoimmune hemolytic anemia was assumed and the malignancy was not felt to be etiologically significant. In the remaining patients etiologic significance was ascribed to an associated systemic lupus erythematosus in two patients and to scleroderma, ulcerative colitis and rheumatoid arthritis each in one patient. Table 68 lists the types of malignancies encountered in association with autoimmune hemolytic anemia. In Table 69 other associated diseases seen in patients with malignancies and autoimmune hemolytic anemia are recorded. It is apparent that multiple disease states were present in many of these subjects.

It is doubtful whether any advantage may be obtained from statistically analyzing this group as if a homogenous population were present. Some basic characteristics, however, deserve emphasis. Seven of

TABLE 68. *Number and variety of malignancies other than reticuloendothelial types seen in 234 patients with autoimmune hemolytic anemia (20 patients studied with 21 malignancies)*

Types of Malignancy and Number			
Type	No.	Type	No.
Carcinoma of cervix	6	Oat cell carcinoma, lung	1
Carcinoma of colon	4	Bronchiogenic carcinoma	1
Carcinoma of uterus*	2	Carcinoma of larynx	1
Carcinoma of kidney	2	Basal and squamous carcinoma, skin	1
Carcinoma of prostate	1	Malignant melanoma	1

Meningioma: 1*

* Both malignancies in the same patient.

TABLE 69. *Type of autoimmune hemolytic anemia and variety of associated diseases found in patients with malignancy other than those involving the reticuloendothelium (20 patients studied)*

1. Idiopathic autoimmune hemolytic anemia	2
2. Autoimmune hemolytic anemia secondary to malignancy	4
Carcinoma of kidney	2
Carcinoma of colon	1
Oat cell carcinoma, lung	1
3. Reticuloendothelial neoplasia in addition to carcinoma	9
Chronic lymphocytic leukemia	3
Acute monocytic leukemia	3
Chronic granulocytic leukemia	1
Lymphosarcoma	1
Thymoma	1
4. Other associated diseases	14
Thyroid disease	4
Lupus erythematosus	2
Scleroderma	1
Ulcerative colitis	1
Pernicious aemia	1
Rheumatoid arthritis	1
Laennec's cirrhosis	1
Amyloidosis	1
Tuberculosis	1
Pancreatitis	1

the 20 patients were males and 16 of the total group have died. The age at time of diagnosis of malignancy ranged from 31 to 80 years with a median and mean of 57 years. In the 16 dead patients the duration of survival following the diagnosis of malignancy ranged from 0.5 to 348 months. Long survivals were common and reflect excellent surgical results obtained in eight patients with carcinoma of the cervix or uterus. The survival of patients after the onset of hemolytic anemia was markedly reduced. A mean of 17 and a median of 10 months were found. In five patients malignancy and autoimmune hemolytic anemia were simultaneously discovered. In 10 patients the malignant state antedated the onset of hemolytic anemia. Long periods of time frequently elapsed between the dis-

covery of malignancy and the development of hemolysis. A median of over 6 years and a mean of 8 years of prior malignancy were found. In five patients, malignancy developed after autoimmune hemolytic anemia. Long periods of preexisting autoimmune hemolytic anemia were also common. These figures are summarized in Table 70.

Clinical Patterns

In four patients an unequivocal relationship existed between malignancy and autoimmune hemolytic anemia. An unsuspected carcinoma of the colon was discovered during laparotomy 16 months after the onset of hemolytic anemia in Case 10. The tumor was not resected and death occurred from coronary occlusion. It is accordingly difficult to prove an etiologic relationship. The following case more clearly illustrates the relationship which may exist between malignancy and positive erythrocyte serologic testing.

Case 87. A 65-year-old white male was hospitalized with urinary obstruction. Physical examination revealed prostatic hypertrophy and a large left renal tumor. The hematocrit was 41

TABLE 70. *Statistical data obtained from 20 patients (13 females, seven males) with autoimmune hemolytic anemia (AHA) and malignancies (CA) other than those involving the reticuloendothelium*

Clinical Data	Statistical Data			
	Total	Range	Mean	Median
Age (years)	20	31–80	57	57
Duration of CA before AHA* (months)	10	4–335	96	75
Duration of AHA before CA* (months)	5	16–53	34	40
Survival with CA, dead (months)	16	0.5–348	67	38
Survival with CA, alive (months)	4	8–132	65	60
Survival with AHA, dead (months)	16	0.5–70	17	10
Survival with AHA, alive (months)	4	43–84	69	74

* Five patients had simultaneous diagnoses of CA and AHA.

per cent and the reticulocyte count was 1.0 per cent. Bone marrow examination was normal. Total bilirubin was 0.09 mg. per cent and serologic tests for syphilis were negative. Urine cultures demonstrated *Escherichia coli*. Routine preoperative cross matches were found to be incompatible. Serologic investigation revealed 2+ direct and indirect antiglobulin and bromelin tests. A clear cell carcinoma of the left kidney was surgically removed. The tumor weighed 2500 gm. and was necrotic. Three units of blood were transfused without difficulty. On the 11th postoperative day both direct and indirect antiglobulin and bromelin tests were positive. By the 21st postoperative day the antiglobulin and bromelin tests had reverted to negative. During this time the hematocrit dropped to 26 per cent and a 30 per cent eosinophilia became apparent. Thrombophlebitis had occurred and heparin as well as antibiotic therapy had been given; these were now discontinued. The patient made an excellent recovery with a return of normal hematologic values. Five months later prostatectomy was performed. Direct and indirect antiglobulin and bromelin tests were negative and the hematocrit was 43 per cent. Surgery was uneventful and transfusions were not given. Followup 84 months after nephrectomy revealed normal hematologic studies. The direct antiglobulin test was negative and the bromelin test was 3+. No other disease state was found.

In this patient positive antiglobulin and bromelin tests were related to adenocarcinoma of the kidney. Surgical removal of the tumor led to disappearance of the positive reactions. No evidence of either hemolysis or anemia was present except for a transient postoperative episode associated with an allergic reaction and infection. After 7 years there is still no evidence of any additional disease which might have been responsible for the positive antiglobulin test. A second patient was also seen with a renal carcinoma. Severe hemolytic anemia was present, as were strong positive antiglobulin tests and an erythrocyte panhemagglutinin. Surgery was not performed and death occurred 2 weeks after diagnosis. Autopsy of this 80-year-old male demonstrated only pulmonary fibrosis and emphysema, in addition to carcinoma of the kidney.

Case 88. A 67-year-old white male had a prostatectomy performed for benign hypertrophy. Two months later he was investigated because of angina and fatigue. Physical examination revealed a spleen 21 cm. below the costal margin. His prior hematocrit of 40 per cent had dropped to 31 per cent with a 2.9 per cent reticulocyte count. The bone marrow appeared hypocellular. Total bilirubin was 1.1 mg. per cent and the A/G ratio was 4.9/2.1 gm. per cent. Serology for syphilis and LE cell preparations were negative. Direct antiglobulin and bromelin tests were positive. A splenic biopsy was performed and metastatic malignancy was diagnosed. Corticosteroid therapy was initiated and the hematocrit progressively rose to 54.5 per cent. Seven subsequent antiglobulin tests were positive. Six months after the start of corticosteroids the antiglobulin test reverted to normal. The hematocrit remained elevated in spite of progressive deterioration of the patient. Death occurred 12 months after splenomegaly was discovered. Autopsy revealed oat cell carcinoma of the lung with extensive metastases. The spleen was heavily invaded with tumor.

In this patient a direct association was apparent between malignancy, anemia and positive antiglobulin tests. Hemolysis was minimal. The anemic state was a minor problem in a clinical course dominated by malignancy. Anemia and positive antiglobulin tests disappeared with corticosteroid therapy without influencing the eventual outcome of the disease.

A clear association between malignancy and autoimmune hemolytic anemia could not be documented in the remaining 16 patients. Carcinoma of the cervix (six cases) or uterus (two cases) was present in eight subjects. The malignancy antedated the hemolytic state by years in many cases. Other associated pathologic conditions became apparent in these subjects and appeared to have greater etiologic significance for autoimmune hemolytic anemia. The same generalization is appropriate for the remaining eight patients. The case histories of nine subjects have already been presented (Cases 6, 17, 28, 39, 60, 61, 63, 65 and 78).

Although a causative association of malignancy with autoimmune hemolytic anemia was not apparent in these cases it is unwarranted to dismiss them as unrelated fortuitous occurrences. The malignant state may be one facet of a complex multisystem

TABLE 71. *Number and variety of benign tumor formation found in 19 patients with auto- immune hemolytic anemia*

Benign Tumors	
Type	No.
Thyroid adenoma	9
Ovarian tumors	5
Thymomas	3
Parotid gland tumor	1
Mycosis fungoides	1
TOTAL	19

disease commonly encountered in these patients (Cases 6, 28, 39, 60, 61, 65 and 78). Nine of these 16 patients also had neoplasia of the reticuloendothelium. Such observations support the suggestion of an aberrant immune apparatus with incompetent immune homeostasis. This defect would permit the survival of cells undergoing somatic mutation, resulting in malignancy. The same abnormality would explain the concomitant association of reticuloendothelial malignancies and the appearance of immunologically mediated multisystem disease (37).

Benign Tumor Formation

Benign tumor formation associated with autoimmune hemolytic anemia was encountered in 19 of the 234 patients of the current series. The involved pathologic states are recorded in Table 71. Several of these have already been described. Thymoma formation is documented in Chapter 6 and thyroid adenoma is documented earlier in this chapter. The one example of mycosis fungoides has been mentioned in connection with associated Hodgkin's disease and ulcerative colitis.

Ovarian Cysts

The association of autoimmune hemolytic anemia and neoplasia of the ovary has been recognized for many years. In 1938 West-Watson and Young (62) reported severe hemolysis in a 44-year-old white female. Splenectomy was ineffectual in controlling the hemolytic process. Laparotomy for an accessory spleen was performed and an

ovarian teratoma was discovered. Correction of the hemolytic state followed removal of the gall bladder and of the ovarian tumor. Watson (63) in 1939 also encountered a patient with a large ovarian cyst and hemolytic anemia. Surgical removal of the cyst did not correct the hemolytic process, but splenectomy resulted in progressive improvement. Singer and Dameshek (64) reported a 47-year-old female who developed severe hemolytic anemia. Splenectomy led to transient improvement. Laparotomy for a presumed accessory spleen was performed and a large dermoid cyst was found and removed. Hematologic remission occurred postoperatively. Jones and Tillman (65) described a patient with dermatomyositis and hemolytic anemia. Removal of a large pseudo-mucinous cyst adenocarcinoma corrected the autoimmune hemolytic anemia. Dermatomyositis did not appear to be involved in the hemolytic process. Additional reports of ovarian tumor formation associated with autoimmune hemolytic anemia have been presented by many investigators (66–80).

In the majority of recorded cases, benign tumor formation has been present. Carcinoma, however, has been noted by Jones and Tillman (65), Norcross (78) and Yam and associates (80). Positive antiglobulin reactions have almost inevitably been present when hemolytic anemia is discovered associated with ovarian tumors. Exceptions to this rule may be found in the cases mentioned by Allibone and Collins (67), Norcross (78) and McAndrew (79). The antiglobulin reaction generally reverts to negative upon correction of hemolytic anemia subsequent to surgical removal of the involved ovary. Splenectomy has been employed therapeutically and in four patients it failed to correct the hemolytic process (63, 64, 66, 74).

Ahrengot (81) has emphasized the role that dermoid cysts or ovarian teratomas may play in autoimmune hemolytic anemia. He suggested that cells with a haploid chromosome content may be produced. Such cells might treat the host as foreign and initiate antibody formation in a graft-host disease syndrome.

Other possibilities must be considered.

It is well known that the A, B, H and P blood group substances are secreted into ovarian cysts. Freiesleben and associates (82) and Lenoel and Soudet (83) reported excessive amounts of such substances concentrated in ovarian cysts. van Loghem (84) suggests, "It seems likely that in these cysts or tumors structurally altered cross-reacting antigens develop, which are responsible for the autoimmune phenomena." Landaw's suggestion (85) that mucin-like material secreted by various tumors might have a cross antigenic relationship to the erythrocyte surface expands this viewpoint. In such cases either an antiglobulin positive hemolytic anemia would result or a termination of tolerance could initiate true autoimmune hemolytic anemia.

A third etiologic mechanism should be considered. Müller and Schubothe (74) reported the development of positive nonspecific serologic tests for syphilis in patients with dermoid cysts. This suggests that ovarian tumors may appear as part of a systemic syndrome characterized by multiple autoantibody formation.

Clinical Patterns

Five patients had benign tumor formation of the ovary or related structures associated with autoimmune hemolytic anemia. One patient had a relatively simple clinical course which resembled the usual pattern reported in the literature.

Case 89. A 28-year-old white female underwent subtotal gastrectomy for an obstructing duodenal ulcer. Three years later anemia was noted during pregnancy. The patient was treated with four transfusions, oral iron and pancreatin. Homologous serum jaundice occurred. Over the next 4 years multiple transfusions were given for persisting anemia. At age 40 an iron deficiency hypochromic microcytic anemia was diagnosed. Physical examination was negative. The hematocrit was 24 per cent and the reticulocyte count was 1.4 per cent. Total bilirubin and the A/G ratio were normal. Serum electrophoresis revealed a broad polyclonal gamma level and a moderately elevated monoclonal spike in the beta range. Kline and Kahn serologic tests for syphilis were weakly positive and the VDRL test was negative. The PBI was reduced to 2.9 μg. per cent. Hypothyroidism was considered

but could not be confirmed. A Schilling test was normal and serum iron was reduced. Direct antiglobulin and bromelin tests were positive. The patient was treated with parenteral iron and the hematocrit rose to 30 per cent with a 6.0 per cent reticulocyte count. Two years later a marginal ulcer was diagnosed and vagotomy was performed. Soon after, a malabsorption syndrome with steatorrhea became apparent. Antiglobulin and bromelin tests remained consistently positive. A Cr^{51} T/2 erythrocyte survival time of 22 days was found. Anemia persisted with the hematocrit approximating 30 per cent. Continual oral iron therapy was given. One year later a hysterectomy was performed for endometriosis. A right salpingo-oophorectomy was also performed for removal of multiple hydatid tube cysts of Morgagni. The hematocrit gradually returned to normal. Antiglobulin and bromelin tests, which had been positive for almost 5 years, became negative. Followup 2 years later revealed hematologic remission with a hematocrit of 40 per cent.

An anemic state with positive antiglobulin tests persisted for 5 years in the above patient. The presence of hydatid cysts was not considered and they were inadvertently discovered during surgery. Removal of the hydatid tumors initiated hematologic remission and the antiglobulin test reverted to negative. The patient's course was complicated by iron deficiency anemia, chronic gastrointestinal blood loss, a malabsorption syndrome and possibly hypothyroidism. Biologically false positive serologic reactions for syphilis and abnormal serum electrophoresis patterns were present. This suggests the possibility of a multisystem immunologically mediated disease.

The remaining four patients with ovarian cysts and autoimmune hemolytic anemia also had widespread disease suggesting multisystem involvement. An additional significant pathologic state was present in all. A fortuitous relationship of ovarian pathology to autoimmune hemolytic anemia therefore could not be excluded. One subject (Case 35) developed autoimmune hemolytic anemia soon after surgical removal of a dermoid cyst. Plasma cell myeloma was subsequently diagnosed, and infectious disease dominated the clinical course. A second patient (Case 28) had an ovarian cyst removed 30 years prior to the development of autoimmune hemolytic anemia. She eventually developed multiple recurrent squamous and basal cell skin carcinomas. Acute monocytic leukemia and autoimmune hemolytic anemia subsequently developed. A third patient (Case 79) developed fulminating ulcerative colitis, autoimmune hemolytic anemia and multiple infections. On autopsy, multinodular thyroid disease and bilateral ovarian cysts were found. The fourth subject had an ovarian tumor removed 28 years prior to the development of autoimmune hemolytic anemia. A thyroid adenoma was simultaneously discovered with the ovarian lesion. This patient subsequently developed chronic lymphocytic leukemia which was complicated 1 year later by autoimmune hemolytic anemia.

All five patients in the current series with ovarian tumor formation and autoimmune hemolytic anemia had evidence suggestive of multiple immunologic aberrations. This suggests that a simple relationship between ovarian tumors and autoimmune hemolytic anemia does not exist. Rather, they both may represent two facets of a multisystem immunologic disease. Additional observations are critically needed in this type of patient.

Parotid Tumor Formation

One patient in the current series had a benign parotid gland tumor associated with autoimmune hemolytic anemia. Unfortunately neither biopsy nor surgical removal of the lesion has been carried out. Accordingly, she has been classified as having idiopathic autoimmune hemolytic anemia.

Case 90. A 77-year-old white female was investigated because of fatigue and abdominal distress. Diabetes was diagnosed and the hematocrit found to be 40 per cent. Positive serologic tests for syphilis were obtained. She returned 1 year later with fatigue, dizziness and intermittent claudication. Jaundice was noted. The spleen was palpated 5 cm. below the costal margin and a firm parotid gland tumor was noted. The hematocrit was 16 per cent and the reticulocyte count was 10.5 per cent. Bone marrow aspiration revealed erythrocytic hyperplasia. A Cr^{51} T/2 of 7.2 days was obtained without splenic sequestration. Total serum bilirubin was 0.4/3.2 mg.

per cent and the A/G ratio and LE cell preparations were normal. Serologic tests for syphilis were still positive. Direct and indirect antiglobulin and bromelin tests were strongly positive. Elution revealed an erythrocyte panhemagglutinin. Prednisone, 60 mg. per day, was started. In 5 days the reticulocyte count reached 46.7 per cent and the hematocrit reached 24.5 per cent. Prednisone was rapidly reduced in view of intensification of diabetes. The hematocrit progressively rose. Fourteen weeks later maintenance prednisone, 10 mg. daily, was employed. Followup 9 months after diagnosis of autoimmune hemolytic anemia revealed an hematocrit of 38 per cent, a reticulocyte count of 3.2 per cent and strong positive direct antiglobulin and bromelin tests. Indirect tests had reverted to normal. The parotid gland tumor was unchanged.

Autoimmune hemolytic anemia promptly responded to prednisone therapy in this patient. The parotid gland tumor was unchanged and its relationship to the hemolytic state is problematical.

Cardiac Surgery with the Insertion of Prosthetic Valves

In recent years surgical procedures have been developed to correct various forms of heart disease by the insertion of prosthetic devices. Hemolytic anemia may result from these procedures. This form of iatrogenic mechanical hemolytic anemia was first noted after insertion of a Hufnagel ball-valve prosthesis (86, 87). Hemodynamic disturbance with turbulence of blood flow was subsequently implicated by several investigators as the most important source of mechanical damage to erythrocytes (88–90). Gross deformities of red cells (schistocytes) supplied morphologic evidence of a relationship of trauma to shortening of the erythrocyte life span (90). An expansion of these studies by Brodeur and associates (91) suggested that the majority of patients with aortic stenosis had a shortening of the erythrocyte survival time prior to the surgical insertion of prosthetic devices. It appears most likely that the hemodynamic state, as it determines the extent of mechanical insult to erythrocytes, is responsible for early death of such cells. Support for this concept is seen in the correlation of mechanical hemolytic anemia with a jet stream resulting from separation, tearing or malposition of the artificial valve. Accordingly, a compensated state of mechanical hemolytic anemia is a common phenomenon with valvular stenosis. The surgical correction of this abnormality may lead to an uncompensated state of overt mechanical hemolytic anemia. Such a complication is seen in approximately 10 per cent of cases in which a Starr-Edwards ball-valve is employed to correct aortic stenosis (92). The physiologic and therapeutic implications of this mechanical form of hemolytic anemia have been recently summarized (92).

In addition to a mechanical etiology for hemolytic anemia in cardiac disease, Pirofsky and associates (93) have suggested that autoimmune mechanisms may be activated. In 1964 Hjeln and associates (94) noted the transient formation of anti-hr″(e) in a hr″(e) patient who had prosthetic aortic valve insertion. There was little to suggest a correlation of autoantibody activity with a hemolytic state. Pirofsky and associates (93) in 1965 reported seven examples of this phenomenon and suggested differences between this state and that seen with mechanical hemolytic anemia. In six of the seven patients positive antiglobulin tests were found. In four patients prednisone therapy aided in correcting hemolysis. Transient hemolysis was noted in these subjects, in contrast to the chronicity of mechanical hemolytic anemia. Schistocytes were not seen with the autoimmune syndrome (95), in contrast to a high incidence of deformed cells in the mechanical variety. Since these initial observations were made, other observers have encountered the same phenomenon. Lustumbo and associates (96) have reported five examples of this syndrome in 127 patients who had had open heart surgery. A transient course was seen with positive antiglobulin tests developing 1 to 2 weeks after surgery and disappearing in 6 months to 1 year. Morse and associates (97) have reported two such cases. In one patient an autoantibody with specificity of anti-hr″ (e) was present and was associated with an isoantibody of anti-rh′(C) specificity. An extensive survey of this problem was recently made by Polesky and associates (98). In a study of 250 patients undergoing cardiac surgical procedures, one-third were found to have positive antiglobulin tests.

Clinical Patterns

Nine subjects in the current series of patients with autoimmune hemolytic anemia presented this syndrome. Rheumatic heart disease with valvular involvement was present in five. In the remaining four patients calcific aortic stenosis was the underlying valvular defect. None of these patients had additional pathologic states suggesting another etiology for the positive antiglobulin test and hemolytic anemia.

Case 91. A 32-year-old white male with rheumatic heart disease underwent open heart surgery. The aortic, mitral and tricuspid valves were replaced with Starr-Edwards prostheses. Four days later an elevation of serum bilirubin was noted. A maximal bilirubin level of 32/20 mg. per cent was reached on the 14th postoperative day. Thereafter a progressive decrease in bilirubin developed. By the 9th postoperative day the hematocrit had dropped to 30 per cent with a 4.0 per cent reticulocyte count. On the 16th postoperative day the hematocrit had reached 25 per cent. Hemolysis continued and on the 18th day the hematocrit was 18 per cent and the reticulocyte count was 5.0 per cent. Direct antiglobulin and bromelin tests were positive and the presence of an autoantibody was discovered in panel studies. Prednisone, 60 mg. per day, was started on the 20th day. Six days later the hematocrit had risen to 31.5 per cent and prednisone was rapidly reduced. The hemolytic syndrome returned and the hematocrit dropped to 24.5 per cent with a reticulocyte count of 8.6 per cent. Fever and abnormal lymphocytes were seen, leading to diagnosis of a febrile lymphocyte-splenomegaly syndrome. Prednisone, 60 mg., was again initiated on the 37th postoperative day, with a rapid rise of the hematocrit to 36 per cent. Reticulocyte counts ranged at the 19 per cent level. Steroid therapy was gradually decreased and by the 76th day it was discontinued. During this time the hematocrit stabilized at approximately 30 per cent. It gradually rose, reaching a level of 38 per cent with a reticulocyte count of 0.8 per cent on the 277th day. Serologic studies revealed positive direct antiglobulin and bromelin tests on the 18th, 19th, 34th and 81st postoperative days.

An unbound erythrocyte autoantibody was also demonstrated in antiglobulin and enzyme procedures. Elution, however, was unsuccessful.

Serologic studies were negative on the 214th, 263rd and 298th days. Open heart surgery with reinforcement of mitral and tricuspid valves was performed 299 days after the first operation. A hemolytic syndrome did not follow this procedure, although positive antiglobulin and bromelin tests were again found on the 127th, 130th and 146th postoperative days. When the patient was last checked 14 months after the first operation and 6 months after the second operative procedure, there was no evidence of a hemolytic state.

Case 92. A 42-year-old white male with congenital calcific aortic stenosis underwent open heart surgery with replacement of the aortic valve by a Starr-Edwards prosthesis. The postoperative course was complicated by acute renal failure and uremia. Three peritoneal dialysis procedures were carried out. The hematocrit dropped to 32.5 per cent on the 3rd postoperative day and to 29 per cent with a 1.5 per cent reticulocyte count 3 days later. Hemolysis became apparent by the 14th postoperative day with an hematocrit of 22 per cent and a 2 per cent reticulocyte count. The hematocrit continued to drop, reaching 17 per cent with a reticulocyte count of 6 per cent on the 27th day. Serum bilirubin values were elevated on the 1st postoperative day and remained elevated until the 9th day. Thereafter it decreased. A blood transfusion was started on the 11th day but was discontinued because of a severe transfusion reaction. Direct antiglobulin and bromelin tests performed on the 13th and 20th postoperative days were negative. On the 23rd day positive direct antiglobulin and bromelin tests were found. Repeated serologic studies performed on the 24th, 30th and 35th days revealed positive direct antiglobulin and bromelin tests. Elution studies were unsuccessful and indirect erythrocyte serology tests were negative. The patient received 8 units of blood between the 14th and 35th postoperative days and two transfusion reactions were encountered. With this therapy the hematocrit was maintained at levels ranging from 28 to 30 per cent. On the 37th postoperative day prednisone, 10 mg. daily, was started. The hematocrit gradually rose. When the patient was last seen 3 months postoperatively, the hematocrit was 35 per cent with a 3.4 per cent reticulocyte count. The antiglobulin and bromelin tests had reverted to normal.

These two patients illustrate some of the clinical variations encountered. In Case **91** a persisting hemolytic state with positive antiglobulin tests responded to corticosteroid therapy after 3 months of severe anemia. Decreasing prednisone resulted in a return of hemolysis. Restarting prednisone at full dosage again induced a hematologic remission. In Case **92** a more abrupt and transient course was present, with correction of the hemolytic state in approximately 1 month.

In seven patients similar clinical patterns were encountered. All seven had placement of a Starr-Edwards artificial aortic valve. In two the mitral and tricuspid valves were also replaced. In one patient mitral valve and aortic valve replacements were performed. Hemolytic anemia was an early clinical complication generally occurring within 2 weeks of the surgical procedure. Hemolysis was overt. Anemia, reticulocytosis and bone marrow erythrocytic hyperplasia were found in all. Hemolytic anemia generally appeared to be transient, but examples of exacerbation and remission were found. Although hemolysis was severe, it did not lead to death or jeopardize cardiovascular benefits resulting from the surgical procedure. The febrile-lymphocyte-splenomegaly syndrome was present in four of these seven patients. An excellent therapeutic result was attained in the four patients who received prednisone therapy.

Hemodynamic studies in these patients suggest that mechanical damage to the erythrocyte may be an important factor. This postulate is supported by the rarity of hemolysis when the mitral valve alone is involved. It is doubtful, therefore, that the prosthesis itself is intrinsically involved in the initiation of the hemolytic state. Rather, it would appear to function by magnifying the mechanical hemodynamic problem. Support for this hypothesis is seen with two additional patients in the current series who presented this syndrome. Positive antiglobulin tests were discovered prior to surgery in both. In one case of calcific aortic stenosis, a moderately severe hemolytic anemia was present. Intermittently positive antiglobulin and bromelin tests were obtained for over 1 year before surgical intervention was employed. The patient tolerated the extensive surgery without difficulty. Washed erythrocytes suspended in albumin were employed for the large number of transfusions needed. Hemolysis did not occur postoperatively and antiglobulin tests were negative. The second patient had severe mitral stenosis with a jet stream noted at surgery. The operative procedure and transfusion of washed, albumin suspended erythrocytes were well tolerated. Death occurred on the 4th postoperative day from cardiac decompensation.

Etiologic Mechanisms

The nature of the erythrocyte coating material leading to positive antiglobulin and bromelin tests is of great interest. Elution of an erythrocyte autoantibody was successful in two cases. The following serologic conclusions can be drawn. Antiglobulin and bromelin reactions are generally weak and commercial antiglobulin serum is highly variable in its ability to detect the erythrocyte autoantibody. Positive serologic reactions may be transient, persisting for only 1 week or so. In other cases it may be demonstrated for over 1 year, even when overt hemolysis is absent. The erythrocyte autoantibodies functioned as panhemagglutinins in our study. In other reports anti-hr″(e) specificity has been found (**94, 97**). The autoantibody was inhibited by streptomycin in a fashion similar to that seen with antirhesus and other erythrocyte autoantibodies (**99**). Treatment of the autoantibody with 2-mercaptoethanol converted the incomplete antibody into a saline acting complete form. A saline titer was found similar to that obtained with antirhesus isoantibodies and other erythrocyte autoantibodies (**99**).

The relationship between autoimmune hemolytic anemia and valvular heart disease and surgery is not immediately apparent. Three suggestions may be made to relate these states. Lymphocytes may survive in transfused blood (**100**). The large amount of fresh blood transfused in such patients introduces the possibility that foreign lymphocytes may survive in the circulation (**101**). A graft-host disease syndrome could then occur with the production of erythrocyte autoantibodies. The transient nature of hemolysis would reflect the reestablishment of immune homeostasis after correction of severe stress with the eventual rejection of foreign lymphocytes and cessation of autoantibody formation. The development of a febrile-lymphocyte-splenomegaly syndrome in four of our patients supports this concept. The survival of foreign lymphocytes does not appear to be a completely adequate explanation. Positive antiglobulin tests do not generally develop in other open heart surgery patients, although similar blood transfusions are given. The development of autoimmune hemolytic anemia preoperatively in cardiac patients not receiving transfusions also minimizes the role of foreign lymphocytes.

A second etiologic hypothesis is dependent on the demonstration that mechanical damage to erythrocytes is present both pre- and postoperatively in patients with valvular heart disease. A mechanical form of hemolytic anemia is frequently present. Mechanical damage to the erythrocyte surface may induce modifications of surface antigenic characteristics (**93**). Erythrocyte antibody formation can then be initiated and may concomitantly act to terminate immune tolerance. The disappearance or diminution in numbers of mechanically damaged erythrocytes would permit reestablishment of a tolerant state. This would be reflected by disappearance of both autoimmune hemolytic anemia and positive antiglobulin tests.

The possibility must always be considered that the positive antiglobulin tests are "false" reactions unrelated to an autoimmune state. Patients undergoing cardiac surgery frequently receive large doses of antibiotics. Both penicillin and cephalothin may lead to positive antiglobulin tests, and such reactions may be misinterpreted as autoimmune hemolytic anemia.

It should be emphasized that hemolytic anemia complicating valvular heart disease and surgical therapy is not always of

TABLE 72. *Number and type of chemical agents having a possible etiologic relationship to autoimmune hemolytic anemia*

Chemical Agents	No.
Dilantin	2
Alpha-methyldopa	2
Sodium cephalothin	1
Butazolidin	1
Quinidine	1
Weed killer	1
Total cases studied	234

the autoimmune variety described above. In most instances a pure mechanical hemolytic state is present. Either iron replacement therapy or surgical correction of a leak, tear or malposition of the valve will correct or compensate for the hemolytic phenomenon. An autoimmune mechanism is relatively uncommon and its true significance and pathogenesis has yet to be determined. An excellent review of the mechanical types of hemolytic anemia seen in heart surgery has been presented by Dacie (61).

Drug Reactions

The development of immunohemolytic anemia as a consequence of drug exposure has been well recognized. Mesantoin (102), stibophen (103), quinidine (104), quinine (105), para-aminosalicylic acid (106, 107), phenacetin (105, 106), chlorpromazine (108), Butazolidin (70), penicillin (109, 110), streptomycin (111), cephalothin (112, 113), alpha-methyldopa (114), L-sarcolysine (115) and insecticides (116) have been reported as initiating such a syndrome. The mechanisms of the action of such chemicals are highly variable and are outlined in Chapter 14. An excellent review of this entire subject has been presented by Dausset and Contu (117). In general an antiglobulin positive type of immunohemolytic anemia is produced, rather than the autoimmune variety.

In the current series of 234 patients with autoimmune hemolytic anemia, a drug or chemical contact relationship was surprisingly infrequent. Only eight patients

and six different chemicals presented this syndrome. Table 72 lists the drugs encountered. An etiologic relationship between drug exposure and autoimmune hemolytic anemia was difficult to document. An unequivocal connection between drug and hemolysis was apparent in only three subjects. In three additional patients an idiopathic form of autoimmune hemolytic anemia was diagnosed, with a possible significant drug exposure noted. In the remaining two patients an additional significant pathologic state was present and was considered more important etiologically than was drug ingestion.

Dilantin Exposure

In 1954 Snapper and associates (102) reported the development of autoimmune hemolytic anemia as a complication of Mesantoin therapy. An etiologic relationship may be challenged in view of concomitant penicillin administration. However, additional reports have noted the induction of hemolysis and erythrocyte metabolic abnormalities upon exposure to anticonvulsive agents. Weiner and associates (118) reported the development of autoimmune hemolytic anemia in an epileptic patient receiving phenobarbital. This patient also received penicillin during the development of positive antiglobulin tests, and an etiologic relationship of phenobarbital and epilepsy is obscure.

In contrast, Dilantin has been clearly shown to lead to a megaloblastic anemia with metabolic abnormalities of the erythrocyte (119). A folic acid deficiency is common and an immunohemolytic anemia is not generally activated. Schwartz and Costea (120), however, noted the association of autoimmune hemolytic anemia with Dilantin administration. Two patients in the current series developed autoimmune hemolytic anemia while receiving Dilantin. One patient (Case 17) had a carcinoma of the cervix removed 4 years prior to the development of hemolytic anemia. A meningioma was diagnosed and surgically removed 3 years later. Mesantoin was given for 1 week and Dilantin therapy was subsequently employed. After receiving Dilantin for 1 year the patient entered with an aplastic bone marrow and positive antiglobulin tests. A response to corticosteroid therapy did not occur and death resulted in 2 weeks. An idiopathic form of autoimmune hemolytic anemia has been assumed. A second example of Dilantin therapy associated with positive antiglobulin tests is presented below.

Case 93. An 8-year-old white child suffered traumatic brain damage and remained permanently in a rest home. Convulsive episodes developed and required Dilantin, 300 mg., and phenobarbital, 60 mg. daily. With this therapy convulsions were absent from age 47 to 55. She was hospitalized at age 55 because of edema. The liver was palpated 2 cm. below the costal margin and inflammatory subcutaneous nodules were felt on the lower extremities. Sigmoidoscopy revealed a submucosal nodule which biopsy proved to be due to benign lymphocytosis. Diabetes was diagnosed. The patient's hematocrit was 38 per cent and this decreased in 1 week to 31.5 per cent. The reticulocyte count was 2.0 per cent. Serum bilirubin was normal and the A/G ratio was 4.1/3.9 gm. per cent. Serum electrophoresis revealed a broad polyclonal elevation of the gamma-globulin. Bone marrow examination was normal. Direct antiglobulin tests were positive and the bromelin test was negative. One week later both the direct antiglobulin and bromelin tests were positive. No therapy was given except oral iron. Phenobarbital, 90 mg. daily, and Dilantin, 300 mg. daily, were continued. The hematocrit rapidly returned to 38 per cent in 10 days. The patient remained asymptomatic except for occassional convulsions.

The exact relationship of Dilantin therapy to the development of positive antiglobulin and bromelin tests in this patient was not determined. A hemolytic state is also equivocal. The possibility of another associated disease must be considered in view of subcutaneous nodules, submucous colonic lymphoid infiltration and an abnormal serum electrophoretic pattern. As yet no definitive diagnosis has been made and followup is continuing.

Alpha-methyldopa Therapy

In 1966 Carstairs and associates (114) called attention to the frequent development of positive antiglobulin tests in patients receiving the antihypertensive drug alpha-methyldopa. This observation has been amply confirmed. Worlledge and associates (121) reported a series of patients in whom autoimmune hemolytic anemia occurred in addition to the positive antiglobulin reaction. The erythrocyte autoantibodies appeared as IgG immunoglobulins with an extremely high incidence of specificity for rhesus agglutinogens. LoBuglio and Jandle (122) reported one erythrocyte autoantibody related to alpha-methyldopa administration which did not react with Rh(null) erythrocytes. Complement does not appear to be involved in these reactions. These reports are summarized in Chapter 14.

In the present series two patients were seen in whom alpha-methyldopa therapy resulted in positive antiglobulin tests and autoimmune hemolytic anemia.

Case 94. A 27-year-old male developed traumatic paraplegia and bladder paresis. Over the next 6 years repeated urinary tract infections occurred with acute and chronic pyelonephritis and hydronephrosis. A right ureterostomy was performed and intermittent uremia with progressive hypertension developed. A persistent *E. coli,* Pseudomonas, and enterococcal urinary tract infection was present. Infectious hepatitis also occurred and spontaneously improved. The patient was placed on alpha-methyldopa therapy for persisting hypertension. Over a 3-month period the hematocrit dropped to 29 per cent with an 8.4 per cent reticulocyte count. Spherocytosis and an 8 per cent eosinophilia were noted in the peripheral blood. Bone marrow aspiration was normal. Direct and indirect antiglobulin and bromelin tests were strongly positive. Elution revealed an erythrocyte panhemagglutinin. Serologic tests for syphilis and LE cell preparations were normal. Alpha-methyldopa therapy was discontinued and the hematocrit rapidly improved. Alpha-methyldopa therapy was again given and the hematocrit rapidly dropped to 22 per cent with marked reticulocytosis. Alpha-methyldopa therapy was discontinued. One week later both direct and indirect antiglobulin and bromelin tests were negative. The hematocrit progressively rose to 30 per cent in spite of persistent uremia. Followup examination is continuing.

In the above case the administration of

alpha-methyldopa therapy resulted in a rapidly developing hemolytic anemia characterized by strong positive antiglobulin and bromelin tests. Cessation of alpha-methyldopa therapy on two occasions corrected the hemolytic state. On the last occasion rapid disappearance of positive antiglobulin and bromelin tests was noted. There is little doubt that alpha-methyldopa ingestion was related both to the hemolytic process and to the development of erythrocyte autoantibodies.

Case 95. A 36-year-old white female developed hyperthyroidism which was treated by thyroidectomy. At age 46 cholelithiasis was diagnosed. At age 54 hypertension was noted and treated with phenobarbital. At age 65 recurrent cystitis developed and was intermittently treated with sulfonamides. Diuril and Serpasil therapy was initiated for persistent hypertension. Throughout this time normal hematologic studies were obtained except for one episode of mild anemia successfully treated with oral iron. At age 71 chronic pyelonephritis was diagnosed and treated with sulfonamides. Several months later two doses of alpha-methyldopa and chlorothiazide were given and discontinued because of syncope. One month later the same agents were again given and maintained with an excellent antihypertensive effect. Seven months later fatigue and anemia were noted which did not respond to iron therapy. Five months later the hematocrit reached 26 per cent with a reticulocyte count of 0.8 per cent. The bone marrow examination, serum bilirubin, WBC and thrombocyte count were all normal. There was free acid in the patient's stomach. LE cell preparations were negative. Gastrointestinal blood loss could not be demonstrated. Direct antiglobulin tests were positive. Alpha-methyldopa and chlorothiazide therapy was discontinued. The hematocrit progressively rose and reached 37 per cent in 3 weeks. Chlorothiazide therapy alone was restarted without affecting the hematologic remission.

The patient was first seen at our laboratories 2 months after the cessation of alpha-methyldopa therapy. Physical examination at that time was essentially normal. The hematocrit was 38 per cent and the reticulocyte count was 0.8 per cent. The WBC was 7,300/mm.³ with a 6 per cent eosinophilia. Thrombocytes were normal. Urinalysis revealed 2+ proteinuria. Direct and indirect antiglobulin and bromelin tests were strongly positive. Elution was successful and an erythrocyte autoantibody acting as a panhemagglutinin was discovered.

The ingestion of alpha-methyldopa and chlorothiazide was followed by progressive anemia and the development of positive antiglobulin tests in this patient. Cessation of therapy while chlorothiazide was maintained resulted in a rapid hematologic remission. Two months after the cessation of alpha-methyldopa, during hematologic remission, antiglobulin and bromelin tests were still strongly positive and an erythrocyte panhemagglutinin could be demonstrated and eluted. Eosinophilia was noted in this case as well as in Case 94, which also presented an alpha-methyldopa induced hemolytic syndrome.

Sodium Cephalothin Therapy

Molthan and associates (113) demonstrated that normal erythrocytes incubated with cephalothin developed positive antiglobulin reactions. They postulated that the effect is dosage related and is due to the chemical combination of cephalothin and one or more plasma proteins to the erythrocyte. It was also observed that cephalthin altered red cell membrane proteins. In a study of 31 patients receiving cephalothin therapy, 25 were found to develop positive antiglobulin reactions. In many cases positive reactions developed from 24 to 72 hours after ingestion of the drug. Such reactions were most commonly found in patients with impaired kidney function. Such states apparently induce blood levels of cephalothin sufficient to react with serum proteins (333 to 666 μg/ ml.).

Gralnick and associates (112) and Gralnick and McGinnis (123) noted that cephalothin treatment of erythrocytes does not lead to positive direct antiglobulin tests. However, almost all normal human sera have the ability to induce agglutination of cephalothin treated erythrocytes. In addition, normal human sera led to positive indirect antiglobulin tests with drug treated erythrocytes. Antipenicillin antibody cross reacts with cephalothin and cephalothin inhibits the action of antipenicillin antibody. These investigators noted that 2-mercaptoethanol reduction of normal sera prevented saline agglutination. Preliminary data strongly suggests that cephalothin modifies the electrical mobility of various serum proteins. A similar observation has been made for streptomycin (124). Neither Gralnick and associates nor Molthan and associates (113) attributed clinical significance to cephalothin induced positive antiglobin tests.

In the current series one patient (Case 49) was encountered who developed hemolytic anemia and positive antiglobulin tests while receiving cephalothin therapy. The subject was an alcoholic with cirrhosis who developed Friedlander's pneumonia. It is accordingly difficult to determine whether the pneumonitis, the cirrhosis or the drug therapy was responsible for the hemolytic state.

Butazolidin

deGruchy (70) in 1954 noted a possible relationship between chronic autoimmune hemolytic anemia and Butazolidin ingestion. One patient in the current series was seen with this association. Only fragmentary studies were carried out and the patient has been lost to followup. The available data are presented below.

Case 96. A 61-year-old white male developed muscle aches and pains. He presented a past history of acute arthritis 16 years prior to this episode. Butazolidin therapy was given for 2 weeks for the current problem with excellent therapeutic results. Two months later fatigue and an upper respiratory infection were noted. Physical examination was entirely negative except for petechiae and purpura. The hematocrit was 30 per cent with a 1.4 per cent reticulocyte count. The WBC was 1,500/mm.³ with 87 per cent of the cells lymphocytes. Spherocytes were seen in the peripheral blood. The thrombocytes were markedly reduced. Bone marrow examination was typical of aplastic anemia. Direct antiglobulin and bromelin tests were positive. A Cr⁵¹ erythrocyte survival time revealed a T/2 of 20 days. Over the next week the hematocrit dropped to 25 per cent with a 2.2 per cent reticulocyte count. The patient returned to his local physician with the advice to initiate corticosteroid therapy. He was subsequently lost to followup.

Butazolidin therapy was subsequently followed by clinical and laboratory evidence of aplastic anemia. A hemolytic component was apparent with spherocytosis, a rapid drop of the hematocrit, a shortened erythrocyte survival time and positive antiglobulin and bromelin tests. The relationship of Butazolidin to the hematologic state is striking. This patient has been classified as having an idiopathic variety of autoimmune hemolytic anemia in view of the lack of followup and detailed studies.

Toxic Chemicals

Muirhead and associates (116) in 1959 reported the development of chronic autoimmune hemolytic anemia following exposure to insecticides. One patient (Case 20) in the current series presented a history of exposure to a toxic chemical prior to the development of autoimmune hemolytic anemia. Pure erythrocyte aplasia developed in this patient after two exposures to a weed killer. A thymoma was subsequently documented. Neither erythrocyte aplasia nor positive antiglobulin tests responded to thymectomy. The relationship of toxic chemical exposure to development of this syndrome is suggestive.

Quinidine

Freedman and associates (104) in 1956 reported the association of quinidine ingestion and autoimmune hemolytic anemia. They postulated a haptenic relationship as discussed in Chapter 14.

In the current series one patient with a hematologic sensitivity to quinidine was seen. The relationship of this drug to autoimmune hemolytic anemia is remote.

Case 97. A 60-year-old white female with a history of hemorrhagic cystitis developed paroxysmal auricular tachycardia. Quinidine therapy was initiated. Three years later acute purpura was noted. Physical examination was negative. The hematocrit was 37 per cent, the WBC was 11,250/mm.³ and thrombocytes were 2,140/mm.³ Quinidine was discontinued and prednisone therapy, 60 mg. daily, was given. Corticosteroid therapy was rapidly decreased and discontinued after 2 weeks. The thrombocyte count reached 490,000/mm.³ 8 days after stopping quinidine. The hematocrit had risen to 41 per cent. Four months later the patient returned with fatigue. Physical examination revealed 2+ axillary lymphadenopathy. The hematocrit was 33 per cent and the reticulocyte count was 0.1 per cent. The WBC was 19,800/mm.³ with 35 per cent eosinophiles and a predominant lymphocyte distribution. The thrombocytes were 300,000/mm.³ Cystitis was apparent. Serum electrophoresis revealed a broad polyclonal elevation of the gamma-globulin. The bone marrow examination was typical of chronic lymphocytic leukemia. Direct and indirect antiglobulin tests were positive and bromelin studies were negative. Elution obtained an erythrocyte autoantibody which functioned as a panhemagglutinin. Antibiotic therapy for the bladder infection was given. The hematocrit dropped to 28 per cent with a 5.3 per cent reticulocyte count, and then it progressively rose. Antiglobulin tests reverted to negative. Five months later the patient was seen with the spleen palpated 3 cm. and the liver 20 cm. below the costal margin. The hematocrit was 25 per cent with a 0.0 per cent reticulocyte count. In spite of prednisone therapy for 10 days, death occurred. Autopsy revealed chronic lymphocytic leukemia, pulmonary thromboembolization and a nodular thyroid gland.

Quinidine sensitivity apparently led to acute thrombocytopenia. This responded to cessation of quinidine therapy and to a short course of corticosteroid therapy. Four months after this episode chronic lymphocytic leukemia and autoimmune hemolytic anemia were simultaneously diagnosed. Autopsy demonstrated nodular thyroid disease also. The exact relationship of quinidine sensitivity to autoimmune hemolytic anemia is not known. This patient has been classified as having autoimmune hemolytic anemia secondary to chronic lymphocytic leukemia. The possibility of a multisystem immunologically mediated disease must also be considered.

A high incidence of marrow depression was noted in the eight patients of the current series with drug contact and autoimmune hemolytic anemia. Aplastic anemia was suggested in two patients and bone marrow erythrocytic aplasia was present in one. This observation strongly suggests that patients with bone marrow depression should be examined serologically for the possible development of autoimmune hemolytic anemia.

Other Drugs

Immunohemolytic anemia has also been reported with penicillin (109, 110), quinine (105), stibophen (103), phenacetin (105, 106), para-aminosalicylic acid (106, 107), streptomycin (111), chlorpromazine (108) and L-sarcolysine (115). These drugs are discussed in detail in Chapter 14. Autoimmune hemolytic anemia following administration of these agents was not encountered in the current series.

Sarcoidosis

Anemia of any type is relatively uncommon in sarcoidosis. In 1939 Hayden (125) studied a patient with sarcoidosis who developed hemolytic anemia. The spleen was not enlarged but bilateral pulmonary involvement was noted. Therapeutic remission of the sarcoid and hemolytic process followed pulmonary radiation therapy. Since this report of the association of hemolytic anemia and sarcoidosis, other investigators have encountered the same phenomenon (41, 126–136). Splenomegaly was frequently noted in these patients but did not appear necessary for the development of hemolysis. Splenectomy had little value in correcting the hemolytic process. A close temporal association between the two states was not always seen. Stats and associates (41) studied a 6-month-old Negro male with hemolytic anemia. At age 7½ sarcoidosis was diagnosed by biopsy during a phase of increased hemolytic activity.

The association of sarcoidosis and autoimmune hemolytic anemia has important theoretical significance. It is well recognized that some patients with sarcoidosis have a deficient immune apparatus and limitations in the ability to initiate delayed hypersensitivity. The premise has been presented that an inability to destroy modified immunocompetent cells because of an aberrant immune homeostasis mechanism may result in multiple autoantibody formation (37). Patients with sarcoidosis would appear to be particularly vulnerable to this sequence of events. The development of leukopenia and thrombocytopenia in sarcoidosis supports this hypothesis. Patients with this combined syndrome were not encountered in the present series. Such cases should be searched for and detailed immunologic studies should be performed.

Gaucher's Disease

Gaucher's disease in association with immunohemolytic anemia is uncommon. No example of this association was seen in the current series. Three reports are available in the literature, however, which indicate that this combination may occur. Mandelbaum and associates (137) in 1942 reported both hemolytic anemia and thrombocytopenia in a patient with Gaucher's disease. Clinical improvement resulted from removal of a massively enlarged spleen. Carling and associates (138) also reported hemolytic anemia with hemoglobinuria in a patient with Gaucher's disease. Wasserman and associates (43) studied one patient with this combined syndrome. Positive antiglobulin tests were obtained in their case. Splenectomy was ineffectual in halting the hemolytic process and corticosteroids had only an equivocal beneficial effect. The patient died with persisting hemolysis.

Kaposi's Sarcoma

Four reports (139–142) of hemolytic anemia associated with Kaposi's sarcoma are available in the literature. This is an uncommon combination and examples were not seen in the current series. In 1932 Greppi and Bettoni (139) noted a hemolytic process complicating the course of a patient with Kaposi's sarcoma involving the skin and genitalia. Hogeman (140) also reported the presence of severe hemolytic anemia in a patient with Kaposi's sarcoma. Unfortunately no data as to either antiglobulin tests or the presence of erythrocyte antibodies are given. Splenectomy was performed without improving the hemolytic process. Martensson and Henrikson (141) in 1954 described a patient with idiopathic autoimmune hemolytic anemia and strong positive antiglobulin reactions. The presence of systemic Kaposi's sarcoma without cutaneous involvement was discovered on autopsy. Splenectomy did

not control the hemolytic process. The investigators suggest that hemolysis may have been potentiated after splenectomy. Corticosteroid therapy was of benefit in reducing hemolysis. Zemek and associates (142) also encountered a patient with autoimmune hemolytic anemia and positive antiglobulin tests. Kaposi's sarcoma had been present 8 years prior to the onset of the hemolytic process.

Hemolytic Anemia in Renal Failure

Anemia is almost invariably seen in severe renal failure. Although many factors may be involved, a hemolytic phenomenon is common. Studies of the erythrocyte life span in patients with renal failure have confirmed the presence of hemolysis. In recent years attention has been paid to several distinctive clinical patterns relating severe hemolysis to acute renal insufficiency. These have been termed hemolytic-uremic syndromes. Three different patient groups are involved: (a) the infant or child, (b) adults with thrombotic thrombocytopenic purpura, and (c) the patient with eclampsia, pre-eclampsia or malignant hypertension. A characteristic abnormality of the erythrocyte has been observed with distorted, fragmented and deformed cells. Brain and associates (143, 144) have termed this state microangiopathic hemolytic anemia, and they relate the morphologic changes to contact of erythrocytes with necrotic and thrombosed small blood vessels.

There is little to suggest an autoimmune pathogenesis for the hemolytic state present in such patients. However, occasional cases with positive antiglobulin tests have been reported (145, 146). It is more probable that mechanical factors, infectious agents or a generalized Schwartzman reaction are important pathophysiologic elements. This entire subject has been thoroughly summarized by Dacie (61).

The Hemolytic-Uremic Syndrome of Infancy

In 1955 Gasser and associates (145) reported five cases of hemolytic anemia with renal failure in infants and children. A fatal course with autopsy evidence of bilateral cortical necrosis was found in all subjects. A positive antiglobulin test was obtained in one patient. Fison (146) reported the association of hemolytic anemia and glomerulonephritis in two siblings. A positive antiglobulin test was found in one. Since these initial observations, a specific clinical syndrome has been formulated. Infants or young children are involved. By 1965 approximately 185 cases had been reported with a mortality of 30 per cent (147). The syndrome is characterized by hemolytic anemia, leukocytosis, thrombocytopenia, reticulocytosis, deformed erythrocytes, elevated serum bilirubin, azotemia, proteinuria, hematuria and cylinduria. Positive antiglobulin tests are rare in spite of the initial observations. A positive antiglobulin test strongly suggests another process simulating the hemolytic-uremic state. Systemic lupus erythematosus should be immediately considered.

Similar observations have been made in the adult forms of this disease, i.e., thrombotic thrombocytopenic purpura and malignant hypertension. Positive antiglobulin tests are not characteristic and their presence suggests another entity. This viewpoint may be modified in the future. Feizi and Woodgate (148) reported the frequent development (12 per cent of 50 cases) of positive antiglobulin tests in patients with hypertension not receiving alpha-methyldopa. Most reactions were of the nongamma variety, but one example of an antigamma antiglobulin reaction was found.

Landry-Guillain-Barré Syndrome

Excellent evidence has been presented implicating autoimmune mechanisms in various neurologic diseases. Ala and Shearman (149) have reported the association of autoimmune hemolytic anemia, thrombocytopenia and a Landry-Guillain-Barré syndrome in a single patient. The direct antiglobulin test was positive and a warm acting erythrocyte autoantibody was found. This combination is interesting. Humoral autoantibody production is generally assumed to account for hemolytic anemia and thrombocytopenia. The neuro-

logic disease either represents a fortuitous association or the activation of autoimmunization through delayed hypersensitivity. The combination of both humoral and tissue autoimmunity in a single patient may assume great importance in the future study of pathogenic mechanisms.

Other Associated Diseases

Various other diseases have been associated with autoimmune hemolytic anemia in our current series of 234 patients. The limited numbers involved and the presence of other significant pathologic states make their significance debatable. However, a relationship either to immunologic or hematologic disease suggests that the occurrence may be more than fortuitous.

Amyloidosis

There is general agreement that the deposition of amyloid results from an immunologic event. Amyloidosis has been induced in experimental animals by prolonged immunization with various antigens (150). Morphologically the deposition of amyloid is accompanied by proliferation of plasma cells. Vazquez and Dixon (151) and Mellors and Ortega (152) have presented immunofluorescent studies suggesting that amyloid may consist of antigen-antibody complexes. Amyloidosis has been found in at least one autoimmune disease, that of the NZB mice (10). In addition, it appears as part of the wasting disease syndrome seen in neonatal thymectomized immunoincompetent animals (153).

In spite of these observations the association of amyloidosis and human autoimmune hemolytic anemia has not been reported. In the current series two patients were seen with this combination. In neither case, however, was amyloidosis assumed to have a significant etiologic relationship to autoimmune hemolytic anemia. One patient had a total laryngectomy for carcinoma of the larynx. Eight years later skin infiltrates were found and diagnosed as lymphosarcoma. One year later amyloidosis of the hilar area of the lung was diagnosed by biopsy. Autoimmune hemolytic anemia developed 3 years later. The second patient, a 63-year-old female, had plasma cell myeloma and autoimmune hemolytic anemia simultaneously diagnosed. Liver biopsy revealed paraamyloidosis.

Gout

There is little to suggest that gout is associated with or results from autoimmune phenomena. In the current series gout was diagnosed in four patients. In each instance, however, a secondary form of gout was present. Two of the patients had chronic granulocytic leukemia and one patient each had chronic lymphocytic leukemia and myelofibrosis with a myeloproliferative syndrome. No clinical correlation between activity of the hemolytic process and gout was observed. No evidence was obtained that the hemolytic process either initiated or magnified the gouty stage.

Pyruvate Kinase Deficiency

One patient was seen with a chronic hemolytic state and a family history of anemia. A pyruvate kinase deficiency was found in the family. The proband appeared to have a heterozygous deficiency of erythrocyte pyruvate kinase. A Cr^{51} T/2 of 5.2 days, with marked splenic sequestration, was found. Spherocytes, reticulocytosis and bone marrow erythrocytic hyperplasia with megaloblastic changes were all demonstrated. Direct antiglobulin and bromelin tests were strongly positive. The indirect bromelin procedure was positive and the indirect antiglobulin test was negative. Elution obtained an erythrocyte autoantibody which functioned as a panhemagglutinin. An excellent therapeutic response resulted from corticosteroid therapy.

This patient has been classified as having idiopathic autoimmune hemolytic anemia. The heterozygous pyruvate kinase deficiency is considered to be fortuitous. This classification may be in error. It is possible that antigenic modification can occur in biochemically defective erythrocytes. This in turn could result in either an antiglobulin positive or autoimmune type of hemolytic anemia. The occasional examples (154–157) of positive antiglobulin reactions found in patients with hereditary spherocytosis may be manifestations of the same phenomenon. In such cases modification of the erythrocyte membrane may be reflected in a change of surface antigens. Mandelli and associates (158) reported the association of autoimmune hemolytic anemia and Hodgkin's disease in a patient with a glucose 6-phosphate dehydrogenase deficiency. The authors suggest that the enzyme deficiency made the erythrocytes more sensitive to the action of erythrocyte autoantibodies.

Iron Deficiency

Hemolysis developing as a complication of iron deficiency is controversial. Gilles and associates (159) and Temperley and Sharp (160) found no evidence of hemolysis in the presence of severe iron deficiency anemia. Layrisse and associates (161) and Huser and associates (162) differ with this view. They demonstrated a shortened erythrocyte life span in the iron deficient state. Many of these studies involved patients with hookworm disease. It is interesting to note that as early as 1907 Widal and associates (163) related ankylostomiasis to hemolytic anemia.

An immunologic mechanism in iron deficiency anemia is not generally considered. In the current series, however, morphologic evidence for iron deficiency was common, particularly in the presence of severe and/or chronic infectious states. Chapter 7 and Cases 45, 56, 58, 72 and 89 should be reviewed for examples of iron deficiency. In addition to these cases, two patients were studied who had a suggestive association of positive antiglobulin tests and iron deficiency. In one patient, a 58-year-old white female, severe hemorrhoidal bleeding resulted in a marked hypochromic microcytic anemia. Reticulocytosis and bone marrow erythrocytic hyperplasia were present. Direct antiglobulin and bromelin tests were positive. After parenteral iron therapy the hematocrit started to rise. The patient has been lost to followup and the possibility of an undiagnosed pathologic state related to the positive antiglobulin test cannot be ruled out. The second patient is presented below.

Case 98. A 53-year-old white male was found to be anemic and received 6 months of oral iron therapy without response. Vitamin B-12 therapy was given parenterally for 1 year without correcting the anemia. The hemoglobin dropped to 5.7 gm. per cent. Three bone marrow examinations demonstrated iron deficiency, erythrocytic hyperplasia and megaloblastic changes. A Schilling test was not diagnostic. Multiple transfusions were given. The physical examination was negative and gastrointestinal studies revealed a huge hiatal hernia and several duodenal ulcers. Serum iron levels were low. The direct antiglobulin test was positive and bromelin test negative. Macrocytosis and hypochromic microcytic changes of the erythrocytes were noted. Diet therapy and oral iron were given. The hematocrit progressively rose from 26 to 43 per cent in 1 month. No other disease process has appeared to explain the positive antiglobulin test. Followup is continuing 26 months since the onset of anemia.

It is too early to state unequivocally that the positive antiglobulin test was related to iron deficiency in the above patient. A hemolytic mechanism contributing to the anemic state is difficult to document in view of intermittent gastrointestinal blood loss. Detailed followup and examination in such cases are obviously needed before a relationship between autoimmune hemolytic anemia and iron deficiency can be clarified. It is interesting to note, however, that Dagg and associates (164) have demonstrated gastric parietal cell autoantibodies in 13 of 64 patients with iron deficiency. The presence of such autoantibodies apparently correlates with achlorhydria. Eleven of the 13 examples were found in 33 of their achlorhydric patients.

Porphyria Cutanea Tarda

In 1963 Bousser and associates (165) reported studies performed on a 38-year-old white female who developed autoimmune hemolytic anemia. A warm acting autoantibody was present. Corticosteroid therapy and multiple transfusions were given and were followed by remission. Six years later porphyria cutanea tarda developed. The possibility of a significant association between these two states was considered. In the current series a similar association was encountered and has been summarized as Case 7. A complex multisystem disease was present. A 45-year-old female developed porphyria cutanea tarda. Sequentially she experienced secondary gout, alopecia, fluid retention, hepatosplenomegaly, hypoalbuminuria, liver disease, scleroderma, thrombocytopenia, pleuritis, pericarditis, positive LE cell tests, a lung abscess, positive antiglobulin tests, lymphadenopathy, Raynaud's syndrome, azotemia and hypergammaglobulinemia. This pattern suggests that porphyria cutanea tarda may appear as part of a systemic immunologic aberration.

Myelosclerosis and Myeloproliferative Syndromes

Abnormal lymphocyte proliferation is considered a characteristic part of autoimmune disease, particularly autoimmune hemolytic anemia. In spite of this, myeloproliferative syndromes can occur in association with autoimmune hemolytic anemia. Seven cases of granulocytic leukemia complicated by autoimmune hemolytic anemia have been presented in Chapter 5 and illustrate this relationship. Patients with nonmalignant myeloproliferative states may also develop autoimmune hemolytic anemia.

Hemolytic processes are commonly found in myeloproliferative syndromes with extramedullary hematopoiesis. Myelosclerosis is particularly likely to show a hemolytic element. Pitcock and associates (166) noted hemolytic anemia in 13 per cent and Bouroncle and Doan (167) hemolysis in 21 per cent of their large series of patients with myeloproliferative disorders. Dacie (61) has summarized the literature and estimates a 16 per cent incidence of overt hemolytic anemia complicating myelosclerosis.

An immunologic pathogenesis for the hemolysis complicating myelosclerosis is uncommon. However, Hennemann and associates (168) encountered two patients with myelosclerosis, hemolytic anemia and positive direct antiglobulin tests. Additional examples are tabulated in the reports of Cassell and Chaplin (169), Yunis and Bridges (170), Pirofsky (171) and possibly the patient studied by Shee (172).

In the current series two patients were seen with a myeloproliferative syndrome, extramedullary hematopoiesis and autoimmune hemolytic anemia. In one patient, a 62-year-old male, hemolytic anemia with positive antiglobulin tests were noted in the presence of massive hepatosplenomegaly and lymphadenopathy. A therapeutic response did not occur with corticosteroid therapy. Death resulted after 6 years of disease with myelosclerosis as the only diagnosis. The second patient is presented below.

Case 99. A 73-year-old white male was hospitalized with complaints of fatigue and a one year history of arthritis. Physical examination demonstrated the spleen palpated 11 cm. and the liver 2 cm. below the costal margins, congestive heart failure and tophi of the hands and ear lobes. The hematocrit was 21 per cent, the reticulocyte count was 8.2 per cent, the WBC was 16,700/mm.^{3} and thrombocytes were elevated. Immature granulocytes and nucleated erythrocytes were found in the peripheral blood. The leukocyte alkaline phosphatase score was greatly elevated. Bone marrow aspiration revealed erythrocytic hyperplasia. Serum bilirubin, the A/G ratio, serum electrophoresis, serologic tests for syphilis and the Bromsulphalein test were all normal. Urine analysis demonstrated proteinuria and serum uric acid was elevated to 16 mg. per cent. Direct antiglobulin and bromelin tests were positive. A diagnosis of myelosclerosis with secondary gout was made and the patient was treated with probenecid and testosterone. Prednisone therapy was initiated for autoimmune hemolytic anemia. The hematocrit progressively rose and was maintained at over 30 per cent on maintenance therapy. The patient's course over the next 3 years was complicated by recurrent arthritis, staphyloccal pneumonia, septicemia and eventually acute renal failure. The hematocrit dropped to 20 per cent with a 6.6 per cent reticulocyte count. Direct and indirect antiglobulin and bromelin tests were now negative. Death occurred, and autopsy revealed myelosclerosis and extramedullary hematopoiesis.

This patient had a myeloproliferative syndrome, extramedullary hematopoiesis and secondary gout. Hemolytic anemia complicated the clinical course and an autoimmune mechanism was suggested by positive antiglobulin and bromelin tests and a hematologic response to prednisone therapy.

Waldenström's Macroglobulinemia

Waldenström's macroglobulinemia is a lymphoproliferative disease characterized by the production of abnormal amounts of gamma M immunoglobulins. An underlying or associated malignancy of the reticuloendothelium may be found. Anemia is typical and has been described in 81 per cent of cases (173). A hemolytic mechanism may be present (173–176). In spite of this, autoimmune hemolytic anemia is uncommon. Only 13 examples of this association have been reported (61, 174, 176–183). Dacie (61) encountered one such case in a series of 250 patients with autoimmune hemolytic anemia. This combined syndrome was not found in the current series. Subsequently, however, two patients were studied with positive antiglobulin tests, hemolytic anemia and macroglobulinemia. This represents a 0.7 per cent incidence of Waldenström's macroglobulinemia in approximately 300 patients with autoimmune hemolytic anemia investigated at our institution.

Waldenström's macroglobulinemia is considered a monoclonal abnormality, with the increased IgM representing the product of one clone of cells (184). Such macroglobulins may be antibodies with the antigen undetected. A positive antiglobulin test could therefore indicate an antigenic status of the erythrocyte, with the macroglobulin functioning as an erythrocyte autoantibody. Bayrakci and associates (185) explored this possibility in one patient. Their studies suggest that an IgG globulin was responsible for the positive antiglobulin test and hemolytic anemia. The IgM macroglobulin appeared as a separate paraprotein. Such observations suggest that Waldenström's macroglobulinemia may not always be a monoclonal process, and that several clones of immunocompetent cells may be involved.

BIBLIOGRAPHY

1. Hektoen, L., Fox, H., and Shulhof, K.: Specificness in the precipitin reaction of thyroglobulin. J. Infect. Dis. **40:** 461, 1927.
2. Witebsky, E., Rose, N. R., Terplan, K., Paine, J. R., and Egan, R. W.: Chronic thyroiditis and autoimmunization. J. A. M. A. **164:** 1439, 1957.

3. Rose, N. R., and Witebsky, E.: Studies on organ specificity. V. Changes in the thyroid gland of rabbits following active immunization with rabbit thyroid extracts. J. Immun. **76**: 417, 1956.

4. Cline, M. J., Selenkow, H. A., and Brooke, M. S.: Autoimmunity in thyroid disease. New Eng. J. Med. **260**: 117, 1959.

5. Roitt, I. M., and Doniach, D.: Human autoimmune thryroiditis: serological studies. Lancet **2**: 1027, 1958.

6. White, R. G.: Immunological investigation of Hashimoto's disease. Proc. Roy. Soc. Med. **50**: 953, 1957.

7. Anderson, J. R., Goudie, R. B., and Gray, K. G.: Complement-fixing autoantibody to thyroglobulin in Hashimoto's disease. Lancet **1**: 644, 1959.

8. Ovary, Z., Randall, H., Witebsky, E., Rose, N. R., Shulman, S., and Metzgar, R.: Thyroid-specific autoantibodies studied by passive cutaneous anaphylaxis of guinea pig. Proc. Soc. Exp. Biol. Med. **99**: 397, 1958.

9. Roitt, I. M., and Doniach, D.: Thyroid autoimmunity. Brit. Med. Bull. **16**: 152, 1960.

10. MacKay, I. R., and Burnet, F. M.: *Autoimmune Diseases*. Charles C Thomas, Publisher, Springfield, Ill., 1963.

11. MacKay, I. R. Weiden, S. and Hasker, J.: Autoimmune hepatitis. Ann. N. Y. Acad. Sci. **124**: 767, 1965.

12. Roitt, I. M., Doniach, D., and Shapland, C.: Autoimmunity in pernicious anemia and atrophic gastritis. Ann. N. Y. Acad. Sci. **124**: 644, 1965.

13. Mellon, J. P., Pay, B. Y., and Green, D. M.: Mongolism and thyroid autoantibodies. J. Ment. Defic. Res. **7**: 31, 1963.

14. Fialkow, P. J., Hecht, F., Uchida, I. A., and Motulsky, A. G.: Increased frequency of thyroid autoantibodies in mothers of patients with Down's syndrome. Lancet **2**: 868, 1965.

15. Hackett, E., Beech, M., and Forbes, I. J.: Thyroglobulin antibodies in patients without clinical disease of the thyroid gland. Lancet **2**: 402, 1960.

16. Hill, O. W.: Thyroglobulin antibodies in 1,297 patients without thyroid disease. Brit. Med. J. **1**: 1793, 1961.

17. Belyavin, G., and Trotter, W. R.: Investigations of thyroid antigens reacting with Hashimoto sera. Evidence for an antigen other than thyroglobulin. Lancet **1**: 648, 1959.

18. Trotter, W. R., Belyavin, G., and Waddams, A.: Precipitating and complement-fixing antibodies in Hashimoto's disease. Proc. Roy. Soc. Med. **50**: 961, 1957.

19. Holborow, J., Brown, P. C., Roitt, I. M., and Doniach, D.: Cytoplasmic localization of "complement-fixing" autoantigen in human thyroid epithelium. Brit. J. Exp. Path. **40**: 583, 1959.

20. Anderson, J. R., Goudie, R. B., and Gray, K. G.: The "thyrotoxic" complement-fixation reaction. Scot. Med. J. **4**: 64, 1959.

21. Pulvertaft, R. J. V., Doniach, D., Roitt, I. M., and Hudson, R. V.: Cytotoxic effects of Hashimoto sera on human thyroid cells in tissue culture. Lancet **2**: 214, 1959.

22. Irvine, W. J.: The cytotoxic factor in thyroid disease. Scot. Med. J. **5**: 511, 1960.

23. Forbes, I. J., Roitt, I. M., Doniach, D., and Solomon, J. L.: The thyroid cytotoxic autoantibody. J. Clin. Invest. **41**: 996, 1962.

24. Chandler, R. W., Blizzard, R. M., Hung, W., and Kyle, M.: Incidence of thyrocytotoxic factor and other antithyroid antibodies in the mothers of cretins. New Eng. J. Med. **267**: 376, 1962.

25. Kite, J. H., Rose, N. R., Kano, K., and Witebsky, E.: Cytotoxicity of human thyroid autoantibodies. Ann. N. Y. Acad. Sci. **124**: 626, 1965.

26. Doniach, D., Roitt, I. M., and Taylor, K. B.: Autoimmunity in pernicious anemia and thyroiditis: a family study. Ann. N. Y. Acad. Sci. **124**: 605, 1965.

27. Hall, R., Owen, S. G., and Smart, G. A.: Evidence for genetic predisposition to formation of thyroid autoantibodies. Lancet **2**: 187, 1960.

28. Irvine, W. J., MacGregor, A. G., Stuart, A. E., and Hall, G. H.: Hashimoto's disease in uniovular twins. Lancet **2**: 850, 1961.

29. Beierwaltes, W. H.: Thyroiditis. Ann. N. Y. Acad. Sci. **124**: 586, 1965.

30. Beare, R. L. B.: Lymphadenoid goitre (Hashimoto's disease). A clinico-pathological study. Brit. Med. J. **1**: 479, 1958.

31. White, R. G., Bass, B. H., and Williams, E.: Lymphadenoid goitre and the syndrome of systemic lupus erythematosus. Lancet **1**: 368, 1961.

32. MacKay, I. R., and Perry, B. T.: Autoimmunity in human thyroid disease. Aust. Ann. Med. **9**: 84, 1960.

33. Buchanan, W. W., Crooks, J., Alexander, W. D., Koutras, D. A., Wayne, E. J., and Gray, K. G.: Association of Hashimoto's thyroiditis and rheumatoid arthritis. Lancet **1**: 245, 1961.

34. Luxton, R. W.: Paget's disease of bone associated with Hashimoto's struma lymphatosa. A clue to the pathogenesis of Paget's disease? Lancet **1**: 441, 1957.

35. Anderson, J. R., Gray, K., Beck, J. S., and Kinnear, W. F.: Precipitating autoantibodies in Sjögren's disease. Lancet **2**: 456, 1961.

36. Wasastjerna, C.: Two autoimmune diseases in one patient. A case of hemolytic anemia and Hashimoto's thyroiditis. Acta Med. Scand. **165**: 299, 1959.

37. Pirofsky, B.: Autoimmune hemolytic anemia and neoplasia of the reticuloendothelium. With a hypothesis concerning etiologic relationships. Ann. Intern. Med. **68:** 109, 1968.

38. Pirofsky, B., and Vaughn, M.: Addisonian pernicious anemia with positive antiglobulin tests; a multiple autoimmune disease syndrome. Amer. J. Clin. Path. **50:** 459, 1968.

39. Bardana, E. J., and Pirofsky, B.: Autoimmune hemolytic anemia and ulcerative colitis; a multisystem immunodeficiency disease? (to be published).

40. Waugh, T. R.: Hemolytic anemia in carcinomatosis of the bone marrow. Amer. J. Med. Sci. **191:** 160, 1936.

41. Stats, D., Rosenthal, N., and Wasserman, L. R.: Hemolytic anemia associated with malignant disease. Amer. J. Clin. Path. **17:** 585, 1947.

42. Paraf, A., and Dausset, J.: Les ictères hémolytiques au cours des affections malignes (leucémies, granulomatose maligne, cancers). Sem. Hop. Paris **28:** 290, 1952.

43. Wasserman, L. R., Stats, D., Schwartz, L., and Fudenberg, H.: Symptomatic and hemopathic hemolytic anemia. Amer. J. Med. **18:** 961, 1955.

44. Brown, G. M.: The pathogenesis of secondary anaemias. Canad. Med. Ass. J. **62:** 472, 1950.

45. Shen, S. C., and Homburger, F.: The anemia of cancer patients and its relation to metastases to bone marrow. J. Lab. Clin. Med. **37:** 182, 1951.

46. Sheets, R. F., Hamilton, H. E., DeGowin, E. L., and Janney, C. D.: Studies with inagglutinable erythrocyte counts. V. Spontaneous and x-ray-induced hemolysis in malignancy. J. Clin. Invest. **33:** 179, 1954.

47. Hyman, G. A., Gellhorn, A., and Harvey, J. L.: Studies on the anemia of disseminated malignant neoplastic disease. II. Study of the lifespan of the erythrocyte. Blood **11:** 618, 1956.

48. Johnston, G. A. W.: Red cell life span in carcinomatosis. Med. J. Aust. **1:** 736, 1956.

49. Hyman, G. A.: The anemia of cancer. Amer. J. Roentgen. **79:** 511, 1958.

50. Ultmann, J. E.: The role of the spleen in the hemolytic anemia of cancer patients. Cancer Res. **18:** 959, 1958.

51. Green, H. N.: An immunological concept of cancer; a preliminary report. Brit. Med. J. **2:** 1374, 1954.

52. Green, H. N., Wakefield, J., and Littlewood, G.: The nature of cancer anaemia and its bearing on the immunological theory of cancer. Brit. Med. J. **2:** 779, 1957.

53. Jordan, W. S., and Dingle, J. H.: Coombs titer variations in acquired hemolytic anemia. J. Lab. Clin. Med. **34:** 1614, 1949.

54. Frumin, A. M., Mendell, T. H., and Meranze,

D. R.: Hematologic manifestations of metastatic gastric malignancy. Gastroenterology **27:** 183, 1954.

55. Renfer, H. R., and Hässig, A.: Über Autoantikörperuntersuchungen bei malignen Tumoren. Klin. Wschr. **33:** 728, 1955.

56. West, C. D., Ley, A. B., and Pearson, O. H.: Myelophthisic anemia in cancer of the breast. Amer. J. Med. **18:** 923, 1955.

57. Sohier, W. D., Juranies, E., and Aub, J. C.: Hemolytic anemia, a host response to malignancy. Cancer Res. **17:** 767, 1957.

58. Jenkins, W. J., and Marsh, W. L.: Autoimmune haemolytic anaemia: three cases with antibodies specifically active against stored red cells. Lancet **2:** 16, 1961.

59. Shibusawa, K.: On autoimmunization. I. Autoimmune hemolytic anemia in patients with cancer. Clin. Surg. (Tokyo) **19:** 80, 1964.

60. Ellis, L. D., and Westerman, M. P.: Autoimmune hemolytic anemia and cancer. J. A. M. A. **193:** 962, 1965.

61. Dacie, J. V.: *The Haemolytic Anaemias, Part III,* Ed. 2. Grune & Stratton, Inc., New York, 1967.

62. West-Watson, W. N., and Young, C. J.: Failed splenectomy in acholuric jaundice, and the relation of toxaemia to the haemolytic crisis. Brit. Med. J. **1:** 1305, 1938.

63. Watson, C. J.: Hemolytic jaundice and macrocytic hemolytic anemia. Certain observations in a series of 35 cases. Ann. Intern. Med. **12:** 1782, 1939.

64. Singer, K., and Dameshek, W.: Symptomatic hemolytic anemia. Ann. Intern. Med. **15:** 544, 1941.

65. Jones, E., and Tillman, C.: A case of hemolytic anemia relieved by removal of an ovarian tumor. J. A. M. A. **128:** 1225, 1945.

66. Lindeboom, G. A.: Rare forms of symptomatic hemolytic anemia. Acta. Haemat. (Basel) **4:** 343, 1950.

67. Allibone, E. C., and Collins, D. H.: Symptomatic haemolytic anaemia associated with ovarian teratoma in a child. J. Clin. Path. **4:** 412, 1951.

68. Wuhrmann, F.: Einige aktuelle klinische probleme aus der humoral pathologie. Bull. Schweiz. Akad. Med. Wiss. **10:** 180, 1954.

69. André, R., Dreyfus, B., and Salmon, C.: Anémie hémolytique et kyste dermoïde de l'ovaire. Bull. Soc. Med. Hop. Paris **71:** 1062, 1955.

70. deGruchy, G. C.: The diagnosis and management of acquired haemolytic anaemia. Aust. Ann. Med. **3:** 106, 1954.

71. Procházka, J.: Symptomatická hemolytická chudokrevnost při dermoidní cystě vaječníku. Vnitrni Lek. **11:** 240, 1956.

72. Barry, K. G., and Crosby, W. H.: Auto-immune hemolytic anemia arrested by removal

of an ovarian teratoma: review of the literature and report of a case. Ann. Intern. Med. **47**: 1002, 1957.

73. Miescher, P., von Rechenberg, H. K., Berger, J., and Holländer, L.: Hämolytische Anämie bei Ovarialtumor. Schweiz. Med. Wschr. **88**: 498, 1958.

74. Müller, W., and Schubothe, H.: Symptomatische hämolytische Anämien bei dermoid Cysten. Folia Haemat. (Frankfurt) **2**: 321, 1958.

75. Heeres, P. A.: Les anémies hémolytiques et les kystes de l'ovaire. Sem. Hop. Paris **36**: 1411, 1960.

76. Szirmai, E.: Symptomatische autoantikörperbedingte hämolytische anämie bei Erkrankungen der weiblichen Genitalien. Wien. Z. Inn. Med. **42**: 320, 1961.

77. Larrain, C., Del Solar, A., and Vargas Molinare, R.: Anemia hemolitica asociada a quiste dermoide del ovario. Sangre (Barc.) **8**: 31, 1963.

78. Norcross, J. W.: Hematologic manifestations of malignant disease. Med. Clin. N. Amer. **47**: 345, 1963.

79. McAndrew, G. M.: Haemolytic anaemia associated with ovarian teratoma. Brit. Med. J. **2**: 1307, 1964.

80. Yam, L. T., Rudgki, C., Busch, S., and Leithold, S. L.: Ovarian neoplasm associated with autoimmune hemolytic anemia. Amer. J. Obstet. Gynec. **95**: 207, 1966.

81. Ahrengot, V.: De serologiske forhold hos en patient med immunologisk haemolytisk anaemi og en antistofholdig abdominal cyste. Nord. Med. **50**: 1570, 1953.

82. Freiesleben, E., Kissmeyer-Nielsen, F., Christensen, J., Jensen Gert, K., and Knudsen Ehlert, E.: Excessive content of blood group substance in serum from patients with ovarian cysts. Vox. Sang. **6**: 1, 1961.

83. Lenoel, J., and Soudet, P.: Un cas de tumeur ovarienne accompagnée d'une forte quantité de substance de group AB circulante. Transfusion (Paris) **6**: 343, 1963.

84. van Loghem, J. J.: Some comments on auto-antibody induced red cell destruction. Ann. N. Y. Acad. Sci. **124**: 465, 1965.

85. Landaw, S. A.: Hemolytic anemia as a complication of carcinoma: a case report and review of the literature. J. Mount. Sinai Hosp. N. Y. **31**: 167, 1964.

86. Rose, J. C., Hufnagel, C. A., Freis, E. D., Harvey, W. P., and Partenope, E. A.: The hemodynamic alterations produced by a plastic valvular prosthesis for severe aortic insufficiency in man. J. Clin. Invest. **33**: 891, 1954.

87. Stohlman, F., Sarnoff, S. J., and Case, R. B.: Hemolytic syndrome following insertion of a lucite ball valve prosthesis in the vascular system. Circulation **13**: 586, 1956.

88. Po-Tum-Fok, F., and Schubothe, H.: Studies on various factors influencing mechanical

hemolysis of human erythrocytes. Brit. J. Haemat. **6**: 355, 1960.

89. Verdon, T. A., Forrester, R. H., and Crosby, W. H.: Hemolytic anemia after open heart repair of ostium primum defects. New Eng. J. Med. **269**: 444, 1963.

90. Sayed, H. M., Dacie, J. V., Handley, D. A., Lewis, S. M., and Cleland, W. P.: Hemolytic anaemia of mechanical origin after open heart surgery. Thorax **16**: 356, 1961.

91. Brodeur, M. T. H., Sutherland, D. W., Koler, R. D., Starr, A., Kimsey, J. A., and Griswold, H. E.: Red cell survival in patients with aortic valvular disease and ball-valve prosthesis. Circulation **32**: 570, 1965.

92. Pirofsky, B.: Hemolysis in valvular heart disease (editorial). Ann. Intern. Med. **65**: 373, 1966.

93. Pirofsky, B., Sutherland, D. W., Starr, A., and Griswold, H. E.: Hemolytic anemia complicating aortic-valve surgery. New Eng. J. Med. **272**: 235, 1965.

94. Hjeln, M., Högman, C. F., Finnson, M., and Malers, E.: Transient auto-antibody formation in case of open heart surgery with no signs of increased red cell destruction. Vox Sang. **9**: 505, 1964.

95. Pirofsky, B.: Aortic valve surgery and autoimmune hemolytic anemia. Amer. Heart J. **70**: 426, 1965.

96. Lustumbo, M. M., Holland, P. V., and Schmidt, P. J.: Isoimmunization after multiple transfusions. New Eng. J. Med. **275**: 141, 1966.

97. Morse, E. E., Davis, S. S., and Charache, S.: Hemolytic anemia following open heart surgery—an auto-immune phenomenon? (abstract). Nineteenth Annual Meeting of the American Association of Blood Banks, Los Angeles, 1966.

98. Polesky, H. F., Smith, R., Weirich, F.: Positive direct anti-human globulin tests in cardiac surgery patients (abstract). Twentieth Annual Meeting of the American Association of Blood Banks, New York, 1967.

99. Pirofsky, B.: The structure and specificity of erythrocyte autoantibodies. Ann. N. Y. Acad. Sci. **124**: 448, 1965.

100. Petrakis, N. L., and Politis, G.: Prolonged survival of viable mitotically competent mononuclear leukocytes in stored whole blood. New Eng. J. Med. **267**: 286, 1962.

101. Scherz, R. G., and Montgomery, R. C.: Survival of transfused donor mononuclear leukocytes during open heart surgery. New Eng. J. Med. **269**: 1236, 1963.

102. Snapper, I., Marks, D., Schwartz, L., and Hollander, L.: Hemolytic anemia secondary to Mesantoin. Ann. Intern. Med. **39**: 619, 1953.

103. Harris, J. W.: Studies on the mechanism of a drug induced hemolytic anemia. J. Lab. Clin. Med. **47**: 760, 1956.

104. Freedman, A. L., Barr, P. S., and Brody, E.: Hemolytic anemia due to quinidine: observations on its mechanism. Amer. J. Med. **20**: 806, 1956.

105. Muirhead, E. E., Halden, E. R., and Graves, M.: Drug dependent Coombs (anti-globulin) test and anemia. Observations on quinine and acetophenetidin (phenacetin). Arch. Intern. Med. (Chicago) **101**: 87, 1958.

106. MacGibbon, B. H., Longhridge, L. W., Hourihane, D. O'B., and Boyd, D. W.: Auto-immune haemolytic anaemia with acute renal failure due to phenacetin and p-aminosalicylic acid. Lancet **1**: 7, 1960.

107. Dausset, J., and Bergerot-Blondel, Y.: Etude d'un anticorps allergique actif en présence de para-amino-salicylate de soude (PAS) contre les hematics, les leucocytes et les plaquettes humaines. Vox Sang. **6**: 91, 1961.

108. Lindberg, L. G., and Norden, A.: Severe hemolytic reaction to chlorpromazine. Acta Med. Scand. **170**: 195, 1961.

109. Ley, A. B., Harris, J. P., Brinkley, M., Liles, B., Jack, J. A., and Cahan, A.: Circulating antibody directed against penicillin. Science **127**: 1118, 1958.

110. Petz, L. D., and Fudenberg, H. H.: Coombs-positive hemolytic anemia caused by penicillin administration. New Eng. J. Med. **274**: 171, 1966.

111. Nachman, R., Javid, J., and Krauss, S.: Streptomycin-induced hemolytic anemia. Arch. Intern. Med. (Chicago) **110**: 187, 1962.

112. Gralnick, H. R., Wright, L. D., and McGinniss, M. H.: Coombs' positive reactions associated with sodium cephalothin therapy. J. A. M. A. **199**: 135, 1967.

113. Molthan, L., Reidenberg, M. M., and Eichman, M. F.: Positive direct Coombs tests due to cephalothin. New Eng. J. Med. **277**: 123, 1967.

114. Carstairs, K. C., Breckenridge, A., Dollery, C. T., and Worlledge, S. M.: Incidence of a positive direct Coombs test in patients on alpha-methyldopa. Lancet **2**: 133, 1966.

115. Eyster, M. E.: Melphalan (Alkeran) erythrocyte agglutinin and hemolytic anemia. Ann. Intern. Med. **66**: 573, 1967.

116. Muirhead, E. E., Groves, M., Guy, R., Halden, E. R., and Bass, R. K.: Acquired hemolytic anemia, exposures to insecticides and positive Coombs test dependent on insecticide preparations. Vox Sang. **4**: 277, 1959.

117. Dausset, J., and Contu, L.: Drug induced hemolysis. Ann. Rev. Med. **18**: 55, 1967.

118. Weiner, W., Whitehead, J. P., and Walkden, W. J.: Acquired haemolytic anaemia. Clinical and serological observations of two cases. Brit. Med. J. **1**: 73, 1956.

119. Klipstein, F. A.: Subnormal serum folate and macrocytosis associated with anti-convulsant drug therapy. Blood **23**: 68, 1964.

120. Schwartz, R. S., and Costea, N.: Autoimmune hemolytic anemia: clinical correlations and biological implications. Seminars Hemat. **3**: 2, 1966.

121. Worlledge, S. M., Carstairs, K. C., and Dacie, J. V.: Autoimmune haemolytic anaemia associated with alpha-methyldopa therapy. Lancet **2**: 135, 1966.

122. LoBuglio, A. F., and Jandl, J. H.: Nature of the methyldopa red-cell antibody. New Eng. J. Med. **276**: 658, 1967.

123. Gralnick, H. R., and McGinniss, M.: Nature of the Coombs positive reaction with sodium cephalothin (abstract). Twentieth Annual Meeting of the American Association of Blood Banks, New York, 1967.

124. Pirofsky, B., Cordova, M. S., and Rigas, D.: The mechanism of streptomycin inhibition of erythrocyte antibodies. Vox Sang. **9**: 653, 1964.

125. Hayden, R. L.: *Principles of Hematology*, 1939, Lea & Febiger, Philadelphia, 1939.

126. Crane, A. R., and Zetlin, A. M.: Hemolytic anemia, hyperglobulinemia, and Boeck's sarcoid. Ann. Intern. Med. **23**: 882, 1945.

127. McCort, J. J., Wood, R. H., Hamilton, J. B., and Ehrlich, D. E.: Sarcoidosis; clinical and roentgenologic study of 28 proved cases. Ann. Intern. Med. **80**: 293, 1947.

128. Wagley, P. F., Shen, S. C., Gardner, F. H., and Castle, W. B.: Studies of destruction of red blood cells; spleen as source of substance causing agglutination of red blood cells by certain patients with acquired hemolytic jaundice by anti-human serum rabbit serum (Coombs serum). J. Lab. Clin. Med. **33**: 1197, 1948.

129. Bruschi, M., and Howe, J. S.: Classification of hematologic variations and abnormalities associated with Boeck's sarcoid; review of literature. Blood **1**: 478, 1950.

130. Schubothe, H.: Antikörperbedingte hämolytische Anämien. Verh. Deutsch. Ges. Inn. Med. **58**: 679, 1952.

131. Davis, A. E., Belber, J. P., and Movitt, E. R.: The association of hemolytic anemia with sarcoidosis. Blood **9**: 379, 1954.

132. Lebacq, E., Tirzmalis, A., Mairiaux, E., and Pluygers, E.: Sarcoïdose de Besnier-Boeck-Schaumann avec anémie hémolytique par auto-immunisation. Bull. Soc. Med. Hop. Paris **72**: 614, 1956.

133. Michon, P., Dornier, R., Kling, C., Larcan, A., and Huriet, C.: Anémie hémolytique avec auto-anticorps et maladie de Besnier-Boeck-Schaumann. Bull. Soc. Med. Hop. Paris **73**: 903, 1957.

134. Garcia, E. L., Garrido, T. A., Lorenzo, E. M., and Guedes, R.: Sarcoidosis con anemia hemolitica sintomatica. Rev. Clin. Esp. **72**: 183, 1959.

135. West, W. O.: Acquired hemolytic anemia

secondary to Boeck's sarcoid. Report of a case and review of the literature. New Eng. J. Med. **261**: 688, 1959.

136. Cox, W. L., and Donald, J. M.: Acquired hemolytic anemia and Boeck's sarcoidosis: review of the literature. Amer. Surg. **30**: 199, 1964.

137. Mandelbaum, H., Berger, L., and Lederer, M.: Gaucher's disease: case with hemolytic anemia and marked thrombopenia; improvement after removal of spleen weighing 6822 gms. Ann. Intern. Med. **16**: 438, 1942.

138. Carling, E. R., Carlett, H., and Pulvertaft, R.: Splenectomy in Gaucher's disease with hemoglobinemia. Proc. Roy. Soc. Med. **26**: 361, 1953.

139. Greppi, E., and Bettoni, I.: Splenomegalia emolitica ed angioendothelioma cutaneo tipo kaposi con associazoni di aggranulocitose sepsi orale. Arch. Ist. Biochem. Ital. **4**: 403, 1932.

140. Hogeman, O.: Hyperhemolysis of nonsplenic origin. Acta Med. Scand. **144**: 247, 1953.

141. Martinsson, J., and Henrikson, H.: Immunohemolytic anemia in Kaposi's sarcoma. Acta Med. Scand. **150**: 175, 1954.

142. Zemek, L., Strom, L., Gordon, G., and Elguezabel, A.: Hemolytic anemia with Kaposi's sarcoma. Report of a case. J. A. M. A. **187**: 232, 1964.

143. Brain, M. C., Dacie, J. V., and Hourihane, D. O'B.: Microangiopathic haemolytic anaemia: the possible role of vascular lesions in pathogenesis. Brit. J. Haemat. **8**: 358, 1962.

144. Brain, M. C., and Hourihane, D. O'B.: Microangiopathic haemolytic anaemia: the occurrence of haemolysis in experimentally produced vascular disease. Brit. J. Haemat. **13**: 135, 1967.

145. Gasser, C., Gautier, E., Steck, A., Siebenmann, R. E., and Oechslin, R.: Hämolytisch-urämische Syndrome: bilaterale Nierenrindennekrosen bei akuten erworbenen hämolytischen Anämien. Schweiz. Med. Wschr. **85**: 905, 1955.

146. Fison, T. N.: Acute glomerulonephritis in infancy. Arch. Dis. Child. **31**: 101, 1956.

147. O'Connell, E. J., Maurer, S. W., and Mills, S. D.: The hemolytic-uremic syndrome of infancy. A recently described syndrome of unknown cause in which hypersensitivity mechanisms have been implicated. Clin. Pediat. (Phila.) **4**: 174, 1965.

148. Feizi, T., and Woodgate, D.: The direct antiglobulin (Coombs' test) in hypertensive patients. Vox Sang. **12**: 273, 1967.

149. Ala, F. A., and Shearman, D. J. C.: A case of autoimmune haemolytic anaemia, thrombocytopenia and Landry-Guillain-Barré syndrome. Acta Haemat. (Basel) **34**: 361, 1965.

150. Giles, R. B., and Calkins, E.: The relation-ship of serum hexosamine, globulins, and antibodies to experimental amyloidosis. J. Clin. Invest. **37**: 846, 1958.

151. Vazquez, J. J., and Dixon, F. J.: Immunohistochemical analysis of amyloid by fluorescence technique. J. Exp. Med. **104**: 727, 1956.

152. Mellors, R. C., and Ortega, L. G.: Analytical pathology. III. New observations on pathogenesis of glomerulonephritis, lipid nephrosis, periarteritis nodosa and secondary amyloidosis in man. Amer. J. Path. **32**: 455, 1956.

153. Kellum, M. J., Sutherland, D. E., Eckert, E., Peterson, R. D. A., and Good, R. A.: Wasting disease, Coombs positivity, and amyloidosis in rabbits subjected to central lymphoid tissue extirpation and irradiation. Int. Arch. Allerg. **27**: 6, 1965.

154. Dameshek, W., and Bloom, M. L.: The events in the hemolytic crisis of hereditary spherocytosis, with particular reference to the reticulocytopenia, pancytopenia and an abnormal splenic mechanism. Blood **3**: 1381, 1948.

155. Singer, K., and Motulsky, A. G.: The developing (Coombs) test in spherocytic hemolytic anemias. J. Lab. Clin. Med. **34**: 768, 1949.

156. Wright, C. S., Dodd, M. C., Bouroncle, B. A., Doan, C. A., and Zollinger, R. M.: Studies of hemagglutinins in hereditary spherocytosis and in acquired hemolytic anemia; their relationship to the hypersplenic mechanism. J. Lab. Clin. Med. **37**: 165, 1951.

157. Young, L. E., and Miller, G.: Differentiation between congenital and acquired forms of hemolytic anemia. Amer. J. Med. Sci. **226**: 664, 1953.

158. Mandelli, F., Deriu, L., DeLaurenzi, A., and Papa, G.: Considerazioni su un caso di anemia emolitica auto-immune in corso di granuloma maligno con difetto completo diglicoso-6-fosfatodeidrogenasi eritrocitaria. Riv. Emoter. Immunoemat. **12**: 71, 1965.

159. Gilles, H., Watson-Williams, E. J., and Ball, P. A. J.: Hookworm infection and anaemia. Quart. J. Med. **33**: 1, 1964.

160. Temperley, I. J., and Sharp, A. A.: The life span of erythrocytes in iron deficiency anaemia. J. Clin. Path. **15**: 346, 1962.

161. Layrisse, M., Linares, S. J., and Roche, M.: Excess hemolysis in subjects with severe iron deficiency anemia associated and unassociated with hookworm infection. Blood **25**: 73, 1965.

162. Huser, H. J., Rieber, E. E., and Berman, A. R.: Experimental evidence of excess hemolysis in the course of chronic iron deficiency anemia. J. Lab. Clin. Med. **69**: 405, 1967.

163. Widal, F., Abrami, P., and Brulé, M.: Pluralité d'origine des ictères hémolytiques; recherches cliniques et expérimentales. Bull. Soc. Med. Hop. Paris **24**: 1354, 1907.

164. Dagg, J. H., Goldberg, A., Anderson, J. R., Beck, J. S., and Gray, K. G.: Autoimmunity in iron deficiency anemia. Ann. N. Y. Acad. Sci. **124**: 692, 1965.
165. Bousser, J., Christol, D., Gajdos, A., Gajdos-Torok, M., Lumbroso, P., and Netter, A.: Porphyrie cutanée de l'adulte apparue apriès une anémie hémolytique à auto-anticorps. Soc. Med. Hop. Paris **114**: 665, 1963.
166. Pitcock, J. A., Reinhard, E. H., Justus, B. W., and Mendelsohn, R. S.: A clinical and pathological study of seventy cases of myelofibrosis. Ann. Intern. Med. **57**: 73, 1962.
167. Bouroncle, B. A., and Doan, C. A.: Myelofibrosis. Clinical, hematologic and pathologic study of 110 patients. Amer. J. Med. Sci. **243**: 697, 1962.
168. Hennemann, G. H., Kunz, G., and Gilbert, K. E.: Symptomatische hämolytische anämie mit positiven Coombs-test bei Oseteomyloretikulose. Acta Haemat. (Basel) **10**: 260, 1953.
169. Cassell, M., and Chaplin, H., Jr.: Studies on anti-eluate sera. II. Comparison of a conventional antiglobulin serum with three anti-eluate sera in the study of 70 patients with acquired hemolytic anemia. Vox Sang. **5**: 43, 1960.
170. Yunis, E. J., and Bridges, R. A.: Blood transfusion problems in auto-immune hemolytic anemias. Minn. Med. **49**: 759, 1966.
171. Pirofsky, B.: Serologic and clinical findings in autoimmune hemolytic anemia. Series Haemat. **9**: 47, 1965.
172. Shee, J. C.: Myelosclerosis. An autoimmune disease. Lancet **1**: 773, 1963.
173. Imhof, J. W., Baars, H., and Verloop, M. C.: Clinical and haematological aspects of macroglobulinaemia Waldenström. Acta Med. Scand. **163**: 349, 1959.
174. Cline, M. J., Solomon, A., Berlin, N. I., and Fahey, J. L.: Anemia in macroglobulinemia. Amer. J. Med. **34**: 213, 1963.
175. Bouroncle, B. A., Purnendu, D., and Frajola, W. J.: Waldenström's macroglobulinemia. J. A. M. A. **189**: 729, 1964.
176. McCallister, B. D., Bayrd, E. D., Harrison, E. G., Jr., and McGuckin, W. F.: Primary macroglobulinemia. Review with a report on thirty-one cases and notes on the value of continuous chlorambucil therapy. Amer. J. Med. **43**: 394, 1967.
177. Wilde, H., and Hitzelberger, A. L.: Macroglobulinemia. Clinical features and differential diagnosis. Blood **9**: 875, 1954.
178. Fankhauser, V. S., Arnold, E., Schaub, F., and Lapp, R.: Hämolytisches Syndrome und Makroglobulinämie Waldenström. Helv. Med. Acta **23**: 645, 1956.
179. Creyssel, R., Charvillat, L., Morel, P., Matray, F., Mendé, P. de, and Croizat, P.: Contribution a l'étude biochimique des myélome multiple et des dysprotéinémies malignes. Rev. Lyon. Med. **1**: 129, 1956.
180. Bousser, J., and Boivin, P.: Macroglobulinémie de Waldenström. A propos de deux nouvelles observations. Rev. Hemat. (Paris) **12**: 100, 1957.
181. Fière, H.: Contribution à l'étude de la macroglobulinémie de Waldenström; à porpos de 8 observations (Dissertation). Presse Med. **65**: 2027, 1957.
182. Kappeler, V. R., Krebs, A., and Riva, G.: Klinik der Makroglobulinämie Waldenström. Beschreibung von 21 Fallen und Übersicht der Literatur. Helv. Med Acta **25**: 54, 1958.
183. Aarseth, S., Ofstad, E., and Torvik, A.: Macroglobulinaemia Waldenström. Acta Med. Scand. **169**: 691, 1961.
184. Waldenström, J.: Macroglobulinemia. In *Immunological Diseases*, edited by M. Samter. Little, Brown and Company, Boston, 1965.
185. Bayracki, C., Bardana, E. J., and Pirofsky, B.: Macroglobulinemia with positive antiglobulin tests, to be published.

Chapter 11

Cryopathic Autoimmune Hemolytic Anemia

Autoimmune hemolytic anemia associated with cold acting erythrocyte autoantibodies may be termed cryopathic autoimmune hemolytic anemia. These varieties may be readily distinguished on clinical and serologic grounds from the warm acting types of autoimmune hemolytic anemia. Cold acting erythrocyte autoantibodies differ from warm acting forms in serologic reactivity, frequency of occurrence, antigenic characteristics, degree of pathogenicity and physical-chemical characteristics. These differences are summarized in Chapters 16 to 20 and Tables 93 to 95. Therapeutic differences also exist between the two broad groups of autoimmune hemolytic anemia and are reviewed in the next chapter.

Cryopathic autoimmune hemolytic anemia may appear in several distinctive clinical patterns. Table 73 lists the specific clinical entities. Classification is similar to that employed with the warm acting types. An idiopathic cold hemagglutinin disease syndrome is assumed if no other significant pathologic state is present. The presence of other disease processes labels the state as a secondary or symptomatic variety. Virus infections have a significant associated relationship and neoplasia of the reticuloendothelium is present with a frequency that appears to be more than fortuitous. Paroxysmal cold hemoglobinuria is classified as a specific entity with distinctive clinical and serologic characteristics.

No attempt has been made at our laboratory to investigate consistently patients with cryopathic autoimmune hemolytic anemia. Accordingly, the majority of clinical material presented below reflects studies performed by other investigators. This is emphasized to encourage the reader to survey other more personal reviews. The presentations by MacKenzie (1), Stats and Wasserman (2), Dacie (3), Schubothe (4, 5), Evans and associates (6) and Levin (7) are excellent and should be reviewed by all students of hemolytic anemia.

Idiopathic Cold Hemagglutinin Disease

Historical Review

Cold acting hemagglutinins were initially demonstrated by Landsteiner (8) in 1903. The hemolytic anemia resulting from such autoantibody activity, however, was consistently confused with two other cryopathic syndromes. Separation of this entity from Raynaud's disease and from paroxysmal cold hemoglobinuria did not occur until the 1930's. Schubothe (5) has summarized many of the early case reports in the 19th century which appear to be examples of cold hemagglutinin disease. He suggests that one of the initial cases reported by Raynaud was a form of cold hemagglutinin disease. The reports of Iwai and Mei-Sai (9), Gonzales Guzman (10), Roth (11), Ernstene and Gardner (12) and Salén (13) did much to clarify the phenomenon of cold hemagglutination. Stats and Wasserman (2) summarized the available knowledge in 1943, and a large number of clinical reports followed. In 1952 Schubothe (14) introduced the term cold hemagglutinin disease (Kalteagglutinin-krankheit). The studies of Dacie (3), Schubothe (4), Gordon (15), Christenson and Dacie (16), and Fudenberg and Kunkel (17) documented many characteristics of cold acting erythrocyte autoantibodies. This permitted separation from the Donath-Landsteiner antibody and established serologic criteria for the diagnosis of cold hemagglutinin disease. The cold acting erythrocyte autoantibody was found to be an IgM immunoglobulin of high titer, with high thermal reactivity. The antibody acts in a monothermic fashion, involves complement and may induce in vivo agglutination and hemolysis. Wiener and associates (18) demonstrated anti-I specificity of the antibody. Cold acting erythrocyte autoantibodies with anti-i specificity were subsequently reported by Marsh (19), van Loghem and associates (20) and Evans and associates (6).

Age, Sex and Incidence

Schubothe (5) noted that cold hemagglutinin disease primarily affects the elderly, with a peak incidence from ages 51 to 60. In Dacie's group (3) of 21 patients, only five were younger than 60 years of age with the peak incidence at ages 70 to 80. Both sexes were involved. In Dacie's experience 76 per cent of cases involved women. Dausset and Colombani (21) noted seven women in their 10 cases. This conflicts with Schubothe's group (5), collected from personal experience and from the literature, which showed a predominantly male involvement.

Idiopathic cold hemagglutinin disease is relatively rare. Dacie (3) studied 175 cases of autoimmune hemolytic anemia. Only 19 examples, an incidence of 10.8 per cent, of idiopathic cold hemagglutinin disease was noted. van Loghem and associates (22) and Dausset and Colombani (21) had similar experiences. Idiopathic cold hemagglutinin disease was present in 7.7 per cent of cases of autoimmune hemolytic anemia in their studies. This syndrome is the most common form of cryopathic autoimmune hemolytic

TABLE 73. *Classification of the cryopathic autoimmune hemolytic anemias*

Cryopathic Autoimmune Hemolytic Anemia
A. Idiopathic cold hemagglutinin disease
B. Secondary cold hemagglutinin disease
1. Associated with virus infection
a. Virus pneumonia
b. Influenza
c. Infectious mononucleosis
d. Other viruses
2. Associated with reticuloendothelial neoplasia
C. Paroxysmal cold hemoglobinuria
1. Luetic type
2. Nonluetic type

anemia. Dacie (3) found 41 per cent and van Loghem and associates (22) found 30 per cent of cryopathic syndromes to be of this idiopathic type.

Clinical Features

A chronic disease is the rule. Dacie (3) describes a patient still living after 14 years of disease, and Schubothe (5) reported a patient still alive after 11 years of illness. Ben-Ishay and associates (23) reported a patient with potent cold hemagglutinins who died 18 years after the onset of disease. A similar patient is reported in this volume (Case 37). Hemolytic anemia with potent cold hemagglutinins was present for 215 months before death occurred from acute monocytic leukemia.

Symptoms in this syndrome are quite variable and may be minimal. When present they usually relate to the anemic state or to intercapillary cold hemagglutination. The symptoms are more marked after exposure to cold, and they generally involve exposed areas such as the fingers, toes, ear lobes and nose. Numbness with minimal pain is typical. A discoloration of the area varying from pale gray to dark blue-violet is characteristic. Reversal of these complaints upon warming is usually noted. These changes are described as Raynaud's phenomenon by Dacie (3) and as acrocyanosis by others. Only one of the 10 patients of Dausset and Colombani (21) had this complaint. Permanent changes with acral gangrene may occasionally develop. Hemoglobinuria can be present. This usually occurs in paroxysms, is related to cold exposure and is not associated with fever, chills or acute renal failure. Dacie (3) states that most of these patients have hemoglobinuria, but Dausset and Colombani (21) noted only one example in their 10 cases.

Physical signs are infrequent and are generally dominated by Raynaud's phenomenon or acrocyanosis as described above. The development of gangrene is associated with edema, ulceration and necrosis of skin and subcutaneous tissue. Pallor and jaundice may be present. Dacie (3) reports that the spleen is palpable in only a minority of patients, but Schubothe (5) states that "usually, the spleen and sometimes the liver are slightly enlarged." Splenomegaly was noted in six of the 10 patients of Dausset and Colombani (21). Hepatomegaly of a mild degree may also be present. The terminal development of a lymphoma in such patients may be associated with massive hepatosplenomegaly. Easy bruising and venous thromboses following venipuncture have been described. Pasero and Muratorio (24) have described a neurohemolytic syndrome relating to cold acting antibodies. Raynaud's phenomenon was present with involvement of the brain, spinal cord and peripheral nerves.

Laboratory Findings

Autohemagglutination of blood samples, which may occur immediately after venipuncture, is characteristic and is frequently the first diagnostic observation. The same phenomenon creates unsatisfactory peripheral blood smears and may prevent chamber counting for red blood cells. These abnormalities are rapidly reversible upon warming to 37°C. This can be employed to distinguish this state from dysproteinemic conditions and from the less prominent autohemagglutination present with warm acting erythrocyte autoantibodies.

Profound anemia is unusual and is less striking than that observed in the warm acting types. The degree of anemia varies with the degree of cold exposure and there-fore may appear seasonal. Anemia may even be absent. Macrocytosis and spherocytosis are less common than in the warm acting autoimmune hemolytic anemias. Nucleated erythrocytes are generally not found in the peripheral blood. Erythrophagocytosis may be observed, particularly in buffy coat preparations or upon performance of an Ehrlich finger test (see below under "Paroxysmal Cold Hemoglobinuria"). Reticulocytosis is slight to moderate and frequently correlates with the degree of anemia. In Schubothe's series (5) it varied from normal to 12.5 per cent. Leukopenia and thrombocytopenia may be observed but are not characteristic. Bilirubinemia of a mild degree is commonly seen. Hemoglobinuria is frequently encountered and generally appears in an intermittent fashion. Urinary hemosiderosis is a more consistent observation.

Diagnosis

The diagnosis of idiopathic cold hemagglutinin disease is dependent on three major criteria. These are: (a) The absence of a significant associated pathologic state such as virus infections and malignancies of the reticuloendothelium. Clinical studies designed to demonstrate hidden lymphomas should be initiated. (b) The absence of paroxysmal cold hemoglobinuria. Differences in serologic reactivity, clinical patterns and the Donath-Landsteiner test can usually separate these two conditions. These reactions are discussed more fully in the section devoted to paroxysmal cold hemoglobinuria. (c) The demonstration of a cold acting erythrocyte autoantibody. All human sera contain cold acting hemagglutinins if a careful examination is performed. The diagnosis of cold hemagglutinin disease is dependent on demonstrating a cold acting erythrocyte autoantibody that differs in two fundamental aspects from those seen in normal human serum. Titers are generally elevated over 500 at 0°C.; in normal serum the cold hemagglutinin titer rarely exceeds 64. In Schubothe's series (5) titers ranged from 1,000 to 256,000 at 0° C. One serum was observed with a titer of one million. In Dacie's series (3) titers at 2 to 4°C.

ranged from 1,024 to 512,000. A titer range from 2,000 to 64,000 was usually found. In general a high thermal reactivity of the pathologic cold acting erythrocyte auto-antibody is also observed. With normal serum agglutination rarely occurs at temperatures over 10 to 15°C. In Dacie's patients (3) with idiopathic cold hemagglutinin disease, striking autoagglutination was observed at temperatures over 20°C. The upper thermal limit, employing normal cells, ranged from 25 to 37°C. Similar observations have been reported by Schubothe (4).

Theoretical Concepts

Cold acting erythrocyte autoantibodies have several distinctive immunologic features. Schubothe (25) has emphasized three unusual characteristics: (a) it is rare for such antibodies to react with their antigen at room temperatures over 32°C., (b) the degree of reactivity of antibody with antigen may increase 100,000-fold by decreasing temperatures from 30 to 0°C., and (c) antibody-antigen union can be completely reversed within seconds of warming the test system. Wiener (26) suggested that such thermal labile characteristics might be produced by cross reacting antibodies exhibiting a poor "fit." Antibody-antigen union may be disrupted by the increased molecular activity present at higher temperatures. Schubothe (25) raises an additional possibility that has important etiologic and theoretical implications. He suggests that cold hemagglutinin immuno-globulins may change their molecular shape under the influence of temperature.

Low temperature polymerization with the production of large complexes may occur in a fashion similar to that seen with cryoglobulins. Studies by Colomb and associates (27), Turro and Straface (28), Gökcen (29) and Harris and Fairley (30) indicate that cold hemagglutinins may appear as cryoglobulins or be associated with cryoglobulin production. Christenson and Dacie (16) demonstrated cryoprecipitation of polymerized cold hemagglutinins. This observation and the IgM nature of cold acting autoantibodies led Schubothe (4),

Mehrotra (31) and Ritzmann and Levin (32) to suggest that they may be para-proteins related to Waldenström's macro-globulinemia.

This concept is supported by three experimental observations. Schubothe hypothesizes that chronic idiopathic cold hemagglutinin disease is a lymphoproliferative syndrome (25). Bone marrow lymphoid proliferation has been observed by several investigators. In an analysis of 14 cases Schubothe (5) noted that nine had bone marrow lymphocyte counts exceeding 25 per cent; in six patients it exceeded 40 per cent. Similar observations have been made by Ritzmann and Levin (32). The bone marrow therefore resembles the changes seen in Waldenström's macroglobulinemia.

Ultracentrifuge studies also supported this concept. The total macroglobulin content is increased in cold hemagglutinin disease. Ritzmann and Levin (32) suggested that the increased macroglobulin is quantitatively identical with cold hemagglutinins. Schubothe (25) investigated this problem, employing the sera of 17 patients with cold hemagglutinin disease. He was unable to correlate titers of cold hemagglutinins and amounts of macroglobulins. Adsorption studies completely removed the cold hemagglutinin; macroglobulin content dropped from 17 to 8.8 per cent. This latter figure is substantially above normal and suggests the production of multiple abnormal macroglobulins in cold hemagglutinin disease.

A third area of research suggests that cold acting autoantibodies found in idiopathic cold hemagglutinin disease may result from a monoclonal process. Franklin and Fudenberg (33) demonstrated that five different cold hemagglutinins all had type K light chains. Studies carried out by Harboe and Deverill (34), Harboe and associates (35), Schubothe (5) and Costea and associates (36) have confirmed this observation. A total of 59 cold hemagglutinins have been examined and all were found to be a type K macroglobulin. van Furth and Diesselhoff-den Dulk (37) demonstrated in bone marrow tissue culture the

production of type K light chain IgM
immunoglobulins in patients with cold
hemagglutinin disease. This strongly suggests a monoclonal origin. The pattern more
closely resembles macroglobulinemia rather
than the usual warm acting erythrocyte
antibody. Franklin and Fudenberg (33)
found a mixture of type K and type L
light chains in isoantibodies directed
against rhesus agglutinogens and rheumatoid factor. Warm acting erythrocyte autoantibodies generally consist of a mixture of
type K and type L chains, although monotypic autoantibodies of either type K or
type L have been described (33, 38, 39).
Not all reported cold hemagglutinins have
fitted into this tidy compartment of an
IgM immunoglobulin with a type K light
chain. Feizi (40) has described three cold
hemagglutinins with L type light chains.
Andersen (41) has studied a cold hemagglutinin classified as an IgA immunoglobulin.

These studies suggest that idiopathic cold
hemagglutinin disease has a close relationship to Waldenström's macroglobulinemia.
Ritzmann and Levin (32) have termed
cold hemagglutinin disease a variety or
variant of macroglobulinemia. Schubothe
(5) "suggests that the chronic cold agglutinin disease belongs not only to the para-
proteinemic lymphoproliferative disorders
but may appear in different variants, partly
perhaps as a monoblastic protein neoplasia, and also as partial manifestation of
a pluriblastic protein neoplasia." It is
suggested (25) that idiopathic cold hemagglutinin disease may be a form of dysproteinemia. It would differ from macroglobulinemia by the "autoaggressive character of
the pathological serum protein" and would
represent a special form of paraproteinemia
(25).

Secondary Cold Hemagglutinin Disease: Virus Related Variety

Virus Pneumonia

In 1918 Clough and Richter (42) studied
the serum of a patient who had virus pneumonia. A cold acting hemagglutinin with a
titer of 500 was found. This dropped to
10 during convalescence. In 1943 a series of

studies confirmed the relationship between
virus pneumonia and high titer cold acting
hemagglutinins. Horstmann and Tatlock
(43) reported high titer hemagglutinins in
27 of 40 patients with virus pneumonia.
Turner and associates (44) studied 83
cases of virus pneumonia. They noted a
peak elevation of cold hemagglutinins in the
period between the 10th to 20th day of disease. Florman and Weiss (45), Young (46)
and Finland and associates (47) reported
that over 50 per cent of patients with virus
pneumonia developed high titer cold hemagglutinins. Finland and Barnes (48)
reported that 22 per cent of patients developing virus pneumonia from 1950 to
1956 had an elevation of cold hemagglutinins. This is substantially reduced from
the incidence previously noted by the same
investigators in the same area, and possibly represents involvement by a different
virus.

In 1943 Peterson and associates (49),
Horstmann and Tatlock (43) and Dameshek (50) each noted two patients with
virus pneumonia, cold hemagglutinins and
acute hemolytic anemia. All of these patients were receiving sulfonamide therapy, and a drug induced hemolysis was
strongly considered. Stats and Wasserman
(2) expressed the prevalent feeling that
"the accumulated evidence favors the view
that the cold hemagglutination in these
cases of hemolytic anemia is not the cause
but may be the result of the anemia."

An increasing number of reports relating hemolytic anemia to virus pneumonia
became available. Many patients did not
receive sulfonamide therapy. The development of high titer cold acting erythrocyte
autoantibodies, with a high thermal level
of activity, appeared significant in relation
to in vivo hemolysis and hemolytic anemia.
The cold acting erythrocyte autoantibody
was subsequently shown to have anti-I
specificity, and its ability to react with host
erythrocytes containing the I antigen appears to be necessary for hemolysis.

Clinical Aspects

There is an extensive literature relating
autoimmune hemolytic anemia to virus

pneumonia. In spite of this, the association of these two states is not common. Dacie (3) encountered 10 cases in a 12-year period but has not seen an additional example in the last 3 years. His total series of cases of autoimmune hemolytic anemia showed an incidence of 6.3 per cent of virus pneumonia. van Loghem and associates (22) noted a 5.3 per cent incidence of such cases in a series of 168 patients with autoimmune hemolytic anemia.

Both males and females may be involved in the combined syndrome. In general, adults are afflicted. A rapid onset of hemolysis is frequently observed. This correlates with the development of high titer cold hemagglutinins in the 2nd or 3rd week of virus pneumonia. Accordingly, the syndrome frequently appears during the convalescent stage after resolution of the infectious disease. Pallor and jaundice are common. Splenomegaly is generally present. Hemoglobinuria has been reported by Dameshek (50), Horstmann and Tatlock (43), Neely and associates (51) and Stuart and Friedlander (52). Acrocyanosis, gangrene or phlebothrombosis with pulmonary emboli have rarely been noted. The prognosis is excellent with spontaneous recovery and cessation of hemolysis after a relatively short course. In this regard it resembles many of the virus induced warm acting autoimmune syndromes described in Chapter 7. Deaths have been recorded by Horstmann and Tatlock (43) and Finland and associates (47) but this is unusual. Recovery is generally complete. Dacie (3) suggests that recovery from the hemolytic state correlates with a change in cold acting erythrocyte antibody activity. Hemolysis terminated with a loss of agglutinating ability at 27°C., although antibody titers at 2°C. were minimally reduced.

Laboratory Findings

Autohemagglutination can immediately occur after venipuncture and is a characteristic observation. It is sufficiently severe to prevent adequate erythrocyte counting and satisfactory blood smears unless warmed specimens and equipment are employed. Severe anemia is not uncommon.

A moderate to marked spherocytosis may be observed and erythrophagocytosis is rarely found. Elevated peripheral blood leukocyte counts are common and Horstmann and Tatlock (43) have reported one patient whose white blood cell count reached 100,000/mm.[3] Moeschlin and associates (53) encountered a patient who developed granulocytopenia and thrombocytopenia. A mild to moderate elevation of serum bilirubin is common and unbound haptoglobins may be absent. Christenson and Dacie (16) reported that serum electrophoresis generally reveals an elevation of gamma- and alpha-globulins.

Diagnosis

Diagnosis is dependent upon demonstration of hemolysis and anemia in a patient recovering from virus pneumonia. Documentation of a high titer cold acting autoantibody with a high thermal level of reactivity is crucial. Titers of cold hemagglutinins at the height of hemolysis have ranged from 512 to 32,000 at 2° to 4°C. Titers obtained in Dacie's series (3) ranged from 2,048 to 8,000 at the height of illness, with agglutination demonstrated at 30°C. in every case tested. The direct antiglobulin test is positive and is of a nongamma variety. Such reactions are found even with specimens collected at 37°C. The cold acting erythrocyte autoantibody may have a lytic potency made more obvious by mild acidification and/or the use of erythrocytes from patients with paroxysmal nocturnal hemoglobinuria.

Theoretical Concepts

The relationship of mycoplasma or pleural pneumonia-like organisms to the development of potent cold acting erythrocyte autoantibodies is an intriguing but still unsettled area of research. No specific serologic differences separate the virus pneumonia type of cold acting erythrocyte autoantibody from that seen in idiopathic cold hemagglutinin diseases or secondarily to neoplasia of the reticuloendothelium. A possible structural difference has been reported by Costea and associates (36). They noted that both K and L type light chains are present in cold hemagglutinins produced in response to mycoplasma infections. Feizi (40) reported a monotypic L type cold hemagglutinin in a patient with *Mycoplasma pneumoniae* infection. This contrasts with the almost exclusive distribution of K type light chains found in cold hemagglutinin disease (33–36).

The cold acting erythrocyte autoantibodies developing after virus pneumonia appear to be similar to those found in all normal human sera. They have an antigenic specificity of anti-I or rarely anti-i. Jenkins and Marsh (54), however, have encountered cold hemagglutinins which they classify as "anti-not I." Schmidt and associates (55, 56) demonstrated that various pleural pneumonia-like organisms may modify the I site of erythrocytes and these authors have described the action of these organisms as secondary invaders in human neoplastic disease. Thomas (57) has suggested that infections with mycoplasma may be implicated in conditions characterized by autoimmune serologic reactions. This is based on the observation that anti-lung tissue antibodies may develop in patients with virus pneumonia. Barile (58) has made a similar suggestion concerning a relationship to autoimmune disease.

It has been suggested by Wiener (26) that cold acting erythrocyte autoantibodies result from heteroimmune stimulation, creating a cross reacting antibody. Costea and associates (59) demonstrated that immunization of rabbits with *Listeria monocytogenes* leads to the production of IgG antibodies directed against the organism and IgM antibodies which appear identical to human cold acting erythrocyte autoantibodies. This experimental animal model system may aid greatly in clarifying the status of cold hemagglutinins.

Influenza Infections

The production of high titer cold hemagglutinins during influenza virus infections has been described by Finland and Barnes (48). Its incidence of occurrence is much less than that recorded with virus pneumonia. These investigators noted that five of 144 patients with proven influenza A or B infections developed high titer cold hemagglutinins. This incidence of 3.4 per cent may be compared to a 22 per cent incidence of elevated cold hemagglutinins found in patients with virus pneumonia studied at the same period of time. Laroche and associates (60) in 1951 reported a patient who developed acute hemolytic anemia during the course of serologically proven influenza A virus infection. High titer cold hemagglutinins were found. A similar association was reported by Ventura and Aresu (61) in 1957. The series of van Loghem and associates (22) contained one patient with "infectious grippe" and hemolytic anemia. Dausset and Colombani (21) encountered five patients with positive Hirst reactions, an influenza-like disease and acute hemolytic anemia. In one patient influenza A was documented. Hemolysins were found in four of the five cases. In all five patients a similar course was seen. A profound anemia (red blood cell count average 1.9 million) developed very rapidly a few days after the initial infection. Recovery was complete in all cases with anemia disappearing in 5 to 25 days. "The average duration of disease was six months, but was undoubtedly overestimated" (21). Puxeddu and associates (62) recorded autoimmune hemolytic anemia complicating an influenza B infection. Springer and Ansell (63) have emphasized the interaction of influenza virus with erythrocytes. They demonstrated destruction of the M, N, Lu^a and Lu^b antigens through such virus activity.

Infectious Mononucleosis

The association of hemolytic anemia and infectious mononucleosis has been reported in 40 patients (64). Such hemolytic states may occur in the absence of demonstrable erythrocyte autoantibodies or be associated with either warm or cold acting autoantibodies. The clinical characteristics of this combined syndrome and examples of the association with warm acting autoantibodies have been presented in Chapter 7.

In 1960 Marsh and Jenkins (19, 65) reported two cases of reticulum cell neoplasia with an associated autoimmune hemolytic anemia. Cold acting erythrocyte autoantibodies were documented and were found to have a specificity of anti-i. Reports of van Loghem and associates (20) and Evans and associates (6) also described cold acting erythrocyte autoantibodies of anti-i specificity associated with hemolytic syndromes. A specific relationship to reticuloendothelial neoplasia was not found. Anti-i antibodies were considered rare until 1965 when Rosenfield and associates (66) reported the association of anti-i and infectious mononucleosis. In an investigation of 38 patients with infectious mononucleosis, 68 per cent were found to have anti-i erythrocyte antibodies. All sera contained heterophile agglutinins which were resistant to adsorption with either guinea pig or horse kidney antigen, but which readily adsorbed with boiled ox cells. Cross adsorption studies clearly separated heterophile and anti-i hemagglutinins and demonstrated their individuality. Other investigators have confirmed this relationship with infectious mononucleosis. Calvo and associates (67) reported the presence of anti-i in 23 of 38 patients. Wollheim and Williams (68) discovered anti-i in 27 of 36 cases of uncomplicated infectious mononucleosis. Jenkins and associates (69) noted anti-i activity in the sera of seven of 85 patients with infectious mononucleosis.

The development of hemolytic anemia in a patient with infectious mononucleosis and anti-i erythrocyte autoantibodies has been described by Jenkins and associates (69). Similar examples have been reported by Calvo and associates (67) and Troxel and associates (70). Kostinas and Cantow (71) found that 10 of 41 patients with infectious mononucleosis had increased in vitro autohemolysis. Neither overt hemolytic anemia nor positive direct antiglobulin tests were found in these patients. All 10 sera, however, gave positive indirect antiglobulin tests and cold hemagglutinins were present in nine. Unfortunately, specificity of the cold acting autoantibodies was not reported.

Infectious mononucleosis resembles virus pneumonia in the frequent production of cold acting erythrocyte autoantibodies. A further similarity is apparent in the rarity of overt hemolytic anemia. However, a major difference exists between these two virus infections. The cold acting erythrocyte autoantibodies found in idiopathic cold hemagglutinin disease and in virus pneumonia generally have anti-I specificity. Worlledge (72) noted that 20 of 21 sera from patients with idiopathic cold hemagglutinin disease contained anti-I erythrocyte autoantibodies. Nine sera obtained from patients with virus pneumonia all contained cold hemagglutinins of anti-I specificity. In contrast, the cold acting erythrocyte autoantibodies found in infectious mononucleosis, whether or not associated with overt hemolytic anemia, have anti-i specificity. The significance of this different antigenic specificity has yet to be determined.

Other Virus Infections

Occasional examples of cold acting autoimmune hemolytic anemia complicating other viral infections have been noted. Betke and associates (73) and Vivell (74) reported this association with Coxsackie virus A. Dacie (3) described formation of a Donath-Landsteiner type of cold acting erythrocyte autoantibody following an attack of measles. Borbolla and Barquet Chediak (75) reported autoimmune hemolytic anemia during recovery from varicella; infectious mononucleosis may also have been present in this case. Unger and associates (76) encountered a case of neonatal hemolytic anemia in an infant with encephalitis. Potent cold hemagglutinins were found in the infant's serum and were absent in the mother. Copps (77) reported the unusual combination of hemolytic anemia, virus pneumonia and erythema multiforme. The relationship of the virus infection to the syndrome is unknown.

Secondary Cold Hemagglutinin Disease: Associated Reticuloendothelial Neoplasia

The association of hemolytic anemia, cold acting erythrocyte autoantibodies and neoplasia of the reticuloendothelium is uncommon. In contrast, warm acting forms of autoimmune hemolytic anemia are not uncommon in the same neoplastic conditions. A cold acting type of hemolytic anemia complicating lymphocytic leukemia was reported by Alexander and Thomson (78) in 1925. Atypical leukemia was implicated in a similar process by Boxwell and Bigger (79) in 1931. Manheims and Brunner (80) in 1933 noted cold acting hemolytic anemia in a patient with granulocytic leukemia. Stats and Wasserman (2) mention one case of lymphosarcoma with persisting low titer cold hemagglutinins in the absence of hemolysis.

The relative infrequency of the combination of cold hemagglutinins, hemolytic anemia and reticuloendothelial neoplasia is apparent in several large published series. The series of Rosenthal and associates (81) of 24 patients with reticuloendothelial neoplasia describes only warm acting varieties of autoimmune hemolytic anemia. In Dacie's series (3) of 175 cases of autoimmune hemolytic anemia, five examples of reticuloendothelial neoplasia and cold hemagglutinins are recorded, an incidence of 3.4 per cent. In the series of van Loghem and associates (22) of 168 cases of autoimmune hemolytic anemia, this is not noted. The series of Dausset and Colombani (21) of 128 cases of autoimmune hemolytic anemia described seven patients (5.4 per cent) with cold hemagglutinins and reticuloendothelial neoplasia. These included two examples of chronic lymphocytic leukemia, two patients with reticulum cell sarcoma, two undiagnosed malignant conditions of the blood and one case of Hodgkin's disease. Ritzmann and associates (82) have also reported the association of cryopathic autoimmune hemolytic anemia and a malignant lymphoma. Yunis and Bridges (83) presented a series of 40 patients with autoimmune hemolytic anemia. Cryopathic forms were found in 24 patients. Four subjects had lymphoproliferative malignancies and one had plasma cell myeloma.

The clinical syndrome resulting from the association of cold hemagglutinins and reticuloendothelial neoplasia is similar to that seen with warm acting varieties. Schubothe (5) states that the course is primarily determined by the activity of the under-

lying malignancy. In Dausset and Colombani's series (21) hemolytic anemia was discovered either simultaneously with or shortly after diagnosis of the neoplastic process. Raynaud's syndrome was found in only one of the seven patients. Hemolysis was demonstrated in two of the four sera examined. A chronic course reflecting progression of the neoplastic process developed with the persistence of the hemolytic stage.

In 1960 Marsh and Jenkins (65) noted hemolytic anemia in two patients with reticulum cell sarcoma and "reticulosis." Cold acting antibodies of anti-i specificity were found. Dacie (3) reported two additional cases of reticulum cell sarcoma and one example of Hodgkin's disease with cold hemagglutinins not having specificity for either I or i. Worlledge (72) working in the same laboratory reported six cases of cryopathic autoimmune hemolytic anemia and neoplasia of the reticuloendothelium. Only three subjects had cold acting erythrocyte autoantibodies of anti-I specificity. The significance of this variation of antigenic specificity is unknown.

Secondary Cold Hemagglutinin Disease: Other Associated Diseases

In the early literature the association of cold hemagglutinins, hemolytic anemia and various pathologic states has been noted. The etiologic significance of such relationships is questionable. Prominent in this group have been trypanosomiasis, relapsing fever, cirrhosis, malaria, infections (particularly septicemia), pernicious anemia and various forms of carcinoma. The pertinent literature has been summarized by Stats and Wasserman (2).

Paroxysmal Cold Hemoglobinuria

Historical Concepts

Paroxysmal cold hemoglobinuria, although exceedingly rare, has a long historical background. It was well documented clinically and serologically before other hemolytic states. The dramatic appearance of hemoglobinuria associated with anemia after cold exposure called attention to this syndrome. MacKenzie (1) and Dacie (3) have summarized much of the older literature. Elliotson (84) in 1832 reported a patient who developed hemoglobinuria "whenever the East wind blew." Cure resulted from quinine therapy, and this may have been a case of malaria hemoglobinuria. Dressler (85) in 1854 described a 10-year-old child with congenital syphilis, intermittent albuminuria and "hematuria." He differentiated hemoglobinuria from hematuria in this patient but failed to recognize the role of chilling or syphilis. The clinical syndrome was accurately described in 1865 by Harley (86), Dickinson (87) and Hassall (88). Harley (86) was unaware of the role of syphilis or the nature of the coloring material in the urine. The term "winter" or "intermittent hematuria" was employed by Hassall (88), and all three authors recognized that the condition was precipitated by cold exposure. They noted that the urine contained free hemoglobin rather than intact erythrocytes. Pavy (89) in 1868 differentiated this disease from the hemoglobinuria of malaria. Gull (90) at approximately the same time recognized the role of chilling and considered it to be one of the several causes of this syndrome. Secchi (91) in 1872 confirmed Dressler's observation (85) that the urine color was due to hemoglobin and introduced the term hemoglobinuria.

Initially, hemolysis was believed to occur in the kidney. Lichtheim (92) first suggested that hemolysis occurred intravascularly with hemoglobin excreted in the urine. An anonymous English physician "D" (93) also suggested a similar mechanism. In 1879 Küssner (94) observed the color of the serum obtained with a cupping glass during attacks of hemoglobinuria. He confirmed Lichtheim's assumption of intravascular hemolysis. Rosenbach (95) at the same time clearly documented the effect of cold by precipitating attacks of hemoglobinuria through immersion of the patient's extremities in ice water. This procedure, the Rosenbach test, assumed diagnostic importance. Ehrlich (96) modified and extended this approach by devising a localized finger test. A ligature was placed around the finger and the member was subsequently chilled in ice water. Serum obtained from this finger was found to contain free hemoglobin. This formed the basis for the diagnostic procedure termed the Ehrlich finger test. Vasomotor phenomena associated with this disease syndrome were recognized by Lichtheim (92), Popper (97), MacKenzie (1) and Murri (98). By 1894 the clinical features of paroxysmal cold hemoglobinuria were well recognized and were summarized in a monograph presented by Chvostek (99).

Very little was known about the pathogenesis of this disease. Götze (100) in 1884 observed a child with congenital syphilis and paroxysmal cold hemoglobinuria. He postulated an etiologic relationship between the two diseases after a thorough review of the literature. Murri (98) in 1885 stated that, of 36 cases previously reported, 15 had concomitant syphilis. Ehrlich and Morgenroth (101) in 1899 suggested an immunologic mechanism for this disorder. The lysis of erythrocytes was assumed to result through an amboceptor-alexin mechanism. Ehrlich had previously shown that the erythrocytes of such patients were not particularly sensitive to cold. He and Morgenroth postulated that the blood vessel walls in specifically disposed individuals produced a ferment under the influence of cold which induced hemolysis. The ability of an extrinsic agent to destroy red cells through an immunological mechanism was therefore proposed. In 1904 Donath and Landsteiner (102) clarified the pathophysiologic process. They described an autohemolysin in the patient's serum which combined with erythrocytes at low temperatures. A biphasic or bithermal sequence was involved. Subsequent warming of such sensitized erythrocytes in the presence of a labile serum factor (alexin or complement) resulted in hemolysis. This classic study presented the first description of an autoantibody. The bithermal action of the Donath-Landsteiner antibody formed the basis for the most frequently employed diagnostic procedure, the Donath-Landsteiner test. These serologic observations were confirmed by Eason (103),

Widal and Rostaine (104) and Langstein (105). The characteristics of the Donath-Landsteiner antibody and its antigenic specificity are discussed in Chapters 19 and 20.

Clinical Characteristics

Paroxysmal cold hemoglobinuria is a rare disease. Jones and Jones (106) found only nine cases in a 30-year period involving 156,000 patients admitted to the Massachusetts General Hospital in Boston. In 74,186 consecutive admissions to the Peter Bent Brigham Hospital in Boston there were three examples of this syndrome (107). Howard and associates (108) noted only two cases in 38 years and 298,878 admissions at the Montreal Hospital. Becker (109) recorded only one case at the University of Chicago clinic in 20 years. This period covered 130,000 hospitalized patients and 382,792 clinic outpatients. Nabarro (110) reported 13 cases which were typical and five which were atypical in a 27-year experience in London. This author has encountered only two cases over a 15-year period at Bellevue Hospital in New York and at the University of Oregon hospitals and clinics. Paroxysmal cold hemoglobinuria is uncommon even in large series of patients with autoimmune hemolytic anemia. Dacie's group of 175 cases (3) contained eight patients or 4.6 per cent with paroxysmal cold hemoglobinuria. van Loghem and associates (22) recorded 17 cases in their series of 168 patients, an incidence of 10 per cent.

Race, Age, Sex

There does not appear to be any particular racial predisposition for the development of paroxysmal cold hemoglobinuria. The Northern European and the American Caucasian and Negro have been commonly reported as suffering from this syndrome. The disease is particularly prevalent in Japan.

Both males and females may be involved. In Becker's series (109) of 38 patients, 74 per cent were males. The age distribution of patients with paroxysmal cold hemoglobinuria differs from that found in idiopathic cold hemagglutinin disease. The young are frequently involved. Becker's series (109) of 38 patients presented an age range from 3 to 56 years, with a median age of 30 years. Ten of the 38 patients were children under age 15. This predisposition for the young reflects the clinical relationship of paroxysmal cold hemoglobinuria to congenital syphilis. In view of the IgG immunoglobulin structure of the Donath-Landsteiner antibody (Chapter 19), erythroblastosis may be anticipated. Hoppe and Witte (111) have reported such a case. Donath-Landsteiner antibodies have also been found by Vos and associates (112) in the sera of patients who frequently abort.

A familial occurrence of this disease has been described. This probably represents transmission of congenital syphilis rather than a genetic abnormality as suggested for warm acting erythrocyte autoantibodies. Matsuo (113) reported two such families. In one, a male proband had a sister and two cousins who were involved. In the second family a father and daughter were involved. Orel (114) observed the disease in twin children. Thurmon and Blain (107) reported two half-brothers with serologic evidence for the Donath-Landsteiner antibody.

Paroxysmal Attacks

Paroxysmal cold hemoglobinuria is a disease characterized by the sudden onset of shaking chills, fever, abdominal distress, nausea and hemoglobinuria developing 4 to 10 hours after exposure to cold. Frequently there is evidence of Raynaud's disease. This description, presented by Becker (109), summarizes the usual clinical pattern seen in paroxysmal cold hemoglobinuria. Dacie (3) has emphasized that the disease process is chronic and comparatively benign. It rarely leads to death or to severe chronic anemia. MacKenzie (1) has presented an excellent review of clinical patterns seen in paroxysmal cold hemoglobinuria. The following description closely follows his observations. The patient's attention to the disease is captured by passage of dark red, brownish or black urine. This frequently follows cold exposure which varies from patient to patient and may be surprisingly slight. The interval between chilling and the development of symptoms ranges from a few minutes to 8 hours. Prodromal symptoms may develop and may include aching pains in the back or legs, abdominal cramps, headaches and malaise. The actual paroxysm is characterized by shaking chills and an elevation of the temperature to values as high as 104°F. Fever may be brief or may persist for several hours. The first urine specimen obtained is dark burgundy red or brownish chocolate black. It contains large amounts of oxyhemoglobin, methemoglobin and hematin. As a rule only the first two urine samples have these characteristics. However, cases have been recorded with hemoglobinuria persisting for 2 to 3 days. Jaundice can develop after severe attacks and may persist for several days. Splenomegaly is common during such paroxysms and transitory hepatomegaly may be demonstrated.

Temperature Sensitivity

The sensitivity of patients to temperature changes and the mode of chilling may vary greatly in subjects. A critical temperature level of 40°F was found in one patient by Macalister (115). Some subjects are susceptible to minimal temperature changes resulting from opening a door into a chilled room. The immersion of the extremities in ice water for 10 to 20 minutes (Rosenbach test) will nearly always induce a paroxysm. Eating ice and inhaling cold air were unsuccessful in inducing paroxysms in some patients. Venous stasis produced by a tourniquet may precipitate an attack in some but was unsuccessful in three subjects tested by MacKenzie (1). Emotional episodes may also precipitate or magnify a paroxysm.

Abortive Attacks

The typical picture presented above may vary greatly. Hemoglobinuria may occur without constitutional manifestations. These have been termed abortive, rudimentary, frustrated or larval attacks. The reverse is also seen. Constitutional symptoms in the absence of hemoglobinuria have been described. Such attacks generally manifest transient albuminuria. Jaundice may also develop in the absence of hemoglobinuria. MacKenzie (1) states that hemoglobinemia can generally be demonstrated even when hemoglobinuria is not present.

Vasomotor Phenomena

Many authors have noted vasomotor disturbances in association with paroxysmal cold hemoglobinuria. Raynaud's syndrome is common. The fingers, toes, tip of the nose, lips or ears may be blanched or may become deeply cyanotic. MacKenzie (1) recorded these changes in two of five patients investigated. Gangrene may also occur. Marked systolic and diastolic blood pressure changes can develop before the start of chills. Nabarro (110) studied 18 patients and reported that blood pressure changes may not occur.

Moss (116) reported cold urticaria as a prodromal manifestation, and Orel (114) also observed this in his affected twin subjects. Harris and associates (117) suggested that cold urticaria may be immunologically mediated through a dermolysin which was cytotoxic in the cold. This phenomenon may be passively transferred and may be reproduced with the application of cold to the skin of the recipient.

Laboratory Studies

MacKenzie (1) found that nearly all patients with paroxysmal cold hemoglobinuria had either moderate or severe anemia during the seasons of the year when attacks occur. The red blood count may drop precipitously following a typical paroxysm. Montagnani (118) reported that the erythrocyte count dropped from 3.8 to 1.8 million after an artifically induced attack in one patient. Donath and Landsteiner (119) noted a drop of hemoglobin from 85 to 55 per cent in one patient and Lazzati and Sorgente (120) reported a patient whose hemoglobin was 80 per cent in the summer and 35 per cent in the winter after repeated attacks. Very rapid recovery with anisocytosis, poikilocytosis, basophilic stippling, polychromatophilia, nucleated erythrocytes, myelocytes and reticulocytosis may be found.

Between paroxysms the total leukocyte count may be normal or slightly elevated.

Widal and associates (121) noted leukopenia soon after chilling. This was accompanied by an increased coagulation time, increased viscosity and a fall in blood pressure. They termed this development "hemoclastic crisis." Uchida (122) found that maximum leukopenia occurred 5 to 20 minutes after chilling. After approximately 2 hours leukocytosis of neutrophilic granulocytes occurred. Montagnani (118) described a reduction of leukocytes from 9,800 to 1,000/mm.[3] and a thrombocyte reduction from 160,000 to 35,000/mm.[3] in an artificially produced attack. Jordan and associates (123) suggested that anaphylaxis, a pyrogen reaction and an alarm or stress reaction all contributed to leukopenia, with erythrophagocytosis aiding in the trapping of leukocytes in capillary beds. This phenomenon is not unique and may occur in all erythrocyte antibody-antigen reactions. The adhesiveness of leukocytes to agglutinated erythrocytes may be involved in this phenomenon in a "mixed agglutination" reaction. The possible presence of P blood group antigens in leukocytes must also be considered. This would permit a direct reaction with the Donath-Landsteiner antibody, inducing leukopenia. Leonardi and Andolfatto-Zaglia (124) described a cold acting leukoagglutinin in paroxysmal cold hemoglobinuria, and this may be important in creating leukopenia.

Erythrophagocytosis was initially described by Ehrlich (125) in blood smears obtained after performance of a finger test. This observation has been repeatedly confirmed. Similar findings are present in buffy coat preparations made after permitting the blood to incubate.

Free hemoglobin is always present in the serum after a paroxysm. Serum bilirubin is elevated and may persist for several days. After a paroxysm and disappearance of hemoglobinuria and albuminuria, the urine may still show hemosiderin.

Relation to Syphilis

Early case reports noted a relationship of syphilis to paroxysmal cold hemoglobinuria. Götze (100) and Murri (98) first emphasized this point. The frequency of the disease in congenital syphilitic children and the lesions of acquired syphilis in many adult patients supported this concept. A large variety of abnormalities were reported which include aortitis, Hutchinson teeth, saddle nose, saber shins, interstitial keratitis, hepatitis, tabes and paresis. The availability of the Wassermann test confirmed earlier clinical impressions. Donath and Landsteiner's review (119) of the literature from 1906 to 1925 revealed evidence of syphilis in 95 of 99 reported cases. A positive Wassermann reaction was demonstrated in 81 patients and a history or clinical evidence of syphilis was found in 24. Donath and Landsteiner (119) and Kumagai and Namba (126) noted that cold hemolysins were present in the sera of patients with latent syphilis, in the absence of clinical manifestations of paroxysmal cold hemoglobinuria. MacKenzie (1) summarized this view by stating that "paroxysmal hemoglobinuria is usually and perhaps always a manifestation of syphilis." He concluded that "a small percentage of patients with late syphilis have the latent form of paroxysmal hemoglobinuria." Becker (109) agreed with this concept. In the 38 cases he reviewed, syphilis was universally present. Burmeister's results and conclusions differed (127). Of 207 examples of paroxysmal cold hemoglobinuria in the literature, he found indications of syphilis in only 79; in 43 cases it was ruled out, in one it was uncertain and in the remainder there was insufficient information. The Wassermann reaction, however, was positive in 95 per cent of cases tested. Burmeister (127) reported that adsorption of the cold acting hemolysin led to disappearance of the Wassermann reaction. In addition, elution of the cold hemolysin from sensitized erythrocytes gave a supernatant capable of inducing a positive Wassermann test. These results have not been confirmed. More recently the elegant techniques employed by Hinz (128) have clearly shown that entirely different substances are involved in cold hemolysis and in the Wassermann reaction.

Acute and chronic forms of paroxysmal cold hemoglobinuria may be found in the absence of syphilis. Such cases have recently been reported by Nelson and Nicholl (129), Dacie (3) and van Loghem and associates (22). In the latter series, six of 17 examples of paroxysmal cold hemoglobinuria occurred in nonluetic patients. The only two cases personally observed by this author occurred in subjects without syphilis.

The nonsyphilitic forms of paroxysmal cold hemoglobinuria may assume various clinical patterns. Figure 11 classifies the types of paroxysmal cold hemoglobinuria and is derived from the classifications employed by van Loghem and associates (22) and Dacie (3). The acute transitory type in the absence of syphilis is generally associated with virus infections. These have included chickenpox, influenza or grippe, infectious mononucleosis, upper respiratory infections, mumps and measles. A chronic variety of nonsyphilitic related paroxysmal cold hemoglobinuria is rare. Dacie (3) reported one patient with a Donath-Landsteiner antibody documented for 8 years. Leonardi and Andolfatto-Zaglia (124) have also presented a similar chronic case with an associated cold leukoagglutinin.

Dacie (3) states that "it seems most logical to consider parxoysmal cold haemoglobinuria as a syndrome of varying aetiology, the connecting link between the different types being the formation of a cold auto-antibody of more or less uniform characteristics." Penicillin therapy and routine premarital and prenatal serologic testing for syphilis have almost eliminated congenital syphilis and tertiary forms of this disease. Accordingly, paroxysmal cold hemoglobinuria of the luetic variety is less apparent and the nonluetic type is assuming greater clinical significance. This changing clinical picture may permit the development of new pathophysiologic and serologic concepts in this disease.

Diagnosis

The classic triad of cold sensitivity, hemoglobinuria and vasomotor phenomena may be seen in all cryopathic autoimmune hemolytic anemias. The diagnosis of par-

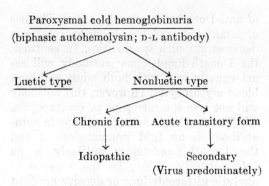

FIGURE 11. Classification of the clinical varieties of paroxysmal cold hemoglobinuria.

oxysmal cold hemoglobinuria is dependent on the presence of typical paroxysms in association with the Donath-Landsteiner antibody. This requires serologic evidence of a cold acting erythrocyte autoantibody fixing to the erythrocyte in the cold and inducing hemolysis when warmed in the presence of complement. Dacie (3) minimizes the significance of this biphasic or bithermal characteristic of the cold acting autoantibody. In contrast, Schubothe (5) and van Loghem and associates (22) employ this characteristic as a major criteria to separate paroxysmal cold hemoglobinuria from other cold hemagglutinin syndromes.

Accurate differentiation among the various cryopathic hemolytic anemias is dependent on documenting the physical, chemical and serologic characteristics of the involved cold acting erythrocyte autoantibody (an outline of these characteristics are presented in Table 95, Chapter 19). Four main serologic features are important and within range of routine laboratory testing. These include: (a) Demonstration of a monothermic or bithermic characteristic by performing a Donath-Landsteiner test. (b) Determination of comparative agglutination and hemolysis titers. The Donath-Landsteiner antibody is a potent hemolysin but a weak hemagglutinin. Agglutination titers are generally below 64. The usual cold acting antibody will have agglutination titers substantially over 500. (c) Demonstration of different antigenic specificity. Cold acting erythrocyte autoantibodies will generally have specificity of anti-I or, less frequently, anti-i. The use of adult and cord blood erythrocytes can demonstrate such specificities. In contrast, the Donath-Landsteiner antibody will react equally well with both adult and cord blood erythrocytes. However, this antibody will not lyse the rare p or p_k erythrocytes. (d) The usual cold acting erythrocyte autoantibody is an IgM immunoglobulin and the Donath-Landsteiner antibody is an IgG antibody (128). In the absence of analytic ultracentrifuge or density gradient studies, disulfide reducing agents may permit differentiation. The use of 2-mercaptoethanol or the less odoriferous Cleland's reagent will destroy immunologic reactivity of cold acting erythrocytes but should not influence the activity of the Donath-Landsteiner antibody in the presence of complement.

BIBLIOGRAPHY

1. MacKenzie, G. M.: Paroxysmal hemoglobinuria. Medicine (Balt.) **8**: 159, 1929.
2. Stats, D., and Wasserman, L. R.: Cold hemagglutination—an interpretive review. Medicine (Balt.) **22**: 363, 1943.
3. Dacie, J. V.: *The Haemolytic Anaemias*, Part II, Ed. 2. Grune & Stratton, Inc., New York, 1962.
4. Schubothe, H.: *Serologie und klinische Bedeutung der autohämantikörper*. S. Karger, Basel, 1958.
5. Schubothe, H.: The cold hemagglutinin disease. Seminars Hemat. **3**: 27, 1966.
6. Evans, R. S., Turner, E., and Bingham, M.: Studies with radioiodinated cold agglutinins of ten patients. Amer. J. Med. **38**: 378, 1965.
7. Levin, W C.: Relation of abnormal proteins to formed elements of blood: effects on erythrocytes, leukocytes and platelets. Ann. Rev. Med. **17**: 323, 1966.
8. Landsteiner, K.: Ueber Beziehungen zwischen dem Blutserum und den Körperzellen. Munchen. Med. Wschr. **50**: 1812, 1903.
9. Iwia, S., and Mei-Sai, N.: Etiology of Raynaud's disease (a preliminary report). Jap. Med. World **5**: 119, 1925.
10. Gonzales Guzman, I.: A proposito de la autoagglutinación. Arch. Lat. Amer. Cardiol. Hemat. **3**: 25, 1932.
11. Roth, G.: Paroxysmal hemoglobinuria with vasomotor and agglutinative features. Proc. Mayo Clin. **10**: 609, 1935.
12. Ernstene, A. C., and Gardner, W. J.: The effect of splanchnic nerve resection and sympathetic ganglionectomy in a case of paroxysmal hemoglobinuria. J. Clin. Invest. **14**: 799, 1935.
13. Salén, E. B.: Thermostabiles, nicht komplexes (Auto)hämolysin bei transitorischer Kältehämoglobinurie. Acta Med. Scand. **86**: 570, 1935.
14. Schubothe, H.: Antikörperbedingte hämolytische Anämien. Verh. Deutsch. Ges. Inn. Med. **58**: 679, 1952.
15. Gordon, R. S.: The preparation and properties of cold hemagglutinin. J. Immun. **71**: 220, 1953.
16. Christenson, W. N., and Dacie, J. V.: Serum proteins in acquired haemolytic anaemia (auto-antibody type). Brit. J. Haemat. **3**: 153, 1957.
17. Fudenberg, H. H., and Kunkel, H. G.: Physical properties of red cell agglutinins in acquired hemolytic anemia. J. Exp. Med. **106**: 689, 1957.
18. Wiener, A. S., Unger, L. J., Cohen, L., and Feldman, J: Type-specific cold auto-antibodies as a cause of acquired hemolytic anemia and hemolytic transfusion reactions: biologic test with bovine red cells. Ann. Intern. Med. **44**: 221, 1956.
19. Marsh, W. L.: Anti-i: a cold antibody defining the Ii relationship in human red cells. Brit. J. Haemat. **7**: 200, 1961.
20. van Loghem, J. J., Peetoom, F., van der Hart, M., van der Veer, M., van der Giessen, M., Prins, H. K., Zurcher, C., and Engelfriet, C. P.: Serological and immunochemical studies in haemolytic anaemia with hightitre cold agglutinins. Vox Sang. **8**: 33, 1963.
21. Dausset, J., and Colombani, J.: The serology and the prognosis of 128 cases of autoimmune hemolytic anemia. Blood **14**: 1280, 1959.
22. van Loghem, J. J., van der Hart, M., and Dorfmeier, H.: Serologic studies in acquired hemolytic anemia. In *Proceedings of the Sixth International Congress of the International Society of Hematology*. Grune & Stratton, Inc., New York, 1958.
23. Ben-Ishay, D., Freund, M., and Groen, J. J.: A case of autoimmune hemolytic anemia with circulating cold agglutinins presenting for many years as "hypersplenism" and terminating in leukemia. Blood **22**: 100, 1963.
24. Pasero, G., and Muratorio, A.: Le sindromi neuroemolitche. Sist. Nerv. **12**: 458, 1960.
25. Schubothe, H.: Current problems of chronic cold hemagglutinin disease. Ann. N. Y. Acad. Sci. **124**: 484, 1965.
26. Wiener, A. S.: Origin of naturally occurring hemagglutinins and hemolysins: a review. J. Immun. **66**: 287, 1951.
27. Colomb, D., Croizat, P., Morel, P., Creyssel, R., Jouvenceaux, A., and Desmonceaux, H.: Reticulolymphoblasto-sarcomatosis with acquired hemolytic anemia caused by cold antibodies and cryoglobulinemia having complicated a paraffinoma after 50 years' development. Lyon Med. **94**: 635, 1962.

28. Turro, O. R., and Straface, R. T.: Anemia hemolitica aguda par crioaglutininas. Arch. Argent. Pediat. **63**: 57, 1965.

29. Gökcen, M.: Cryoglobulins behaving as "cold autoantibodies." Postgrad. Med. **39**: 68, 1966.

30. Harris, G., and Fairley, C. H.: Immunological identification of a cryomacroglobulin in a patient with acquired hemolytic anemia associated with a cold antibody. Nature (London) **194**: 1090, 1962.

31. Mehrotra, T. N.: Immunological identification of the pathological cold auto-antibodies of acquired hemolytic anemia as $beta_2$ M globulin. Immunology **3**: 265, 1960.

32. Ritzmann, S. E., and Levin, W. C.: Cold agglutinin disease, a type of primary macroglobulinemia. Texas Rep. Biol. Med. **20**: 236, 1962.

33. Franklin, E. C., and Fudenberg, H. H.: Antigenic heterogeneity of human Rh antibodies, rheumatoid factors, and cold agglutinins. Arch. Biochem. **104**: 433, 1964.

34. Harboe, M., and Deverill, J.: Immunochemical properties of cold haemagglutinins. Scand. J. Haemat. **1**: 223, 1964.

35. Harboe, M., van Furth, R., Schubothe, H., Lind, G., and Evans, R. S.: Exclusive occurrence of kappa chains in isolated cold haemagglutinins. Scand. J. Haemat. **2**: 259, 1965.

36. Costea, N., Yakulis, V., and Heller, P.: Light-chain heterogeneity of cold agglutinins. Science **152**: 1520, 1966.

37. van Furth, R., Diesselhoff-den Dulk, M.: The formation in vitro of cold auto-hemagglutinins with anti-I specificity. J. Immun. **96**: 920, 1966.

38. Leddy, J. P., and Bakemeier, R. F.: Structural aspects of human erythrocyte autoantibodies. I. L chain types and electrophoretic dispersion. J. Exp. Med. **121**: 1, 1965.

39. Eyster, E. M., Nachman, R. L., Christenson, W. N., and Engle, R. L.: Structural characteristics of red cell autoantibodies. J. Immun. **96**: 107, 1966.

40. Feizi, T.: Lambda chains in cold agglutinins. Science **156**: 1111, 1967.

41. Andersen, B. R.: Gamma-A cold agglutinin. Importance of disulfide bonds in activity and structure. Science **154**: 281, 1966.

42. Clough, M. C., and Richter, I. M.: A study of an autoagglutinin occurring in a human serum. Johns Hopkins Hosp. Bull. **29**: 86, 1918.

43. Horstmann, D. M., and Tatlock, H.: Cold agglutinins: a diagnostic aid in certain types of primary atypical pneumonia. J. A. M. A. **122**: 369, 1943.

44. Turner, J. C., Nisnewitz, S., Jackson, E. B., and Berney, R.: Relation of cold agglutinins to atypical pneumonia. Lancet **1**: 765, 1943.

45. Florman, A. L., and Weiss, A. B.: Serologic reactions in primary atypical pneumonia. J. Lab. Clin. Med. **30**: 902, 1945.

46. Young, L. E.: The clinical significance of cold hemagglutinins. Amer. J. Med. Sci. **211**: 23, 1946.

47. Finland, M., Peterson, O. L., Allen, H. E., Samper, B. A., Barnes, M. W., and Stone, M. B.: Cold agglutinins. I. Occurrence of cold isohemagglutinins in various conditions. J. Clin. Invest. **24**: 451, 1945.

48. Finland, M., and Barnes, M. W.: Cold agglutinins. Arch. Intern. Med. (Chicago) **101**: 462, 1958.

49. Peterson, O. L., Ham, T. H., and Finland, M.: Cold agglutinins (autohemagglutinins) in primary atypical pneumonias. Science **97**: 167, 1943.

50. Dameshek, W.: Cold hemagglutinins in acute hemolytic reactions in association with sulfonamide medication and infection. J. A. M. A. **123**: 77, 1943.

51. Neely, F. L., Baria, W. H., Smith, C., and Stone, C. F.: Primary atypical pneumonia with high titer of cold hemagglutinins, hemolytic anemia and false positive Donath-Landsteiner test. J. Lab. Clin. Med. **37**: 383, 1951.

52. Stewart, J. W., and Friedlander, P. H.: Haemoglobinuria and acute haemolytic anaemia associated with primary atypical pneumonia. Lancet **2**: 774, 1957.

53. Moeschlin, S., Siegenthaler, W., Gasser, C., and Hässig, A.: Immunopancytopenia associated with incomplete cold hemagglutinins in a case of primary atypical pneumonia. Blood **9**: 214, 1954.

54. Jenkins, W. J., and Marsh, W. L.: Glandular fever and cold agglutinins. Lancet **1**: 1158, 1966.

55. Schmidt, P. J., Barile, M. F., and McGinniss, M. H.: Mycoplasma (pleuropneumonia-like organisms) and blood group I. Associations with neoplastic disease. Nature (London) **205**: 371, 1965.

56. Smith, C. B., McGinniss, M. H., and Schmidt, P. J.: Changes in erythrocyte I agglutinogen and anti-I agglutinins during mycoplasma pneumoniae infection in man. J. Immun. **99**: 333, 1967.

57. Thomas, L.: Circulating autoantibodies and human disease. With a note on primary atypical pneumonia. New Eng. J. Med. **270**: 1157, 1964.

58. Barile, M. F.: Mycoplasma (PPLO), leukemia and autoimmune disease. In *Methodological Approaches to the Study of Leukemias*. Wistar Institute Press, Philadelphia, 1965.

59. Costea, N., Yakulis, V., and Heller, P.: Experimental production of cold agglutinins in rabbits. Blood **26**: 323, 1965.

60. Laroche, C., Milliez, P., Dreyfus, B., Dausset, J., and Leprat, J.: Ictère hémolytique aigu post-grippal. Bull. Soc. Med. Hop. Paris **67**: 779, 1951.

61. Ventura, S., and Aresu, G.: Grave anemia immuno-emolitica in decorso di influenza cosidetta "asiatica." Rass. Med. Sarda **59**: 609, 1957.

62. Puxeddu, A., Colonua, A., Nenci, G. G., et al.: Su di un raro caso di anemia emolitica autoimmune da virus influenzale B. Haematologica **50**: 1073, 1965.

63. Springer, G. F., and Ansell, N. J.: Inactivation of human erythrocyte agglutinogens M and N by influenza viruses and receptor-destroying enzyme. Proc. Nat. Acad. Sci. USA **44**: 182, 1958.

64. Fekete, A. M., and Kerpelman, E. J.: Acute hemolytic anemia complicating infectious mononucleosis. J. A. M. A. **194**: 1326, 1965.

65. Marsh, W. L., and Jenkins, W. J.: Anti-i: a new cold antibody. Nature (London) **188**: 753, 1960.

66. Rosenfield, R. E., Schmidt, P. J., Calvo, R. C., and McGinniss, M. H.: Anti-i, a frequent cold agglutinin in infectious mononucleosis. Vox Sang. **10**: 631, 1965.

67. Calvo, R., Stein, W., Kochwa, S., and Rosenfield, R. E.: Acute hemolytic anemia due to anti-i: frequent cold agglutinins in infectious mononucleosis. J. Clin. Invest. **44**: 1033, 1965.

68. Wollheim, F. A., and Williams, R. C.: Studies on the macroglobulins of human serum. 1. Polyclonal immunoglobulin class M (IgM) increase in infectious mononucleosis. New Eng. J. Med. **274**: 61, 1966.

69. Jenkins, W. J., Koster, H. G., Marsh, W. L., and Carter, R. L.: Infectious mononucleosis: an unsuspected source of anti-i. Brit. J. Haemat. **11**: 480, 1965.

70. Troxel, D. B., Innella, F., and Cohen, R. J.: Infectious mononucleosis complicated by hemolytic anemia due to anti-i. Amer. J. Clin. Path. **46**: 625, 1966.

71. Kostinas, J. E., and Cantow, E. F.: Studies on infectious mononucleosis. II. Autohemolysis. Amer. J. Med. Sci. **252**: 296, 1966.

72. Worlledge, S. M.: Serologic aspects of the auto-immune haemolytic anaemia. In *Autoimmunity,* edited by R. W. Baldwin and J. H. Humphrey. Blackwell Scientific Publications Ltd., Oxford, 1965.

73. Betke, K., Richerz, H., Schubothe, H., and Vivell, O.: Beobachtungen zu Krankheitsbild, Pathogenese und Ätiologie der akuten erworbenen häemolytischen Anämie (Lederer-anämie). Klin. Wschr. **31**: 373, 1953.

74. Vivell, O.: Ergebnisse virologischer Studien bei Fällen von akuter hämolytischer Anämie (Lederer-Brill). Mschr. Kinderheilk. **102**: 113, 1954.

75. Borbolla, L., and Barquet Chediak, A.: Anemia hemolítica de etiología viral (revisión de la literatura). Presentación de un caso en la convalescencia de una varicela con Coombs positivo. Rev. Cubana Pediat. **25**: 557, 1953.

76. Unger, L. J., Wiener, A. S., and Dolan, D.: Anémie autohémolytique chez un nouveauné. Rev. Hemat. (Paris) **7**: 495, 1952.

77. Copps, S. C.: Primary atypical pneumonia with hemolytic anemia and erythema multiforme. Clin. Pediat. (Phila.) **3**: 491, 1964.

78. Alexander, H. L., and Thompson, L. D.: Autohemagglutination in chronic leukemia. Report of a case. J. A. M. A. **85**: 1707, 1925.

79. Boxwell, W., and Bigger, J. W.: Autohemagglutination. J. Path. Bact. **34**: 407, 1931.

80. Manheims, P. J., and Brunner, E. K.: Faulty blood grouping due to autoagglutinins; an unusual case. J. A. M. A. **101**: 207, 1933.

81. Rosenthal, M. C., Pisciotta, A. V., Komninos, Z. D., Goldenberg, H., and Dameshek, W.: The auto-immune hemolytic anemia of malignant lymphocytic disease. Blood **10**: 197, 1955.

82. Ritzmann, S. E., Lang, P. H., and Levin, W. C.: Multiple paraproteinemia with cold agglutinin syndrome in malignant lymphoma. Texas Rep. Biol. Med. **20**: 251, 1962.

83. Yunis, E. J., and Bridges, R. H.: Blood transfusion problems in auto-immune hemolytic anemia. Minnesota Med. **49**: 759, 1966.

84. Elliotson, J.: Diseases of the heart united with ague. Lancet **1**: 500, 1832.

85. Dressler, Dr.: Ein Fall von intermittierender Albuminurie und Chromaturie. Virchow. Arch. Path. Anat. **6**: 264, 1854.

86. Harley, G.: On intermittent haematuria. Med. Chir. Trans. **48**: 161, 1865.

87. Dickinson, W. H.: Notes on four cases of intermittent haematuria. Lancet **1**: 568, 1865.

88. Hassall, A. H.: On intermittent, or winter, haematuria. Lancet **2**: 368, 1865.

89. Pavy, F. W.: On paroxysmal haematuria. Lancet **2**: 33, 1868.

90. Gull, W. W.: Intermittent haematinuria. Guy Hosp. Rep., Third Ser. **12**: 381, 1866.

91. Secchi, –.: Ein Fall von Hamoglobinurie. Berlin. Klin. Wschr. **9**: 237, 1872.

92. Lichtheim, L.: Ueber periodische Hämoglobinurie. Sammlung. Klin. Vortrage **134**: 1147, 1876.

93. "D" (anonymous): Periodic hemoglobinuria. Med. Times Gaz. **1**: 215, 1879.

94. Küssner, B.: Paroxysmale Hämoglobinurie. Deutsh. Med. Wschr. **5**: 475, 1879.

95. Rosenbach, O.: Beitrag zur Lehre von der periodischen Hämoglobinurie. Berlin. Klin. Wschr. **17**: 132, 157, 1880.

96. Ehrlich, P.: Ueber paroxysmale Hämoglobinurie. Deutsch. Med. Wschr. **7**: 224, 1881.

97. Popper, M.: Nervöse Hämoglobinurie. Ostrei. Z. Prakt. Heilk. **14**: 657, 1868.

98. Murri, A.: Emoglobinuria e sifilide. Rev. Clin. Bologna, Ser. 3, **241**: 321, 1885.

99. Chvostek, F.: *Über das Wesen der Parox-*

ysmalen Hämoglobinurie. Franz Deuticke, Wien, 1894.

100. Götze, L.: Beitrag zur Lehre von der paroxysmalen Hämoglobinurie. Berlin. Klin. Wschr. **21**: 716, 1884.
101. Ehrlich, P., and Morgenroth, J.: Ueber Hämolysine. Zwiete Mittheilung. Berlin. Klin. Wschr. **36**: 481, 1899.
102. Donath, J., and Landsteiner, K.: Ueber paroxysmalen Hämoglobinurie. Munchen. Med. Wschr. **51**: 1590, 1904.
103. Eason, J.: The pathology of paroxysmal haemoglobinuria. J. Path. Bact. **11**: 167, 1906.
104. Widal, F., and Rostaine, –.: Sérothérapie préventive de l'attaque d'hémoglobinurie paroxystique. C. R. Soc. Biol. (Paris) **58**: 397, 1905.
105. Langstein, L.: Paroxysmale Hämoglobinurie und Hämaturie im Kindesalter. Med. Klin. **45**: 1140, 1905.
106. Jones, B. B., and Jones, C. M.: Paroxysmal hemoglobinuria. In *Nelson Loose-Leaf Living Medicine*, **4**: 173A. Thomas Nelson & Sons, New York, 1920–1929.
107. Thurmon, F., and Blain, D.: Paroxysmal hemoglobinuria; Observations based upon study of three cases. Amer. J. Syph. **15**: 350, 1931.
108. Howard, C. P., Mills, F. S., and Townsend, S. R.: Paroxysmal hemoglobinuria with report of case. Amer. J. Med. Sci. **196**: 772, 1938.
109. Becker, R. M.: Paroxysmal cold hemoglobinurias. Arch. Intern. Med. (Chicago) **81**: 630, 1948.
110. Nabarro, D.: *Congenital Syphilis*. Eward Arnold Publishers Ltd., London, 1954.
111. Hoppe, H. H., and Witte, A.: Hämolytische Erkrankung eines Neugeborenen bei paroxysmaler Kältehämoglobinurie der Mutter. Vox Sang. **5**: 425, 1960.
112. Vos, G. H., Celano, M. J., Falkowski, F., and Levine, P.: Relationship of a hemolysin resembling anti-Tjᵃ to threatened abortion in Western Australia. Transfusion **4**: 87, 1964.
113. Matsuo, J.: Über die Klinischen und serologischen Untersuchungen der paroxysmalen Hämoglobinurie, zugleich ein Beitrag zur Kenntnis der Isolysine. Deutsch. Arch. Klin. Med. **107**: 335, 1912.
114. Orel, H.: Kältehämoglobinurie bei Zwillingen. Z. Kinderheilk. **41**: 756, 1926.
115. Macalister, G. H. K.: The pathology of paroxysmal haemoglobinuria. A critical review. Quart. J. Med. **2**: 368, 1908.

116. Moss, W. L.: Paroxysmal hemoglobinuria; blood studies in three cases. Johns Hopkins Hosp. Bull. **22**: 238, 1911.
117. Harris, K. E., Lewis, T., and Vaughan, J. M.: Haemoglobinuria and urticaria from cold occurring singly or in combination: observations referring especially to the mechanism of urticaria with some remarks on Raynaud's disease. Heart (London) **14**: 305, 1929.
118. Montagnani, M.: Crise hémoclassique et hémoglobinurie paroxystique. Presse Med. **29**: 1017, 1921.
119. Donath, J., and Lansteiner, K.: Ueber Kältehämoglobinurie. Ergebn. Hyg. Bakt. **7**: 184, 1925.
120. Lazzati, T., and Sorgente, P.: Ueber einen Fall von paroxysmaler Hämoglobinurie. Klinische Beobachtungen und experimentelle Untersuchungen. Arch. Kinderheilk. **32**: 183, 1901.
121. Widal, F., Abrami, P., and Brissaud, E.: Recherches sur l'hémoglobinurie paroxystique "a frigore." Sem. Med. **33**: 585, 1913.
122. Uchida, H.: Über die Erythrophagozytose der Leukozyten, besonders bei der paroxysmalen Hämoglobinurie. Mitt. Med. Fak. Tokio **26**: 503, 1921.
123. Jordan, W. S., Prouty, R. L., Heinle, R. W., and Dingle, J. H.: The mechanism of hemolysis in paroxysmal cold hemoglobinuria. III. Erythrophagocytosis and leukopenia. Blood **7**: 387, 1952.
124. Leonardi, P., and Andolfatto-Zaglia, G.: Emoglobinuria parossistica a frigore non luetica da anticorpo bifasico tipo Donath e Landsteiner. Minnerva Med. **51**: 453, 1960.
125. Ehrlich, P.: Ueber paroxysmale Hämoglobinurie. In *Farbeanalytische Untersuchungen zur Histologie und Klinik des Blutes*. Hirschweld, Berlin, 1891.
126. Kumagai, T., and Namba, M.: Weitere Beiträge zur Kenntnis der paroxysmalen Hämoglobinurie. Dutsch. Arch. Klin. Med. **156**: 257, 1927.
127. Burmeister, J.: Ueber paroxysmale Hämoglobinurie und Syphilis; Zugleich ein Bietrag zum Problem der Erkältungskrankheiten. Z. Klin. Med. **92**: 19, 1921.
128. Hinz, C. F.: Serologic and physicochemical characterization of Donath-Landsteiner antibodies from six patients. Blood **22**: 600, 1963.
129. Nelson, M. G., and Nicholl, B.: Paroxysmal cold haemoglobinuria. Irish J. Med. Sci., Sixth Ser. **410**: 49, 1960.

Chapter 12

Therapy of the Autoimmune Hemolytic Anemias

The autoimmune hemolytic anemias are not a homogeneous disease entity. Variations exist in the magnitude and rapidity of hemolysis, in the association of additional pathologic states and in the comparative clinical influences of these two factors. This heterogeneity is particularly apparent in devising efficient therapeutic procedures. A large number of approaches have been advocated. This in itself indicates the unavailability of a completely satisfactory therapy.

Corticosteroid Therapy

Historical Review

In 1944 Dougherty and associates (1) described a lympholytic effect of pituitary-adrenal cortical activity. Fischel and associates (2) confirmed this and noticed a slight fall in circulating antibody titer. In 1951 Dameshek and associates (3) applied these observations to autoimmune hemolytic anemia. They investigated the effect of adrenocorticotrophic hormone (ACTH) administration in five patients. A therapeutic remission was induced in four, although the antiglobulin test remained positive. The oral administration of cortisone was also found to be efficacious. Numerous workers confirmed the therapeutic benefits of corticosteroid therapy.

In 1956 Dameshek and Komninos (4) summarized the effect of corticosteroid therapy in 43 consecutive cases of autoimmune hemolytic anemia. Twenty-one cases were idiopathic and 22 were of a secondary variety (18 examples of chronic lymphocytic leukemia, two cases of systemic lupus erythematosus, one case each of polyarteritis nodosa and cirrhosis). An initial response to corticosteroid therapy was noted in 40 patients. In 28 the remission was complete and in 12 it was partial with the persistence of anemia and reticulocytosis. Corticosteroid therapy was discontinued in 23 patients presenting a satisfactory initial therapeutic response. Fifteen relapsed while eight remained in remission. Twenty-three patients were placed on maintenance therapy and 15 continued in remission. Adequate serologic followups were obtained with 24 patients. In 16 the antiglobulin test was reduced in titer and degree. In three it became negative, only to return to positive in two. In five patients the antiglobulin test persisted unchanged. In 19 of 35 patients the indirect antiglobulin test was positive at the start of therapy. After therapy it became negative or only weakly positive in eight. In the remaining 11 patients it persisted at a lower titer. Dameshek and Komninos (4) summarized their data as follows. An initial therapeutic response to corticosteroids may be anticipated in 90 per cent of cases of autoimmune hemolytic anemia. In 65 per cent a complete remission is seen and in 25 per cent a definite but not spectacular response is noted. Complete failure occurs in less than 10 per cent of cases. When corticosteroid therapy is discontinued a high relapse rate involving two-thirds of the group may be anticipated.

Horster (5) reported the effect of corticosteroid therapy in 167 cases of idiopathic autoimmune hemolytic anemia. A therapeutic response was obtained in 83 per cent of cases with therapeutic failure in 17 per cent. In 6.8 per cent a "cure" was obtained. In an additional 31.7 per cent remission persisted for over 1 year after discontinuation of corticosteroid therapy. In 51 per cent remission continued only while therapy was maintained.

Analysis of Present Series

Adequate clinical data are available for 230 patients of the current series. Of these, 158 or 69 per cent received corticosteroid therapy. In eight patients the effect of corticosteroids could not be determined because of inadequate time (less than 3 days) or because of simultaneous administration of other therapies. The 150 patients with sufficient data were analyzed as to the type of initial response obtained after the start of corticosteroids. Responses were classified as *excellent* if complete remission occurred, *good* if remission occurred in the face of continuing clinical evidence of hemolysis, *poor* if a response could be documented but was inadequate to control the disease process, and *none* if complete therapeutic failure was present. These figures have also been combined into a *therapeutic response* group which includes the *excellent* and *good* categories and *therapeutic failure* group incorporating patients who had *none* or a *poor* response. Table 74 summarizes the results obtained. Of these patients, 57.3 per cent had a therapeutic response to corticosteroid therapy and 42.7 per cent had therapeutic failures. These values are poorer than anticipated in reviewing the literature. Reasons for this discrepancy are apparent when disease categories are separately analyzed.

Response of Idiopathic Autoimmune Hemolytic Anemia

Corticosteroid therapy was highly efficient in combatting idiopathic autoimmune hemolytic anemia. A therapeutic response was obtained in 76 per cent of patients, with a complete remission in 25 of 33 cases. A corticosteroid failure was present in only six cases. It is striking that these six failures included two cases each of the pancytopenic, the aplastic and the erythrocytic aplastic varieties. In the more common erythrocytic and Evans syndrome types, an excellent therapeutic response was almost universal.

Other Categories with Therapeutic Response

An excellent therapeutic response was noted in systemic lupus erythematosus. Of these cases, 75 per cent were considered as excellent or good responders and complete failures were not recorded. Therapeutic responses following corticosteroid therapy were also commonly observed in infectious disease and heart surgery patients. Success rates of 80 and 100 per cent, respectively, were obtained. These latter figures are deceptive and should not be misinterpreted. Only a small number of patients in each category received corticosteroid therapy. In most subjects clinical remission occurred without corticosteroids. Accordingly, a spontaneous remission or remission related to other therapies must be considered, and the outstanding success rate observed with corticosteroids should be minimized. A similar interpretation is indicated for the 61.5 per cent therapeutic success rate recorded in the "other secondary forms" category.

Reticuloendothelial Neoplasia

The therapeutic response obtained in patients with an associated reticuloendothelial neoplasia was poor in contrast with that seen in idiopathic autoimmune hemolytic anemia. A 50 per cent response rate to corticosteroid therapy was obtained in chronic lymphocytic leukemia. Less satisfactory results were encountered in other forms of reticuloendothelial malignancies. A 60 per cent failure rate was found in this patient category. Treatment of the lymphomas with corticosteroids was moderately successful. However, the other forms of leukemia associated with auto-

TABLE 74. *Therapeutic effect of corticosteroid therapy in autoimmune hemolytic anemia (AHA)**

Diagnosis, AHA	Patients Who Received Steroids	Therapeutic Response					
		Excellent	Good	Poor	None	Success	Failure
							%
Idiopathic	*33*†	*25*	0	*2*	*6*	76	24
Secondary varieties							
Chronic lymphocytic leukemia	*40*	*11*	*9*	*3*	*17*	50	50
Acute lymphocytic leukemia	9	2	1	1	5	33	67
Granulocytic leukemia	5	0	1	1	3	20	80
Acute monocytic leukemia	10	0	1	0	9	10	90
Hodgkin's disease	10	2	4	2	2	60	40
Lymphosarcoma	4	1	2	0	1	75	25
Reticulum cell sarcoma	3	3	0	0	0	100	0
Giant follicular lymphoma	1	0	0	0	1	0	100
Plasma cell myeloma	5	2	0	1	2	40	60
Reticuloendothelial neoplasia, total	*47*	*10*	*9*	*5*	*23*	40	60
Infections	*5*	*4*	0	0	*1*	80	20
Lupus erythematosus	*8*	*3*	*3*	*2*	0	75	25
Heart surgery	*4*	*2*	*2*	0	0	100	0
Other secondary forms	*13*	*5*	*3*	*1*	*4*	62	38
ENTIRE TOTAL	150	60	26	13	51	57	43

* Patient load:

> 234 patients had autoimmune hemolytic anemia
> 230 patients had adequate clinical data
> 158 patients received prednisone
> 150 patients were evaluated for prednisone effect
> 72 patients did not receive prednisone

† Figures in italics are those contributing to the entire total.

immune hemolytic anemia were generally resistant to this therapeutic approach.

Current Status of Corticosteroid Therapy

The above studies suggest that corticosteroid therapy is valuable in autoimmune hemolytic anemia. Its effectiveness, however, is not universal. Its inadequacy is particularly apparent with secondary forms of autoimmune hemolytic anemia. The suggestion that autoimmune hemolytic anemia is only one manifestation of a systemic immunologic deficiency disease supplies some rationale for these results. In the relatively uncomplicated stage of this syndrome (idiopathic autoimmune hemolytic anemia), corticosteroid therapy is effective. With additional defects reflecting multiple autoantibody formation, the efficacy of such therapy is less impressive. If malignancy results from the same immune deficient state this dominates the overall clinical prognosis with corticosteroids appearing less effective.

Type of Corticosteroid Preparation

ACTH therapy was rarely employed in the current series. Cortisone was initially used in several patients and hydrocortisone was given in a larger number. The great majority of patients were treated with prednisone, with significant numbers receiving prednisolone, triamcinolone and dexamethasone. The following general conclusions may be drawn. All forms of corticosteroid therapy were mutually interchangeable. The observation of Dameshek and Komninos (4) that prednisone and cortisone might have variable clinical effects at equilibrant doses was not confirmed. Dacie's observation (6) that ACTH might rarely be more efficient was not duplicated in the current series. A crucial factor is the establishment of equilibrant doses of various corticosteroid preparations. In our laboratory the following dose levels have had comparable effects in autoimmune hemolytic anemia: cortisone 300 mg., hydrocortisone 240 mg., prednisone 60 mg., prednisolone 60 mg., triamcinolone 48 mg. and dexamethasone 9 mg.

Side Effects

Undesirable side effects were universally encountered during effective corticosteroid therapy. Differences have been observed with various preparations and such differences may dictate the preferable agent. Cortisone is undesirable with extreme cushingoid changes, a high incidence of osteoporosis, fluid retention, gastric ulcers and psychosis. Hydrocortisone had a similar distribution but less marked incidence of side effects. Prednisone and prednisolone were similar. Cushingoid changes and fluid retention are less than with cortisone, and psychosis is extremely rare with these two drugs. Unfortunately, osteoporosis and gastric ulcers are common. Neither triamcinolone nor dexamethasone has solved this problem. Occasionally we have seen less fluid retention with triamcinolone. This benefit has been overshadowed by the occasional development of quadriceps myopathy. Dexamethasone had effects similar to those of prednisone and prednisolone. Accordingly, on a cost basis the current drug of choice is prednisone. However, the clinician must accept cushingoid changes, osteoporosis, fluid retention, susceptibility to infections and gastric ulcers at the dose level employed in the initial treatment of autoimmune hemolytic anemia. Weight gain, hyperactivity, nervousness, irritability, purpura, myopathy and poor wound healing are all commonly seen in various combinations with the above side effects.

One additional complication deserves emphasis. There is a high incidence of latent and overt diabetes in patients with autoimmune hemolytic anemia. Whether this reflects the age distribution of involved patients or whether it is a significant part of the immune aberration is still to be determined. The clinician must be aware of this relationship and should closely observe patients receiving corticosteroid therapy for activation or intensification of diabetes. Routine urine analysis must be performed if severe ketosis is to be avoided.

Dosage of Corticosteroids

High levels of corticosteroids are required for the treatment of autoimmune hemolytic anemia. Initial therapy almost always requires 60 mg. of prednisone daily. An attempt to reduce this dosage after remission must be made and generally can be accomplished. The reduced level necessary to maintain remission is highly variable. In some patients therapy may be discontinued and a clinical "cure" may result. More commonly, maintenance therapy will have to be given. In most patients maintenance requires 10 to 30 mg. of prednisone daily. It is doubtful whether daily maintenance doses of 2.5 to 5.0 mg. are of value, although the author has frequently employed them. If relapse occurs, 45 mg. of prednisone daily will generally induce remission. In some cases a return to the daily 60-mg. level is required. Failure to induce remission, initially or after relapse, with 60 mg. of prednisone daily is a disastrous prognostic sign. High levels of dosage, e.g., of 80, 90 and 120 mg., have been employed by many investigators. In the author's experience this approach has little if any value. In a few instances remissions were induced with higher levels of dosage. It is probable that a continuation of prednisone at the 60-mg. level would have resulted in the same remission.

Characteristics of the Remission State

Symptomatic improvement frequently occurs before a hematologic response is apparent. This usually involves a loss of malaise, improvement of appetite, increased strength, less fatigue, disappearance of fever and a feeling of well being. The clinician should be cautioned from

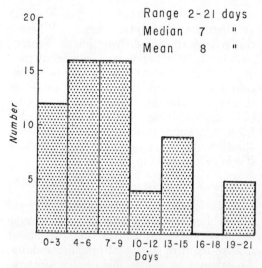

FIGURE 12. The time in days for an initial therapeutic response to corticosteroid therapy in 62 patients with autoimmune hemolytic anemia. Only six subjects required longer than 14 days to initiate a response.

placing too much significance on these symptomatic benefits. A mild euphoric state is commonly seen with corticosteroid therapy. It is not uncommon to observe symptomatic improvement in the face of hematologic evidence of a therapeutic failure.

Remission is interpreted as hematologic evidence of reduced hemolysis. Reticulocytosis is frequently the first evidence of a therapeutic response. This observation is less significant when high levels of reticulocytes are found prior to therapy. In such cases reversal of a rapidly falling hematocrit is the first observation. Stabilization of the hematocrit, even at a low level, generally indicates that an elevation will shortly occur. Serum bilirubin values are of less significance and decrease slowly after the hematocrit and reticulocyte counts indicate remission.

The time of onset of the initial response to corticosteroids is rapid but variable. Pertinent data were available in 62 of the 86 patients in the current series who underwent therapeutic remission. The data are summarized in Figure 12. A range extending from 2 to 21 days was seen, with a median response rate of 7 and a mean of

8.1 days. In only six patients was a therapeutic response delayed for longer than 2 weeks. Although therapeutic effects have occasionally been observed after 21 days of therapy, the response is generally poor and the patient requires persistently high prednisone dosages. It is wise to consider such cases as therapeutic failures and to arrange for more efficient therapy. A lack of therapeutic response after 3 weeks is usually an ominous prognostic sign. The following case history illustrates a delayed therapeutic response followed by remission.

Case 100. A 22-year-old white female developed weakness, pallor, tinnitus, anorexia, palpitations and jaundice. Physical examination revealed retinal hemorrhages and a spleen palpated 4 cm. below the costal margin. The hematocrit was 13.5 per cent, the red blood cell count was 940,000/mm.[3] and the reticulocyte count was 4.8 per cent. The serum bilirubin was 2.4/4.6 mg. per cent, the albumin-globulin (A/G) ratio was 5.0/3.6 gm. per cent and serum electrophoresis revealed a broad elevation of the gamma-globulin. Lupus erythematosus (LE) cell tests and serologic tests for syphilis were negative. Bone marrow aspiration demonstrated erythrocytic hyperplasia with megaloblastic changes. The Schilling test was negative. A Cr^{51} half-life (T/2) of 8.9 days, without splenic sequestration, was found. Strong positive direct and indirect antiglobulin and bromelin tests were obtained. Eluates revealed a panhemagglutinating erythrocyte autoantibody. Prednisone, 60 mg. daily, was given. The hematocrit dropped to 11.5 per cent and the reticulocyte count elevated to 12.2 per cent. For the next 21 days the hematocrit and the reticulocyte count remained at this level. Transfusions were withheld and strict bedrest was maintained. Three weeks after the start of prednisone the hematocrit rapidly rose to 20.5 per cent and continued to rise. One week later it reached 27 per cent and 11 weeks after the start of therapy it reached 39.5 per cent. Prednisone was reduced at the start of remission and was gradually decreased over the next 6 months when it was discontinued. Marked migratory polyarthritis developed with each reduction of prednisone therapy. Such episodes only persisted for 2 to 3 days. The spleen remained palpable. Remission continued without corticosteroids for 6 months. At that time abdominal trauma occurred with left upper quadrant pain. A splenectomy was performed. Hematologic remission has continued for an additional 6 months of followup without prednisone therapy. Direct and indirect antiglobulin tests became negative 11 months after therapy, but direct and indirect bromelin tests are still strongly positive.

As a general rule normal or stable hematocrit and reticulocyte values will be found 30 to 90 days after the initiation of therapy. Pertinent data are available for 56 patients of the current series and are summarized in Figure 13. A range of time for stabilization of the hematocrit extended from 6 to 150 days. The mean and median time for stabilization was approximately 2 months. In only six patients was stabilization delayed for longer than 3 months.

Remission hematocrit values were available for 77 of the 86 patients in the current series who showed a therapeutic response. In 53 patients (68.8 per cent) normal hematocrit values were ultimately obtained. In the remaining 24 patients the hematocrit was still reduced but was over 30 per cent.

Hematologic remission frequently occurs while direct antiglobulin tests remain positive and splenomegaly persists. The effect of corticosteroid therapy on hepatosplenomegaly and lymphadenopathy is highly variable. Such organ enlargement is generally corrected in idiopathic autoimmune hemolytic anemia, although delays as long as 6 months are not unusual. Transient improvements may also be seen in secondary types. When leukemia or lymphoma is present, reduction of organomegaly frequently parallels a tumorcidal effect of corticosteroids, rather than correction of the hemolytic process. Persisting splenomegaly and lymphadenopathy in idiopathic autoimmune hemolytic anemia 6 months after hematologic remission are an indication to search for an associated pathologic state.

Characteristics of the Relapse Stage

Relapse after discontinuation of or while receiving maintenance prednisone therapy almost always occurs within 6 months. Careful observation is important during this period of time. In the current series adequate data were available in 75 of the 86 patients who had a therapeutic response to corticosteroids. Thirty-nine patients (52

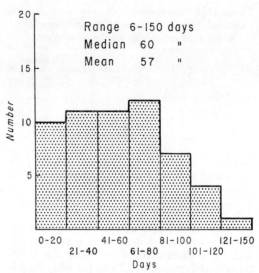

FIGURE 13. The time in days required for stabilization of the therapeutic response to corticosteroid therapy in 56 patients with autoimmune hemolytic anemia. Only six subjects required longer periods than 3 months for stabilization.

per cent) relapsed. In nine, relapse occurred after discontinuation of corticosteroids. In the remaining 30, relapse developed while they were receiving maintenance drug therapy. The median and mean dose level of prednisone at the time of relapse approximated 20 mg. daily. Table 75 summarizes these figures. Relapse seldom develops precipitously, although it can so occur. The following patient, seen through the courtesy of Dr. M. S. Cordova, illustrates a severe relapse presenting as hemolytic crisis.

Case 101. A 51-year-old Mexican female was hospitalized with abdominal pain, anorexia, malaise, chills, fever and jaundice. Physical examination revealed only jaundice and pallor. The hematocrit was 14 per cent, the hemoglobin was 4.3 gm. per cent and the reticulocyte count was 83.4 per cent. Spherocytes and nucleated erythrocytes were found in the peripheral blood. Serum bilirubin was 1.74/4.12 mg. per cent, the A/G ratio was 4.8/2.6 gm. per cent and a normal serum electrophoresis was present. LE cell preparations and serologic tests for syphilis were negative. Direct and indirect antiglobulin and bromelin tests were strongly positive. A panhemagglutinating erythrocyte autoantibody and iso-anti-E were demonstrated in eluates. Complete hemolysis occurred with the autoantibody

TABLE 75. *Characteristics of the corticosteroid induced remission in autoimmune hemolytic anemia (75 patients in remission analyzed)*

Group	No. of Patients	Prednisone Therapy		Corticosteroid Therapy (Amount of Prednisone Continued)		
		Discontinued	Continued	Range	Mean	Median
				mg.		
Relapse	39	9	30	2.5–60	23	20
Continued re-mission	36	20	16	2.5–40	14	10

and test erythrocytes at pH 6.5. Cold hemagglutinins were not found. Prednisone, 150 mg. daily, was started. After 24 hours the hemoglobin had decreased to 2.7 gm. per cent. Prednisone was increased to 240 mg. daily and one transfusion was given without reaction. Two days later the hematocrit reached 17 per cent and the reticulocyte count reached 51.5 per cent. Nine days after the start of prednisone therapy, progressive reduction in dosage was initiated. Thirty-two days later prednisone, 20 mg. daily, was being given, and the hematocrit was 42 per cent with a 1.8 per cent reticulocyte count. Hematologic remission was still apparent 3 weeks later with a stable hematocrit. Prednisone was decreased and finally discontinued 76 days after the start of therapy. Two days later malaise and fatigue were noted. Four days later fever and jaundice became apparent. The hematocrit had dropped to 13 per cent and the reticulocyte count was 59 per cent. Nucleated erythrocytes and spherocytes were common in the peripheral blood. Direct and indirect antiglobulin and bromelin tests were negative and the acid hemolysin could no longer be demonstrated. Bone marrow aspiration revealed erythrocytic hyperplasia. Serum bilirubin was 1.0/1.5 mg. per cent. Prednisone, 240 mg. daily, was started and 2 days later the patient was asymptomatic with a rapidly rising hematocrit. Followup 1 month after restarting therapy demonstrated a hematocrit of 44 per cent and a reticulocyte count of 4 per cent. Prednisone, 40 mg. daily, was being administered.

Several interesting observations are present in this patient. Rapidly decreasing and finally discontinuing prednisone therapy in 76 days resulted in a precipitous drop of the hematocrit from 42 to 13 per cent. Symptoms developed within 2 days of stopping prednisone therapy. The second hemolytic crisis, which appeared identical with the initial episode, developed in the absence of demonstrable autoantibodies. Fortunately, remission was again induced with corticosteroid therapy.

Relapse is usually gradual, with a sufficient hematologic warning to the clinician. Gradual reduction of the hematocrit and an elevation of the reticulocyte count is generally observed. A decrease of the hematocrit to 30 per cent or lower is an indication that higher doses of prednisone are needed. Elevation of the reticulocyte count while the hematocrit remains stable is considered to indicate relapse. However, the episode may be transient and increased therapy may be withheld until the hematocrit falls. Infectious disease may frequently precipitate this pattern. An infectious process may also initiate a rapid fall of both the reticulocyte count and the hematocrit.

Corticosteroid Induced "Cures"

In the current series relapse did not occur in 36 patients after a remission induced by corticosteroids. In 20 patients, remission continued after prednisone therapy was discontinued. In 14 of these 20 patients idiopathic autoimmune hemolytic anemia or a secondary type involving infectious disease or aortic valve prosthesis was present. Of the remaining six patients, four had malignancies and one each had ulcerative colitis and thyroiditis. It is difficult to classify any of these cases as "cured," with the exception of the heart surgery and infectious disease patients. All four patients with malignancies died less than 6 months after remission without a return of hemolytic anemia. One of the idiopathic cases (Case 73) died 46 months after discontinuation of prednisone without relapse; autopsy, however, revealed toxic hepatitis. Several patients have been free of hemolytic anemia for over 5 years since discontinuation of prednisone. Considering such patients as "cured" is questionable. Case 62 illustrates a typical patient in whom relapse of hemolytic anemia has not occurred 83 months after discontinuation of prednisone. However, the patient has developed discoid lupus erythematosus. It is probable that a fundamental immunologic aberration is still present and has not been corrected by prior corticosteroid therapy.

In 16 patients hematologic remission has continued while receiving maintenance prednisone therapy. The drug dosage employed varies from 2.5 to 40 mg. of prednisone daily, with a mean of 14 and a median of 10 mg. It is striking that the dosages of prednisone sufficient to maintain remission are lower than values permitting relapse in other patients. These data are summarized in Table 75.

Remission and Antiglobulin Tests

Two major serologic observations may be made during a corticosteroid induced remission. Direct antiglobulin tests generally remain positive for a variable period of time in spite of excellent hematologic remissions (4, 6–9). The degree of agglutination in the direct antiglobulin test may be reduced. Evans and associates (10) emphasized that, although positive direct antiglobulin tests are usually observed, less autoantibody is bound to the erythrocyte surface. It is common to find positive direct antiglobulin tests 6 months and even 1 year after hematologic remission. Positive direct bromelin tests may persist in spite of negative direct antiglobulin tests years after remission. The significance of such persisting reactions is unknown. The clinician should therefore not rely on the direct antiglobulin test to evaluate the state of remission and the necessity of starting or increasing corticosteroid therapy.

Several investigators have noted that clinical remission may be associated with reduction or disappearance of positive indirect antiglobulin tests (4, 6, 7, 9). In the current series indirect bromelin tests tended to persist longer and at higher titers than indirect antiglobulin tests, although parallel results were seen. The significance of this observation is unknown. Dausset and Colombani (9) emphasized the prognostic significance of the indirect antiglobulin test. In their patient group which re-

TABLE 76. *Serologic data obtained in 147 patients with autoimmune hemolytic anemia who received corticosteroid therapy (82 patients had a therapeutic response and 65 patients had a therapeutic failure)*

Testing	Therapeutic Response Group		Therapeutic Failure Group	
	No. positive/ no. tested	Positive	No. positive/ no. tested	Positive
		%		%
Initial				
Direct				
Antiglobulin	78/82	95	64/65	99
Bromelin	66/78	85	44/61	72
Indirect				
Antiglobulin	30/54	56	10/31	32
Bromelin	34/49	69	11/25	44
Followup				
Direct				
Antiglobulin	38/74	51	9/40	23
Bromelin	33/63	52	15/36	42
Indirect				
Antiglobulin	33/52	64	4/24	17
Bromelin	19/50	38	8/23	35

sponded to therapy ("cured groups"), 18.5 per cent had positive indirect antiglobulin tests and 61.5 per cent had positive indirect trypsin tests. In contrast, patients with autoimmune hemolytic anemia who died had a 53 per cent incidence of positive indirect antiglobulin tests and an 85 per cent incidence of indirect trypsin tests.

The significance of the indirect antiglobulin test could not be confirmed in the current study. Serologic data were available in 147 patients who received corticosteroid therapy. The analysis of this group is presented in Table 76. Eight-two of these patients had a therapeutic response classified as excellent or good. Sixty-five patients were considered as therapeutic failures. Serologic studies at the start of therapy gave no indication of the therapeutic response subsequently obtained. The group who responded had stronger direct antiglobulin reactions and a higher incidence of positive indirect antiglobulin and bromelin tests than did patients who subsequently presented therapeutic failures. After prednisone therapy direct antiglobulin tests reverted to normal in 49 per cent of those patients showing a therapeutic response and in 36.5 per cent of the therapeutic failure group. Indirect antiglobulin and bromelin tests became negative at approximately the same rate in both therapeutic groups. These data partially reflect the presence of a chronic disease. It is obvious that disappearance and reappearance of serologic tests are in part a function of time. Continual followup examinations may substantially modify these figures as further relapses and remissions develop.

Mechanism of Action of Corticosteroid Therapy

The mode of action of corticosteroids in autoimmune hemolytic anemia is unknown. Five mechanisms may be postulated as acting individually or in combination. (a) Stimulation of the bone marrow: increased erythrocyte delivery to the peripheral blood may reflect an increase of erythropoiesis, premature release of cells from the bone marrow, a delay in maturation of reticulocytes or a redistribution of erythrocytes from sinusoidal pools (11). (b) Effect on associated pathologic states: corticosteroid therapy may reduce organomegaly in approximately 50 per cent of patients with neoplasia of the reticuloendothelium. This may reduce the number of abnormal cells involved in autoantibody formation. In addition, a decrease in splenomegaly may remove hypersplenism from contributing to the hemolytic process. (c) Prevention of autoantibody formation: the lympholytic action of corticosteroids may result in a reduction of the numbers of immunocompetent cells capable of antibody formation. (d) Interference with antibody-antigen union: this theorized effect may result from action of corticosteroids on either the antibody molecule or the erythrocyte surface. (e) Interference with the release of lysosomal enzymes by making cell lysosomes more resistant to antibody and/or complement action (12). The relative importance of these five postulated mechanisms of action has not been determined. Additional studies in these areas are needed.

Therapeutic Regime

Prednisone (15 mg. four times a day) is the therapy of choice. If oral medication cannot be given, hydrocortisone (80 mg. three times a day) or dexamethasone (3 mg. three times a day) is employed intravenously or intramuscularly. Potassium bicarbonate (0.5 gm. three times a day), a salt poor diet and milk between meals are given to all patients at the start of therapy. These adjuvants are continued while corticosteroid therapy is maintained. Testosterone (400 mg. intramuscularly) is frequently given every 6 weeks in order to minimize osteoporosis.

The patient's hematocrit and reticulocyte count are determined daily at the start of therapy. Elevation of the reticulocyte count and/or hematocrit, or stabilization of a falling hematocrit, indicates the start of hematologic remission. A therapeutic failure of prednisone may be assumed if remission is not apparent in 3 weeks. Two different procedures may then be used. Prednisone therapy may be increased to 120 mg. daily or ACTH or dexamethasone may be employed. This approach generally will not induce remission, and it is wiser to terminate prednisone therapy. A slow reduction entails the withdrawal of 10 mg. of prednisone weekly. When necessary, prednisone may be completely discontinued over a 5- to 7-day period without employing ACTH therapy. It is crucial to establish a time limit for therapeutic failure of corticosteroids. This prevents the prolonged administration of large doses of corticosteroids, with its severe side effects, in the face of therapeutic failure. It also establishes the necessity of initiating other therapies in a potentially dangerous clinical situation. A therapeutic failure of corticosteroids is a poor prognostic sign requiring the initiation of alternate therapies.

If remission is induced with prednisone, progressive but slow reduction of drug intake is indicated. The minimal level maintaining hematologic remission is to be determined. Small changes in drug doses must be followed by adequate periods of observation before additional changes are made. Prednisone may be reduced to 50 mg.

daily upon initiation of remission. The hematocrit and reticulocyte count are then determined weekly. After 1 week and a continuation of remission, a further reduction of 10 mg. of prednisone may be made. If remission persists for an additional week, reduction of prednisone by 10 mg. is again indicated. Accordingly, 3 weeks after remission the patient will be receiving 30 mg. of prednisone daily. If relapse is to occur it will generally develop at levels below 30 mg. of prednisone daily. At this point a change of drug dosage must not be made more frequently than every 2 weeks. Prednisone should not be reduced more rapidly than 5 mg. in each 2-week period. Hematologic examinations may now be performed every 2 weeks. A continuing remission will permit the sequential reduction of prednisone by 5 mg. every 2 weeks. If the hematocrit has not reached normal levels but does not drop, prednisone is maintained an additional 2 weeks at the existing dose. When the prednisone dosage reaches 10 mg. daily, a 1-month waiting period is employed before a further reduction to 5 mg. daily. A similar 1-month waiting is employed before reducing prednisone to 2.5 mg. daily. After 1 month without relapse, prednisone may be discontinued. If relapse does not occur, the patient is periodically seen every 2 to 3 months for routine evaluation.

Relapse at any time during this procedure is a signal to return to either 60 or 45 mg. of prednisone daily to reinitiate remission. The dosage is then even more slowly lowered until the level is reached at which relapse occurred. This dosage is maintained a minimum of 3 months before further reduction is attempted.

With this therapeutic schedule the patient will eventually be classified into one of four categories. One group represents failure to respond to prednisone in 3 weeks and another therapeutic procedure must be employed. A second patient group will stay in remission after prednisone is discontinued. Such "cures" may persist for many years. The majority of patients present a pattern between these two extremes. A therapeutic remission is present with relapse developing below a specific prednisone level. The critical drug dosage is variable and must be determined in each patient. The clinician has to make an important decision with such patients and will eventually classify them into one of two groups. Only rough guidelines may be offered. If the hematocrit can be maintained at 30 per cent or higher with prednisone levels of 15 mg. daily or less, maintenance prednisone therapy is continued. If 30 mg. daily or more of prednisone is necessary to maintain the hematocrit at 30 per cent, an additional therapeutic procedure such as splenectomy should be considered. The decision is particularly difficult in the patient group requiring 15 to 30 mg. of prednisone daily to maintain remission. The dangers of long term steroid therapy must be individually balanced against the potential dangers of other therapies in the specific patient.

This outline of therapeutic approaches is particularly suited to idiopathic autoimmune hemolytic anemia; it also should be employed in secondary varieties. Remissions are common, although "cures" are unusual in the presence of reticuloendothelial neoplasia. Relapse frequently develops and hemolysis may progress irrespective of the clinical activity of the associated malignancy. Such relapses may not respond a second time to the same therapeutic approach. Complete failure of prednisone eventually may occur. Other therapeutic approaches are then indicated, but they seldom induce more than a transient response.

The therapeutic approach outlined above is designed for use in warm acting forms of autoimmune hemolytic anemia. Most investigators agree that corticosteroid therapy is of little use in cryopathic autoimmune hemolytic anemia (6, 9, 13).

Splenectomy

The study of experimental splenectomy by Banti (14, 15) led to its application in human diseases characterized by destruction of formed blood elements. The first description of splenectomy in acquired hemolytic anemia is credited to Micheli (16) in 1911 in Turin. In more recent years Jandl and associates (17, 18) have emphasized the mechanical role of the spleen in sequestering damaged erythrocytes. The exact role of the spleen in autoimmune hemolytic anemia is still unknown. In addition to mechanical sequestration, erythrophagocytosis and splenic antibody production may be involved in hemolysis. These concepts are discussed in Chapter 21.

Effectiveness of Splenectomy in Autoimmune Hemolytic Anemia

Micheli's initial report (16) described the beneficial results of splenectomy in acquired hemolytic anemia. Antonelli in 1913 (19) and Noble and Steinebach in 1914 (20) reported similar benefits. In 1940 Dameshek and Schwartz (21) reviewed the literature, collected 19 splenectomized cases and added four of their own. A therapeutic response was recorded in 20 of the 23 patients. Dameshek (22) expanded his personal experience and recorded the beneficial results of splenectomy in 10 of 18 patients with autoimmune hemolytic anemia. Welch and Dameshek in 1950 (23) reported 34 patients with idiopathic autoimmune hemolytic anemia who were splenectomized. Fifty per cent obtained complete remission. Eighteen patients with secondary autoimmune hemolytic anemia were also treated by splenectomy. Remissions were found in 33 per cent of cases. Unsatisfactory results were obtained in four patients with chronic lymphocytic leukemia and in two patients with Hodgkin's disease.

Other investigators have reported essentially similar results. Hansmann (24) reported a 15-year remission following splenectomy for autoimmune hemolytic anemia. Dausset and Malinvaud (25) studied 14 patients after splenectomy. Three postoperative deaths were recorded. A rapid cure was seen in two patients, a clinical cure in four and transient improvement in five. Young and associates (26) described a beneficial effect of splenectomy in approximately 65 per cent of patients. Goldberg and associates (27) noted that 52 per cent of 182 patients were improved by splenectomy. Veeger and associates (28)

studied 53 patients with autoimmune hemolytic anemia. Twenty-six had splenectomy with three deaths. A beneficial effect was found in 17 patients. Crosby and Rappaport (29) reported two immediate postoperative deaths and death in nine additional patients from various causes within 1 year of splenectomy. Seventeen patients in their series had a good to fair therapeutic response and only one patient had a poor response. Dausset and Colombani (9) noted that 58 per cent of splenectomized patients improved clinically with either permanent or temporary correction of hemolysis. They observed that splenectomy performed within 6 months of the diagnosis of disease led to a death rate similar to that obtained in patients not treated with splenectomy. The death rate was increased when surgery was performed after 1 year of disease. Splenectomy had been performed in 52 per cent of patients who died. Of the patients still living, 30 per cent had had splenectomy. In Dacie's series (6) 13 patients were treated by splenectomy alone. A clinical cure resulted in seven and compensated hemolysis resulted in one. Uncompensated hemolysis persisted in five cases. Thirteen patients received corticosteroids in addition to splenectomy. No clinical cures occurred. Compensated hemolysis was found in seven with uncompensated hemolytic anemia persisting in six. Accordingly, splenectomy led to clinical improvement in 15 of 26 patients. Three immediate postoperative deaths were noted.

Present Experience

The current series has been collected during the corticosteroid era of autoimmune hemolytic anemia. During this time splenectomy was relegated to a relatively unimportant role in the management of autoimmune hemolytic anemia. In the present series splenectomy was performed in only nine of 234 cases. Such selection makes it impossible to draw sound conclusions concerning the potential value of this procedure.

In three patients idiopathic autoimmune hemolytic anemia was present. Splenectomy was performed in one (Case 100) because of abdominal trauma suggesting splenic rupture. A prednisone induced hematologic remission was present and continued after splenectomy. In a second patient (Case 12) relapse developed after a 44-month corticosteroid induced remission. Hemolysis was unresponsive to further corticosteroid therapy. Splenectomy induced a remission which has persisted for over 7 years. In a third patient prednisone failed to induce remission of a pancytopenic form of idiopathic autoimmune hemolytic anemia. Splenectomy was performed and pancytopenia persisted. However, bleeding disappeared and transfusions were no longer required. This limited response has continued for 24 months. All three patients are still living.

Secondary forms of autoimmune hemolytic anemia were present in the remaining six patients. These included chronic lymphocytic leukemia, plasma cell myeloma (Case 3), scleroderma (Case 66), hyperthyroidism (Case 86), postnecrotic cirrhosis (Case 70) and cold hemagglutinin disease terminating in acute monocytic leukemia (Case 37). One postoperative death occurred because of generalized bleeding. In one patient splenectomy was performed for portal hypertension prior to active hemolysis. It did not influence the subsequent development of autoimmune hemolytic anemia. In another patient splenectomy was performed with little effect after 7 years of cold hemagglutinin disease. The patient survived 131 months after splenectomy and died from acute leukemia. The two patients with malignancy of the reticuloendothelium did poorly after surgery. No therapeutic response was noted and death occurred 2 and 5 months after splenectomy. The patient with hyperthyroidism was in therapeutic remission on maintenance prednisone. Splenectomy was performed as an elective procedure and remission has continued for 53 months without corticosteroids.

Side Effects of Splenectomy

Splenectomy in autoimmune hemolytic anemia is considered to be a formidable procedure. Postoperative deaths are common. Dameshek and Schwartz (21) reported four deaths in 10 cases, Crosby and Rappaport (29) reported two deaths in 27 cases and Lorie and Patsiora (30) reported five deaths in 21 patients. Welch and Dameshek (23) and Dausset and Colombani (9) all emphasized the poor results seen with malignancies of the reticuloendothelium. The latter group reported two postoperative deaths in five cases. Dacie (6) encountered three postoperative deaths in 26 splenectomized patients with autoimmune hemolytic anemia.

In addition to the immediate surgical mortality of splenectomy, several other harmful effects may be encountered. Thrombocytosis frequently follows splenectomy. This in turn may lead to in vivo thrombosis (30). Careful management is required and may involve the postoperative use of anticoagulants. Thrombocytosis and leukocytosis may be prominent and persist many years after splenectomy. It is not unusual to see such patients unnecessarily in consultation for leukocytosis. Such referrals are frequently made to rule out leukemia or idiopathic thrombocytosis. Patients having splenectomy may become particularly susceptible to overwhelming attacks of infectious disease. Children are particularly vulnerable. The data are conflicting on the reality of this problem. Hematologic relapse may develop following splenectomy after a variable period of time. Progressive and sometimes rapid hepatomegaly can develop. The prognosis is poor and survival is generally limited with this complication.

Systemic lupus erythematosus is frequently associated with autoimmune hemolytic anemia and idiopathic thrombocytopenic purpura. After splenectomy has been performed for autoimmune hemolytic anemia, systemic lupus erythematosus may become apparent (4, 31). Dameshek (31) suggested that the spleen may inhibit systemic lupus erythematosus or that splenectomy may disturb immune homeostasis maintaining a quiescent stage. He therefore advises avoidance of splenectomy in autoimmune hemolytic anemia. Best and Darling (32) have examined this premise in detail, analyzing 107 cases from the literature and 13 of their own patients.

They concluded that no evidence existed that splenectomy disseminated or made overt latent systemic lupus erythematosus. On the contrary, splenectomy frequently had a beneficial effect.

Splenectomy may be followed by a decrease in erythrocyte autoantibody production. This is reflected in negative or weakened direct and indirect antiglobulin tests. In spite of hematologic remission, however, such serologic tests may remain positive for long periods of time. Dacie (6) analyzed seven of 26 splenectomized patients. The antiglobulin test eventually became negative in five but persisted as positive in two.

When to Employ Splenectomy

Corticosteroid therapy is the treatment of choice for autoimmune hemolytic anemia. The high surgical mortality of splenectomy adds weight to this conclusion. This recommendation is supported by Dausset and Colombani (9) who emphasize that splenectomy neither cures nor affects the eventual outcome of autoimmune hemolytic anemia.

It is premature, however, to discard splenectomy as an effective therapy. Crosby (33) reported its effectiveness and emphasized the severe side effects of prolonged corticosteroid therapy. He suggests that splenectomy may induce remission in 75 per cent of patients who fail to have a lasting benefit from corticosteroids. Of this group, 50 per cent may obtain complete remission and 25 per cent may obtain partial improvement.

There is little doubt that the author has been too conservative in performing splenectomy in the current series. Retrospective analysis clearly indicates that the disastrous side effects of prolonged corticosteroid therapy were minimized and were not appreciated. Many patients were maintained in partial remission by prolonged administration of prednisone at dose levels over 15 mg. daily. This is an undesirable approach. Splenectomy offers an excellent method to avoid this problem. The high mortality reported for splenectomy in autoimmune hemolytic anemia is not an intrinsic part of the disease or of the operative procedure. Improvement in surgical techniques and the pre- and postoperative management of such patients has removed many of these objections. The availability of a team of surgeons experienced in splenectomy, working closely with the hematologist, has corrected most technical problems.

A rational therapeutic approach to autoimmune hemolytic anemia can be suggested. This requires initiation of corticosteroid therapy. If permanent remission with hematocrits of 30 per cent or higher cannot be induced or maintained with prednisone at dose levels of 15 mg. daily or less, splenectomy should be strongly considered. The degree of side effects and the patient's sensitivity to corticosteroid therapy should be considered. The performance of splenectomy as a last desperate therapeutic approach must be avoided. If at all possible the operation should be performed electively during complete or partial remission induced by prednisone. Parenteral corticosteroids should be used during the operative and immediate postoperative periods. Economic factors may help dictate which patients undergo splenectomy. The cost of continual corticosteroid and ancillary therapy and the necessity for continual medical followup while the patient is receiving such drugs must be considered. The expense of drug therapy may be minimized if the clinician orders prednisone specifically, rather than various trade name preparations.

Several criteria exist which may aid in selection of splenectomy candidates. Dausset and Colombani (9) and Dacie (6) have emphasized that patients with warm acting erythrocyte autoantibodies are most likely to have a beneficial effect from splenectomy. Such antibodies are incomplete agglutinins and do not cause hemolysis in vitro. A sequestrational type of splenic hemolysis is generally found. Cr^{51} external body scintillation counting may be performed. The studies of McCurdy and Rath (34) suggest that documentation of splenic sequestration may be employed to predict a successful splenectomy. Kinlough and associates (35) studied nine patients who failed to respond to corticosteroids. All patients had a shortened Cr^{51} T/2 and splenic sequestration. A lasting remission following splenectomy was seen in eight. An inability to demonstrate splenic sequestration by body surface counting does not indicate that splenectomy will fail to induce remission. In the report of Veeger and associates (28) one patient with normal sequestration had an excellent response to splenectomy. A reduced Cr^{51} T/2 may be of more prognostic significance. Goldberg and associates (27) performed splenectomy in 13 patients with a shortened erythrocyte survival time, with good results in 11. Evidence of liver sequestration is a poor prognostic sign suggesting severe erythrocyte damage (Chapter 21). Jandl (36) suggests that splenectomy offers little benefit in such cases.

Splenectomy in Cold Acting Autoimmune Hemolytic Anemias

Splenectomy is generally not indicated in cryopathic autoimmune hemolytic anemia. Cold acting autoantibodies usually are complete hemagglutinins, are complement dependent and lead to either circulatory hemolysis or hepatic sequestration hemolysis. Splenectomy offers little in correcting hemolysis induced by such agents. This serologic limitation to splenectomy is supported by the clinical data of various investigators (37, 38). Dacie (6), however, suggests that splenectomy may benefit patients with mild cold hemagglutinin disease in the absence of Raynaud's phenomenon and hemoglobinuria. In the current series, one patient with idiopathic cold hemagglutinin disease had splenectomy performed (Case 37). No obvious clinical benefit was noted. Prednisone was given with equivocal results for 5½ years.

Splenic Irradiation

Splenectomy is an efficient therapy for autoimmune hemolytic anemia. Its major limitation involves the operative risk. It is therefore rational to investigate procedures having the same potential benefits without the surgical danger. Radiation induced splenectomy may accomplish this. Heni and Blessing (39) in 1954 and Sokal (40) in 1957 noted that splenic irradiation intensified hemolysis. Jandl (36) reported that splenic irradiation is of no benefit, but he does not supply data supporting this statement. Scott (41) in 1957 and Galton and associates (42) in 1961 applied this procedure to hemolytic anemia and reported some success. Diamond (43), without giving examples, stated that the hemolytic anemia present in chronic lymphocytic leukemia may be controlled by administering 1,000 to 2,000 r in 3 weeks at 250 kv., at 70 TSD (target skin distance), through appropriately sized splenic portals.

Djaldetti and associates (44) investigated this therapeutic approach. Eight patients with chronic lymphocytic leukemia and severe hemolytic anemia were studied. A therapeutic failure with steroids and leukemic therapy was noted in all. Splenomegaly was universal. Direct antiglobulin tests were negative but adequate laboratory evidence for hemolysis was present. The patients received a total splenic radiation dose ranging from 200 to 700 r. A daily dose of 100 r (in air) was given at a tension of 200 kv., with a filtration of 0.5 mm./cu. and a focus-skin distance of 50 cm. Two opposite fields, abdominal and dorsal, were applied. All patients had elevated leukocyte counts. Irradiation was continued until the total white blood cell count (WBC) dropped to half the initial value. Splenic irradiation induced remission of hemolysis in five of the eight patients. The hemoglobin rose to over 10 gm. per cent in 1 to 2½ months. A decrease in splenomegaly was noted in four of the five cases showing a therapeutic response.

In the current series, 12 patients received splenic irradiation therapy. Malignancy of the reticuloendothelium and a secondary form of autoimmune hemolytic anemia were present in all. Nine patients had chronic lymphocytic leukemia, two patients had chronic granulocytic leukemia and one patient had Hodgkin's disease. Four patients received splenic radiation prior to the development of autoimmune hemolytic anemia. The durations of time between radiation and hemolytic anemia were 17, 22, 31 and 39 months, respectively.

Splenic irradiation was administered to eight patients during severe hemolytic ane-

294 CLINICAL ASPECTS

mia unresponsive to prednisone therapy. In three, no therapeutic effect was noted. One patient received 778 r and died 1 month later with transition of chronic to acute lymphocytic leukemia. A second patient (Case 29) received 302 r and died 4 months later with chronic granulocytic leukemia. The third patient (Case 21) received only small doses of radiation and died in 5 days with extensive chronic lymphocytic leukemia.

In the remaining five patients, a good to equivocal therapeutic response was noted with control of the hemolytic process. One patient with Hodgkin's disease died 1 month after irradiation. However, the hemolytic process was less severe. In the remaining four patients splenic radiation decreased hemolysis or else acted synergistically with corticosteroids. The following protocol illustrates a typical patient.

Case 102. A 53-year-old asymptomatic Negro male had an annual physical examination. He was found to have a spleen palpated 10 cm. below the costal margin and 2+ generalized lymphadenopathy. The hematocrit was 38.5 per cent, the reticulocyte count was 1.2 per cent, the WBC was 125,000/mm.³ and the thrombocytes were 136,000/mm.³ The peripheral blood and bone marrow were typical of chronic lymphocytic leukemia. With chlorambucil therapy the WBC dropped to 11,000/mm.³ and the spleen decreased to 5 cm. below the costal margin. Six weeks after the start of chlorambucil, fatigue, angina, jaundice and dark urine developed. The hematocrit had dropped to 21 per cent and the reticulocyte count was 7.1 per cent. Direct and indirect antiglobulin and bromelin tests were strongly positive. Elution revealed a panhemagglutinating erythrocyte autoantibody. A Cr^{51} T/2 of 4 days was found with marked splenic sequestration. Prednisone, 60 mg. daily, was given. The hematocrit precipitously dropped to 12 per cent. Over the next 27 days 20 units of blood were transfused. Each 2-unit transfusion elevated the hematocrit to 18 per cent. However, in 1 to 2 days it had again decreased to 12 per cent. Reticulocyte counts remained at approximately 10 per cent. Marked angina complicated the clinical course. After 10 days of prednisone therapy without response, splenic irradiation was started. A total of 275 r was given in 8 days. Five days after the start of radiation the reticulocyte count rose to 18 per cent and progressively rose to 23 per cent. Ten days after the

last dose of radiation the hematocrit reached 24 per cent; transfusions had been discontinued 2 days before. Prednisone was progressively decreased. The hematocrit reached 46 per cent 9 weeks after the start of remission. Maintenance prednisone, 2.5 mg. daily, has been given. Relapse of hemolytic anemia has not occurred in the 27 months since remission. Direct antiglobulin and bromelin tests are still positive. The indirect bromelin test has remained positive, although the indirect antiglobulin test is negative.

It is difficult to determine whether hematologic remission would have occurred in this patient without splenic irradiation. Ten days of prednisone therapy did not correct the problem. Severe hemolysis, persisting angina and the necessity of continually transfusing incompatible blood indicated the need for additional therapy. Splenic irradiation appeared to answer this need.

Only a short hematologic remission was obtained after splenic radiation therapy in the remaining three patients. The therapeutic effect appeared to be similar to the type of response frequently seen with corticosteroids in chronic lymphocytic leukemia. Case 23 illustrates a typical pattern. Splenic irradiation was employed three times in a 60-month period, with a beneficial effect noted on each occasion.

The data presented above are not sufficiently conclusive to warrant a final statement of the role of splenic irradiation in autoimmune hemolytic anemia. No experience has been accumulated with the idiopathic varieties. This reflects the general efficiency of corticosteroid therapy in such states. When neoplasia of the reticuloendothelium is complicated by autoimmune hemolytic anemia, however, failure of prednisone therapy may be anticipated at some time during the clinical course. Splenectomy does not hold much promise for such patients. Splenic irradiation may frequently be of aid. This appears to be a valid therapeutic procedure deserving critical clinical investigation. It is relatively safe and simple to perform, and preliminary data suggest that it may be of aid in selected patients.

Other forms of irradiation have been employed with some success. Evans and

Duane (45) reported transient hematologic remission following thorotrast administration; the patient was in relapse after splenectomy. Abdominal irradiation induced a longer remission in the same subject but was unsuccessful in another case.

Tocantins and Wang (46) reported a beneficial effect from the intravenous administration of 10 to 20 mc. of radioactive gold (Au^{198}). Dameshek (47) mentions that this is ineffective. This is a complex and potentially dangerous therapy. The authors advised this procedure only after failure of corticosteroids, splenectomy and transfusions.

Immunosuppressive Drug Therapy

Accumulated evidence suggests that autoimmune hemolytic anemia is an immunologically mediated disease. Therapeutic procedures have therefore been devised which attempt to decrease antibody production. Dameshek (47) employed Congo red in order to saturate or block the reticuloendothelium. This was unsuccessful in treating autoimmune hemolytic anemia. Nitrogen mustard was similarly employed (47–49). A therapeutic response occurred in one of four patients treated by Dameshek and Rosenthal (48). In general the results were not striking and frequent bone marrow depressive effects were noted. Triethylene melamine, urethane and radioactive gold were employed on the same rationale by Dameshek and associates (47, 48) and were generally unsuccessful.

In 1957 Sterzl and Holub (50) suggested that 6-mercaptopurine might interfere with antibody synthesis. This was independently confirmed in extensive studies by Schwartz and associates (51, 52). They demonstrated that this agent would suppress antibody formation in rabbits immunized with purified proteins. In addition, 6-mercaptopurine could induce a state of immunologic unresponsiveness in adult rabbits and could suppress transplantation rejection of skin grafts (53, 54). In 1960 these studies were expanded to include cases of human autoimmune hemolytic anemia and a favorable therapeutic effect was noted (55).

Since these initial observations, immuno-suppressive drug therapy employing 6-mercaptopurine, 6-thioguanine and azathioprine has been employed. Varying degrees of success have been noted in immunologically mediated syndromes such as systemic lupus erythematosus, nephrosis, transplantation rejection and autoimmune hemolytic anemia (56–59). Lambert and associates (59) reported their experience with 15 patients. Stiehm and associates (60) noted the inhibitory effect of immunosuppressive agents on measles vaccination. Berenbaum and Brown (61) studied various immunosuppressive agents in mice following TAB vaccine. Immune inhibition was most marked with cyclophosphamide, amethopterin, 6-thioguanine and 6-mercaptopurine. Vincaleukoblastine and triethylene melamine were less effective. An excellent review of the various immunosuppressive agents has been presented by Hitchings and Elion (62).

The effect of 6-mercaptopurine and thioguanine in autoimmune hemolytic anemia has been reported by Schwartz and Dameshek (63). Fourteen patients with autoimmune hemolytic anemia were studied. The series contained six cases of an idiopathic variety, two cases associated with lupus erythematosus, and single cases associated with myxedema, hepatitis, chronic lymphocytic leukemia, Dilantin ingestion, virus infection and rheumatoid arthritis. Two patients were exclusively treated with immunosuppressive drugs. Remissions occurred in both and did not require maintenance therapy. Nine patients initially received corticosteroids. An adequate therapeutic response either did not occur (no response in 10 to 14 days or more than 100 mg. of prednisone per week required) or serious side effects precluded continuation of therapy. Immunosuppressive therapy led to a good response in four, a partial response in one and a poor response in four patients. Three additional patients were initially treated with immunosuppressive drugs and subsequently with corticosteroids. One patient did not respond to thioguanine but did well on prednisone. In the remaining two patients adequate responses to both drugs were recorded. Three patients developed severe bone marrow depression at the recommended dose (2.5 mg./kg.). Five patients had mild to severe gastrointestinal side effects. The authors concluded that "the eventual role of 6-mercaptopurine and its analogs in the treatment of autoimmune hemolytic anemia is difficult to assess at this time." They suggest its use in patients exhibiting therapeutic failure to corticosteroids or to corticosteroids and splenectomy. It may be used in patients with severe toxic reactions to corticosteroids or as an adjuvant to corticosteroids, permitting a reduction in dosage of both drugs.

Taylor (64) described a patient with autoimmune hemolytic anemia and possible Hodgkin's disease who failed to respond to corticosteroids and splenectomy. Over the next 6 years remissions of the hemolytic state were induced with triethylene melamine, chlorambucil and cyclophosphamide.

Hitzig and Massimo (65) reported the use of azathioprine in three cases of childhood autoimmune hemolytic anemia. A complete remission was seen in one patient and in the remaining two patients a marked decrease in steroid dosage resulted. Corticosteroids have severe side effects on growth and metabolism in the young. Accordingly, this therapy may be valuable. Azathioprine, 2.5 mg./kg., was employed and the investigators suggested that the dose can be doubled.

Analysis of Present Series

Immunosuppressive drugs were not specifically employed for treatment of autoimmune hemolytic anemia in the current series. However, patients with various leukemias and lymphomas received many immunosuppressive drugs either individually or in multiple combinations during hemolysis. The following drugs were employed in individual patients during the stage of active autoimmune hemolytic anemia: chlorambucil, 40 patients; P^{32}, 22; 6-mercaptopurine, 19; vincristine, 17; nitrogen mustard, 15; cyclophosphamide, 13; methotrexate, eight; vinblastine, seven; spray x-ray irradiation, five; triethylene melamine, four; L-sarcolysine, three; busulfan, two; Colcemid, two; urethane, one;

and streptonigrins, one. In almost all instances corticosteroid therapy was concomitantly administered. It is accordingly difficult to determine specifically the effect of immunosuppressive therapy. However, the poor response rate to corticosteroids previously described for autoimmune hemolytic anemia associated with leukemias and lymphomas is applicable to this group. Analysis of these cases did not indicate that the immunosuppressive therapy described above either initiated or acted synergistically with corticosteroids in producing remission. Continual use of immunosuppressive therapy at levels designed to control the malignancy did not reduce the prednisone dosage necessary for induction or maintenance of hematologic remission.

These observations are not presented to suggest that immunosuppressive therapy has no value in autoimmune hemolytic anemia. A highly selected group of patients was employed in a confusing therapeutic regime. The study was not primarily designed to demonstrate the effect of such therapy on autoimmune hemolytic anemia. All patients had reticuloendothelial malignancy with immunosuppressive therapy administered in an attempt to halt the relentless progress of neoplasia. The clinical patterns of most of these patients were dominated by the malignancy with autoimmune hemolytic anemia appearing as a complication. Death resulted from the underlying disease in many subjects less than 6 months after administration of immunosuppressive therapy. In such patients immunosuppressive therapy was unimpressive in controlling the hemolytic process. This observation simply emphasizes that the associated disease generally dominates and determines the prognosis in secondary forms of autoimmune hemolytic anemia.

Heparin Therapy

In 1949 Owren (66) treated a patient with severe hemolytic anemia for 7 days with 350 mg. of heparin daily. No therapeutic effect was noted. When heparin was increased to 800 mg. daily, hemolysis decreased. Cessation of heparin therapy led to a return of severe hemolysis. Roth (67) in 1954 reported that heparin inhibited the in vitro agglutination of erythrocytes sensitized with autoantibodies. Storti and associates (68) in 1956 described the results of heparin therapy in a patient with idiopathic autoimmune hemolytic anemia without demonstrable erythrocyte auto-antibodies. Heparin, 750 mg. intravenously daily, was given for 30 days. Hemolysis markedly decreased. Discontinuation of heparin resulted in a return of the hemolytic process. Roth and Frumin (69) in the same year reported that a single 50-mg. intravenous dose of heparin reduced the direct antiglobulin titer, serum bilirubin and plasma hemoglobin in a patient with autoimmune hemolytic anemia. The effect was rapid and could be demonstrated 6 hours after heparin administration.

McFarland and associates (70) observed therapeutic benefits from heparin in autoimmune hemolytic anemia associated with Hodgkin's disease. Corticosteroids and splenectomy had failed in this patient. Heparin, 150 mg. daily subcutaneously, led to striking improvement of the hemolytic process. Positive direct and indirect antiglobulin tests reverted to negative. Hematologic remission continued with maintenance heparin, 20 mg. daily, for 3 months. When heparin was increased to 50 mg. daily, severe thrombocytopenia was partially corrected. Discontinuation of heparin was followed by a return of severe thrombocytopenia and hemolysis.

Hartman (71) reported a patient with autoimmune hemolytic anemia in whom corticosteroid therapy failed. Heparin, 100 mg. twice a day, was given. Within two hours of the initial heparin dose the direct antiglobulin test became negative. This was subsequently followed by hematologic remission. Heparin, 25 mg. daily for 3 months, maintained the remission.

TenPas and Monto (72) have presented an excellent summary of the heparin literature. They reported a patient with a small cell lymphoma and autoimmune hemolytic anemia. The hemolytic process responded poorly to cyclophosphamide, corticosteroids and splenectomy. Heparin, 100 mg. subcutaneously three times a day, induced hematologic remission. The antiglobulin test became negative 2 days after the start of heparin therapy. Maintenance heparin, 25 mg. b.i.d., and prednisone, 10 mg. daily, were continued and remission persisted for eight months.

Reports of Roth (67), Roth and Frumin (69), McFarland and associates (70), Hartman (71) and TenPas and Monto (72) indicate that heparin can modify the antiglobulin test in vitro and in vivo. In addition Johnson and Bencze (73) noted that heparin in excess of 1 mg./ml. would inhibit the LE cell and antinuclear factor tests. The mechanism of these actions is unknown.

The dramatic reports of the beneficial effect of heparin indicate that further experimental and clinical studies are desired. TenPas and Monto (72) suggest that case selection of appropriate patients may involve the in vitro demonstration of reversal of the antiglobulin test after incubation with heparin. The presence of a low serum complement level in a patient with autoimmune hemolytic anemia also suggests a potential benefit from heparin therapy.

In the current series heparin was not specifically employed as a treatment for autoimmune hemolytic anemia. Only two patients received the drug during the stage of hemolysis. One patient (Case 87) received transient heparin therapy for thrombophlebitis. This was discontinued after an allergic reaction and intensification of hemolysis. A second patient had idiopathic thrombocytoses in addition to autoimmune hemolytic anemia. Subcutaneous heparin therapy was given and was followed by severe bleeding at the injection site. Death occurred 6 days after the start of bleeding. The effect of heparin on hemolysis could not be determined because of multiple transfusions administered during bleeding. However, it was noted that direct antiglobulin and bromelin tests became negative at the first repeat erythrocyte serologic testing carried out 5 days after heparin was given.

The author's limited and unfortunate experience with heparin should not discourage the reader from attempting this therapeutic approach. Insufficient data are currently available to evaluate the role of heparin in autoimmune hemolytic anemia. The reports described by other workers are striking and clinical evaluation of this form of therapy is urgently needed. The theoretical rationale for heparin therapy is discussed in Chapter 17.

Thymectomy and Thymic Irradiation

The thymus gland plays a critical role in establishing a normal immune apparatus. Its participation in immune and autoimmune phenomena is explored in Chapter 22. The relationship of human thymic abnormalities to autoimmune hemolytic anemia is unclear. Burnet and MacKay (74) pointed out that thymic abnormalities may occur in patients with myasthenia gravis, rheumatoid arthritis, thrombotic thrombocytopenic purpura and systemic lupus erythematosus. The association of a thymoma with autoimmune hemolytic anemia has been recorded by several investigators (75–79). Three such patients (Cases 6, 20 and 36) are discussed in Chapter 6.

Such observations suggest that a surgical or radiation induced thymectomy may have some therapeutic value in autoimmune hemolytic anemia. This therapeutic approach has been applied in two clinical situations.

Thymectomy in the Presence of a Thymoma

In 1954 Ross and associates (75) performed a thymectomy in a patient with a thymoma, erythrocytic aplasia and autoimmune hemolytic anemia. The surgery did not influence the hemolysis, positive antiglobulin tests or erythrocytic aplasia. A similar patient was investigated in the current series (Case 20). Thymectomy also failed to correct hemolysis, positive erythrocyte serologic studies or erythrocytic asplasia. Halperin and associates (77) studied a patient with a thymoma, myasthenia gravis and autoimmune hemolytic anemia. Hematologic remission was induced with prednisone. Thymectomy was performed with improvement of myas-

thenia gravis. Prednisone was discontinued and the antiglobulin test remained weakly positive. The effect of thymectomy on the hemolytic process could not be determined, and death occurred soon after. Mongan and associates (79) reported a patient who developed autoimmune hemolytic anemia 80 months after thymectomy.

Thymectomy in the Absence of a Thymoma

Richmond and associates (80) studied a patient with an Evans' syndrome type of autoimmune hemolytic anemia. Splenectomy and corticosteroid therapy failed. Radiation (500 r) was directed at the thymus gland and immediate improvement of hemolysis was noted. The therapeutic effect was transient. A second course of 500 r directed to the thymus did not influence hemolysis. Remission was induced with azathioprine and actinomycin-C. Wilmers and Russell (81) reported a $2\frac{1}{2}$-month-old infant with autoimmune hemolytic anemia unresponsive to splenectomy or corticosteroids. Thymectomy induced hematologic remission. The antiglobulin test was still positive 8 weeks after surgery but reverted to negative 11 weeks after thymectomy. The thymus gland appeared entirely medullary with disappearance of the cortex. Hancock (82) and Karaklis and associates (83) reported successful thymectomies in infants with autoimmune hemolytic anemia. This procedure failed in the case reported by Oski and Abelson (84).

These studies suggest that thymectomy is of little value in correcting hemolysis when a thymoma and autoimmune hemolytic anemia are present. Erythrocytic aplasia magnifies this problem. In contrast, idiopathic autoimmune hemolytic anemia in the infant may respond to thymectomy. There are insufficient data to evaluate the effect of thymectomy in the adult with autoimmune hemolytic anemia. Surgical and radiation induced thymectomy must be considered to be experimental treatments. One aspect deserves emphasis. Thymectomy is technically easier than splenectomy and should be accompanied by a lower mortality rate. It is obvious that additional studies are required.

Spontaneous Improvement and Treatment of Associated Diseases

The therapeutic procedures previously discussed are drastic, have severe side effects and may induce substantial morbidity or mortality. In addition, there is no evidence that available therapeutic procedures can induce "cures" with any degree of predictability. Such therapies must be considered to be symptomatic procedures, although they may be life saving and may significantly prolong survival. A pertinent question must therefore be raised. Is specific therapy for autoimmune hemolytic anemia always indicated? A rational answer is dependent on whether or not any of three situations occurs with regularity. These include spontaneous remission, remission following control of associated diseases and establishment of a stable state with mild hemolysis.

Spontaneous Remission

Lederer (85, 86) called attention to a fulminating hemolytic anemia characterized by an abrupt onset, fever and rapid remission following transfusion therapy. There is little to support Lederer's original concept of a curative effect of transfusions. Rather, such cases of Lederer-Brill's anemia possibly represent antiglobulin positive immunohemolytic anemia related to infection. Remission probably occurs spontaneously with improvement of the associated virus infection. It may therefore be suggested that therapy, other than transfusions, is not indicated when a relationship to virus disease is documented. Cases 41 and 42 illustrate spontaneous remissions without therapy in infectious mononucleosis. Case 43 related to measles and Case 1 with cytomegalic disease are examples of the employment of corticosteroid therapy with excellent immediate results. The urgency of the clinical state must dictate whether such therapy is required.

Antiglobulin positive immunohemolytic anemia following cardiac surgery may also exhibit spontaneous remission without specific therapy. Remission may reflect clearance of transfused foreign lymphocytes or disappearance of mechanically damaged erythrocytes which initiated the termination of tolerance. Spontaneous remission is seen with sufficient regularity to warrant the withholding of potentially dangerous therapy if a delay in remission is not life threatening.

In idiopathic or other secondary forms of autoimmune hemolytic anemia, spontaneous remissions are occasionally noted. These are frequently transient and do not occur with regularity. Accordingly, withholding specific therapy in order to await spontaneous remission is unwarranted and potentially dangerous. Hemolytic crisis may suddenly develop. It is therefore advisable to initiate prednisone therapy for severe anemia and hemolysis in all such patients.

Stable State with Mild Hemolysis and Anemia

In some patients with autoimmune hemolytic anemia, erythrocyte production may increase sufficiently to balance the increased rate of destruction. A stable clinical state can result. Low grade anemia is frequently present and mild hemolysis may be documented. In other patients mild anemia and positive antiglobulin tests may be present in the absence of clinical evidence of hemolysis. In the current series such states were found with regularity in patients with systemic lupus erythematosus, rheumatoid arthritis, scleroderma, various forms of liver disease, ulcerative colitis and occasionally in patients with leukemia or lymphoma. Specific therapy to correct autoimmune hemolytic anemia may not be indicated in such patients. In many subjects the intent would be merely to correct a positive direct antiglobulin test. To risk the increased morbidity and mortality associated with antihemolysis therapy does not appear to be worthwhile.

The clinician electing not to treat such states must assume two obligations. An ostrich viewpoint is to be avoided. Withholding of therapy is not indicated in order to await spontaneous remission. Remission generally does not occur. In addition, careful followup of patients must be continued. Intensification of hemolysis or diminution of erythrocyte production resulting from infection or renal insufficiency may suddenly magnify the anemic state or even result in hemolytic crisis. Such crises may also occur spontaneously. Therapy must be immediately initiated at adequate levels.

A similar attitude is to be taken during the stage of remission induced by therapies for autoimmune hemolytic anemia. A stable hematocrit approximating 30 per cent is acceptable, even with persistence of hemolysis and positive antiglobulin tests. If stability can be maintained without therapy, it should be discontinued, or minimal maintenance doses should be employed in order to avoid side effects. Vigorous therapy employed to elevate the hematocrit to normal, while assuming additional risks from the augmented therapy, is not indicated. The precautions mentioned above should also be observed; relapse may appear at any time.

Remission Following Control of Associated Diseases

Two different therapeutic relationships exist between autoimmune hemolytic anemia and associated pathologic states. In some conditions the associated disease and autoimmune hemolytic anemia appear to be clinically and therapeutically independent. This is particularly evident with the leukemias and lymphomas. Substantial evidence indicates that therapies designed to control the neoplastic state, even when successful, have little effect in correcting the hemolytic process. Autoimmune hemolytic anemia occurring in patients with such neoplasia is best treated as a separate entity. This combined state is to be approached as if two unrelated disease processes were present. A similar observation is valid in cases of myelosclerosis.

Other secondary forms of autoimmune hemolytic anemia show a distinct relationship between hemolysis, positive antiglobulin tests and associated disease processes. Therapy directed toward the associated process may lead to hematologic and serologic remission. The clinician is urged to avoid specific therapy for autoimmune hemolytic anemia and to direct therapeutic attention to the associated abnormality. Immunohemolytic anemia "cures" are not unusual in this group.

The most striking example of this relationship is seen in the antiglobulin positive type of hemolytic anemia which may occur secondarily to drug therapy. Penicillin, alpha-methyldopa, quinine, quinidine, stibophen, cephalothin and anticonvulsives are the more common drugs involved in this process. Simple cessation of drug therapy will correct the hematologic problem. Corticosteroids, splenectomy or immunosuppressive drug therapy should be avoided as needlessly hazardous.

Surgical removal of various lesions may also lead to permanent hematologic and serologic remission in some secondary forms of autoimmune hemolytic anemia. The removal of ovarian cysts, dermoid cysts, teratomas, infected gall bladders, the prostate gland, carcinoma of the kidney and possibly other malignancies may be "curative" when such abnormalities are associated with autoimmune hemolytic anemia.

Specific therapy for infectious diseases, when associated with autoimmune hemolytic anemia, may lead to permanent hematologic remission and to "cure." Urinary tract infections and pneumonia are prominent in this group (see Chapter 7). Active pulmonary and miliary tuberculosis also demonstrate this relationship. The control of active tuberculosis through drug or surgical therapy will frequently correct associated autoimmune hemolytic anemias. The initiation of specific antihemolytic therapy is dependent on the degree of hemolysis. If the process is rapid and the anemia profound, such therapy may have to be employed. Sufficient time usually is available to warrant the withholding of such therapy while awaiting remission of the infectious process.

Various hematologic diseases also appear in a similar relationship. Positive antiglobulin tests, with or without evidence of hemolysis, may be observed in Addisonian pernicious anemia, folic acid deficiency and iron deficiency anemia. Replacement of the deficient material not only results in hematologic remission but may lead to disappearance of positive antiglobulin tests. Therapies designed to correct autoimmune hemolytic anemia are not only unnecessary but may be ineffectual. Thyroid disease was found to have a similar relationship in at least one patient (Case 85).

Miscellaneous Therapies for Autoimmune Hemolytic Anemia

Various other therapies have been employed for autoimmune hemolytic anemia. These approaches either have been insufficiently evaluated or have been proved unsuccessful.

Venom Antiserum

Singh and Bird (87) in 1960 presented a remarkable paper indicating the therapeutic efficacy of concentrated polyvalent anti-snake venom serum in autoimmune hemolytic anemia. The antiserum used was prepared against cobra, common krait, Russell's viper and saw scaled viper venom. Twenty-seven patients with autoimmune hemolytic anemia were treated, all successfully. In four, the process was acute and in 23 it was chronic. No information was supplied as to an idiopathic or secondary nature or warm or cold acting type of hemolytic anemia. Twenty ml. of antiserum were given intravenously and 20 ml. intramuscularly. The intramuscular injection was repeated on the 3rd, 7th and 14th days. The intravenous dose was used only in acute cases. The authors frequently noted rapid and dramatic hematologic remission. Some antiglobulin tests reverted to normal. Side effects of this therapy are not mentioned. The mechanism of action of venom antiserum is unknown, but the reagent did not inhibit the antiglobulin test in vitro. No confirmatory reports on this therapy are available.

Exchange Transfusions

In 1950 Piney (88) reported the use of a 15 liter exchange transfusion in a 29-year-old female with autoimmune hemolytic anemia. A satisfactory result occurred but re-lapse soon developed. In 1951 Cattan and associates (89) and Milliez and associates (90) employed partial exchange transfusion with 5½ and 6 liters of blood, respectively, in the treatment of autoimmune hemolytic anemia. Results were generally poor without lasting remission. Wingstrand and Selander (91) utilized exchange transfusions in two patients with autoimmune hemolytic anemia. In a 2-year-old child an immediate and complete remission occurred and persisted for 12 months. The possibility of spontaneous remission starting before exchange transfusion could not be ruled out. In a second patient 3½ liters of washed erythrocytes were employed. Immediate improvement with weaker direct antiglobulin tests was noted. Hemolysis and strong positive antiglobulin tests rapidly returned. Cortisone had been started 1 day prior to exchange transfusion, and remission soon occurred.

There is little rationale for the use of hazardous exchange transfusions in autoimmune hemolytic anemia. The basic process of erythrocyte autoantibody production is not affected by this procedure. It is difficult to conceive of any benefits that would not be obtained by simple transfusion therapy. Dacie (6) states that "exsanguination transfusions do not appear often to be justified by the results." The author would concur with this viewpoint.

Salicylate Therapy

Bateman (92) and Craddock (93) have both reported the use of salicylate therapy in autoimmune hemolytic anemia. No apparent beneficial effects were noted. Formijne (94) employed Na 5-iodosalicylic acid for the same purpose. One of four treated patients appeared to improve. Currently, salicylate therapy is not generally considered to be an .accepted therapeutic remedy.

Epsilon-Aminocaproic Acid Therapy

Epsilon-aminocaproic acid functions as an esterase inhibitor. It may therefore inhibit complement through blockade of C'1-proesterase. This suggests that epsilon-aminocaproic acid may have a beneficial effect in complement dependent forms of autoimmune hemolytic anemia. Unpublished studies in our laboratory are incomplete and have not demonstrated the efficacy of this concept. However, only patients with warm acting forms of autoimmune hemolytic anemia and one patient with paroxysmal nocturnal hemoglobinuria were studied. This therapy deserves evaluation in complement dependent reactions such as cold hemagglutinin disease and paroxysmal cold hemoglobinuria.

Transfusion Therapy

Blood transfusion therapy for autoimmune hemolytic anemia is a time honored procedure presenting many frightening clinical aspects. Lederer (85, 86) described remissions following blood transfusion and considered it to be a specific, curative procedure. There is little reason to perpetuate this myth. In the current series there were no examples of curative transfusion therapy in autoimmune hemolytic anemia. The complacency in ordering this therapy in the past reflects the lack of serologic procedures and knowledge that such transfusions are almost universally incompatible.

The clinician faces a difficult problem in deciding whether or not to employ transfusion therapy. He may be dealing with a desperately ill patient whose hematocrit is below 15 per cent. When a blood transfusion is requested the laboratory will report positive antiglobulin tests and the absence of compatible blood. The clinician may attempt to avoid the problem. The author has studied one case in which the clinician responsible was informed that cross matches in saline and albumin were compatible but that the antiglobulin test was incompatible. In an attempt to avoid transfusion of incompatible blood the clinician requested the laboratory to discontinue the antiglobulin test and to examine compatibility only in saline and albumin procedures. This irrational approach is more a therapy for the physician than for the patient.

Management of this problem is based on two fundamental observations. (a) As a general rule all blood transfusions will be incompatible in a patient with autoimmune hemolytic anemia. The problem is magnified to the extent that accurate ABO and rhesus blood typing may be impossible. (b) Corticosteroid therapy may induce a therapeutic remission in 1 week or less in a large number of patients with autoimmune hemolytic anemia.

The physician must therefore employ clinical judgment as to the relative dangers of permitting a patient to remain severely anemic for a limited period of time or transfusing incompatible blood. As a general rule the severe anemic state found in autoimmune hemolytic anemia is well tolerated, even in the elderly, if complete bedrest is employed. This reflects acclimatization occurring during slow but progressive hemolysis. There is no reason for the clinician to treat a blood count and to ignore the clinical status of the patient. In most instances all that is necessary is careful clinical and laboratory study while awaiting a therapeutic response to prednisone. This viewpoint must be balanced by the observation that some patients have severe difficulties even at higher hematocrits. The development of a semicomatose stage, coma, angina, peripheral edema, pulmonary edema or other evidence of cardiac decompensation is a medical emergency. The hazards of transfusion must then be assumed irrespective of the degree of hemolysis.

If remission with corticosteroid therapy is not obtained in a reasonable period of time (maximum, 21 days) transfusion therapy will have to be employed. However, this should not represent the sole therapy. Transfusions are purely palliative and aid the clinician in obtaining sufficient time to induce remission through additional procedures. Splenectomy may be considered. The mortality of desperation splenectomy is high. The wise surgeon will avoid accepting such anemic patients in whom compatible blood for transfusion is not available. Immunosuppressive drug therapy, splenic irradiation, heparin administration and even thymic irradiation appear to be better suited in such cases.

Several important characteristics of blood transfusion therapy in patients with autoimmune hemolytic anemia must be considered in order to evaluate its potential danger. The clinician should not expect any aid from the laboratory. The choosing of "less incompatible" blood through various in vitro test procedures is of doubtful value in warm acting autoimmune hemolytic anemia. Incompatible blood resembles pregnancy in the sense that a woman is not "a little pregnant." A meaningful correlation between degrees of in vitro incompatibility and in vivo hemolysis is not present. Even when specificity of an autoantibody is demonstrated, the variation in test tube "fit" versus in vivo "fit" of the antibody to the erythrocyte antigen is such that freedom from hemolysis cannot be guaranteed. In most instances a panhemagglutinating erythrocyte autoantibody is present in addition to the specific autoantibody (95). If specificity is found, sensitization of the patient to the compatible blood may develop with the production of an isoantibody directed against the originally compatible antigen. Such a sequence has been reported by Ley and associates (96).

It is more sound for the clinician to face directly the problem of transfusing incompatible blood. This is usually obvious. Transfusions generally result in a rise of the hematocrit which persists for only 1 or 2 days and is then followed by a return to the original low level. Increased evidence of hemolysis, as indicated by a rise of bilirubin or intensification of jaundice, may follow such transfusion. The palliative nature of transfusions becomes evident and repeated transfusions must be administered. Transfusion reactions consisting of fever are common; shock occurs less often. Two types of hemolysis may be encountered. In the most common reaction transfused erythrocytes are destroyed at the same or at an increased rate as are the patient's own cells. A sequestrational type of hemolysis is usually seen. Unbound erythrocyte autoantibodies or dissociation of bound autoantibodies and subsequent reattachment to transfused erythrocytes probably is responsible for this type of reaction.

A reversed sensitivity to transfused plasma may also be observed. This may take the form of a pyrogenic reaction (97) and most likely reflects the presence of leukoagglutinins (98). Hemolytic crisis represents a greater potential danger. Massive lysis of the patient's own cells may result from the transfusion of complement into a patient whose hemolytic state has stabilized because of complement depletion. A circulatory type of hemolysis will then occur. Most of the above mentioned difficulties may be avoided by the transfusion of washed erythrocytes. It has been found sufficient in our laboratory to centrifuge the blood and to remove plasma without washing. The residual 10 per cent or so of plasma generally does not produce difficulties. The packed erythrocytes may be resuspended in 5 per cent albumin to permit a more efficient transfusion.

The current discussion has emphasized the hazards of transfusion therapy in autoimmune hemolytic anemia. However, it would be an error for the clinician to avoid transfusions altogether. In the present series transfusions were frequently given. In spite of many reactions and only transient palliation, only one death was directly attributable to transfusion therapy (Case 47). In this patient the diagnosis was not recognized and cross matches failed. Acute renal failure resulted from transfusions administered during surgery. In contrast, transfusion therapy was life saving in several cases, and in many more it protected the patient while awaiting a therapeutic response to more efficient procedures (e.g., Case 102). In surgical conditions such as heart valve replacement and portacaval shunt procedures, large volumes of washed and resuspended blood were transfused without difficulty in the face of incompatible cross matches (Case 66).

These suggestions may be summarized as follows. Transfusion therapy should only be employed in life saving situations with the realization that responses are palliative and that incompatible blood is being employed. Transfusions should not be employed to treat either the physician or the hematocrit. The patient's clinical state must determine the necessity of risking a transfusion reaction. The physician must rely on clinical judgment and not expect valuable help from the laboratory in choosing "compatible" blood. The tran-

sient benefit of transfusion therapy should
be approached only when it cannot be
avoided, and then only to gain time while
other therapeutic procedures are utilized.

The Treatment of Cryopathic Autoimmune Hemolytic Anemia

Therapy for the cold acting autoimmune
hemolytic anemias is unsatisfactory. For
chronic hemolytic states, prophylaxis consisting of the avoidance of chills and maintenance of a constant warm temperature
are the most satisfactory procedures. Dacie
(6) has emphasized that simple bedrest in
a constant environment corrects anemia
and improves general health to a similar
extent as attained by corticosteroids. In
the acute virus related secondary forms of
cold hemagglutinin disease, palliation while
awaiting spontaneous recovery is the only
indicated therapy.

Various therapeutic approaches have
been tried and found to be unsuccessful.
The failure of splenectomy and corticosteroids has already been discussed. No
data are available for splenic irradiation,
heparin administration or thymectomy.

In devising rational therapeutic procedures for cryopathic autoimmune hemolytic
anemia, the physical, biologic and pathophysiologic characteristics of cold acting
erythrocyte autoantibodies must be considered. These are presented in Chapter
19. Cold acting erythrocyte autoantibodies
differ from warm acting erythrocyte autoantibodies in two critical aspects. They
are complement dependent and they usually
induce a circulatory or hepatic sequestration type of hemolysis (see Chapter 21).
The dependence of cold acting autoantibody
damage on complement fixation suggests
a focus amenable to therapy. Employment of a protease inhibitor (epsilon-
aminocaproic acid) which will block C'1 or
other agents which inhibit complement
(heparin and other anticoagulants acting
on C'3) deserve evaluation for possible
therapeutic benefits.

Disulfide Reduction Therapy

The cold acting erythrocyte autoantibodies, with the exception of the Donath-

Landsteiner antibody, are IgM immunoglobulins. In 1957 Deutsch and Morton
(99) and Fudenberg and Kunkel (100)
demonstrated that in vitro treatment of
such macromolecules with mercaptanes
would depolymerize the macromolecule and
destroy immunologic activity. These observations were confirmed by Mehrotra
and Charlwood (101). Walshe (102) employed the mercaptane penicillamine as a
chelating agent to remove copper in hepatolenticular degeneration (Wilson's disease). Bloch and associates (103) used
penicillamine in the treatment of Waldenström's macroglobulinemia and noted in
vivo depolymerization of the macroglobulin.

These studies formed the basis for Ritzmann and Levin's therapeutic trial of
penicillamine in cold hemagglutinin disease
(104). They reported clinical improvement
and reduction of cold acting hemagglutinins and hemolysins with the use of dl-penicillamine, 1.5 gm. daily by mouth for 10
days, and mercaptopyridoxine, 0.6 gm.
daily intravenously. They suggested that
cysteamine and penicillin G potassium
might have a similar beneficial effect. A
therapeutic response in cold hemagglutinin
disease was recorded by Edwards and
Gengozian (105) using d-penicillamine. In
contrast, Dacie (6) noted the failure of
dl-penicillamine in two patients. Schubothe
(106) noted the failure of mercaptopyridoxine to correct the cold hemagglutinin
syndrome in three patients, and he quotes
Krug as also reporting negative results.
Lind and associates (107) confirmed the
observation of Ritzmann and Levin (104)
of the in vitro action. However, an in vivo
effect was lacking and therapeutic failure
resulted in two patients. They employed
d-penicillamine at a 1.5-gm. daily dose for
10 days in one patient and a 3.0-gm. daily
dose for 11 days in another patient without
success. Evans and associates (10) also
noted the failure of in vivo penicillamine
therapy in a patient with cold hemagglutinin disease. Schubothe (106) states that a
plasma level of 0.25 per cent mercaptopyridoxine would be necessary for the destruction of cold hemagglutinin reactivity:

such a level would be produced by 12.5 gm. daily, a toxic dose. Accordingly, the current status of mercaptane therapy for cold hemagglutinin disease is confused and needs further study.

Jaffe (108) employed d-penicillamine therapy in rheumatoid arthritis and noted a significant reduction of rheumatoid factor titers. Jaffe's studies suggested that mechanisms other than in vivo depolymerization of IgM immunoglobulins may be involved. These possibilities include: (a) mercaptanes may have a preferential reaction with "tissue pool" macroglobulins; (b) mercaptanes may inhibit macroglobulin production through an anti-vitamin B-6 action; and (c) mercaptanes may directly affect the disease process itself.

Cytotoxic Drug Therapy

Schubothe (106) has emphasized the similarity of cold hemagglutinin disease to Waldenström's macroglobulinemia and the resemblance of cold autoantibody formation to paraprotein formation. Klemm and Schubothe (109) utilized cyclophosphamide therapy in Waldenström's macroglobulinemia and noted reduction of macroglobulin formation. Cyclophosphamide was accordingly employed in several cases of cold hemagglutinin disease (106). A reduction in cold hemagglutinin titer was noted in two patients. In two additional patients no reduction in cold antibody titer was noted after short courses; therapy had to be discontinued because of complications.

Other cytotoxic drugs have been utilized in an attempt to reduce the titer and the activity of cold hemagglutinins. Dacie (6) mentioned disappointing results with 6-mercaptopurine. Oleson (110) reported one patient in whom chlorambucil therapy led to reduction of cold hemagglutinin titers with prolonged therapy.

The use of potentially dangerous marrow depressing agents in cold hemagglutinin disease is limited by the chronicity of the ailment. In addition, a warm, constant environment is an effective means of prophylaxis to prevent severe attacks. Accordingly, only a safe cytotoxic agent that may be employed for many years is indicated. Such an agent is not yet available.

Therapy of Paroxysmal Cold Hemoglobinuria

The prophylactic avoidance of cold or of an abrupt drop in temperature is the major therapy for paroxysmal cold hemoglobinuria. The Donath-Landsteiner antibody differs from other cold acting erythrocyte autoantibodies. It is an IgG immunoglobulin, and a relationship to paraproteins has not been described. Accordingly, there is no rationale to apply either disulfide reduction therapy or cytotoxic agents in this chronic disease.

Other than prophylaxis, the major therapeutic approach in this syndrome is eradication of associated syphilitic infections. Kumagai and Namba (111) as early as 1927 reported a clinical cure in 10 of 14 patients after antiluetic therapy. Penicillin therapy for syphilis has also been effective (112), although Milic (113) reported failure in one case.

Additional therapies have been suggested. Becker (114) in 1948 noted that antihistamines would correct cold urticaria without influencing hemoglobinuria. Carey and associates (115) reported a similar effect of short term ACTH therapy.

If syphilis is absent, no specific therapy is available other than prophylaxis. In acute secondary forms, palliation may be employed. In chronic idiopathic types, avoidance of cold is the only satisfactory approach.

Future Therapies

The large amount of material presented in this chapter emphasizes that a completely satisfactory therapy for all cases of autoimmune hemolytic anemia is not available. Cure is initiated in a relatively small number of cases that may differ in pathogenesis from the majority of patients with autoimmune hemolytic anemia. These patients possibly have antiglobulin positive immunohemolytic anemia rather than a true autoimmune disease.

Efficient therapy depends on an understanding of the fundamental pathophysiologic mechanisms involved in autoimmune hemolytic anemia. Current therapy of autoimmune hemolytic anemia reflects the premise that the disease process results from abnormal antibody production directed against the erythrocyte. It is designed primarily to reduce antibody production or the erythrocyte destruction resulting from such antibody action. Therapy is therefore directed against the end stage phenomenon, rather than the basic disease process.

It has been suggested that an aberrant immune apparatus may be present in certain patients (116). Such individuals are immunologically deficient and their systems may permit the survival and growth of modified immunocompetent cells. Antibodies can be produced against various host constituents including the erythrocyte. Therapy initiated to reduce antibody production in such patients would have two results. Overt evidence of the disease process may be decreased as autoantibody production is reduced. However, the primary defect in the patient, i.e., an inability to marshal a normal immune response, would not be corrected and in actuality would be magnified. It is possible that current therapies in autoimmune hemolytic anemia have a beneficial short term effect and a detrimental long term action. Future therapy of this disease syndrome may reverse current approaches, and it may consist of methods to increase antibody production. Specific therapies correcting an immune deficient state are highly desirable. Such therapies are not at present available.

Current therapeutic procedures have a major flaw. All attempts to reduce antibody formation are nonspecific. A shotgun approach is used which affects the entire immune apparatus. In addition to the beneficial depression of erythrocyte autoantibodies, a concomitant harmful depression of all immune responses may develop. This may act synergistically with the increased susceptibility to infection exhibited by these patients. The ideal therapy would be specific suppression of erythrocyte autoantibody formation. Therapy should be designed to create (or reestablish) a state of immune tolerance of the host to the erythrocyte. This approach does not appear to be impossible or incompatible with current immunologic theory. Evidence has accumulated that humoral antibody formation involves a feedback mechanism (117). Manipulation of this system offers the potential to specifically shut down the formation of one antibody without affecting the synthesis of other antibodies. The observations of Denman and associates (118) with NZB mice appears to be important. It was found that antilymphocyte globulin started at 2 months of age suppressed the development of positive antiglobulin tests and hemolytic anemia. Such therapy had no effect in adult mice with active disease.

The ideal therapy is correction of the primary immunologic abnormality or, failing this, establishment of an immunologic unresponsive state for the erythrocyte. Other approaches should be considered. The immunochemist is approaching the degree of knowledge necessary to neutralize specifically antibodies after they are formed. It may be possible to synthesize compounds able to fix to antibodies and to change the molecular conformation leading to steric obstruction of the antibody site. The action of basically charged hexosamine antibiotics on erythrocyte autoantibodies is an example of this phenomenon (119). More specific approaches are desirable. Elucidation of the physical-chemical nature of erythrocyte antigenic determinants may permit the synthesis of antigenic analogs able to compete efficiently with the erythrocyte for humoral autoantibodies.

Four theoretical approaches are therefore available for the design of future therapies. These include: (a) restoration of a normal immune homeostatic mechanism, (b) creation of immune tolerance, (c) specific shut down of erythrocyte autoantibody production, and (d) neutralization of circulating autoantibodies. It is safe to predict an exciting and ultimately satisfying future for the study and management of autoimmune hemolytic anemia.

BIBLIOGRAPHY

1. Dougherty, T. F., and White, A.: Influence of hormones on lymphoid tissue structure and

function. The role of the pituitary adreno-
trophic hormone in the regulation of the
lymphocytes and other cellular elements
of the blood. Endocrinology **35**: 1, 1944.
2. Fischel, E. E., LeMay, M., and Kabat, E. A.:
Effect of adrenocorticotrophic hormone and
x-ray on amount of circulating antibody. J.
Immun. **61**: 89, 1949.
3. Dameshek, W., Rosenthal, M. C., and
Schwartz, L. I.: The treatment of acquired
hemolytic anemia with adrenocorticotrophic
hormone (ACTH). New Eng. J. Med. **244**:
117, 1951.
4. Dameshek, W., and Komninos, Z. D.: The
present status of treatment of autoimmune
hemolytic anemia with ACTH and cortisone. Blood **11**: 648, 1956.
5. Horster, J. A.: *Die Korticosteroid-behandlung
hämatologischer und verwandter Erkrankungen.* Georg Theime Verlag KG., Stuttgart, 1961.
6. Dacie, J. V.: *The Haemolytic Anaemias, Part
II,* Ed. 2. Grune & Stratton, Inc., New York,
1962.
7. Evans, R. S.: Autoantibodies in hematologic
disorders. Stanford Med. Bull. **13**: 152, 1955.
8. Pisciotta, A. V., and Hinz, J. E.: Detection
and characterization of autoantibodies in acquired auto-immune hemolytic anemia.
Amer. J. Clin. Path. **27**: 619, 1957.
9. Dausset, J., and Colombani, J.: The serology
and the prognosis of 128 cases of autoimmune hemolytic anemia. Blood **14**: 1280,
1959.
10. Evans, R. S., Bingham, M., and Turner, E.:
Autoimmune hemolytic disease: observations of serological reactions and disease activity. Ann. N. Y. Acad. Sci. **124**: 422, 1965.
11. Baikie, A. G., and Pirrie, R.: The effect of
ACTH and cortisone in experimental
haemolytic anaemias in guinea pigs. Studies
on anaemias due to heterologous anti-red
cell-serum and on the anaemia of chronic
lead poisoning. Scot. Med. J. **3**: 264, 1958.
12. Weissman, G., and Thomas, L.: Studies on
lysosomes. I. The effects of endotoxin, endotoxin tolerance and cortisone on the release
of acid hydrolases from a granular fraction
of rabbit liver. J. Exp. Med. **116**: 433, 1962.
13. Pisciotta, A. V.: Cold hemagglutination in
acute and chronic hemolytic syndromes.
Blood **10**: 295, 1955.
14. Banti, G.: La splenomegalia emolitica anemopoietica (anemia emolitica splenomegalica
anemopoietica). Sperimentale **67**: 323, 1913.
15. Banti, G.: Splenomégalie hémolytique anhémopoiétique; le rôle de la rate dans
l'hémolyse. Sem. Med. **33**: 313, 1913.
16. Mitcheli, F.: Unmittelbare Effekte der Splenektomie bei einem Fall von erworbenen
hämolytischen splenomegalischen Ikterus,
typus Hayem-Widal. Wien. Klin. Wschr.
24: 1269, 1911.
17. Jandl, J. H., Jones, A. R., and Castle, W. B.:
The destruction of red cells by antibodies in

man. I. Observations on the sequestration
and lysis of red cells altered by immune
mechanisms. J. Clin. Invest. **36**: 1428, 1957.
18. Jandl, J. H., Simmons, R. L., and Castle, W.
B.: Red cell filtration and the pathogenesis
of certain hemolytic anemias. Blood **18**:
133, 1961.
19. Antonelli, G.: Intorno agli itteri emolitici.
Effetti della splenectomia su di una par-
ticulare forma di ittero emolitico acquisato
con anemia a tipo perniciosa. Policlinico
(Med.) **20**: 97, 170, 193, 1913.
20. Nobel, E., and Steinebach, R.: Zur Klinik der
Splenomegalie im Kindersalter. Z. Kinderheilk. **12**: 75, 1914.
21. Dameshek, W., and Schwartz, S. O.: Acute
hemolytic anemia (acquired hemolytic icterus, acute type). Medicine (Balt.) **19**: 231,
1940.
22. Dameshek, W.: The management of acute
hemolytic anemia and the hemolytic crisis.
Clinics **2**: 118, 1943.
23. Welch, C. S., and Dameshek, W.: Splenectomy in blood dyscrasias. New Eng. J. Med.
242: 601, 1950.
24. Hansmann, H.: Fifteen-year follow-up of acquired hemolytic anemia of the auto-antibody type after splenectomy. Klin. Wschr.
40: 755, 1962.
25. Dausset, J., and Malinvaud, G.: Les anémies
hémolytiques acquises avec auto-anticorps.
Evolution, prognostic et traîtement d'après
l'étude de 54 cas. Sem. Hop. Paris **30**: 3130,
1954.
26. Young, L. E., Miller, G., and Swisher, S. N.:
Treatment of hemolytic disorders. J.
Chronic Dis. **6**: 307, 1957.
27. Goldberg, A., Hutchison, H. E., and MacDonald, E.: Radiochromium in the selection of
patients with haemolytic anaemia for splenectomy. Lancet **1**: 109, 1966.
28. Veeger, W., Woldring, M. G., van Rood, J. J.,
Eernisse, J. G., Leeksma, C. H., Verloop,
M. C., and Nieweg, H. O.: The value of the
determination of the site of red cell sequestration in hemolytic anemia as a prediction
test for splenectomy. Acta Med. Scand.
171: 507, 1962.
29. Crosby, W. H., and Rappaport, H.: Autoimmune hemolytic anemia. I. Analysis of
hematologic observations with particular
reference to their prognostic value. A survey
of 57 cases. Blood **12**: 42, 1957.
30. Lorie, I. I., and Patsiora, M. D.: The treatment of acquired hemolytic anemias. Probl.
Hemat. Blood Transf. **3**: 1, 1958.
31. Dameshek, W.: Systemic lupus erythematosus: a complex auto-immune disorder.
Ann. Intern. Med. **48**: 707, 1958.
32. Best, W. R., and Darling, D. R.: A critical
look at the splenectomy-SLE controversy.
Med. Clin. N. Amer. **46**: 19, 1962.
33. Crosby, W. H.: Aspects of treatment of autoimmune hemolytic anemia. In *Proceedings
of the Seventh International Congress of the*

International Society of Hematology. **II**
Pensiero Scientifico, Rome, **1959.**

34. McCurdy, P. R., and Rath, C. E.: Splenectomy in hemolytic anemia. Results predicted by body scanning after injection of Cr^{51} tagged red cells. New Eng. J. Med. **259:** 459, 1958.

35. Kinlough, R. L., Bennett, R. C., and Lander, H.: The place of splenectomy in haematological disorders: the value of 51 Cr techniques. Med. J. Aust. **2:** 1022, 1966.

36. Jandl, J. H.: Current concepts in therapy. Hemolytic anemia. New Eng. J. Med. **268:** 482, 1963.

37. Baumgartner, W.: Die Kälteagglutininkrankheit. Schweiz. Med. Wschr. **85:** 1157, 1955.

38. Lewis, S. M., Szur, L., and Dacie, J. V.: The pattern of erythrocyte destruction in haemolytic anaemia, as studied with radioactive chromium. Brit. J. Haemat. **6:** 122, 1960.

39. Heni, F., and Blessing, K.: Beschreibung zweier schwerer erworbener idiopathischer hämolytischer Anämien. Klin. Wschr. **32:** 481, 1954.

40. Sokal, G.: Hypersplénisme hémolytique. Présence d'un anticorps aux caractères inhabituels. Rev. Belg. Path. **26:** 95, 1957.

41. Scott, R. B.: Leukaemia. Lancet **1:** 1162, 1957.

42. Galton, D. A. G., Wiltshaw, E., Szur, L., and Dacie, J. V.: The use of chlorambucil and steroids in the treatment of chronic lymphocytic leukaemia. Brit. J. Haemat. **7:** 73, 1961.

43. Diamond, H. D., and Miller, D. G.: Chronic lymphocytic leukemia. Med. Clin. N. Amer. **45:** 601, 1961.

44. Djaldetti, M., DeVries, A., and Levie, B.: Hemolytic anemia in lymphocytic leukemia. Arch. Intern. Med. (Chicago) **110:** 449, 1962.

45. Evans, R. S., and Duane, R. T.: Observations on the effect of irradiation in chronic acquired hemolytic anemia exhibiting hemolytic activity for transfused erythrocytes. Blood **2:** 72, 1947.

46. Tocantins, L. M., and Wang, G.: Radioactive colloidal gold in the treatment of severe acquired hemolytic anemia refractory to splenectomy. Progr. Hemat. **1:** 138, 1956.

47. Dameshek, W.: Acquired hemolytic anemia. Physiopathology with particular reference to autoimmunization and therapy. In *Proceedings of the Third International Congress of the International Society of Hematology.* William Heinemann, Ltd., London, 1951.

48. Dameshek, W., and Rosenthal, M. C.: The treatment of acquired hemolytic anemia. With a note on the relationship of periarteritis nodosa to hemolytic anemia. Med. Clin. N. Amer. **35:** 1423, 1951.

49. Meyers, M. C., Miller, S., Linman, J. W., and Bethell, F. H.: The use of ACTH and cortisone in idiopathic thrombocytopenic purpura and idiopathic acquired hemolytic anemia. Ann. Intern. Med. **37:** 352, 1952.

50. Sterzl, J., and Holub, M.: The influence of 6-mercaptopurine on antibody formation. Folia Biol. (Praha) **4:** 59, 1958.

51. Schwartz, R., and Dameshek, W.: Drug induced immunological tolerance. Nature (London) **183:** 1682, 1959.

52. Schwartz, R., Eisner, A., and Dameshek, W.: The effect of 6-mercaptopurine on primary and secondary immune responses. J. Clin. Invest. **38:** 1394, 1959.

53. Schwartz, R., and Dameshek, W.: The effects of 6-mercaptopurine on homograft reactions. J. Clin. Invest. **39:** 952, 1960.

54. André, J. A., Schwartz, R. S., Mitus, W. J., and Dameshek, W.: The morphologic responses of the lymphoid system to homografts. I and II. Blood **19:** 313, 334, 1962.

55. Dameshek, W., and Schwartz, R.: Treatment of certain "autoimmune" diseases with antimetabolites; a preliminary report. Trans. Ass. Amer. Physicians **73:** 113, 1960.

56. Calne, R. Y.: Rejection of renal homografts inhibition in dogs by 6-mercaptopurine. Lancet **1:** 417, 1960.

57. Demis, D. J., Brown, C. S., and Crosby, W. H.: Thioguanine in treatment of certain autoimmune, immunologic and related diseases. Amer. J. Med. **37:** 195, 1964.

58. Shearn, M. A.: Mercaptopurine in the treatment of steroid-resistant nephrotic syndrome. New Eng. J. Med. **273:** 943, 1965.

59. Lambert, P. H., and Salmon, J.: Traitement immuno-suppressif chez 15 patients atteints d'affections auto-immunes ou de maladies ayant une pathogénie immunologique. Acta Clin. Belg. **21:** 171, 1966.

60. Stiehm, E. R., Ablin, A., Kushner, J. H., and Zoger, S.: Measles vaccination in patients on immunosuppressive drugs. Immune response to certain hematologic patients to inactivated measles vaccine. Amer. J. Dis. Child. **111:** 191, 1966.

61. Berenbaum, M. C., and Brown, I. N.: Dose-response relationships for agents inhibiting the immune response. Immunology **7:** 65, 1964.

62. Hitchings, G. H., and Elion, G. B.: Chemical suppression of the immune response. Pharmacol. Rev. **15:** 365, 1963.

63. Schwartz, R., and Dameshek, W.: The treatment of autoimmune hemolytic anemia with 6-mercaptopurine and thioguanine. Blood **19:** 483, 1962.

64. Taylor, L.: Idiopathic autoimmune hemolytic anemia. Response of a patient to repeated courses of alkylating agents. Amer. J. Med. **35:** 130, 1963.

65. Hitzig, W. H., and Massimo, L.: Treatment of autoimmune hemolytic anemia in children with azathioprine (Imuran). Blood **28:** 840, 1966.

66. Owren, P. A.: Acquired hemolytic jaundice. Scand. J. Clin. Lab. Invest. **1:** 41, 1949.

67. Roth, K. L.: Interaction of heparin with auto-agglutinins in idiopathic acquired

hemolytic anemia. Proc. Soc. Exp. Biol. Med. **86:** 352, 1954.

68. Storti, E., Vaccari, F., and Baldini, E.: Studies on the relationship between anticoagulants and hemolysis. Parts I and II. Acta Haemat. (Basel) **15:** 12, 106, 1956.

69. Roth, K. L., and Frumin, A. M.: Effect of intramuscular heparin on antibodies in idiopathic acquired hemolytic anemia. Amer. J. Med. **20:** 968, 1956.

70. McFarland, W., Galbraith, R. G., and Miale, A.: Heparin therapy in autoimmune hemolytic anemia. Blood **15:** 741, 1960.

71. Hartman, M. M.: Reversal of serologic reactions by heparin: Therapeutic implications. II. Idiopathic acquired hemolytic anemia (IAHA). Ann. Allerg. **22:** 313, 1964.

72. TenPas, A., and Monto, R. W.: The treatment of autoimmune hemolytic anemia with heparin. Amer. J. Med. Sci. **251:** 63, 1966.

73. Johnson, G. D., and Bencze, G.: The effect of heparin on nuclear immunofluorescence. Bibl. Haemat. **23:** 40, 1965.

74. Burnet, F. M., and MacKay, I. R.: Lympho-epithelial structures and autoimmune disease. Lancet **2:** 1030, 1962.

75. Ross, J. F., Finch, S. C., Street, R. W., and Strieder, J. W.: The simultaneous occurrence of benign thymoma and refractory anemia. Blood **9:** 935, 1954.

76. Janbon, M. M., Bertrand, L., and Bonnet, H.: Sarcome du thymus avec anémie hémolytique par autoanticorps. Montpelier Med. **49:** 161, 1956.

77. Halperin, I. C., Minogue, W. F., and Komninos, Z. D.: Autoimmune hemolytic anemia and myasthenia gravis associated with thymoma. New Eng. J. Med. **275:** 663, 1966.

78. Jacox, R. F., Mongan, E. S., Hanshaw, J. B., and Leddy, J. P.: Hypogammaglobulinemia with thymoma and probable pulmonary infection with cytomegalovirus. New Eng. J. Med. **271:** 1091, 1964.

79. Mongan, E. S., Kern, W. A., and Terry, R.: Hypogammaglobulinemia with thymoma, hemolytic anemia, and disseminated infection with cytomegalovirus. Ann. Intern. Med. **65:** 548, 1966.

80. Richmond, J., Woodruff, M. F. A., Cumming, R. A., and Donald, K. W.: A case of idiopathic thrombocytopenia and autoimmune hemolytic anemia. Lancet **2:** 125, 1963.

81. Wilmers, M. J., and Russell, P. A.: Autoimmune haemolytic anaemia in an infant treated by thymectomy. Lancet **2:** 915, 1963.

82. Hancock, D. M.: Autoimmune haemolytic anaemia in an infant treated by thymectomy. Lancet **2:** 1118, 1963.

83. Karaklis, A., Valaes, T., Pantelakis, S. N., and Doxiadis, S. A.: Thymectomy in an infant with autoimmune haemolytic anaemia. Lancet **2:** 778, 1964.

84. Oski, F. A., and Abelson, N. M.: Autoimmune hemolytic anemia in an infant. Report of a case treated unsuccessfully by thymectomy. J. Pediat. **67:** 752, 1965.

85. Lederer, M.: A form of acute hemolytic anemia probably of infectious origin. Amer. J. Med. Sci. **170:** 500, 1925.

86. Lederer, M.: Three additional cases of acute hemolytic (infectious) anemia. Amer. J. Med. Sci. **179:** 228, 1930.

87. Singh, I., and Bird, G. W. G.: Autoimmune haemolytic anaemia treated with venom antiserum. Lancet **1:** 92, 1960.

88. Piney, A.: Acquired haemolytic anaemia. Sang **21:** 229, 1950.

89. Cattan, R., Frumasan, P., Dausset, J., and Trélat, R.: Ictère hémolytique acquis traité notamment par deux exsanguinotransfusions. Bull. Soc. Med. Hop. Paris **67:** 45, 1951.

90. Milliez, P., Larouche, C., Dubost, C., Dreyfus, B., Dausset, J., and Moreau, L.: Maladie neuro-hémolytique apparemment acquise. Bull. Soc. Med. Hop. Paris **67:** 771, 1951.

91. Wingstrand, H., and Selander, S.: Exchange transfusion in cases of acquired acute hemolytic anemia. Acta Med. Scand. **167:** 309, 1960.

92. Bateman, J. C.: Symptoms attributable to cold hemagglutination. Report of two cases. Arch. Intern. Med. (Chicago) **84:** 523, 1949.

93. Craddock, C. G.: Acute idiopathic hemolytic anemia; report of a severe fatal case with immunologic observations. Ann. Intern. Med. **35:** 912, 1951.

94. Formijne, P.: Clinical applications of 5-iodo-salicylic acid in acquired hemolytic anemia and other diseases. Verh. Akad. Wet. Amst. (Ser. C) **59:** 335, 1956.

95. Dacie, J. V., and Cutbush, M.: Specificity of auto-antibodies in acquired haemolytic anaemia. J. Clin. Path. **7:** 18, 1954.

96. Ley, A. B., Mayer, K., and Harris, J. P.: Observations on a "specific autoantibody". In *Proceedings of the Sixth Congress of the International Society of Blood Transfusion.* S. Karger, Basel, 1958.

97. Dameshek, W., and Neber, J.: Transfusion reactions to plasma constituent of whole blood: their pathogenesis and treatment by washed red blood cell transfusions. Blood **5:** 129, 1950.

98. Payne, R.: The association of febrile transfusion reactions with leukoagglutinins. Vox Sang. **2:** 233, 1957.

99. Deutsch, H. F., and Morton, J. I.: Dissociation of human serum macroglobulins. Science **125:** 600, 1957.

100. Fudenberg, H. H., and Kunkel, H. G.: Physical properties of red cell agglutinins in acquired hemolytic anemia. J. Exp. Med. **106:** 689, 1957.

101. Mehrotra, T. N., and Charlwood, P. A.: Physico-chemical characterization of the cold auto-antibodies of acquired haemolytic anaemia. Immunology **3:** 254, 1960.

102. Walshe, F. M.: Penicillamine, a new oral

therapy for Wilson's disease. Amer. J. Med. **21**: 487, 1956.

103. Block, H. S., Prasad, A., Anastasi, A., and Briggs, D. R.: Serum protein changes in Waldenström's macroglobulinemia during administration of a low molecular weight thiol (penicillamine). J. Lab. Clin. Med. **56**: 212, 1960.

104. Ritzmann, S. E., and Levin, W. C.: Effect of mercaptanes in cold agglutinin disease. J. Lab. Clin. Med. **57**: 718, 1961.

105. Edwards, C. L., and Gengozian, N.: Autoimmune hemolytic anemia treated with d-penicillamine. Ann. Intern. Med. **62**: 576, 1965.

106. Schubothe, H.: The cold hemagglutinin disease. Seminars Hemat. **3**: 27, 1966.

107. Lind, K., Mansa, B., and Olesen, H.: Penicillamine treatment in the cold hemagglutinin syndrome. Acta Med. Scand. **173**: 647, 1962.

108. Jaffe, I. A.: Comparison of the effect of plasmapheresis and penicillamine on the level of circulating rheumatoid factor. Ann. Rheum. Dis. **22**: 71, 1963.

109. Klemm, D., and Schubothe, H.: Zytostatische Langzeitbehandlung makroglobulinämischer Erkrankungen. In *Proceedings of the Tenth International Congress of the International Society of Hematology*, Stockholm, 1964.

110. Olesen, H.: Chlorambucil treatment in the cold agglutinin syndrome. Scand. J. Haemat. **1**: 116, 1964.

111. Kumagai, T., and Namba, M.: Weitere Beiträge zur Kenntnis der paroxysmalen Hämo-globinurie. Deutsch. Arch. Klin. Med. **156**: 257, 1927.

112. Nichols, F. T., and Williams, C. J.: Paroxysmal cold hemoglobinuria associated with dementia paralytica. Report of treatment with penicillin. J. A. M. A. **140**: 1322, 1949.

113. Milic, N.: Paroxysmal cold hemoglobinuria with positive treponema immobilization test. Report of a case. Blood **12**: 907, 1957.

114. Becker, R. M.: Paroxysmal cold hemoglobinurias. Arch. Intern. Med. (Chicago) **81**: 630, 1948.

115. Carey, R. A., Harvey, A. M., Howard, J. E., and Wagley, P. F.: The effect of adrenocorticotrophic hormone (ACTH) and cortisone on drug hypersensitivity reactions. Bull. Hopkins Hosp. **87**: 354, 1950.

116. Pirofsky, B.: Autoimmune hemolytic anemia and neoplasia of the reticuloendothelium. With a hypothesis concerning etiologic relationships. Ann. Intern. Med. **68**: 109, 1968.

117. Wigzell, H.: Antibody synthesis at the cellular level. Antibody induced suppression of 7S antibody synthesis. J. Exp. Med. **124**: 953, 1966.

118. Denman, A. M., Denman, E. J., and Holborow, E. J.: Suppression of Coombs positive haemolytic anaemia in NZB mice by antilymphocyte globulins. Lancet **1**: 1084, 1967.

119. Pirofsky, B., Cordova, M., and Rigas, D.: The mechanism of streptomycin inhibition of erythrocyte antibodies. Vox Sang. **9**: 653, 1964.

Part II
THEORETICAL AND SEROLOGIC
ASPECTS

Chapter 13

The Self-Recognition Phenomenon and Autoimmunization

Autoimmunization and immunologic self-recognition, as theoretical principles, are undergoing constant changes and modifications. In recent years fundamental discoveries have changed such concepts from biologic curiosities into major experimental fields. Information obtained in this area is of profound medical interest with unlimited possibilities for application to human disease. For example, the ability to manipulate self-recognition offers the most logical approach for the correction of autoimmune diseases, malignancies and homotransplantation rejection.

In its simplest form autoimmunization is a violation of immunologic self-recognition. The principle of self-recognition must therefore form the basis for any meaningful discussion of autoimmune hemolytic anemia. The various theories of antibody formation supply a crucial link in such an analysis. Unfortunately the scope of this volume does not permit a review of current experimental studies in antibody formation. Only an abbreviated summation of basic observations involving self-recognition can be presented. An attempt will be made to supply the clinician with the background and the semantic tools to approach autoimmunization. The reader should supplement this brief summary. Several excellent reviews presenting the concepts of "instruction" and "selection" theories of antibody formation are available (1–10).

The Self-Recognition Phenomenon

In 1900 Ehrlich and Morganroth initiated a set of experiments documenting the self-recognition state (11, 12). These studies have been summarized by Dacie (13) in terms of autoimmune hemolytic anemia. The experimental system involved the production of hemolysins in the goat. Laked blood from donor goats was injected intraperitoneally into recipient goats. The sera were then examined for the presence of hemolysins. Ehrlich and Morganroth found that erythrocytes of recipient goats, in whose sera the hemolysin had been formed, were not lysed by that specific hemolysin. Two types of hemolysin, an isolysin and an autolysin, could be postulated. The *isolysin* appeared as an immune hemolysin capable of reacting with the erythrocytes of members of the same species but not with those of the animal producing the antibody. The *autolysin* would be capable of lysing the erythrocytes of the test animal producing the antibody. Landsteiner's discovery of naturally occurring anti-A and anti-B in the sera of normal individuals appeared as an example of the same phenomenon (14). He demonstrated that an individual's serum does not react with his own erythrocytes.

The data obtained acted as a puzzle and a challenge to Ehrlich and Morganroth (11, 12). The dilemma the immunologist faces today was clearly stated. A natural law indicated that a living organism always responded to the injection of blood cells from a foreign species by the production of a specific hemolysin. How could this natural law be suspended when the erythrocytes injected were those of the recipient animal? It was of "the highest pathologic importance to determine whether the absorption of its own body material can excite reactive changes in the organism, and what the nature of the change is." Ehrlich and Morganroth speculated that the living organism must have regulatory contrivances to prevent formation of antibodies directed against its own body constituents. Such antibodies would appear as autotoxins and would be detrimental to the organism. The possibility that anti-autolysins were developed to neutralize autolysins was considered. If homeostatic mechanisms preventing the development of such autotoxins failed, damage to the living organism could result. In 1906 Ehrlich (12) confirmed their initial impression that elements of a living creature did not elicit the expected immune response in that organism. "Further investigations made by us have confirmed this view, so that one might be justified in speaking of a 'horror autotoxicus' of the organism."

The self-recognition and "horror autotoxicus" phenomena are illustrated in Figure 14. If human serum is injected into a horse, the horse's system will respond with the production of antibodies directed against human serum. If horse serum is

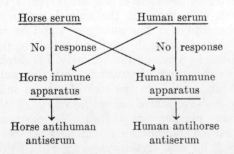

FIGURE 14. The "horror autotoxicus" or self-recognition phenomenon. Horse serum is antigenic when injected into the human. Human serum is antigenic when injected into the horse. Both the human and the horse are good antibody producers. However, neither the human nor the horse produce antibodies against their own sera.

similarly injected into a human, the human system will produce antibodies directed against horse serum. In immunologic terms, therefore, human serum and horse serum are both potentially antigenic, i.e., they can lead to the production of specific antibodies. In addition, both the horse and the human are good antibody producers when placed in parenteral contact with serum. Why doesn't the horse or the human, therefore, form antibodies against his own serum? Through what means or mechanism does the human antibody producing system distinguish its own serum from that of a foreign serum?

The problems raised are of critical importance to many clinical syndromes. The rejection of a foreign tissue or organ graft is an example of the normal self-recognition mechanism. The experimental production of immune tolerance in the immature and an immune paralysis state in the adult are examples of artificially created self-recognition for foreign substances. In such conditions of immune unresponsiveness, antibody formation directed against the foreign material is not initiated. Malignancies, within this framework, may be considered to represent a spontaneous failure of the self-recognition mechanism or the immune response. "Foreign" malignant tissue may be recognized as "self," or else it may elicit an ineffectual immune response which results in the survival of the abnormal tissue. Autoimmune diseases appear at the other end of the spectrum. The failure of the immune apparatus results in recognition of "self" antigens as foreign, with eventual production of an immune response directed against host constituents. An autotransplantation rejection state against normal body constituents occurs. The interrelation between the self-recognition phenomenon and transplantation rejection, tolerance and paralysis, malignancies and autoimmunization is diagrammatically summarized in Figure 15.

Immunologic Unresponsiveness

For many years autoimmunization was considered to be an unlikely theoretical concept. It seemed improbable that the neces-

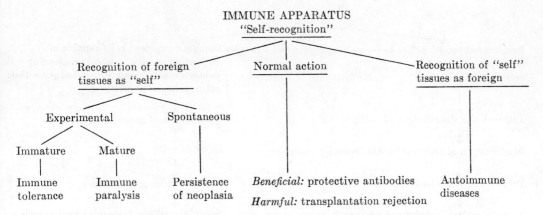

FIGURE 15. Normal and abnormal expressions of the self-recognition phenomenon. Experimental forms of specific immunologic unresponsiveness, malignancies and auto-immune disease reflect different aberrations of self-recognition. The homotransplantation rejection phenomenon appears as a normal expression of self-recognition.

sary failure of self-recognition could occur. This attitude reflected the general acceptance of "instruction" theories of antibody formation. Such concepts required antigenic determinants to enter immunocompetent cells and physically modify the molecular conformation of the forming antibody (8). In this fashion antibodies with a specific structure complementary to the molecular conformation of a specific antigenic determinant could be created. There appeared to be no place within such hypotheses for a failure of self-recognition. Burnet and Fenner (1) were aware of this discrepancy. They postulated the presence of cellular "self-markers" to explain self-recognition and incorporated this concept as an integral part of their adaptive enzyme theory of antibody formation.

The development of the natural selection (4) and clonal selection (2, 3) theories of antibody formation supplied the necessary theoretical matrix for self-recognition. The clonal selection hypothesis relied on antigenic selection of immunocompetent cells capable of producing antibody of the required molecular conformation. With such "selection" theories the antigen initiated the process by choosing the appropriate reacting cell. It also functioned as a mitogenic agent stimulating growth and division. The end result of this process was a clone of daughter cells all producing the

same antibody, without the necessity of further antigenic action. Self-recognition was dependent on the inhibition or destruction during embryonic life of cells capable of producing antibody against host antigens. Throughout this volume concepts and terms derived from clonal selection theories of antibody formation are employed. The role of the thymus gland, the presence of forbidden clones, the committed cell, the immunologically competent cell and immune unresponsiveness are a few of the more important concepts useful in discussing autoimmunization. Figure 16 presents a simplified version of the instruction and selection theories of antibody formation.

Immune Tolerance

The original adaptive enzyme theory predicted that embryonic exposure to foreign antigenic material would lead to self-recognition of the foreign agents (1). This would result in immune unresponsiveness when the adult was again exposed to the antigen. Medawar and associates (15, 16) tested this postulate experimentally. They transplanted foreign cells into an inbred group of embryonic homozygous mice. The adult mice were subsequently challenged with tissue transplants from the foreign donors. The foreign tissue was recognized as "self" and homotransplant rejection did not result. The state of immune unrespon-

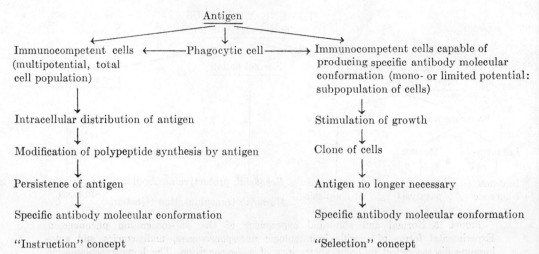

FIGURE 16. Contrasts between "instruction" and "selection" concepts of antibody formation. Differences in the role of the antigen and the population and potential of immunocompetent cells are prominent.

siveness was immunologically specific. The term immune tolerance or actively acquired tolerance was given to this phenomenon.

In addition to predicting a state of immune unresponsiveness, clonal selection implied two major characteristics of such unresponsiveness. (a) The immune tolerant state would be permanent. This reflected destruction or elimination of specific mesenchymal cells possessing the ability to produce antibodies directed against the specific antigens. (b) The embryonic or neonatal state was essential for the establishment of self-recognition. Immunoincompetent animals would therefore have to be employed in establishing experimentally produced actively acquired tolerance. Although the original postulate is valid, both assumptions have now been found to be incorrect.

The mechanisms through which experimental immune tolerance and natural self-recognition are established remain obscure. If experimental systems can be equated to normal physiologic states, certain conclusions seem valid. It is apparent that immune tolerance is not necessarily permanent. Transplantation of lymphocytes from a homologous animal immunized against a cellular antigen, into a homologous animal tolerant to the cellular antigen, will terminate the tolerant state. Presumably the sensitized lymphocytes, being homologous,

can proliferate, producing antibodies and ending tolerance. A break of tolerance, however, may be initiated without the addition of new antibody producing cells. Hanan and Oyama (17) studied rabbits injected with a soluble antigen in the immediate neonatal period. Antibodies were not produced when the animals had matured and were reinjected with the original antigen. Smith and Bridges (18) demonstrated that persistence of tolerance to soluble antigens was dependent on continual availability of antigen. Rabbit tolerance to bovine serum albumin led to immunologic unresponsiveness for approximately 3 months. If bovine serum albumin was reinjected before tolerance was lost, the tolerant state could persist indefinitely. Prolonging the time before exposure to bovine serum albumin led to antibody formation, rather than to a persistence of tolerance. Immune tolerance of newborn rabbits was lost when circulating antigen (BSA) dropped below 10^{12} molecules per animal. Humphrey (19) found tolerance to persist when the antigen concentration was 10^3 molecules or less in rabbits.

Such studies indicate that immune tolerance is not the result of a permanent loss of cells capable of producing antibody. Similar conclusions can be drawn from Weigle's studies (20). Immune tolerance induced with bovine serum albumin may be terminated by immunizing with a related albumin. If the albumin used is closely related serologically, e.g., sheep albumin (75 per cent cross reactivity), neither immunization nor a break in tolerance occurs. A moderately foreign albumin, such as pig albumin (32 per cent cross reactivity), may lead to immunization against pig albumin without a break in tolerance to bovine albumin. With appropriate cross reacting material, e.g., horse or human albumin (15 per cent cross reactivity), antibody formation against horse and human albumin occurs. Concomitantly, tolerance established for bovine albumin is broken. Weigle has also noted that a break in tolerance may be produced by denaturing the original antigen prior to reinjection.

Immune Paralysis

The unique nature of the embryonic state in establishing immune unresponsiveness must also be challenged. Felton and associates (21, 22) in 1949 and 1955 demonstrated a state of immune unresponsiveness in adult mice immunized with an excess of pneumococcal polysaccharide S III. He noted the persistence of polysaccharide antigen in injected animals for many months. The persistence of antigen resulted from a lack of enzymes which might degrade the polysaccharide. Felton designated this state of immune unresponsiveness as immunologic paralysis. In 1955 Dixon and Mauer (23) attempted to immunize rabbits with huge doses of bovine serum albumin. They encountered the same phenomenon. Five to ten milligrams of bovine serum albumin is generally adequate to stimulate rabbit antibody production. These investigators initiated immunization with 500 mg. of bovine serum albumin, using as much as 20 gm. with some rabbits. A state of immune unresponsiveness specific for bovine serum albumin resulted.

Characteristics of Immunologic Unresponsiveness

Most investigators now assume that immune tolerance and immune paralysis are manifestations of the same process. A char-

acteristic common to both phenomena is an excess of antigenic material. This results in an inability either to produce antibodies or to permit their passage into the circulation. A relatively small amount of antigen is required to induce the tolerant stage in the embryo or newborn. This possibly reflects a limited ability to produce antibody at the time of initiating the tolerant state. Throughout this volume these two important states are discussed according to the following definitions:

Immune tolerance: Specific immune unresponsiveness exhibited by a host animal to antigenic material. Unresponsiveness is induced by exposure of the host to small amounts of antigen during early life.

Immune paralysis: Specfic immune unresponsiveness exhibited by a host animal to antigenic material. Unresponsiveness is induced by exposure of the host to large amounts of the antigen during adult life.

The antigen concerned may be either replicating or soluble. The following observations, modified from Smith (24), summarize the characteristics of the immunologic unresponsive state established against both cellular and soluble antigenic material. (a) Immune unresponsiveness results from the failure of the induction or recognition phase of the immune response. (b) The productive phase of the immune response is also inhibited. (c) A continuation of tolerance is dependent on the continued presence of antigenic determinants in critical sites. (d) The critical sites appear to be intracellular. (e) With soluble, nonliving antigens, continual replacement is necessary to maintain the tolerant stage. (f) With "living" antigens, replication may supply the necessary critical amount of antigenic determinants. (g) As long as tolerance exists, antigenic determinants have the same relation to or same access to these critical areas as upon initial exposure. (h) Tolerance is as specific as the immunologic response. Immunologic unresponsiveness is therefore specific for each antigenic determinant rather than for the entire antigen. (i) All immunocompetent cells able to respond to a specific determinant, as well as their daughter cells, must be tolerant if complete unresponsiveness is to persist. (j) A return of immunologic responsiveness occurs when antigen is eliminated from the critical sites.

The number of antigenic molecules necessary to induce the unresponsive state is variable. Nossal and associates (25) have demonstrated that zones of antigenic concentration exist for the establishment of immune tolerance or antibody production in mice. Employing polymers of flagellin obtained from Salmonella, dose orders of 10^{-3} μg. per day or more, and 10^{-7} μg. per day or less, led to tolerance. Antigenic concentrations between these extreme ranges, e.g., 10^{-5} μg. per day, led to sensitization. Accordingly, there exists a biphasic curve of antigenic concentration resulting in either unresponsiveness or immunization. Thorbecke and Benacerraf (26) have noted that the sequential administration of antigen at doses too small to be immunogenic may also induce tolerance in adult rabbits.

In both forms of immune unresponsiveness the ability to form antibody gradually reappears. The initial state of complete immune unresponsiveness is followed by a stage in which antibody formation begins. Exposure to the antigen at this point leads to a typical secondary response. In the next stage, circulating antibody against the injected antigen may be found in the serum.

Why an antigen induces tolerance in a newborn animal, although it initiates antibody formation in the adult, is not fully understood. Haurowitz (8) states that the amount of retained antigen in the embryo or newborn is not very different from that of the adult. Several suggestions have been made. These include the possibility that excess or persisting antigen blocks the formation of antibody. An alternate suggestion would implicate antigen as interfering with maturation of embryonic cells into antibody producing cells. The reverse should also be considered. Antigen may function as a potent mitogenic agent converting all embryonic cells into mature, nonreplicating units. Jerne (27) has suggested that release of antibody from a producing cell may involve an enzyme such as a hydrolase. From this viewpoint, toler-

ance may be considered as the result of inactivation of the enzyme by a repressor. This sequence would prevent the release of antibody. Phagocytosis of antigen by macrophages is an early, necessary step for antibody production. The macrophage activity of newborn animals has been shown to be poorly developed. Martin (28) suggests that the ease of inducing tolerance in the newborn is a reflection of immaturity of macrophage activity.

Nossal and Ada (29) and Nossal (30) have investigated cellular mechanisms involved in the tolerant state. Soluble and particulate antigens are actively phagocytosed by cells of the reticuloendothelium. Such antigens may persist in tissues for long periods of time. In a normal animal recognition of the foreign nature of an antigen depends on its phagocytosis by macrophages. Interaction of the antigen containing macrophages with primitive lymphoid cells then occurs. This is followed by the proliferation of lymphoid germinal centers and an increase in the number of plasma cells. Antibody formation appears as the eventual result of these cellular interactions. Figure 17 diagrammatically depicts the postulated pathways. Nossal (30) reports that a tolerant animal presents a different sequence of events. Phagocytosis of the foreign antigen occurs in a pattern apparently similar to that seen with immunized animals. The next step in the immune reaction, however, does not occur. Primitive lymphoid cells do not make contact with the antigen laden macrophages, and lymphoid germinal center and plasma cell proliferation do not occur. Nossal has emphasized that this sequence of events separates normal self-recognition of host antigens from experimentally induced immune unresponsiveness. The critical first stage of macrocytic phagocytosis is present in actively induced tolerance. It is absent in the normal animal tolerant to self-antigens.

Autoimmune Diseases

Autoimmunization is of theoretical importance to both the clinician and the basic scientist. Extensive studies designed to determine the pertinent pathophysiologic mechanisms have resulted from this interest. Many of these studies have led to confusion. In part this reflects a lack of agreement as to what is meant by the term autoimmunization. The uncritical assumption of an autoimmune pathogensis in human disease syndromes illustrates the problem. Table 77 lists the more than 50 disease states variously reported as autoimmune. In many instances grossly inadequate criteria have been employed in arriving at such an etiology.

Characteristics of the Autoimmune State

An accurate study of a pathophysiologic mechanism is dependent on a generally accepted definition of the process. In addition, minimum criteria permitting documentation of the state must be formulated. MacKay and Burnet (31) have provisionally defined autoimmune disease as *"any condition in which clinical symptoms or functional changes result from immunologic reactions of immunologically competent cells or antibodies, produced by the individual, with normal components of the body."* This definition is excellent. Several critical aspects of autoimmunization are emphasized. The immunologic nature of the process is clearly stated. The definition permits the postulation of immune mechanisms other than circulating antibody in the establishment of an autoimmune state. The application of delayed hypersensitivity in autoimmunization is implicit. Finally, the definition states the dependence of autoimmunization on the host production of agents capable of reacting with normal host self constituents. This latter statement is sufficiently broad to incorporate the various theoretical possibilities of autoimmunization without limiting the investigator to only one hypothesis.

How may the clinician recognize a case of autoimmunization? This is a complex problem when the vast variety of possible anatomic abnormalities are considered. MacKay and Burnet (31) have listed characteristics commonly observed, which may be present in all autoimmune conditions. These include: (a) serum gamma-globulin

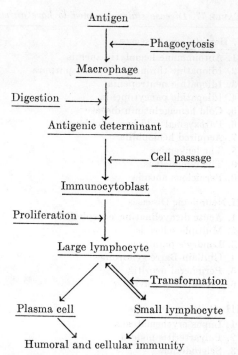

FIGURE 17. Schematic representation of the postulated sequence of cellular events through which an antigen stimulates antibody formation.

level above 1.5 gm. per cent, (b) the presence of demonstrable autoantibody against a body component, (c) the deposition of denatured gamma-globulin or its derivatives, which probably include amyloid, at sites of election, (d) accumulations of lymphocytes and plasma cells in damaged tissues, (e) a significant transient or lasting benefit from treatment with corticosteroid drugs, and (f) evidence of multiple unrelated autoimmune processes.

Although such criteria are helpful, they suffer from the same deficiencies as do the less formally stated criteria used by most clinicians. The nondiagnostic character of elevated serum globulins, fibrinoid degeneration, infiltration of lymphocytes and plasma cells and response to corticosteroids is well known.

It is essential that the basic immunologic process involved in autoimmunization be incorporated in any set of criteria used to establish the presence of an autoimmune disease. Witebsky (32) has employed a list of principles reminiscent of Koch's postu-

TABLE 77. *Disease states assumed to have an etiologic or secondary relationship to autoimmunization*

I. Hematologic Diseases
1. Autoimmune hemolytic anemia
2. Idiopathic thrombocytopenic purpura
3. Idiopathic neutropenia
4. Idiopathic pancytopenia
5. Cold hemagglutinin disease
6. Paroxysmal cold hemoglobinuria
7. Acquired hemophilia
8. The leukemias
9. The lymphomas
10. Pernicious anemia

II. Neurologic Diseases
1. Acute demyelinating encephalitis
2. Multiple sclerosis
3. Landry's paralysis
4. Guillain-Barré syndrome
5. Peripheral neuritis
6. Myasthenia gravis

III. Collagen Diseases
1. Lupus erythematosus
2. Polyarteritis nodosa
3. Scleroderma
4. Dermatomyositis
5. Sjögren's disease
6. Rheumatoid arthritis
7. Rheumatic fever
8. Thrombotic thrombocytopenia
9. Erythema nodosa
10. Stevens-Johnson syndrome

IV. Endocrine Diseases
1. Thyroiditis
2. Thyrotoxicosis
3. Addison's disease
4. Aspermatogenesis
5. Diabetes?

V. Gastrointestinal Diseases
1. Portal cirrhosis
2. Acute hepatitis
3. Chronic active hepatitis
4. Lupoid hepatitis
5. Biliary cirrhosis
6. Ulcerative colitis
7. Regional enteritis
8. Pancreatitis

VI. Miscellaneous Diseases
1. Glomerulonephritis
2. Basement membrane disease
3. Sympathetic ophthalmia
4. Phacoanaphylactic endophthalmitis
5. Postcardiotomy syndrome
6. Postinfarction syndrome
7. Psychogenic states
8. Postaortic valve prosthesis
9. Id reaction
10. Exfoliative dermatitis
11. Psoriasis
12. Behcet's syndrome

lates. (a) Free circulating antibody must be demonstrated by direct means, or cell bound antibody must be demonstrated by indirect means. (b) A specific antigen must be recognized against which the antibody is directed. (c) Antibody must be produced against the same antigen in experimental animals. (d) The pathologic changes in the corresponding tissue of an actively sensitized experimental animal must be basically similar to those found in the human disease.

Probably a blend of clinical criteria as presented by MacKay and Burnet (31) and the immunologic requirements as suggested by Witebsky (32) should be considered. The following outline for establishing a syndrome as autoimmune can be suggested:

1. Evidence Suggestive of an Immunologic Event: The markers of autoimmunization suggested by MacKay and Burnet (31), as well as other nonspecific findings, are included. These include hypergammaglobulinemia, fibrinoid degeneration, infiltration by monocytes, plasma cells and lymphocytes, eosinophilia, evidence of other immunologic disease, response to corticosteroid or immunosuppressive therapy, etc.

2. Evidence of Antibody Formation in the Host: Circulating antibody formation or delayed hypersensitivity initiated by the host must be demonstrated. Multiple methods of detecting antibodies should be employed. Reliance on only one immunologic procedure is extremely precarious. The simple demonstration of either precipitation, hemagglutination of tanned erythrocytes or complement fixation, when crude reagents are used, should not be considered to constitute proof of antibody formation.

3. Identification of the Antigen as a Host Constituent: Host cells, tissues or extracts of these materials may be used in *preliminary* studies of antigenicity. Cells and tissues contain hundreds of antigenic constituents. Any complete analysis of an autoimmune state requires an attempt to determine specific antigenic substances. An expansion of this approach should be carried out. Involved antigens should be analyzed as to their "normal" state or possible modification by environmental or disease processes.

4. Specificity of Host Antibody for Host Antigen: Two separate and independent requirements are included in this category. The host antibody must react specifically with the host antigen. An unrelated immunologic event such as the adsorption of foreign antigens or immune complexes onto innocent bystander cells should be ruled out. The second requirement is frequently forgotten. An antibody is an immunoglobulin whose structure is oriented for combination with a specific antigenic group. An autoantibody must also have specificity for the documented antigen. Demonstrating that serum of a patient either binds complement or induces precipitation, in the presence of tissue extracts, does not prove specificity. Other tissue extracts of the host should be shown not to have similar reactivity. If such reactivity is present, the investigator must identify the specific antigen. Its cross reactivity or distribution in other tissues has to be demonstrated before the diagnosis of autoimmunization, or even of an immune reaction, can be accepted.

5. Evidence that Host Autoantibody Damages Host Tissues: Tissue damage is not crucial for the proof of autoimmunization. Classifying a disease as autoimmune, however, carries the tacit assumption that autoimmunization is related to the pathologic process. The investigator must relate autoantibody production to the clinical syndrome before the disease can be considered autoimmune. Milgrom (33) has stated "it should be stressed ... that formation of autoantibodies is by no means synonymous with an autoimmune disease."

Lawrence (34) similarly accepts this view. Accordingly, a complete picture of an autoimmune disease requires clarification of the relationship between autoantibodies and tissue damage.

It is realized that several items of this list, particularly categories 3 and 4, are beyond the scope of usual clinical investigations. This should encourage the clinician to collaborate more fully with the immunologist in his approach to these disease states. These criteria should not be considered complete. They are suggested as a checklist for the clinical investigator in his approach to confusing disease syndromes. A great deal of the fascination of immune mediated diseases results from the broad spectrum of anatomic and physiologic abnormalities. They reflect the ubiquitous bodywide action of immunologic phenomena. The distinctive characteristics of specific autoimmune reactions will introduce distinctive criteria. Whenever possible immunologic techniques should be expanded to study more satisfactorily the disease state. The application of passive transfer procedures should be encouraged. Evidence is accumulating that circulating autoantibodies may not necessarily be related to the actual clinical syndrome (35). A search for delayed hypersensitivity should therefore be included in immunologic investigations even though circulating autoantibodies are documented (35, 36). The development of satisfactory model animal systems is of major importance. This may involve the selective breeding of animals with spontaneous autoimmunization or the experimental development of specific animal analogs. Table 78 summarizes some animal systems currently in use.

The reader should review Table 77, in which suggested autoimmune diseases are listed. By applying the criteria outlined above, only a small number of these diseases would satisfy the requirements to prove autoimmunization. The studies of Witebsky (32) may be used to illustrate procedures that should be employed in arriving at an autoimmune diagnosis. This does not imply that autoimmunization is a rare phenomenon. Our current status has

TABLE 78. *Experimental animal systems employed as models for autoimmune diseases*

Human Disease	Experimental Disease	Tissue Involved
Postinfectious encephalomyelitis	Allergic encephalomyelitis	Central nervous system myelin
Multiple sclerosis	Allergic neuritis	Peripheral nerve myelin
Landry's paralysis, Guillain-Barré syndrome, peripheral neuritis	Allergic neuritis	Myelin
Thyroiditis	Allergic thyroiditis	Thyroglobulin
Sympathetic ophthalmia, postinfectious iridocylitis	Allergic uveitis	Uvea
Phacoanaphylactic endophthalmitis	Phacoanaphylactic endophthalmitis	Lens
Mumps orchitis, aspermatogenesis	Allergic orchitis	Germinal cells
Adrenal hypotrophy	Allergic adrenalitis	Cortical cells
Autoimmune hemolytic anemia	NZB mice: hemolytic anemia	Erythrocyte
Systemic lupus erythematosus	NZB mice: lupus nephritis	Kidney
Autoimmune hemolytic anemia	Dog: hemolytic anemia	Erythrocyte
Evans' syndrome	Dog: hemolytic anemia and thrombocytopenia	Erythrocyte and thrombocyte
Systemic lupus erythematosus	Dog: lupus nephritis	Kidney

resulted from investigations primarily oriented toward humoral antibody production. It is anticipated that new theoretical and laboratory approaches involving cellular immune reactions will aid in the understanding of autoimmune diseases. Delayed hypersensitivity as a pathophysiologic mechanism will undoubtedly swell the ranks of autoimmune diseases.

Theories of Autoimmunization

The theory of autoimmunization first received serious consideration in clinical medicine. This concept was applied to syndromes characterized by tissue damage and gamma-globulin fixation. The assumption was made that globulin functioned as an antibody specifically reacting with host antigens, i.e., that it was an autoantibody. This assumption is no longer valid. The characteristic findings may result from many different pathologic sequences. Although a similar end stage develops, the underlying etiology may vary greatly. Clinical syndromes currently considered to be induced by autoimmunization may involve mechanisms that are neither autoimmune nor even immune. An attempt has been made to document the various means through which tissue damage associated with gamma-globulin deposition occurs. Thirteen different mechanisms must be

considered. The relevant concepts are broadly discussed within three main categories: (a) a nonimmunologic pathogenesis, (b) an immunologic but not autoimmune pathogenesis, and (c) an autoimmune pathogenesis. Table 79 summarizes the groups and specific mechanisms discussed below. Excellent reviews of the same subject with a diversity of viewpoints have been presented in a symposium edited by Trentin (37) and in the publications of MacKay and Burnet (31), Glynn and Holborow (38), Dameshek (39) and Gras (40).

A Nonimmunologic Pathogenesis

Immunologic self-recognition is an important physiologic mechanism of all vertebrates possessing an antibody forming capacity. Investigators have therefore been reluctant to accept an abnormality of this homeostatic system. Clinical and experimental studies, however, have clearly shown that an individual's serum components may react with his own tissue. Damage to tissue may occur during such reactions. This phenomenon deserves an explanation. It may be postulated that the serum components are not antibodies and that a nonimmunologic pathologic sequence has occurred. Two theoretical mechanisms should be considered.

1. The Specificity of the Nonspecific: Specificity for an antigenic determinant is characteristic of antibody reactivity. Many but not all abnormal serum reacting substances demonstrate specificity for various host tissues. Any nonimmunologic pathogenesis must therefore contain an explanation for such specificity. It should not be assumed that specificity is unique for antibody. Enzymes may have the same exquisite specificity for substrate. In addition, nonantibody substances have documented specificity for individual antigenic determinants. This phenomenon is illustrated in the reaction of various plant lectins with human erythrocytes. Reagents able to specifically agglutinate red cells of type A_1, A_2, M, N and H have been prepared. The similarity in reactivity between such lectins and known blood group isoantibodies is remarkable. There is no suggestion, however, that the plant has been immunized with specific human erythrocytes in order to produce a specific antibody molecule.

It may be postulated that autoantibodies are analogous substances. They possibly represent the fortuitous production of protein molecules with a molecular structure complementary to specific antigenic determinants. This concept of the "specificity of the nonspecific" has been well summarized by Boyd (41). Applying this rationale, autoimmune syndromes would be a form of dysgammaglobulinemia. This viewpoint might be dismissed as simply an exercise in semantics, but a fundamental question is at stake. Exactly what constitutes antibody must be defined. In terms of natural selection theories of antibody formation, such substances may be considered as antibodies. This problem will continue to exist until the exact function of antigen in antibody formation is clarified.

2. Nonimmune Clonal Formation: A similar problem is encountered in another possible nonimmune pathogenesis. Antigenic determinants may be considered as mitogenic agents which "select" appropriate immunocompetent cells without "instructing" in the establishment of a specific globulin molecular conformation. This

TABLE 79. *Pathophysiologic mechanisms leading to autoimmune and simulated autoimmune diseases (all mechanisms may lead to tissue damage and deposition of gamma-globulin)*

Pathogenesis	Specific Mechanism
Nonimmunologic	1. Specificity of the non-specific 2. Monoclonal dysgamma-globulinemia

Immune but not autoimmune	1. Exogenous antigens
	   a. Innocent bystander
	   b. Immune complex
	   c. Cross reacting antibody
	 2. Modified autologous antigens
	   a. Denaturation
	   b. Hapten formation

Autoimmune	1. Immunologic quarantine 2. Unusual propensity 3. Foreign clone 4. Forbidden clone 5. Immune deficiency state 6. Termination of tolerance

introduces the possibility of antibody formation occurring without the influence of antigenic material. Indeed the theories of both Ehrlich (12) and Jerne (4) concerning antibody formation are based on the assumption that antibody exists independently of antigenic action. The possibility that nonimmune mitogenic activity may simulate antibody formation deserves evaluation.

One such example immediately comes to mind. Will malignancy involving an immunocompetent cell result in antibody production without antigenic stimulation? Rapid division of such cells should create a clone of cells with the same end product of protein metabolism. Studies in plasma cell myeloma indicate that clones of cells do arise, all producing the same immunoglobulin. Current biochemical investigations suggest that similar molecular structures are present among antibodies and myeloma proteins. Are such immunoglobulins "abnormal" proteins resulting from monoclonal dysgammaglobulinemia? Shall they be thought of as antibodies produced without antigenic stimulation, with specificity for an unidentified antigen? Experimental tolerance studies indicate that host cells with the capacity to produce antibodies against host tissues are not destroyed in embryonic life, but that rather they are inhibited (18–20, 24). Is it too unlikely that inhibition can be overcome, with a break in immune tolerance, under malignant and other forms of mitogenic stimulation? Is the process then to be considered autoimmunization or monoclonal dysgammaglobulinemia? Cold hemagglutinin disease illustrates this dilemma. Characteristically there is a monoclonal production of immunoglobulins with anti-I or anti-i specificity (see Chapters 19 and 20).

The relationship of nonspecific "specific" globulins and monoclonal dysgammaglobulinemia to autoimmunization still must be clarified. Agreement as to the fundamental nature of antibody formation is crucial. However, it is unlikely that such mechanisms explain the vast array of presumed autoimmune disease. The frequent and almost predictable occurrence of autoantibodies, as seen in thyroid surgery and radiation, makes the possibility of a fortuitous occurrence unlikely. Many autoimmune states are unrelated to malignant transformation. Accordingly, nonimmune clonal stimulation is unlikely as a universal mechanism. Even with a malignant syndrome, little proof of this postulate is available. A direct search for autoantibodies in lymphocyte extracts from patients with chronic lymphocytic leukemia complicated by autoimmune hemolytic anemia demonstrated hemagglutinins and hemolysins but no autoantibodies (42, 43).

Immunologic But Not Autoimmune Pathogenesis

Most investigators accept the premise that antibody formation is a part of autoimmune syndromes. This does not imply, however, that the involved antibody is an autoantibody or that the process is truly autoimmunization. The type of antigen permits distinction between autoimmune,

and immune but not autoimmune, processes. Two unrelated immunologic sequences may be concerned in the production of tissue damage, with an incorrect assumption of autoimmunization.

A. Foreign Antigens

Within this subheading three major mechanisms must be considered. In all three, antibody formation is initiated against foreign antigenic determinants that are not host constituents. Specificity of the antibody is misinterpreted as a result of incomplete documentation of antigen. Involvement of host tissues in the immune reaction occurs. The erroneous assumption is then made that host antigens are the primary target against which the antibody is directed.

1. The Innocent Bystander: Many in vivo interactions occur between soluble antigen and antibody without overt evidence of immunologic activity. Antibody formation acts in such states as an immunologic homeostatic mechanism removing foreign materials from the host. This relatively simple process would be drastically modified if a foreign substance were to initiate antibody formation and also bind to various tissues. Antibody-antigen union could then take place on the cellular surface. The kinetics of such a reaction would differ from that seen in the soluble state. The association and dissociation rate of soluble antigen to cell surface would introduce a variable. The avidity of antibody for such cell bound antigen would also differ from that in the soluble state. Theoretically, the reverse situation is also possible. Globulin molecules are continually coating cells and dissociating. Antibody bound to cell surfaces in such a nonimmunologic fashion may retain its ability to react immunologically with soluble antigen. The results of immunologic union under the conditions of cellular adsorption of either antibody or antigen are difficult to predict. Cellular injury or death could occur during this process. Complement fixation during antibody-antigen union may have a significant role in the resulting cellular injury.

In the situation described above the cell functions as an innocent bystander. It simply offers a favorable surface environment for the interaction of a totally unrelated immunologic event. During such immunologic activity the innocent bystander sustains sufficient injury to be clinically detected. Without identifying the antigen, specificity for the cell can be erroneously interpreted as antigen specificity. Autoantibody formation is incorrectly assumed. This sequence occurs in the penicillin induced forms of immunohemolytic anemia. The host antibody reacting with penicillin bound to erythrocytes can be demonstrated in an antiglobulin procedure and may simulate an autoimmune state.

2. Antigen-antibody Complexes: The vertebrate with an immune apparatus is surrounded by a foreign antigenic evironment. The in vivo interaction of soluble antigen and antibody is a continual process. Immune complexes formed are rapidly cleared from the circulation, broken down and eventually excreted. Accordingly, tissues with a filtration apparatus and large circulation would be expected to encounter such complexes.

The deposition of immune complexes in various tissues may lead to tissue damage. It is generally obvious that an immunologic event has occurred. Localization of damage to an organ or cell system may be interpreted as antigenic specificity and autoimmunization may be assumed. In reality a foreign antigen has combined with an autologous antibody and has been deposited in an immunologically unrelated tissue. Dixon and associates (44) investigated such a system. Rabbits sensitized to bovine serum albumin were studied. Challenging these animals with large amounts of bovine serum albumin resulted in serum sickness. However, a similar group of animals received repeated small doses of antigen without significant depletion of circulating antibody. Chronic glomerulonephritis developed in such animals. Electron microscopy and labeled antibody identified the areas of fibrinoid degeneration as depositions of bovine albumin and rabbit globulin (44, 45). Immune complexes had been deposited in the renal tubular areas, resulting in tissue damage and glomerulonephritis. Fish and asso-

ciates (46) have confirmed many of these observations using a single dose of antigen. It is not too difficult to visualize a comparable clinical situation. With an unidentified antigen, the obvious immunologic reaction may suggest autoimmunization. The autologous antibody is erroneously assumed to be an autoantibody reacting with host renal tissue.

Dixon (47, 48) has summarized the properties of antigen-antibody complexes which may induce pathologic changes. He emphasizes that these complexes are formed by the combination of molecules which separately do not damage tissue. As the result of their combination, biologic activity is developed against various unrelated tissues and organs. The toxic properties of immune complexes are probably due to distortion of antibody molecules. The mechanism appears similar to that described by Ishizaka and associates (49) for the toxic effect of gamma-globulin modified by various chemical and physical methods. Dixon (48) lists the following characteristics of immune complexes: (a) the complexes themselves may be toxic; (b) complexes formed in moderate antigen excess show the greatest biologic activity; (c) most active complexes have an affinity for tissues and are able to interact with complement; (d) the biologic activity of the complex is dependent on antibody properties, rather than on the antigen; (e) complement fixation and tissue fixation properties of immune complexes are dependent on the Fc portion of the antibody molecule; and (f) biologic activity of immune complexes is associated with a change in their optical rotation.

Antigen-antibody complexes may initiate tissue damage by reacting with various serum components. They can activate part of the C'1 component of complement to an active esterase. In addition, they will cause the formation of fibrinolysin, anaphylatoxin and active peptides such as bradykinin. On a cellular level Dixon (48) describes the following reactions: (a) degranulation of mast cells with liberation of various amines, (b) attachment of complexes to leukocytes and thrombocytes with agglutination, (c) contraction of smooth muscles, (d) increase of vascular permeability, (e) endothelial proliferation, (f) chemotactic attraction of mature granulocytes in the presence of complement, and (g) the production of degenerative, hyaline changes in various tissues.

It is apparent that immune complexes possess the ability to induce cellular damage in tissues unrelated to either the antibody or the antigen. If the antigen involved is not identified, the immunologic reaction may be interpreted as a host antibody reacting with a self-antigen, i.e., autoimmunization. This process occurs in thrombocytopenia induced by quinine and quinidine and in hemolytic anemia induced by stibophen. In both of these examples, autoimmunization was assumed until Schulman (50) documented the fixation of immune complexes to thrombocytes and erythrocytes, respectively. Miescher and associates (51) had previously shown that thrombocytes offered a reacting surface for the adsorption of unrelated immune complexes. Pulmonary fibrinoid degeneration observed in children with circulating antibody against cow's milk is a possible human counterpart of Dixon's study (44). Such patients have a daily intake of milk in the presence of humoral antibody directed against milk components. It is apparent that immune complexes must be considered whenever autoimmunization is suggested. Precise delineation of the antigen is required to clarify this problem.

3. Cross Reacting Antibodies: A living vertebrate is exposed to a vast array of foreign antigenic material. It is reasonable to assume that some foreign materials contain antigenic determinants with a structural relationship to various host antigens. For example, material analogous to human blood group A substance has a wide distribution in nature. The production of "naturally" occurring anti-A in the human is probably the result of such heteroimmune stimulation (52). In general, antibody formation does not follow exposure to a foreign antigen when host antigens are closely related. Accordingly, only individuals of blood group O or B will produce "naturally" occurring anti-A.

It may be postulated that structural resemblances between foreign and self antigenic determinants are sufficiently distinctive to permit antibody formation. The antibody formed could appear as a cross reacting substance. It would have the ability, depending on the degree of antibody-antigen fit, to react with self-antigens. This cannot be considered as autoimmunization. Stadsbaeder (53) has elegantly presented this viewpoint in describing heterogeneous antiinfectious agent antibodies which cross react with erythrocytes and simulate autoantibodies. Antibody formation is directed against foreign antigenic determinants, rather than host self-antigens. Normal immune tolerance is violated to some degree by production of such cross reacting antibody. However, host antigens do not initiate the process and possibly do not interact with the antibody in vivo.

Two examples may be used to illustrate this process in relation to autoimmunization. Wiener (52) suggested that cold acting erythrocyte autoantibodies present in all human sera result from heteroimmune stimulation. Antigens structurally related to human erythrocyte antigens may be supplied by various infectious states and through the ingestion of foods. He visualized such cross reacting cold autoagglutinins as poor "fitting" antibodies with a relatively low avidity for human red cells. The poor fit permits the dissociation of antigen-antibody union by thermal agitation, resulting in a cold acting autoantibody. This concept is supported by the studies of Costea and associates (54). They demonstrated that rabbits immunized with *Listeria monocytogenes* of serotype 4b produced cold acting erythrocyte autoantibodies reactive against both rabbit and human erythrocytes. Smith and associates (55) have demonstrated the production of anti-I cold hemagglutinins in human volunteers subsequent to immunization with *Mycoplasma pneumoniae*.

Kaplan and Meyeserian (56) have applied these principles to rheumatic fever in the human. Their studies indicate that antigenic constituents of streptococcal cells, group A Tripp, Lancefield type 5, contain an antigenic constituent immunologically cross reactive with human heart tissue. The antigen is localized to the cell wall of streptococci. It appears to be a protein unrelated to M protein. Antiserum against this antigen reacts with human heart tissue suspensions in complement-fixation tests. Immunofluorescence procedures suggest that the reactive antigen is localized in the sarcolemma and smooth muscle elements of cardiac vessels and endocardium. Kaplan (57) has demonstrated the presence of reacting antibodies in the sera of patients with acute rheumatic fever, inactive rheumatic heart disease and acute glomerulonephritis. Immunoglobulins and complement components have been described in sarcolemma or subsarcolemma sites in hearts obtained from patients suffering from rheumatic fever. This further supports the postulated immunologic etiology. Kaplan suggests that continual production of the cross reacting antibody may result from stimulation by autologous heart antigens. If this could be demonstrated, a true state of autoimmunization would exist. Goldstein and associates (58) have studied a similar system. They suggest a cross reacting relationship between group A streptococcus polysaccharide and glycoprotein fractions present in heart valvular structures.

B. Modified Autologous Antigens

Other states may simulate autoimmunization through an immunologic but not autoimmune pathogenesis. This represents an area of probable controversy. How autoimmunization is defined appears to be crucial for classification. Autoimmunization may be considered as antibody formation initiated against any host constituent, whether normal or modified. If antibody formation is directed toward modified host constituents, this process would involve recognition of the induced foreign state of the host antigen. Antibody formation would represent the normal physiologic pathways activated in immune homeostasis. Such an immune reaction would differ fundamentally from that induced by normal, unmodified self-antigens. The similarity between these

two mechanisms is related to the end stage observation of antibodies reacting with host tissues.

Autoimmunization, however, may be classified by the mechanism which initiates antibody formation, rather than by the end stage process. The living vertebrate is surrounded by a mass of self-antigens which have the potential ability to stimulate antibody formation. Self-recognition and natural immune tolerance prevent the production of such antibody. Autoimmunization within this concept is considered as a new immunologic relationship. Antibody formation initiated against normal self-antigens occurs through a termination of natural immune tolerance. The underlying abnormality is therefore a loss of self-recognition. The author prefers this latter classification. Autoimmunization is considered to be the host production of antibodies with specificity for normal, unmodified host antigens.

Considering syndromes as immunologic but not autoimmune does not minimize their clinical significance. The terminology is employed to emphasize the diversity of mechanisms which result in immunologically mediated tissue damage. Perhaps the majority of syndromes now classified as autoimmune are initiated through immunologic but not autoimmune pathways. Modified autologous antigens may produce this state in two distinct ways.

1. Modification of the Antigen: The simplest explanation for autoimmune syndromes, without resorting to autoimmunization, is to assume a change in the cellular antigen. Autoimmune diseases generally occur in patients with profound illness. Such disease states could induce sufficient changes of involved cells to produce foreign components. Relatively minor changes may be involved and may still permit the self-recognition system to recognize them as foreign. Modification of cellular self-antigens sufficient to elicit a response implies either acquisition of new specificity to which the organism is not tolerant, or the loss of those features of the self-antigen against which the tolerant state was established. Perpetuation of the disease process maintains the continual production of modified cellular components, leading to continual production of antibodies. The antibody produced could have a narrow reactivity, with its action restricted to the modified cell or components. An antibody with a broader reactivity might also result, capable of cross reacting with normal cells or cell components. Such a possibility has been entertained by Shulman and Witebsky (59) and Asherson and Dumonde (60).

The changes described above are dependent on a disease state followed by antibody formation. Self-reacting antibody would result from, rather than initiate, the disease process. An experimental system illustrating this sequence has been studied by McClusky and associates (61). They demonstrated autoantigenicity of autologous rabbit and guinea pig gamma-globulin after protein denaturation by alkali treatment. This interpretation does not minimize the role of the antibody in the symptom complex. Modification of cells or cellular components by minor and unrecognized environmental factors is possible. The initiating process may be asymptomatic and only the end stage of antibody formation may be apparent. Somatic mutation, various drugs, bacteria, bacterial products, viruses and mechanical trauma are some of the means by which normal cellular components may be modified. Antibody formation initiated in this fashion could result in an immunologic disease syndrome. Many of these factors are discussed in greater detail in the section on antiglobulin positive hemolytic anemia (Chapter 14).

2. The Formation of Haptens: The antibody producing organism has been visualized as surviving in an environment of foreign antigenic substances. For the human in particular, one legacy of civilization has been the expansion of this foreign environment through contact with drugs and chemicals. Such chemicals can combine with protein. This can produce a complex antigen with immunogenicity due to the protein moiety and specificity to the nonprotein moiety. The nonprotein moiety, previously nonimmunogenic but now directing specificity, is known as a hapten. It may be postulated that an in vivo or cellular counterpart of hapten formation exists. The new antigen resulting from hapten for-

mation would initiate antibody production. The antibody or antibodies produced may have specificity for the hapten, for the protein carrier or for both. It is obvious that an unrecognized haptenic state with an autologous protein carrier could be misinterpreted as specificity of host antibodies for host antigens, i.e., as autoimmunization.

Studies by Cinader and Dubert (62) suggest that antibody formation cannot result with such haptens when a state of immune tolerance exists for the carrier protein. Hapten formation with autologous proteins is insufficient in itself to terminate tolerance and permit antibody formation. Two possibilities may be suggested to overcome this objection. The combination of hapten with a protein carrier may in itself introduce modifications in the carrier which have immunologic significance. The fixation of picryl chloride to various proteins illustrates how haptens may modify proteins. Hapten formation arising from a reversal of the involved reagents must also be considered. Host constituents may act as haptens binding to foreign proteins. Glynn and Holborow (38) have emphasized the possible role of bacteria in this latter mechanism.

Ackroyd (63) in 1949 first suggested the role of a hapten state as an etiologic mechanism in autoimmunization. He postulated that Sedormid functioned as an exogenous hapten combining with host thrombocytes and creating a complex antigen. Thrombocytopenia followed the subsequent ingestion of Sedormid. Antibodies produced were specific and reacted with the complex but not with normal thrombocytes in the absence of Sedormid. A similar hapten explanation was used by Harris (64) to explain hemolytic anemia occurring during stibophen therapy. Skillman and associates (65) also employed the hapten concept to relate prior beta hemolytic streptococci infections to the development of rheumatic fever. All of these studies deserve reevaluation. Immune complex and cross reacting antibody systems have been suggested to explain the same syndromes.

Autoimmune Pathogenesis

The above discussion has outlined mechanisms which explain events generally considered as autoimmune within a framework of more classically recognized immunologic systems. The postulates are similar in that the self-recognition system of the living organism is not at fault. Antibody formation appears as a normal response of the immune homeostatic apparatus initiated by intrinsic or extrinsic substances foreign to the host. If we limit autoimmunization to conditions in which normal unmodified host constituents appear foreign to the self-recognition system of a host, additional theoretical principles are necessary. Six such systems can be postulated at this time.

A. Immunologic Quarantine

Classification of this category is difficult. The mechanism is autoimmune if the process is defined as the development of host antibodies with specificity for unmodified self-antigens. The difficulty arises because antibody formation is initiated against host self-antigens without loss of self-recognition or termination of immune tolerance. The semantic difficulty in discussing autoimmunization is again apparent.

Antigenic materials are immunogenic only if they are available in an appropriate form to stimulate antibody formation. Their solubility and access to lymphatic drainage are characteristics necessary to their function as antigens. The other end of the immune spectrum must also be considered. For antibody-antigen interaction to occur, it is not sufficient merely to produce an antibody. An arterial blood supply is necessary to deliver antibody to fixed tissue antigens.

One or more of the above criteria may not be met in vivo. Host antigens not capable of reacting with antibody producing cells are "foreign" to the immune apparatus. Such host constituents may be thought of as existing in a state of immunologic quarantine. This may arise in several ways. Anatomic and physiologic peculiarities may prevent a host's tissues from interacting with the immune apparatus during embryonic and neonatal life. Self-recognition therefore cannot occur and normal immune tolerance will not be created. Even if contact of self-antigens with the immune apparatus initially occurs, self-recognition may be lost with further growth and development. Ex-

perimental studies have clearly shown that a continual supply of antigen is necessary to maintain the state of immune unresponsiveness (18, 24). The isolation of host constituents from the immune apparatus because of anatomic or physiologic considerations would terminate natural immune tolerance. Contact of such self-antigens with the immune system in later life would lead to recognition of them as foreign and to initiation of antibody formation. This process may be termed autoimmunization. There are four major methods by which termination of immunologic quarantine may initiate autoimmunization.

1. Anatomic Peculiarities: A limited number of tissues may be considered as existing in a state of immunologic quarantine (66, 67). These include the nervous system, the lens of the eye, aqueous humour, the cornea, the uveal tract, the testis, the adrenal gland, fat tissue and the cheek pouch of the hampster. Such tissues have anatomic similarities. In many cases they are separated from the vascular bed by more or less impermeable cellular barriers. Such barriers may be found in the lens capsule, the pia-glia membrane of the central nervous system and the basement membrane of the seminiferous tubule. The absence of effective lymphatic drainage from these tissues is significant. This anatomic peculiarity creates self-antigens which are foreign in relation to the immune apparatus. Such systems are discussed in great detail by Waksman (66).

2. Late Developing Antigens: The testes present an interesting modification of the concept of immunologic quarantine. Self-recognition and the establishment of immune tolerance occur in a definitive and finite period of time in the embryonic and immediate neonatal period. Certain host antigenic substances may not be present in this critical period. Several tissues in the body, particularly the sex organs, are incompletely developed during the stage when self-recognition generally occurs. Spermatozoa are an example of this phenomenon. Such cells are not present until puberty, a time well past the establishment of normal immune tolerance. Spermatozoa may accordingly appear as a normal, unmodified host tissue which is "foreign" to the immune system. The basement membrane of the seminiferous tubules and the poor lymphatic drainage establish immunologic quarantine of these cells. Sterility resulting from aspermatogenesis in the presence of circulating antispermatocyte autoantibodies may reflect a break in immunologic quarantine (68).

3. Intracellular Quarantine: Various intracellular components may be entirely confined to the intracellular state. Their passage through the cell membrane or their release upon disruption of the cell membrane usually results in destruction or modification of the intracellular constituent. Host constituents which are normally present in an exclusive intracellular distribution may therefore be considered as foreign in relation to the immune apparatus. They exist in a state of immunologic quarantine. Thyroglobulin is an example of such an intracellular material. This material exists only within the secretory thyroid cell. Upon transmembrane passage into the circulation, thyroglobulin is converted into triiodothyronine. Witebsky (32) and his group have clarified many of the problems related to autoimmunization, using the thyroglobulin system. These investigators found that removal of part of the thyroid gland, homogenization of the gland with Freund's adjuvant and injection of this material into the donor animal result in the production of antibodies directed against the remaining thyroid tissue. The specific antigenic substance was determined to be thyroglobulin. It is possible to visualize the counterpart of this experimental state. Disease, surgery or radiation may release sufficient unmodified thyroglobulin to initiate antibody formation.

4. A Change in Molecular Structure: The concept of host antigens existing in immunologic quarantine can be further expanded. Proteins have a specific molecular conformation with certain portions of the molecule exposed and functioning as antigenic determinants. Other parts of the molecule may be unavailable and therefore may not evoke self-recognition or create immune tolerance. Such portions of a protein molecule exist in immunologic quarantine. If the molecular conformation could be modified to expose unavailable antigenic determinants, antibody formation directed against the new determinants could be initiated. Experimental studies by Najjar and Fisher (69) suggest that such a sequence can occur with immunoglobulins. These workers have postulated that during antibody-antigen union modification of the antibody globulin molecular structure occurs. Modification of autologous globulin molecules result in the exposure of previously inaccessible antigenic determinants. Antibody formation directed against the modified antibody globulin may now be initiated with the formation of *antiantibodies*. Milgrom and Dubiski (70) and Milgrom (71) have expanded these observations into a proposed system of autoimmunization. This concept is presented in detail in Chapter 14. The theoretical basis for the development of anti-antibody has been summarized by Najjar (72).

The four mechanisms outlined above differ greatly on anatomic and physiologic grounds. A similarity is apparent, however, when they are examined from the viewpoint of autoimmunization. In all cases host antigens are normally unavailable to the antibody producing system. This creates a group of antigenic substances to which a state of normal immune tolerance has not been established. It is helpful to consider these materials as existing in a state of immunologic quarantine. A break in this quarantine and the exposure of such antigens to the immune apparatus may lead to antibody formation. This mechanism opens an almost unlimited vista for potential immunologic reactivity in the host. The autoantibody produced upon violation of immunologic quarantine appears as the result of a pathologic state, rather than as the etiologic agent causing the primary disease syndrome. For example, a vast number of intracellular substances exist in a state of immunologic quarantine. Normal enzymatic degradation during metabolism and cellular death maintains their inaccessible nature in relationship to the immune apparatus. Disease states or even therapeutic procedures may produce a sudden and massive release of unmodified intracellular components. Autoantibody formation can be anticipated without prior establishment of a self-recognition state. Thyroiditis, thyroid surgery and radiation, pancreatitis, hepatitis, the postmyocardial infarct syndrome and the postcardiotomy syndrome are a few clinical examples which may be involved in this category. Although autoantibody formation may not initiate the pathophysiologic state, its occurrence as a secondary phenomenon can dominate the clinical picture.

B. Enhanced Sensitivity of the Immune Apparatus

Host antigens are constantly changing through metabolism and under the influence of nonhost factors. Antibody formation may be initiated if modification of a host antigen is sufficient to produce a foreign state or if a previously inaccessible host antigen is presented to the immune system. A change of immunogenicity must involve either a loss of the antigenic determinant groups which established self-recognition or else creation of new antigenic determinants not involved in a tolerant state. At what point, however, will the immune apparatus recognize modifications of host antigens as foreign? The immune apparatus is a biologic system subject to individual variations. Variations in the capacity of individual immune systems to recognize such changes appear to be innate. There are species and interspecies differences. There are "good" antibody producers and "poor" antibody producers. The human system presents a spectrum of ability to recognize antigenic determinants as foreign and to produce antibodies against such determinants. A theoretical system of autoimmunization may be formulated by applying these concepts to self-antigens continually changing through growth, metabolism and catabolism. Changes induced in this fashion, which are nonimmunogenic in the large majority, may be of sufficient magnitude to initiate antibody formation in a select few. These individuals with an enhanced propensity to produce antibodies may then form autoantibodies.

This proposed mechanism requires antigenic modification as a prerequisite for antibody formation. However, such changes are normal for the host and do not result in a loss of self-recognition or antibody production. Antibody formation appears to be an abnormal variation of the reticulo-endothelium which permits the immune apparatus to recognize normal modifications. In other words, self-recognition is lost and the normal state of immune tolerance is terminated in the select few. A true state of autoimmunization may accordingly be postulated. This concept is expanded in Chapter 15 in terms of autoimmune hemolytic anemia.

C. The Establishment of a Foreign Clone

Dameshek (39) has emphasized the high incidence of lymphocytic abnormalities in autoimmune diseases, particularly those related to the blood and the blood forming organ. This suggests that autoimmunization may reflect the establishment of a foreign clone of cells, leading to a graft versus host reaction. This mechanism does not involve modification of antigenic constituents but rather an abnormality of the antibody producing system. The following sequence of events may be proposed. An abnormality of an immunocompetent cell occurs. This may take the form of a permanent somatic mutation leading to malignancy, or it may be temporary, derived from an environmental factor such as a virus. Unrestricted proliferation of the modified immunocompetent cell occurs. A clone of daughter cells containing the same foreign state in reference to the host is created. A situation analogous to experimental runt disease could then occur. The established clone of modified host cells, derived from immunocompetent cell precursors, possesses the ability to recognize foreign tissue and to produce antibodies. In the situation proposed above, host tissues may appear foreign. Antibody formation could then occur, initiated against foreign constituents which are normal, unmodified antigens.

Several assumptions are necessary to allow this mechanism to work. A clone of cells foreign to the host organism must persist and proliferate. This would require either a defect in the self-recognition mechanism, or a growth rate of the clone sufficient to overcome the immunologic handicap. There is also difficulty in relating this view to the original clonal selection theory of antibody formation (2). Theoretically, the immunocompetent cell undergoing malignancy and clonal formation would be limited to the formation of a single or at the most two or three preselected specific antibodies. In addition, the antigenic determinant could not be a host constituent, as cells able to react with such self-antigens are presumed to be eliminated during embryonic life. This clonal selection view is incompatible with the disastrous regularity of autoimmune hemolytic anemia complicating chronic lymphocytic leukemia. A 25 per cent incidence effectively eliminates the chance involvement of a specific cell, previously inhibited, with the exclusive potential to produce antibodies directed against host erythrocytes. A multipotential antibody producing cell must be assumed. Dameshek (73) has postulated just such a cell, which he terms the immunocyte or immunoblast.

The subcellular hypothesis of Szilard (7) offers a model system applicable to the above mechanism. Predilection for erythrocyte autoantibodies would be accounted for by assuming the production of a clone of cells with the protein synthesizing mechanism "unlocked" during malignant proliferation. Such cells would be immediately exposed to large amounts of erythrocyte antigenic material in view of the juxtaposition of both cell types in the circulation and reticuloendothelium. The "locking" of these cells with antibody formation directed toward the erythrocyte would then result in typical autoimmune hemolytic anemia.

D. The Concept of the Forbidden Clone

Burnet (74) has also suggested that autoimmunization results from an abnormality of the antibody producing mechanism. The postulated defect in the immune apparatus involves the persistence of cells which have been termed forbidden clones. These cells carry a pattern of immunologic reactivity corresponding to accessible self-constituent antigenic determinants. It is postulated that such cells are inhibited or eliminated during embryonic development in order for self-recognition to occur. MacKay and Burnet (31) proposed that a functional abnormality of the lymphoid tissue, which allowed the development of such forbidden clones, would result in autoantibody production and autoimmune disease. The development of such clones is dependent on mutations, with persistence occurring through a failure of immunologic homeostasis. "Probably the most satisfactory way to look at autoimmune disease is as a failure at some point of the normal homeostatic mechanisms that prevent the emergence of forbidden clones." Persistence and growth of such forbidden clones would give rise to a self-perpetuating disease. Autoantibody formation would induce cellular damage which in turn would release further antigenic material. A vicious cycle of antibody production and cellular damage would then ensue.

This concept is supported by evidence of a familial predisposition in many autoimmune syndromes. The development of a murine form of autoimmune hemolytic anemia in the NZB mouse strain offers an excellent experimental model. This is discussed in detail in Chapter 22. Such studies suggest that a genetically inherited weakness in the immunologic homeostatic mechanism has been selected by inbreeding, which permits the emergence of forbidden clones. Vertical transmission of viruses may modify this view (75).

The forbidden clone concept is vulnerable from two aspects. The abnormality must involve the specific cell with a capability to produce the specific autoantibody. The frequency of complicating autoimmune disease in various clinical entities makes it unlikely that pure chance is involved. This suggests that simple persistence of a forbidden clone is an insufficient explanation. The problem is magnified when the time relationship of autoimmune syndromes is examined. If a forbidden clone has persisted and is available, autoantibody formation may be anticipated simultaneously with the capacity to produce immunoglobulins. This generally does not occur. It is apparent that additional precipitating factors and homeostatic mechanisms are involved in the maintenance of the state of self-recognition.

E. The Immunodeficient State

The forbidden clone, foreign clone and graft-host disease postulates have supplied valuable theoretical tools in the study of autoimmunization. By themselves, however, they appear inadequate to explain all clinical manifestations. A combination of these hypotheses should be considered. Burnet's suggestion of a defect in immune homeostasis (74) and Dameshek's concept of an immunocyte functioning in a graft-host syndrome (39) are particularly pertinent. The following pathogenesis may occur. An individual may have a basic defect in his immune apparatus which limits the capacity to initiate normal immune responses. There is some evidence that this aberration is genetically mediated. Such individuals are poor antibody producers. The immunodeficiency would prevent the establishment of normal immune homeostatic mechanisms. Abnormal cells produced in vivo, which normally are recognized as foreign and destroyed, may survive because of this malfunction. Permanent somatic mutations or virus modifications can be involved in the creation of such foreign host cells. Reticuloendothelial cells would be particularly vulnerable because their growth and turnover rate is of the highest magnitude. Survival and replication of modified immunocompetent cells (immunocyte) would result in a foreign clone capable of initiating a graft-host reaction. A single clone involved in this process presumably produces a single autoantibody. This static state is probably unusual. It is more reasonable that multiple modified clones of cells are produced sequentially and persist throughout the natural history of the disease. The result would be complex syndromes characterized by multiple autoantibody formation in varying multisystem patterns (76). This concept of a vulnerable immunodeficient individual is particularly valuable in considering the autoimmune hemolytic anemias, and it is discussed in Chapter 15.

F. A Termination of Immune Tolerance

Immune tolerance experimentally induced to soluble antigens is not permanent (18, 24). This observation suggests a possible analogy to natural tolerance and self-recognition. If natural immune tolerance to host antigens is similarly impermanent, the living organism is perpetually faced with the possible development of autoimmunization. On a cellular basis this suggests that immunocompetent cells with the potential to produce antibodies against self-constituents are not eliminated or destroyed. The forbidden clones of Burnet are always present. Proliferation of such cells and autoantibody formation must be actively inhibited.

Accordingly, immune tolerance and self-recognition are considered to be a temporary condition requiring a continual and active mechanism to maintain the state of inhibition. This may be accomplished by the saturation of receptor sites, by the "locking" of the cell protein synthesizing apparatus into other pathways or by other means not as yet delineated. However, the potential to "unlock" the cell and to initiate synthesis of autoantibodies is always present. Weigle (20) has pointed out that the tolerant state may be terminated by formation of cross reacting antibody or by immunization with the original antigen in a denatured form.

The above concepts may be formulated into a sequence of events leading to autoimmunization. Disease states or environmental factors such as drugs, bacteria, bacterial products, viruses and physical conditions may modify a host's antigenic structures sufficiently to induce antibody formation. The antibody produced could be directed specifically against the now foreign self-antigen. However, it may have a broader range of activity and may appear as a cross reacting antibody. This mechanism has been described as an immune but not autoimmune pathogenesis. One further step may be postulated to lead to autoimmunization. Antibody formation initiated against modified self-constituent antigenic determinants may terminate the temporary state of natural immune tolerance. Autoantibody formation would result. This hypothesis would suggest that autoantibody formation and autoimmunization are a normal immune response. It is activated after removal of the inhibition which establishes a temporary state of unresponsiveness. This postulate makes it unnecessary to search for a continually active pathologic process producing autoantibodies. In addition there is no reason to presuppose an abnormality of the antibody producing apparatus which permits autoantibody formation to occur.

Although this proposed hypothesis is compatible with observed immunologic findings, several critical questions must still be answered. How is the state of natural immune tolerance initiated and maintained? Why is autoimmunization comparatively rare when tissue antigen modification is a continual process? Exactly how do modified antigens and the production of cross reacting antibodies result in a termination of immune tolerance? This subject is extensively reviewed by Weigle (20).

Summary of Mechanisms Involved in Autoimmunization

The 13 mechanisms discussed above may lead to an apparent state of autoimmunization. They have been briefly reviewed from a theoretical viewpoint. Chapters 14 and 15 greatly expand these concepts and illustrate their application to a specific autoimmune syndrome, autoimmune hemolytic anemia. The number of possible mechanisms make it apparent that no single postulate has received universal acceptance.

It appears to the author that a stubborn denial of autoimmunization, with the necessity of resorting to concepts such as a fortuitous occurrence of nonspecific materials, is an evasion of the fundamental problem posed by innumerable experimental studies. More disastrously, it limits investigational studies and prevents the development of new approaches in an area with unlimited possibilities for investigation. The opponents of autoimmunization, however, can make a sound case against much that has been written in this field. A superficial assumption that any self-destructive immunologic event occurring in a living organism represents autoimmunization is as harmful as denying the existence of such a process. Inexact terminology and semantics have contributed to this confusion.

Tissue damage associated with fixation of globulin molecules occurs in many diversified clinical conditions. It is unlikely that a single pathophysiologic mechanism will suffice to explain all of these states. What we now term autoimmunization is actually an end stage phenomenon. Tissues have a limited number of ways to respond after damage. A similarity in the final response pattern should not be interpreted as being synonymous with identical etiologic pathways. This confusion can be eliminated by considering autoimmunization as the result of an immunologic loss of self-recognition for normal host antigens. There is no reason to suppose that this state can arise through only one mechanism. Rather, multiple etiologies acting alone or in interrelation are probably present. In one condition, a genetic predisposition may result in the emergence of a forbidden clone. In another, the production of a cross reacting antibody to a modified self-antigen may terminate natural immune tolerance. In a third instance, an immunodeficient individual may be involved. Malignancy might establish a foreign clone of cells, leading to a graft-host syndrome in another patient. Disease states may disrupt immunologic quarantine of an intracellular host antigen in other patients. There is no reason to consider any one of these five examples as more representative or as the prototype of all cases of autoimmunization.

Two suggestions can clarify current approaches in autoimmunization. An investigator should clearly define his terminology and preferably he should limit "autoimmunization" to cases which satisfy the criteria discussed above. In addition, the end stage nature of the phenomenon should be realized and an attempt should be made to document the one or more mechanisms involved. With this approach no single mechanism should be employed as an exclusive and limiting criterion. Rather, the multiple possible sequences may aid in developing more definitive theoretical, diagnostic and therapeutic approaches.

BIBLIOGRAPHY

1. Burnet, F. M., and Fenner, F.: *The Production of Antibodies*. MacMillan & Company, Melbourne, 1949.
2. Burnet, F. M.: *The Clonal Selection Theory of Acquired Immunity*. Vanderbilt University Press, Nashville, 1959.
3. Burnet, F. M.: Theories of immunity. In *Conceptual Advances in Immunology and Oncology*. Hoeber Medical Divison, Harper & Row, Publishers, New York, 1963.
4. Jerne, N.: The natural selection theory of antibody formation. Proc. Nat. Acad. Sci. USA **41**: 849, 1955.
5. Talmage, D. W.: Allergy and immunology. Ann. Rev. Med. **8**: 239, 1957.
6. Lederberg, J.: Genes and antibodies. Science **129**: 1649, 1959.
7. Szilard, L.: The molecular basis of antibody formation. Proc. Nat. Acad. Sci. USA **46**: 293, 1960.
8. Haurowitz, F.: Antibody formation. Physiol. Rev. **45**: 1, 1965.
9. Lennox, E. S., and Cohn, M.: Immunoglobulins. Ann. Rev. Biochem. **36**: 365, 1967.
10. Nossal, G. J.: Mechanisms of antibody production. Ann. Rev. Med. **18**: 81, 1967.
11. Ehrlich, P., and Morganroth, J.: Ueber Hämolysine. Dritte Mittheilung. Berlin. Klin. Wschr. **37**: 453, 1900.
12. Ehrlich, P.: *Collected Studies on Immunity*, translated by C. Bolduan. John Wiley & Sons, Inc., New York, 1906.
13. Dacie, J. V.: *The Haemolytic Anaemias, Part II*, Ed. 2. Grune & Stratton, Inc., New York, 1962.
14. Landsteiner, K.: Zur Kenntnis der antifermentativen, lytischen und agglutinierenden Wirkungen des Blutserums und der Lymphe. Zbl. Bakt. **27**: 357, 1900.
15. Billingham, R. E., Brent, L., and Medawar, P. W.: "Actively acquired tolerance" of foreign cells. Nature (London) **172**: 603, 1953.
16. Medawar, P. W.: Immunological tolerance. Science **133**: 303, 1961.
17. Hanan, R., and Oyama, J.: Inhibition of antibody formation in mature rabbits by contact with the antigen at an early age. J. Immun. **73**: 49, 1954.
18. Smith, R. T., and Bridges, R. A.: Immunologic unresponsiveness in rabbits produced by neonatal injection of defined antigens. J. Exp. Med. **108**: 227, 1958.
19. Humphrey, J. H.: In *Mechanisms of Antibody Formation*, edited by M. Holub and L. Jarósková. Czechoslovakian Academy of Science, Prague (Academic Press, New York), 1960.
20. Weigle, W. O.: *Natural and Acquired Immunologic Unresponsiveness*. World Publishing Company, Cleveland, 1967.
21. Felton, L. D.: Significance of antigen in animal tissues. J. Immun. **61**: 107, 1949.
22. Felton, L. D., Kauffmann, G., Prescott, B., and Ottinger, B.: Studies on the mechanism of the immunological paralysis induced in mice by pneumococcal polysaccharides. J. Immun. **74**: 17, 1955.
23. Dixon, F. J., and Mauer, P. H.: Immunologic unresponsiveness induced by protein antigens. J. Exp. Med. **101**: 245, 1955.
24. Smith, R. T.: Immunological tolerance of nonliving antigens. Advances Immun. **1**: 67, 1961.
25. Nossal, G. J. V., Shortman, K. D., Miller, J. F. A. P., Mitchell, G. F., and Haskill, J. S.: The target cell in the induction of immunity and tolerance. Cold Spring Harbor Symposia on Quantitative Biology **32**: 369, 1967.
26. Thorbecke, G. J., and Benacerraf, B.: Tolerance in adult rabbits by repeated non-immunogenic doses of bovine serum albumin. Immunology **13**: 141, 1967.
27. Jerne, N. K.: Selective theories on antibody formation. Arb. Ehrlich Inst. **57**: 1, 1962.
28. Martin, W. J.: The cellular basis of immunological tolerance in newborn animals. Aust. J. Exp. Biol. Med. Sci. **44**: 605, 1966.
29. Nossal, G. J. V., and Ada, G. L.: Recognition of foreignness in immune and tolerant animals. Nature (London) **201**: 580, 1964.
30. Nossal, G. J. V.: Self-recognition. Ann. N. Y. Acad. Sci. **124**: 37, 1965.
31. MacKay, I. R., and Burnet, F. M.: *Autoimmune Diseases*. Charles C Thomas, Publisher, Springfield, 1963.
32. Witebsky, E.: Historical roots of present concepts of immunopathology. In *Immunopathology, First International Symposium*, edited by P. Grabar and P. Miescher. Schwabe and Company, Basel, 1959.
33. Milgrom, F.: When does self-recognition fail? Series Haemat. **9**: 17, 1965.
34. Lawrence, H. S.: Transfer factor and autoimmune disease. Ann. N. Y. Acad. Sci. **124**: 56, 1965.
35. Hall, R.: Immunologic aspects of thyroid function. New Eng. J. Med. **266**: 1204, 1962.
36. Roitt, I. M., and Doniach, D.: Delayed hypersensitivity in auto-immune disease. Brit. Med. Bull. **23**: 66, 1967.
37. Trentin, J., editor: *Cross-reacting Antigens and Neoantigens*. The Williams & Wilkins Company, Baltimore, 1967.
38. Glynn, L. E., and Holborow, E. J.: *Autoimmunity and Disease*. F. A. Davis Company, Philadelphia, 1965.
39. Dameshek, W.: Theories of autoimmunity. In *Conceptual Advances in Immunology and Oncology*. Hoeber Medical Division, Harper & Row, Publishers, New York, 1963.
40. Gras, J.: Los estados de no respuesta imunológica y su interés en la discusión de los teorías sobre la formación de anticuerpos, especialmente en relación a la interpretación

de los mecanismos de formación de auto-anticuerpos. Rev. Clin. Esp. **95**: 205, 1964.

41. Boyd, W. C.: The specificity of the nonspecific. J. Immun. **85**: 221, 1960.

42. Pirofsky, B.: Studies on leukemic leukocyte extracts. I. Lack of antigenic relationship in acquired hemolytic anemia. II. The demonstration of a hemolysin and agglutinin. J. Lab. Clin. Med. **48**: 745, 1956.

43. Pirofsky, B.: Studies on the hemolysin and agglutinin of leukemic leukocytes. Blood **12**: 620, 1957.

44. Dixon, F. J., Feldman, J. D., and Vazquez, J. J.: Experimental glomerulonephritis. The pathogenesis of a laboratory model resembling the spectrum of human glomerulonephritis. J. Exp. Med. **113**: 899, 1961.

45. Adres, G. A., Seegal, B. C., Hsu, K. C., Rothenberg, M. S., and Chapeau, M. L.: Electron microscopic studies of experimental nephritis with ferritin-conjugated antibody. Localization of antigen-antibody complexes in rabbit glomeruli following repeated injections of bovine serum albumin. J. Exp. Med. **117**: 691, 1963.

46. Fish, A. J., Michael, A. F., Vernier, R. L., and Good, R. A.: Acute serum sickness nephritis in the rabbit. Amer. J. Path. **49**: 997, 1966.

47. Dixon, F. J.: The role of antigen-antibody complexes in disease. Harvey Lect. **58**: 21, 1962–1963.

48. Dixon, F. J.: Antigen-antibody complexes and autoimmunity. Ann. N. Y. Acad. Sci. **124**: 162, 1965.

49. Ishizaka, K., Ishizaka, T., and Campbell, D.: Biological activity of aggregated γ-globulin. III. Production of Arthus-like reactions. J. Immun. **86**: 220, 1961.

50. Schulman, N. R.: Mechanism of cell destruction in individuals sensitized to foreign antigens and its implication in autoimmunity: combined clinical staff conference at National Institutes of Health. Ann. Intern. Med. **60**: 506, 1964.

51. Miescher, P., Cooper, N. S., and Hurez, D.: The "in vitro" action of antigen-antibody complexes on thrombocytes and erythrocytes. In *Cellular Aspects of Immunity,* edited by G. E. W. Wolstenholme and M. O'Connor. Little, Brown and Company, Boston, 1959.

52. Wiener, A. S.: Origin of naturally occurring hemagglutinins and hemolysins; a review. J. Immun. **66**: 287, 1951.

53. Stadsbaeder, S.: Discussion critique de l'auto-immunization au cours des anémies hémolytiques acquises. Acta Clin. Belg. **14**: 480, 1959.

54. Costea, N., Yakulis, V., and Heller, P.: Experimental production of cold agglutinins in rabbits. Blood **26**: 323, 1965.

55. Smith, C. B., McGinniss, M. H., and Schmidt, P. J.: Changes in erythrocyte I agglutinogen and anti-I agglutinins during *Mycoplasma*

pneumoniae infection in man. J. Immun. **99**: 333, 1967.

56. Kaplan, M. H., and Meyeserian, M.: Immunological relation of streptococcal and tissue antigens. I. Properties of an antigen in certain strains of group A streptococci exhibiting an immunologic cross-reaction with human heart tissue. J. Immun. **90**: 595, 1963.

57. Kaplan, M. H.: Autoantibodies to heart and rheumatic fever: the induction of autoimmunity to heart by streptococcal antigen cross-reactive with heart. Ann. N. Y. Acad. Sci. **124**: 904, 1965.

58. Goldstein, I., Halpern, B., and Roberts, L.: Immunological relationship between Streptococcus A polysaccharide and the structural glycoprotein of heart valve. Lancet **1**: 44, 1967.

59. Schulman, S., and Witebsky, E.: Studies on organ specificity. IX. Biophysical and immunochemical studies on human thyroid autoantibody. J. Immun. **85**: 559, 1960.

60. Asherson, G. L., and Dumonde, D. C.: Characterization of autoantibodies produced in the rabbit by the injection of rat liver. Brit. J. Exp. Path. **43**: 12, 1962.

61. McClusky, R. T., Miller, F., and Benacerraf, B.: Sensitization to denatured autologous gamma-globulin. J. Exp. Med. **115**: 253, 1962.

62. Cinader, B., and Dubert, J. M.: Acquired immune tolerance to human albumin and the response to subsequent injections of diazo human albumin. Brit. J. Exp. Path. **36**: 515, 1955.

63. Ackroyd, J. F.: The cause of thrombocytopenia in recurrent purpura. Clin. Sci. **7**: 249, 1949.

64. Harris, J. W.: Studies on the mechanism of a drug induced hemolytic anemia. J. Lab. Clin. Med. **47**: 760, 1956.

65. Skillman, R. K., Spurrier, W., Friedman, I. A., and Schwartz, S. O.: Rheumatic fever activity determination by two correlative methods. Arch. Intern. Med. (Chicago) **96**: 51, 1955.

66. Waksman, B. H.: Experimental allergic encephalomyelitis and the "auto-allergic" diseases. S. Karger, Basel, 1959.

67. Billingham, R. E., and Silvers, W. K.: Studies on cheek pouch skin homografts in the Syrian hamster. In *Transplantation,* edited by G. E. W. Wolstenholme and M. P. Cameron. Little, Brown and Company, Boston, 1962.

68. Rümke, P.: Autospermagglutinins: a cause of infertility in men. Ann. N. Y. Acad. Sci. **124**: 696, 1965.

69. Najjar, V. A., and Fisher, J.: Mechanisms of antibody-antigen reaction. Science **122**: 1272, 1955.

70. Milgrom, F., and Dubiski, S.: Antigenicity of

antibodies of the same species. Nature (London) **179**: 1351, 1957.

71. Milgrom, F.: Antibodies to denatured autologous antigens. Ann. N. Y. Acad. Sci. **124**: 118, 1965.

72. Najjar, V. A.: Some aspects of antibody-antigen reactions and theoretical considerations of the immunologic response. Physiol. Rev. **43**: 243, 1963.

73. Dameshek, W.: "Immunoblasts" and "immunocytes"—an attempt at a functional nomenclature. Blood **21**: 243, 1963.

74. Burnet, F. M.: Autoimmune Disease. II. Pathology of the immune response. Brit. Med. J. **2**: 720, 1959.

75. Mellors, R. C., and Huang, C. Y.: Immunopathology of NZB/Bl mice. VI. Virus separable from spleen and pathogenic for Swiss mice. J. Exp. Med. **126**: 53, 1967.

76. Pirofsky, B.: Autoimmune hemolytic anemia and neoplasia of the reticuloendothelium. With a hypothesis concerning etiologic relationships. Ann. Intern. Med. **68**: 109, 1968.

Chapter 14

The Antiglobin Positive Hemolytic Anemias

Clinical data previously presented strongly suggest that autoimmune hemolytic anemia is not a specific disease entity. Rather, various pathophysiologic processes may have a similar end stage characterized by erythrocyte damage and positive antiglobulin tests. Nonimmune, immune but not autoimmune and autoimmune pathways may be involved in creating such reactions.

The etiologic mechanisms concerned in hemolysis and positive antiglobulin tests must be delineated. The prognosis of the disease process as well as the therapeutic approach depends on such information. Etiologic mechanisms which involve nonimmune and immune but not autoimmune phenomena should be distinguished from autoimmune hemolytic anemia. Antiglobulin positive hemolytic anemia has been employed as a descriptive term to categorize these nonautoimmune hemolytic processes. The pertinent criteria and definitions have been presented in Chapter 1. Tables 2 and 4 relate this group to the extracellular hemolytic anemias and specifically to the immunohemolytic anemias. This chapter is designed to evaluate the nonautoimmune pathologic states which may function in human immunohemolytic disease.

A Nonimmunologic Etiology

Several investigators have challenged the concept that the erythrocyte coating material demonstrated in the antiglobulin test is an erythrocyte autoantibody. Roth (1), Roth and Frumin (2) and Pirofsky (3) investigated the reactivity of such substances with heparin, protamine and antiglobulin serum, respectively. The erythrocyte coating material was found to differ from erythrocyte isoantibodies. Witebsky (4), on immunologic grounds, objected to the uncritical assumption of an autoantibody status for such erythrocyte coating materials.

The Specificity of the Nonspecific

The antiglobulin test simply demonstrates globulin molecules fixed to the erythrocyte surface in a particular molecular conformation. Nonimmunologic events may be involved in such globulin reactivity with the erythrocyte. In addition, various substances may fix to the erythrocyte, leading to agglutination. These include such unlikely materials as plant lectins (5), eel serum (6), body fluid from mollusks (7) and various chemicals (8). Some of these exhibit exquisite specificity for erythrocyte isoantigens.

Adequate studies are now available to eliminate this nonspecific mechanism from general consideration in the autoimmune hemolytic anemias. This does not imply that all positive antiglobulin reactions are due to binding of antibodies to the erythrocyte surface. Several uncommon situations have been described in which positive antiglobulin tests are created in the absence of immunologic action.

Sutherland and Eisentraut (9) studied the effect of lead on erythrocytes. They demonstrated positive antiglobulin tests and hemolytic anemia in man and in the dog as the result of lead intoxication. The reaction was not immunologically mediated. It was suggested that lead salts affect the lipoprotein envelope of erythrocytes, leading to microscopic denaturation. This results in a loss of membrane elasticity and the premature death of the cell. Globulin groups may be exposed by disruption of the normal membrane. Alternatively, globulin may be deposited on such damaged erythrocytes. Watanabe (10) found that the antiglobulin test did not correlate with the degree of hemolysis. However, it did correlate with cellular damage as represented by Heinz body formation.

Jandl and Simmons (11) studied the effect of metallic cations such as ferric and chromic ions on the erythrocyte membrane. They found that basically charged metallic ions had the ability to fix to polyanionic erythrocyte surfaces. When erythrocytes coated with such cations were suspended in serum, globulin was adsorbed, presumably by its negatively charged groups. Antiglobulin serum would react with such erythrocytes, leading to positive antiglobulin tests.

Brown and associates (12) produced hemolytic anemia and positive direct and indirect antiglobulin tests in rats exposed to trypan blue. Leukopenia, thrombocytopenia, splenomegaly and lymphadenopathy developed. Splenectomy did not correct the syndrome. Heating the serum to 56°C. did not inactivate indirect antiglobulin tests. Positive indirect antiglobulin tests could be produced in vitro. It was suggested that serum proteins in contact with trypan blue treated erythrocytes led to positive antiglobulin tests and erythrocyte damage. Norlind and associates (13) found that a similar reaction was produced by the azo dyes benzo sky blue 2B, chlorazol sky blue FF, Evans blue, Niagara blue 2B, Niagara sky blue 4B and Niagara sky blue 6B. Anemia was most profound in 9 to 11 days, with positive antiglobulin reactions always associated with free dye in the serum.

Similar nonimmunologically induced antiglobulin reactions have been reported following the administration of phenylhydrazine (14), lipoid solvents (15) and cephalothin (16, 17). The action of such materials on the erythrocyte membrane or serum proteins is thought to result in the positive antiglobulin test (see Chapter 18).

Dysgammaglobulinemia

In 1961 Brody and Finch (18) questioned the antibody status of erythrocyte autoantibodies. Employing immune adherence procedures, they found that serum factors obtained from leukemia and lymphoma patients did not react as erythrocyte antibodies. It was suggested that erythrocyte autoantibodies were abnormal globulins with an affinity for the erythrocyte surface. Positive antiglobulin tests would therefore represent manifestations of dysgammaglobulinemia rather than autoimmunization. Osgood (19) has agreed with this suggestion without supplying experimental validation.

Hinz and Boyer (20) reported studies on a woman with immunohemolytic anemia. Anti-N was discovered in her serum and this reacted with her own MM erythrocytes. The patient was found to have multiple serum protein abnormalities. The investigators suggested that anti-N formation was a chance occurrence reflecting a dysproteinemic state characterized by hepatosplenomegaly and macroglobulinemia.

Shapiro (21) studied an interesting family which supports this concept. The proband had acute hemolytic anemia and the clinical state resembled graft-host disease. He was $Rh_o(D)$ positive and his serum contained anti-$Rh_o(D)$. Four siblings also had clinical evidence of immunologic disease. Both the parents and the siblings had multiple serum protein abnormalities. It was suggested that asymptomatic dysgammaglobulinemia was present in heterozygotes and that a lethal dysgammaglobulinemia was present in homozygotes. Anti-$Rh_o(D)$ formation was considered as the fortuitous production of an abnormal protein specifically reacting with the $Rh_o(D)$ antigen.

A similar familial distribution of dysgammaglobulinemia and immunologic abnormalities was reported by Fialkow and associates (22) and Pirofsky (23). Cases 3, 4 and 5 summarize the protocols of the three siblings studied at our institution. These two investigating groups, however, have interpreted their family studies as indicating a genetic predisposition to develop autoimmune abnormalities, rather than a nonimmunologic dysgammaglobulinemia.

Immunologic But Not Autoimmune Pathogenesis

Most investigators have discarded a nonimmunologic pathogenesis for hemolytic anemia associated with positive antiglobulin tests. Examples of dysgammaglobulinemia and chemically induced positive antiglobulin tests are rare. There is almost universal agreement that the erythrocyte coating material is an antibody. This does not imply, however, that autoimmunization is etiologically involved in all instances of hemolytic anemia and positive antiglobulin tests. If a foreign antigen, or an autologous antigen modified sufficiently to appear foreign, is immunogenic, true autoimmunization is not present. A lack of self-recognition is not involved and autoantibodies are not produced. Five mechanisms through which such antigens may initiate tissue damage and the deposition of globulin have been described in Chapter 13. In reference to the erythrocyte, immunohemolytic anemia characterized by positive antiglobulin tests may result from such immune but not autoimmune phenomena.

All suggested mechanisms involve a foreign antigen. These include modified host antigens, hapten formation with host antigens, exposure to cross reacting foreign antigens, an innocent bystander adsorption of foreign antigens and the effects of immune complexes. The erythrocyte is particularly susceptible to such immunologic sequences. Its ubiquitous distribution, proximity to the environment, long survival with aging, and membrane characteristics are unique. Activation of any of these mechanisms involving the erythrocyte can result in hemolytic anemia and positive antiglobulin tests. Various environmental states

may initiate these pathologic processes, resulting in antiglobulin positive hemolytic anemia. These include disease states, drugs, bacteria and bacterial products, viruses and physical factors. Such conditions would have a similar end stage and may be clinically indistinguishable at that point from autoimmune hemolytic anemia.

The Effect of Disease

The damage, modification or denaturation of erythrocyte antigens by disease states may lead to immunogenicity in a host. Campbell (24) emphasized that autologous proteins could become antigenic if they contained faulty or abnormal configurations. Autologous erythrocytes may become antigenic through synthesis of faulty protein structures or by adsorption of abnormal antigenic fragments. Dubert (25) has made similar suggestions in reference to modified normal body constituents.

Such "foreign" antigens would be expected to initiate antibody formation directed specifically against the modified host tissue. This is generally not the case in the antiglobulin positive and autoimmune types of hemolytic anemia. The eluted anti-erythrocyte antibody most often functions as a panhemagglutinin and reacts with normal unmodified erythrocytes. Accordingly, if this process does occur, it must be assumed that the antibody produced has low specificity and is capable of cross reacting with normal erythrocyte antigenic determinants. This mechanism has been considered by Gear (26), Stats and Wasserman (27) and Dubert (25). There is no firm evidence that this sequence of events occurs. Attempts to produce this state in animals have given contradictory results. Hamamoto and Yoshikawa (28) reported the production of both specific and cross reacting antibodies when formalin treated erythrocytes were used to immunize rabbits.

Most investigators now minimize the role of disease initiated antigenic modifications as the stimulus for erythrocyte antibody production. This may be premature. In the clinical section of this volume, 234 cases of autoimmune hemolytic anemia are reviewed. Eighty-two per cent of these appeared in association with additional significant pathologic states. The number and variety of these associated conditions are impressive. Although a fortuitous juxtaposition of common diseases undoubtedly exists, a possible cause and effect relationship must be considered.

Five patients with Addisonian pernicious anemia had positive antiglobulin tests (Cases 6 and 80 to 83). Treatment of pernicious anemia with vitamin B-12 resulted in hematologic remission and disappearance of positive antiglobulin tests. The association of two such autoimmune states has been interpreted as evidence for an aberrant immune apparatus (29). Another explanation is possible. Erythrocyte abnormalities are characteristic of untreated Addisonian pernicious anemia. Such defects may extend to various antigenic determinants. This may create immunologically foreign erythrocytes in a host, resulting in an antiglobulin positive hemolytic anemia. A similar phenomenon may be involved in the positive antiglobulin tests occasionally observed in hereditary spherocytosis (30–32) and in the one patient in the current series with a heterozygotic erythrocyte pyruvate kinase deficiency (Chapter 10).

The association of ovarian cysts with immunohemolytic anemia may represent a similar pathogenesis. Various blood group substances are secreted, stored and possibly concentrated in cyst fluid. These include the A, B, H and P substances. Such materials, as well as others not yet identified, might undergo structural changes during storage in cyst fluid. Modified blood group substances could appear as foreign and could stimulate antibody production. Disappearance of positive antiglobulin tests and correction of hemolytic anemia occur after surgical removal of the ovarian cyst. This further suggests the presence of a foreign material involved in antibody formation.

At this time there is no clear proof that systemic or hematologic diseases can induce antiglobulin positive hemolytic anemia by modification of erythrocytes. If this process does occur, antibody formation would represent a secondary phenom-

enon. This secondary role does not imply that such a sequence is not responsible for serious or chronic hemolytic anemia. A self-perpetuating disease may even develop through continual modification of erythrocytes by erythrocyte antibody.

The Effect of Drugs

Modification of host erythrocyte immunogenicity by disease appears speculative. No question exists, however, as to the influence of drugs in initiating an antiglobulin positive hemolytic anemia. An extensive literature has accumulated documenting the association of hemolytic anemia, positive antiglobulin tests and exposure to various drugs. Dausset and Contu (33) have presented an excellent review of this entire field. Two different pathophysiologic processes may be involved. Drugs or chemicals may induce erythrocyte damage and positive antiglobulin reactions through nonimmunologic pathways. Several examples of this mechanism have been discussed above. In addition an antiglobulin positive hemolytic anemia may be precipitated through several immunologic but not autoimmune processes. Five distinctly different mechanisms appear to be involved in this latter relationship.

Erythrocyte Damage

In the 1940's several reports of hemolytic anemia associated with drug ingestion were published. Dacie (34) reviewed these cases which were primarily related to sulfa therapy. He concluded that the underlying disease syndrome could not be eliminated from etiologic responsibility in initiating hemolytic anemia. In 1953 Snapper and associates (35) reported the association of hemolytic anemia and positive antiglobulin tests following ingestion of Mesantoin. Leukopenia and thrombocytopenia were also noted. All abnormalities disappeared with discontinuation of therapy and recurred with administration of the drug. The authors suggested that Mesantoin produced erythrocyte membrane damage. This created modified erythrocyte antigens and led to the production of antibodies with a low specificity or cross reactivity. Figure 18 diagrammatically presents the

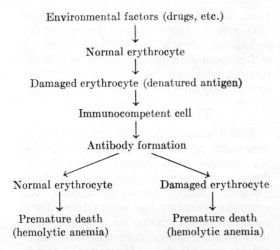

FIGURE 18. Antiglobulin positive hemolytic anemia. The modification of autologous antigens by environmental factors.

proposed sequence of events. The influence of Mesantoin in this particular case must now be questioned. The patient received penicillin concomitantly with Mesantoin therapy.

Hapten Formation

Ackroyd in 1949 (36) suggested the role of hapten formation in Sedormid induced thrombocytopenia. This reaction became a prototype to explain the etiologic influence of various drugs on autoimmune thrombocytopenic purpura. Harris (37) in 1956 reported hemolytic anemia following the ingestion of the tri-antimony compound stibophen (Fuadin). Stibophen and patient's serum were both necessary to induce positive antiglobulin tests and hemolysis. A hapten state for stibophen in relationship to erythrocyte antigens was postulated. Stibophen presumably created a new antigenic substance by functioning as a hapten with erythrocyte surface antigens. Antibodies formed against this antigen complex had specificity for the stibophen hapten. Other investigators have confirmed this relationship of stibophen to an antiglobulin positive hemolytic anemia (38). Figure 19 illustrates the mechanism of erythrocyte antibody formation resulting from a hapten state.

Development of an antiglobulin positive hemolytic anemia on the basis of the two above mechanisms has been ascribed to other drugs. These include Butazolidin (39), anticonvulsants, phenacetin (40, 41), para-aminosalicylic acid (41, 42), quinine (40), quinidine (43), melphalan (44) and chlorpromazine (45). Muirhead and associates (46) reported a case of chronic hemolytic anemia precipitated by exposure to chlorinated hydrocarbon insecticides. Hemolytic anemia was associated with thrombocytopenia and leukopenia. The disease responded to splenectomy, underwent exacerbation when reexposure to the insecticide occurred and was associated with positive antiglobulin tests. The chronicity of hemolytic anemia reported in this case is unusual. Drug induced hemolytic anemia is generally corrected upon removal of the involved substance. However, the authors emphasize that such insecticides are deposited and stored in adipose tissue. A prolonged but gradual release of the offending agent is possible, leading to a chronic hemolytic process.

Immune Complexes

The validity of these early studies suggesting a hapten pathogenesis for drug induced antiglobulin positive hemolytic ane-

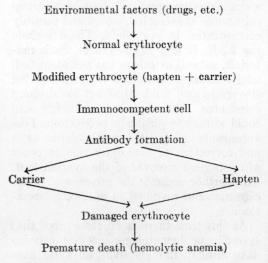

FIGURE 19. Antiglobulin positive hemolytic anemia. The creation of a new antigen through hapten formation.

mia must be challenged. Miescher and associates (47) demonstrated that soluble antibody-antigen complexes could adsorb to the thrombocyte surface. Schulman expanded these studies in 1964 (48). He employed both thrombocytes and erythrocytes in his test system. It was shown that drugs adsorbed onto cells were easily washed off and that they did not form a stable hapten combination with surface proteins. Schulman demonstrated that drug antigen-antibody complexes differed from the drugs alone. Immune complexes were firmly bound to sensitized cells. During adsorption of immune complexes, serum components were adsorbed. These serum complexes were demonstrated to be complement. It was suggested that complement adsorption aided in producing hemolysis or cell destruction. The sensitized cell simply acted as an innocent bystander for deposition of an unrelated immune complex. Figure 20 illustrates the role of immune complexes and complement in creating an antiglobulin positive type of drug induced hemolytic anemia.

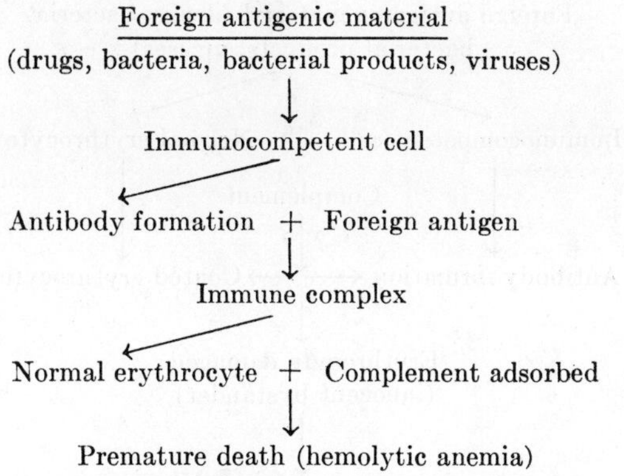

Employing this test system Schulman (48) demonstrated that quinine and quinidine purpurae and stibophen hemolytic anemia were due to adsorption of immune complexes onto thrombocytes and erythrocytes, respectively. The following mechanism was postulated. A drug antigen interacts with antibody directed against it, forming an immune complex. Sequentially, the immune complex is adsorbed onto the cellular surface, and complement components are bound to the cell. The fixation of complement plays a critical role in the process. Absence or reduction of complement fixation produces loosely adsorbed immune complexes which may be easily eluted. An adequate amount of complement fixation also seems to be necessary for cellular damage. Elution of immune complexes will not remove complement which is irreversibly bound to the erythrocyte surface. Positive antiglobulin reactions are directly related to the presence of complement. These reactions are usually of the non-gamma variety (see Chapter 17). Complement alone will produce positive antiglobulin tests, depending on the nature of

Foreign antigenic material
(drugs, bacteria, bacterial products, viruses)
↓
Immunocompetent cell
←
Antibody formation + Foreign antigen
↓
Immune complex
←
Normal erythrocyte + Complement adsorbed
↓
Premature death (hemolytic anemia)

FIGURE 20. Antiglobulin positive hemolytic anemia. The formation of immune complexes and their adsorption onto the erythrocyte surface, leading to hemolytic anemia.

the antiglobulin serum. Schulman (48) has shown that erythrocytes bound with sublytic amounts of complement may survive in the circulation for as long as 50 days. Persistently positive antiglobulin reactions will then be present after discontinuation of drug therapy and correction of the hemolytic anemia.

Such studies have great theoretical importance in the investigation of autoimmunization. They emphasize that documentation of the antigen is critical in any immune reaction. Only in this fashion can the erythrocyte be removed as an integral part of the immune state. The presence of a clinical syndrome and an obviously immune reaction are insufficient evidence of autoimmunization or antibody formation.

Innocent Bystander

Ley and associates (49) reported that a humoral antibody directed against penicillin would agglutinate normal erythrocytes previously exposed to penicillin. Shortly thereafter many reports appeared documenting the occurrence of hemolytic anemia in individuals receiving penicillin (50–52). The daily administration of large amounts of parenteral penicillin was characteristic in these cases.

Penicillin initiated hemolytic anemia involved a different mechanism from that involved in the three forms of drug reactions discussed above. Penicillin contrasted with

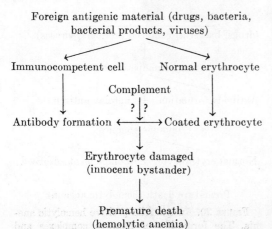

FIGURE 21. Antiglobulin positive hemolytic anemia. The "innocent bystander" role of the erythrocyte in adsorbing foreign antigens. Hemolytic anemia results from the interaction of antibody with antigen bound to the erythrocyte.

the drugs investigated by Schulman (48) by firmly binding to the erythrocyte surface. Thiel and associates (53) employed tritium labeled penicillin and noted that erythrocytes exposed to penicillin could not be washed free of the drug. The erythrocyte in vivo or in vitro will fix penicillin to its surface in a firm bond. Circulating antibodies directed against penicillin are necessary for the development of hemolytic anemia. The reaction of humoral antipenicillin antibodies with surface bound penicillin results in erythrocyte damage and premature death of the red cells. Immune complexes do not appear involved in this reaction. The adsorption of complement is not necessary for erythrocyte damage. The positive antiglobulin test is due to penicillin antibodies rather than to complement components. As yet there is no satisfactory explanation for erythrocyte damage resulting from an unrelated immunologic event taking place on its surface. Figure 21 illustrates the proposed sequence of events.

Swanson and associates (52) eluted penicillin antibodies from antiglobulin positive erythrocytes. IgG and IgM immunoglobulins were demonstrated. The eluate would only sensitize penicillin coated erythrocytes. They postulated an innocent bystander role of the erythrocyte in the positive antiglob-

ulin test and hemolytic anemia. Petz and Fudenberg (51) thoroughly investigated this system. The IgG nature of the involved antibody was shown and found to have a direct relationship to penicillin and positive antiglobulin tests. The authors emphasized that identification of the antigen is critical before a process is classified as autoimmune.

Unknown Mechanisms

A fifth drug related hemolytic anemia system has recently been described. No satisfactory description of the involved mechanisms has been reported. In 1966 Carstairs and associates (54) noted the association of hemolytic anemia, positive antiglobulin tests and ingestion of the hypotensive drug alpha-methyldopa. These investigators studied three patients with positive antiglobulin tests; two developed anemia, whereas the third was asymptomatic. This observation was expanded with an analysis of 202 consecutive hypertensive patients receiving alpha-methyldopa therapy. Of these 202 cases, 41 were found to have positive antiglobulin tests, an incidence of 20 per cent. This observation has been confirmed by numerous other reports of positive serologic tests found in patients receiving similar therapy. In the series of Carstairs and associates (54) no selectivity was noted on the basis of age and sex. The development of positive antiglobulin reactions seemed to be related to drug dosage. The incidence of positive antiglobulin tests increased from 11 per cent, when the dosage was below 1 gm. daily, to 19 per cent at a dose level of 1 to 2 gm. daily. It reached 36 per cent when the daily dose was over 2.0 gm. Positive antiglobulin tests were uncommon when alpha-methyldopa had been taken for less than 6 months. After 1 year of therapy the development of positive serologic reactions was rare if it had not occurred previously. Anemia was absent in these 202 cases. Six patients had an elevated reticulocyte count and a mild compensated hemolytic anemia was assumed. Lupus erythematosus cells were absent in 12 cases and thyroid antibodies could not be found in 13 cases. Splenomegaly and lymphade-nopathy were not encountered.

Worlledge and associates (55) studied 25 cases of hemolytic anemia developed during alpha-methyldopa therapy. They estimate a hemolytic anemia incidence of 0.02 per cent in patients receiving such therapy. This preliminary estimate is undoubtedly low and an increased incidence can be anticipated. There were 11 men and 14 women in the reported series. The intake of alpha-methyldopa varied from 3 to 37 months with 10 patients receiving the drug for 1 year or less. Eighteen patients received 1 gm. or less of the drug daily. Splenomegaly was found in eight of 13 examined patients. In seven patients cessation of drug therapy improved the anemia. The remaining 18 patients received prednisone therapy with some response. Positive antiglobulin tests persisted for long periods after the cessation of alpha-methyldopa. Case 94 in the current series describes the rapid disappearance of positive erythrocyte serologic tests upon the cessation of drug therapy. Serologic studies demonstrated an IgG type of immunoglobulin in all cases. Two examples (Cases 94 and 95) of an antiglobulin positive hemolytic anemia secondary to alpha-methyldopa were encountered in the present series.

Carstairs and associates (54) noted similar serologic findings in 28 patients. The antibody was demonstrated with enzyme treated erythrocytes in all patients. Eleven had positive indirect antiglobulin tests. Elution of the antibody was successful in all cases. Sixteen of the 28 eluates had specificity for rhesus agglutinogens. In the group of Worlledge and associates (55) elution was attempted in 18 cases and antibody was obtained in 13. A high incidence of specificity was found with anti-hr'(c) and anti-hr"(e) activity prominent. The relationship of such autoantibodies to the rhesus blood group was further shown by LoBuglio and Jandl (56). They noted that eluted autoantibodies, without apparent rhesus specificity, did not react with Rh (null) cells.

Worlledge and coworkers (55) studied the role of alpha-methyldopa and other related drugs in the serologic reaction. Antibody activity was not inhibited by the addition of drugs. Sensitivity of red cells to antibodies was not enhanced by previous exposure to the drugs. Similar results were obtained by LoBuglio and Jandl. Wurzel and Silverman (57) reported a different experience. They noted that alpha-methyldopa could directly affect the erythrocyte surface. Their studies included alpha-methyldopa and 10 metabolites of methyldopa or closely related catecholamines. After incubation of erythrocytes with these drugs for several days, positive direct antiglobulin tests were obtained. Accordingly, these authors postulate a nonimmunologic reaction with positive antiglobulin tests developing in the absence of antibodies.

These studies separate alpha-methyldopa induced hemolytic anemia from those reactions previously reported for drugs. A drug hapten state, the adsorption of immune complexes and complement and the innocent bystander role of the erythrocyte can apparently be ruled out. The high incidence of autoantibody specificity makes it unlikely that membrane damage with a modified or denatured antigen is present. Worlledge and associates (55) suggest that the drug or a derivative may be incorporated into immature erythrocytes, creating a subtle alteration of red cell antigens. A termination of normal immune tolerance must also be considered. Two puzzling observations deserve particular attention. Why are erythrocytes not damaged in many subjects when potent autoantibodies are present with specificity directed against the patient's erythrocytes? The patients of Worlledge and associates (55) developed hemolytic anemia with relatively low dosages of alpha-methyldopa. Is there a particular predisposition in certain patients for this syndrome? Breckenridge and associates (58) noted positive antinuclear factor tests in 15 per cent of patients treated with alpha-methyldopa. Systemic lupus erythematosus did not develop and the significance of this observation is unknown.

Drugs, cosmetics and chemicals are playing an increasingly prominent role in our modern civilization. Man may be consid-

TABLE 80. *Development of hemolytic anemia and/or positive antiglobulin tests concomitantly with exposure to various drugs and chemicals*

Drug	Investigator	Year
	Immunologic Mechanisms	
Mesantoin	Snapper et al. (35)	1953
Stibophen	Harris (37), Schulman (48)	1954, 1964
Butazolidin	deGruchy (39)	1954
Quinidine	Freedman et al. (43)	1956
Quinine	Muirhead et al. (40)	1958
Acetophenetidine	Muirhead et al. (40), MacGibbon et al. (41)	1958, 1960
Penicillin	Ley et al. (49)	1958
Chlorinated hydrocarbon insecticides	Muirhead et al. (46)	1959
Para-aminosalicylic acid	MacGibbon et al. (41), Dausset et al. (42)	1960, 1961
Chlorpromazine	Lindberg and Norden (45)	1961
Alpha-methyldopa	Carstairs et al. (54)	1966
Melphalan	Eyster (44)	1967
	Nonimmunologic Mechanisms	
Lead	Sutherland and Eisenstraudt (9)	1956
Metallic cations	Jandl and Simmons (11)	1957
Trypan blue	Brown et al. (12)	1961
Phenylhydrazine	Muirhead et al. (14)	1954
Lipoid solvents	Muirhead and Groves (15)	1956
Cephalothin	Molthan et al. (17), Gralnick et al. (16)	1967

ered as existing in a rapidly changing chemical environment. We must be aware of the potentially harmful side effects of this exposure and of the creation of new iatrogenic disease syndromes. The development of antiglobulin positive hemolytic anemia frequently may reflect our chemical environment. Table 80 lists our current knowledge in this area. In the future we may anticipate an expansion of this knowledge concerning both nonimmunologic and immunologic mechanisms.

The Effect of Bacteria and Bacterial Products

The effect of bacteria and bacterial products in creating an antiglobulin positive type of hemolytic anemia deserves detailed consideration. The clinical relationship of infectious disease to autoimmune hemolytic anemia is striking, particularly in children. This has been summarized in Chapter 7. Neter (59), in a masterly review of microbial agglutination and hemolysis,

has summarized the methods by which bacteria and their products may affect the erythrocyte. He describes eight mechanisms through which hemagglutination and hemolysis may be initiated. Table 81 summarizes these mechanisms. At least six of the postulated sequences could be involved in the development of an antiglobulin positive form of hemolytic anemia.

Indirect Microbial Hemagglutination

Approximately 35 bacteria have been identified as possessing antigenic constituents capable of fixing to the surface of normal erythrocytes. Table 82 lists the organisms implicated by Neter (59). Almost all of these antigenic constituents are polysaccharide in nature. Prominent in this group are the common gram negative organisms frequently responsible for chronic subclinical infections (*Escherichia coli, Aerobacter aerogenes, Proteus* sp., Pseudomonas, etc.). The tuberculosis organism may also be involved in the same process

TABLE 81. *Production of hemagglutination (HA) by bacteria and bacterial products**

Mechanism	Reaction			
	First stage	Second stage	Third stage	End stage
Direct microbial he-magglutination	Bacterium + RBC†			HA
Indirect microbial hemagglutination	Bacterial antigen + RBC	Coated RBC + Bac-terial antibody		HA
Immune complex	Microbial antigen + microbial antibody	Immune complex + RBC		HA
Hapten formation	Microbial antigen + complexing chemical	Hapten complex + RBC	Coated RBC + micro-bial antibody	HA
Surface modifications	Chemical (tannic acid) + RBC	Modified RBC + mi-crobial antigen	Coated RBC + micro-bial antibody	HA
RBC linked antigen	Microbial antigen + incomplete RBC antibody	Antigen-RBC anti-body complex + RBC	Coated RBC + homol-ogous antibody	HA
Huebener-Thomsen-Friedenreich phe-nomenon	Bacterium (enzyme) + RBC	Modified RBC + RBC antibody (anti-T)		HA
Bacteriogenic hemag-glutination	Bacterium + serum	Modified serum + RBC		HA

* Modified from Neter (59).
† RBC, red blood cells.

TABLE 82. *Bacterial species containing antigens capable of adsorbing on erythrocytes and being subsequently agglutinated by exposure to homologous bacterial antibodies**

Species	Antigen	Species	Antigen
Micrococcus sp.	Polysaccharide	*Proteus* OX$_{19}$, OXK	Polysaccharide
Diplococcus pneumonia	Polysaccharide	*Pseudomonas aeruginosa*	Lipopolysaccharide
Streptococcus sp.	Crude polysaccharide	*Pseudomonas* sp.	Crude antigen
Neisseria meningitides	Polysaccharide	*Vibrio comma*	Crude antigen
Neisseria gonorrhoeae	Polysaccharide	*Pasteurella pestis*	Protein?, polysac-charide
Escherichia coli	Lipopolysaccharide, V$_1$-acidic polymer		
		Pasteurella multocida	Capsular antigen
Escherichia freundii	Crude antigen, crude V$_1$	*Pasteurella tularensis*	Lipopolysaccharide, polysaccharide
Aerobacter aerogenes	Polysaccharide		
Aerobacter cloacae	Polysaccharide	*Brucella* sp.	Lipopolysaccharide, polypeptide
Paracolobactrum sp.	Crude antigen		
Salmonella typhosa	O (polysaccharide, lipo-polysaccharide) crude V$_1$, H.? protein	*Malleomyces mallei*	Crude antigen
		Haemophilus influenzae	Polysaccharide
		Haemophilus pertussis	Crude antigen
Salmonella sp.	Polysaccharide, lipopoly-saccharide	*Corynebacterium diph-theriae*	Polysaccharide
Shigella sp.	Polysaccharide	*Mycobacterium tuberculo-sis*	Crude fractions, polysaccharide
Sorratia marcoscons	Lipopolysaccharide		
Proteus sp.	Lipopolysaccharide	*Mycobacterium paratu-berculosis*	Crude antigen
		Mycobacterium phlei	Crude antigen
		Leptospira sp.	Crude antigen

* Modified from Neter (59).

and has been implicated in immunohemo-lytic anemia (Cases 51 to 54 and 81).

Keogh and associates (60) in 1947 de-scribed the role of such bacterial products in hemagglutination. The erythrocyte func-tioned as an innocent bystander in the postulated sequence of events. Antigenic materials released from various bacteria have two actions. Such substances are ad-sorbed onto the surface of erythrocytes. Simultaneously, antibody production is initiated against the bacterial antigen. Humoral antibody may now react with its antigen which is firmly bound to the eryth-rocyte surface. Hemagglutination, cellular damage and premature death of the eryth-rocyte can occur. The similarity of this process to that described with penicillin is striking. Autologous antibody directed against the erythrocyte bound bacterial antigen and/or complement components create positive direct antiglobulin tests. Without documenting antigen and antibody specificity, the resulting hemolytic anemia may be classified as autoimmune. This re-flects an erroneous assumption of autoanti-body formation directed against erythro-cytes.

Some experimental evidence supports this speculative concept. Ceppellini and DeGregorio (61) demonstrated rapid hemol-ysis of autologous erythrocytes exposed to the V_1 *Salmonella ballerup* antigen, when such cells were reinjected into a rabbit im-munized against the V_1 antigen. Although these authors failed to produce in vivo coating of the erythrocyte with the V_1 anti-gen, Boyden (62) demonstrated in vivo adsorption of tuberculin. DeGregorio (63) later succeeded in producing in vivo coat-ing of the same V_1 antigen. Studies by Schumway and associates (64) and Suzuki and associates (65) confirmed this mech-anism. Schumway's group used the O and V_1 antigens (64) and Suzuki and associates used the enterobacterial antigens (65). These workers demonstrated lysis of au-tologous cells coated with antigens when erythrocytes were reinjected into immunized animals. Skillman and associates (66) had postulated a similar indirect microbial he-magglutination mechanism in another pre-sumed autoimmune disease. They submit

evidence implicating streptococci infection in man in the development of rheumatic fever. Stormont and associates (67) and Cohen and Norins (68) have presented data indicating that circulating antibodies di-rected against various common bacteria are frequently present in the sera of hu-mans and animals.

Direct Microbial Hemagglutination

Bacteria may be directly adsorbed onto the erythrocyte surface. Hemagglutination can ensue and has been termed direct mi-crobial hemagglutination (59). Such a proc-ess may be involved in an antiglobulin positive type of acquired hemolytic anemia. Somatic bacterial antigens may stimulate antibody formation as well as coat the erythrocyte. Erythrocyte damage and posi-tive antiglobulin reactions may result in a fashion similar to that outlined for indirect microbial hemagglutination.

Immune Complexes

Boyden and Anderson (69) in 1955 per-formed a series of pertinent studies utiliz-ing tuberculin. They found that bacterial antigen-antibody complexes were adsorbed onto the erythrocyte surface. Hemagglu-tination resulted from this process. They also noted that complement could enter into this reaction and lead to lysis. Normal human serum inhibited this reaction. This latter observation is similar to the experi-ence of Dameshek and Schwartz (70) and Farrar and associates (71). They noted that warm acting hemolysis resulting from eryth-rocyte autoantibodies could be inhibited by normal human serum.

Complexing Chemicals

The number of bacteria interacting with erythrocytes may be increased greatly by incorporating an additional substance in the reacting system. Various chemicals possess the ability to complex with bac-terial antigenic material. Antigens pre-viously unable to fix to the erythrocyte surface may, through such complexes, ac-quire this ability. In this fashion a se-quence similar to indirect microbial hemag-glutination can develop with erythrocyte damage and positive antiglobulin tests.

The Uncovering of Antigenic Material

Bacterial enzymes may induce changes of the erythrocyte surface. The Huebener-Thomsen-Friedenreich phenomenon (72–74) is an example of this process. It is suggested that all human erythrocytes contain a latent receptor or antigenic determinant termed the T antigen. This antigenic site may be "activated" or uncovered by various bacterial products. In vitro demonstration of this process is accomplished through the action of corynebacteria. Chu (75) has also indicated that products obtained from pneumococci, streptococci and *Staphylococcus albus, aureus* and *citreus* uncover the T antigen. Erythrocytes so treated undergo agglutination when exposed to normal human serum. This appears related to the presence of an antibody with anti-T specificity. Anti-T is present to a variable degree in all adult human sera. Polyagglutination is accordingly characteristic. Anti-T does not appear in the infant's serum until age 6 months. The antibody has maximal reactivity at room temperature. Figure 22 illustrates the proposed anti-T mechanism of action.

Friedenreich (74) first demonstrated that these events can occur in vivo. Polyagglutinability may occur at any age but is more frequent in the young. Poulsen (76) analyzed 40 patients and found five in the first year of life. Jørgensen (77) studied one patient with neonatal jaundice. Polyagglutinability apparently had its onset in fetal life. The uncovering of the T antigen can result in hemolysis as well as hemagglutination. This was experimentally demonstrated by Ejby-Poulsen (78), using pneumococcal type XIX enzymes. Enzymes such as the receptor destroying enzyme, trypsin and papain similarly induce a shortened red cell survival time in experimental animals.

Polyagglutination characterizing the Huebener-Thomsen-Friedenreich phenomenon is usually transient. Freiesleben and associates (79), however, have reported permanent polyagglutinability in a normal subject. Dausset and associates (80) described a case of polyagglutination of erythrocytes associated with chronic hemolytic

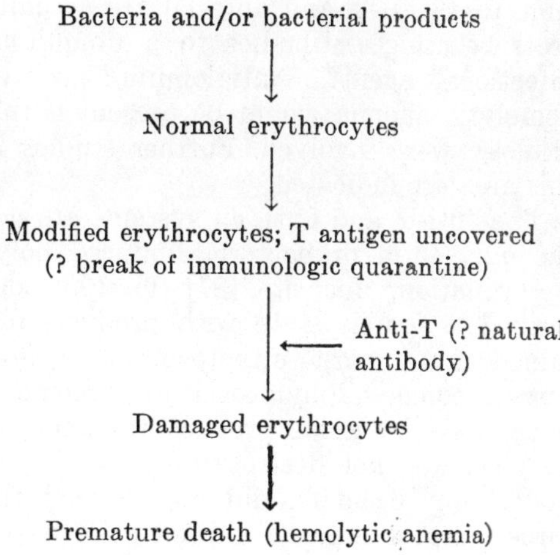

Bacteria and/or bacterial products

↓

Normal erythrocytes

↓

Modified erythrocytes; T antigen uncovered (? break of immunologic quarantine)

↓ ← Anti-T (? natural antibody)

Damaged erythrocytes

↓

Premature death (hemolytic anemia)

FIGURE 22. The Huebener-Thomsen-Friedenreich phenomenon. The "hidden" antigen T is uncovered by bacterial action. Hemolytic anemia results from the action of "natural" anti-T on the modified erythrocytes.

anemia of 12-year duration. These workers postulated that a new antigen, Tn, had been created. Anti-Tn was found in 490 normal human sera tested, and it appeared to be distinct from anti-T. van der Hart and associates (81) have described two additional cases of anti-Tn induced polyagglutination of erythrocytes.

Several aspects of the T-anti-T and Tn-anti-Tn systems are intriguing. If bacterial substances uncover antigenic sites of erythrocytes, autoimmune hemolytic anemia presumably results from a violation of immunologic quarantine. However, why are anti-T and anti-Tn present in all normal human sera if the antigen is unavailable? Are such substances "natural" antibodies as postulated in the Jerne theory of natural selection (see Reference 4, Bibliography, Chapter 13)? May such antibodies appear as the result of heteroimmune stimulation as suggested by Wiener (82) for anti-A and cold hemagglutinins? Stadsbaeder (83) has suggested that anti-infectious antibodies form cross reacting systems with erythrocytes. Similar results have been obtained by Costea and associates (84) and Smith and associates (85). Goldstein and associates (86) postulate that streptococcal polysaccharides have a cross reacting relationship with heart glycoproteins. Is it possible that anti-T and anti-Tn are actually cross reacting antibodies to a ubiquitous infectious agent? Antiglobulin positive hemolytic anemia would be present if this etiology were involved. Further studies in this area are indicated.

The anti-T and anti-Tn systems are not the only form of bacterial induced poly-agglutination. Jochem (87) in 1958 described a similar state with products obtained from most streptococci, *Bacillus cereus*, some staphylococci and pneumococci. The bacterial product was not an enzyme, was not destroyed by heating to 100°C. for 6 hours, did not destroy the virus receptor site and did not function by activating the T receptor or antigen. Poly-agglutination of treated red cells by all normal human sera was noted. Polyagglutination could be prevented by exposing human serum to the specific filtrate employed in sensitizing erythrocytes.

Evans and associates (88, 89) have described an excellent experimental system for the investigation of polyagglutination in the rabbit. The hemolytic system became apparent in weaning rabbits 5 to 8 weeks old. It was associated with mucoid enteritis characterized by bloody, mucoid or watery diarrhea. The erythrocyte abnormality responsible for polyagglutinability was resistant to trypsin and papain and persisted in heated stroma. Filtrates of mixed cultures of bowel organisms produced a similar abnormality. It was postulated that the cellular lesion resulted from the adsorption of a bacterial polysaccharide or that a bacterial enzyme uncovered or altered a polysaccharide cell antigen. Factors inducing agglutination and hemolysis are present in normal rabbit sera but are depleted in the sera of rabbits with polyagglutinable cells. van der Hart and associates (81) noted the same exhaustion phenomenon with erythrocyte polyagglutinability induced by anti-T and anti-Tn. The agglutinating factor in the rabbit system is heat stable at 56°C., whereas the hemolytic factor is heat labile. Although complement is fixed when normal rabbit serum is reacted with erythrocyte stroma, the hemolytic factor appears distinct from complement and properdin.

A similar modification of erythrocyte antigens may occur in the absence of bacterial products. Brendemoen (90) described a patient whose serum contained an incomplete cold acting erythrocyte antibody active only against stored erythrocytes. This may be termed the *stored blood syndrome*. Erythrocyte modification could be produced by heat treatment. It was postulated that the antigen arose by denaturation of the receptor site. Hougie and associates (91) and Stratton and associates (92) reported the same phenomenon with warm acting erythrocyte antibodies. The latter investigators confirmed that heating could transform the erythrocyte. Jenkins and Marsh (93) described three patients with hemolytic anemia who had erythrocyte antibodies reactive only against stored erythrocytes. All patients improved with corticosteroid therapy. Brief exposure of erythrocytes to ficin would make the antigen available. A T antigen was not involved. They suggested that the antigen arises during storage by the action of erythrocyte intracellular enzymes. The erythrocyte autoantibody presumably reacts with a basic substrate normally present in all erythrocytes.

Modified Erythrocytes and Bacteriogenic Hemagglutination

Bacterial products may directly modify erythrocytes or serum proteins. It is conceivable that such substances induce in vivo erythrocyte surface changes. This may permit a nonimmunologic fixing of globulin molecules to the erythrocyte surface, producing cell damage and positive antiglobulin tests. This sequence is analogous to the in vitro treatment of erythrocytes with tannic acid as described by Boyden (94). It has also been demonstrated that enzymes such as bromelin may modify erythrocytes sufficiently to induce agglutination in the absence of antibodies. Bromelin treated erythrocytes will agglutinate when they are suspended in the following solutions: bovine albumin 15 per cent, human albumin 12.5 per cent, human gamma-globulin 2.5 per cent, dextran 1.5 per cent and polyvinylpyrrolidone 1 per cent (95).

Davidsohn and Toharsky (96) in 1940 demonstrated that bacterial products could directly affect serum proteins. They noted that 69 per cent of human sera incubated with *Corynebacterium H* agglutinated normal erythrocytes. Induction of panhemagglutination was due to the formation of a substance called anti-h. Further studies indicated that filtrates of *Corynebacterium H* could induce anti-h formation in 24 hours; plasma was more easily converted than sera. This process was termed bacteriogenic hemagglutination. A similar phenomenon may be involved with basic charged antibiotics. Streptomycin has been shown to react with serum proteins, changing their net charge (97). Cephalothin similarly affects serum proteins and may then cause binding to the erythrocyte surface, leading to positive antiglobulin tests (98). The cephalothin reaction apparently does not damage the erythrocyte.

The means by which enzymes or other bacterial products induce erythrocyte surface changes are obscure. It was initially assumed that proteolytic enzymes expose hidden erythrocyte receptor groups. This explanation was employed to explain the ability of incomplete antibodies to directly agglutinate enzyme treated erythrocytes. The availability of more antigen presumably permitted agglutination. However, Pirofsky and associates (99), employing bromelin, and Masouredis (100), using papain, demonstrated that agglutination of enzyme treated cells was unrelated to increased antibody uptake. Ficin apparently exhibits a similar phenomenon (101). An increased cellular uptake of antibody was noted with all three enzyme preparations. Pirofsky and associates (99) postulated that a change in erythrocyte surface charge results from enzymatic action. This permitted agglutination to occur in the presence of lesser numbers of antibody molecules.

The relationship of bacterial infections and bacterial products to antiglobulin positive hemolytic anemia is still speculative. The widespread nature of such infections and the many possible mechanisms by which bacterial products may react with the erythrocyte all suggest a fruitful area

for experimental studies. An extensive clinical relationship exists between infections and immunohemolytic anemia and should not be ignored.

Bacteria are not unique in their ability to react with erythrocytes. The influence of viruses is discussed in the following section. In addition, rickettsiae (102) trypanosomes (103), schistosomes (104), candidae (105), histoplasma (106) and trichomonas (107) have all been implicated in this erythrocyte relationship. It is possible that the long forgotten and debunked idea of "autointoxication" may rise again and even replace "autoimmunization."

The Effect of Viruses

The clinical association of virus infections and hemolytic anemia has been frequently noted. Such hemolytic anemias are often characterized by erythrocyte autoantibodies and positive antiglobulin reactions.

In 1943 high titer cold acting erythrocyte autoantibodies were first noted to develop in primary atypical virus pneumonia. Acute hemolytic anemia was also encountered as a rare complication of such pneumonias. A similar relationship has since been observed with infectious mononucleosis, influenza A and B infections, Coxsackie virus A, measles, mumps, varicella, encephalitis, herpes simplex, Newcastle disease virus and cytomegalic inclusion disease, and during vaccination against measles, smallpox and poliomyelitis. Both cold acting and warm acting autoantibodies have been described. The clinical syndromes have been presented in Chapters 7 and 11. The ability of viruses to interact with the normal erythrocyte surface focused attention on the influence of infectious agents in hemolytic syndromes. The theoretical mechanisms through which viruses can initiate hemolytic anemia are essentially similar to those postulated for bacteria and bacterial products in Table 81.

Direct Viral Hemagglutination

In 1941 Hirst (108) and McClelland and Hare (109) independently noted the ability of influenza A virus to induce hemagglutination by fixing to the erythrocyte surface. Hemagglutination could be specifically inhibited by homologous viral antisera. Many viruses possess this hemagglutination ability; the mumps-influenza group appears to be particularly significant. Profound effects on erythrocytes have been demonstrated by virus action in vitro (110). Hemagglutination results from a complex enzymatic sequence. The first step involves adsorption of enzyme or virus onto the erythrocyte surface. A specific chemical compound on the surface of red cells serves as receptor. Enzymatic change of this receptor site occurs. Elution of virus or enzyme follows enzymatic modification of red cell receptors; this elution never appears to be complete. The altered erythrocyte no longer can adsorb virus or enzymes, and erythrocytes remained agglutinated even after partial elution of virus. The agglutinated erythrocytes may be dispersed by treating the erythrocytes with antiserum specific for the virus.

Hemolysis of erythrocytes can also occur as a result of such virus action. The study of Chu and Morgan (111) indicated that hemagglutination and hemolytic characteristics of the mumps virus were separate. Kilham (112), however, suggests that these two actions are similar in the Newcastle disease virus. Springer and Ansell (113) reported that agglutination of erythrocytes by influenza virus was accompanied by destruction of M, N, Lu^a and Lu^b antigens. Neuraminidase is apparently involved in this process.

Indirect Virus Hemagglutination

Burnet (114) in 1946 pointed out that virus induced erythrocyte agglutination could occur through a different mechanism. A sequence essentially similar to that described for bacterial indirect microbial hemagglutination was postulated. Burnet demonstrated that red cells exposed to hemotoxic viruses would undergo agglutination by specific antiviral immune serum.

Viral Effect on Erythrocytes

Stewart and associates (115) showed that canine erythrocytes modified in vitro by influenza A virus have a significantly shortened survival time. Premature death of red cells was due to a serum polyhemag-

glutinin and to modification of the erythrocyte by virus. Wright and Gardner (116) reported that erythrocytes treated with viruses exhibited a number of important changes. These included a change of antigenicity, an increased susceptibility to phagocytosis and a shortened survival time. The possibility that such erythrocyte surface changes might produce modified erythrocyte antigens and initiate antibody formation deserves evaluation. Vivell (117) and van Loghem (118) both feel that this theoretical possibility may be important in the etiology of hemolytic anemia. Burnet (119), however, suggests that modification of antigenicity by viruses is unlikely to have significance in human disease. Experimental studies are unfortunately lacking in this area. Motulsky and Crosby (120) immunized guinea pigs with erythrocytes modified by Freund's adjuvant or influenza virus. A positive antiglobulin test was obtained with both sets of animals. Such reactions disappeared upon cessation of injections. In some cases positive antiglobulin tests recurred when further injections were given. Hemolytic anemia did not occur.

Application of Viral Theories

There is no question that viruses can induce profound changes in erythrocytes. As Dacie (34) states, however, "there is also no doubt but that the vast majority of human subjects who suffer from virus infections do *not* develop hemolytic anemia in consequence." In order to relate virus infection to immunohemolytic anemia, one or several of the above described mechanisms must be shown to occur in vivo. In turn, this must be related to both hemolytic anemia and the development of erythrocyte antibodies. A series of papers reporting such a relationship was published by Moolten and associates (121–123). They initially reported a patient with hemolytic anemia induced by warm acting hemagglutinins. Newcastle disease virus was isolated from the patient's blood. The antiglobulin test was consistently negative at the start and at the height of the patient's illness. Weak positive antiglobulin tests were eventually obtained with the patient's blood and with that of her husband. The authors invoked the mechanisms of in vivo hemagglutination, hemolysis, modification of erythrocyte antigenicity and autoantibody formation to explain their findings. A series of patients with various underlying diseases having the common finding of hemagglutination were studied. Viruses such as that of Newcastle disease and herpes simplex were isolated in a substantial number.

The studies of Moolten and associates (121–123) have not been confirmed. Accordingly, the relationship of virus infection to human immunohemolytic anemia is problematical. Morgan (124, 125) carried out an extensive search for similar viruses in the blood and spleens of 14 patients with acquired hemolytic anemia. Entirely negative results were obtained. Eyquem and Dausset (126) examined the sera of 129 anemic patients for virus hemagglutination antibodies. Seven sera had the ability to neutralize Newcastle disease virus hemagglutination; in three the antibody appeared to be potent. Only one of these patients had acquired hemolytic anemia. These negative studies for many years discouraged investigations of the relationship of viruses to hemolytic anemia.

Cappell and McFarlane (127) and Wyatt and associates (128) reported a hemolytic syndrome in the newborn or infant associated with a virus infection. This syndrome has been termed cytomegalic inclusion disease. Zuelzer and associates (129) investigated children with autoimmune hemolytic anemia and noted a relationship between respiratory infections, lymphadenopathy and intensification of the hemolytic process. Lymph node biopsy on four occasions over a 2-year period in one patient consistently revealed cytomegalic virus. It was noted that hemolysis primarily correlated with virus activity. A retrospective pathologic analysis of the childhood type of immunohemolytic anemia indicated a significant incidence of cytomegalic virus disease.

The ubiquitous nature of cytomegalic virus makes it possible that such viruses simply represent proliferation in severely ill, debilitated patients. However, the one case that our laboratory has studied (Case 1) does not indicate a fortuitous relationship. This patient was born with a hemolytic syndrome which was characterized as antiglobulin positive at 2 months of age. Hemolysis was controlled but death occurred soon after with widespread cytomegalic virus disease as the only pathologic abnormality.

Zuelzer and associates (129) have developed an integrated etiologic theory for childhood immunohemolytic anemia. Twenty-two children were studied; 18 had positive antiglobulin tests. The following major conclusions were reached. (a) The presence of cytomegalic virus in immunohemolytic anemia is not fortuitous. An etiologic relationship exists. (b) Hemolysis in such cases, whether acute, intermittent or chronic, is due to the activity of cytomegalic or other latent viruses. Such viral activity develops in infants with a physiologically or pathologically impaired immune response. (c) The pathogenesis of immunohemolytic anemia involves the presence of circulating virus or viral products. Virus infections of the reticuloendothelium permit the passage of virus or viral products into the circulation, creating hemolysis. (d) The frequency of such viruses in immunohemolytic anemia, in the presence or absence of erythrocyte antibodies, suggests an etiologic status. Erythrocyte antibody formation appears as a variable secondary response unrelated to the disease.

Several important aspects of this theory deserve emphasis. Zuelzer and associates (129) reject autoimmunization as the pathogenesis of childhood immunohemolytic anemia. Erythrocyte antibody production is considered to be a secondary phenomenon without clinical significance. How erythrocyte antibody formation is initiated is unknown. The viral antibodies are not cross reactive. Zuelzer and colleagues speculate that they may be related to the formation of new antigens created by virus action on cells. Lymphadenopathy is not related to a "lymphoproliferative" syndrome as has been suggested in autoimmune hemolytic anemia. Rather, it is an accurate clinical index of the degree of virus infection involving the reticuloendothelium.

This hypothesis would discard autoimmunization as functioning in immunohemolytic anemia. In addition, the concept of antiglobulin positive hemolytic anemia would serve little value. The presence or absence of erythrocyte antibodies would no longer retain importance. Acceptance or rejection of this fascinating hypothesis seems to depend on clarification of the role of erythrocyte autoantibodies. Why are they produced in association with cytomegalic virus infections? What influence do they have on erythrocyte survival and hemolysis? If erythrocyte autoantibodies do not damage erythrocytes, how does cytomegalic virus initiate hemolysis?

In spite of adequate evidence that viruses have a profound effect on erythrocytes, their role in immunohemolytic anemia is still unclear. There is little doubt that occasional cases of antiglobulin positive hemolytic anemia may result from virus infections. Several examples are presented in Chapter 7. The influence of viruses in the majority of cases of autoimmune hemolytic anemia must still be determined. The widespread distribution of overt and subclinical virus infection suggests a fruitful area for experimental study.

The Effect of Physical Factors

Physical factors acting on the erythrocyte may induce a change in the molecular conformation of surface antigens. An erythrocyte modified in this fashion may appear foreign to the host's immune apparatus. If antibody formation is initiated, an antiglobulin positive hemolytic anemia may result. The capacity of the erythrocyte antibody to cross react with unmodified erythrocytes could determine the degree and chronicity of hemolytic anemia.

Experimental data to support this hypothesis are limited and contradictory. Freund's adjuvant may denature proteins because of the interaction of hydrophobic and hydrophilic groups. It may therefore serve as an experimental model for the effect of erythrocyte surface modifications.

The mixing of erythrocytes with Freund's adjuvant will lead to the production of positive antiglobulin tests (120, 130, 131). However, hemolytic anemia either does not occur or is uncommon. Anemia was observed in two of Stadsbaeder's animals (131), but its significance is questionable. Both animals concomitantly developed pneumococcal infections.

There are three clinical observations which suggest that physical factors acting on the erythrocyte surface may have etiologic significance in the development of antiglobulin positive hemolytic anemia. Liu and Evans (132) noted an antiglobulin positive state following intraperitoneal hemorrhage. Physical or chemical damage to the erythrocyte membrane in its extravascular distribution may have significantly modified the cells, leading to erythrocyte antibody formation.

Eng and Suinadurai (133) reported a strange sequence of events in a patient struck by lightning. Abnormal red cells suggesting the presence of di Guglielmo's disease were noted. An antiglobulin positive type of hemolytic anemia developed. The patient died soon after with acute monocytic leukemia. The time sequence of the lightning injury and hematologic abnormality suggested a cause and effect relationship.

Pirofsky and associates (134) have suggested that hemodynamic abnormalities may damage the erythrocyte surface, resulting in an antiglobulin positive hemolytic anemia. They noted transient hemolytic anemia and positive antiglobulin tests in several patients who had a Starr-Edwards aortic valve prosthesis (Cases 91 and 92). Lustumbo and associates (135) and Polesky and associates (136) have encountered similar groups of patients. Spontaneous recovery developed or improvement followed corticosteroid therapy. Pirofsky and associates (134) suggested that mechanical damage to the erythrocyte surface resulted from aortic stenosis and/or valve prosthesis. This created a "foreign" antigen structure, eventually leading to antibody formation. A termination of tolerance could also arise from this sequence and initiate true autoimmune hemolytic anemia. A graft-host or runt disease status resulting from multiple transfusions and preservation of foreign lymphocytes was also considered.

Anti-Antibody Formation

Milgrom (137) has suggested an ingenious blending of two different mechanisms which together can result in an antiglobulin positive hemolytic anemia. It is difficult to classify this hypothesis, which is known as anti-antibody formation. Both autoimmune and immune but not autoimmune pathways are involved. A termination of immunologic quarantine is essential for this sequence. However, the erythrocyte is not primarily involved in the immune reaction and functions only as an innocent bystander offering an adsorbing surface. Accordingly, the resulting anemia is considered as antiglobulin positive rather than autoimmune hemolytic anemia.

Najjar and Fisher (138) postulated that molecular conformation of an antibody might change during antibody-antigen interaction. This change in molecular shape could make available antigenic determinants previously inaccessible to the immune apparatus. Antibody-antigen union may therefore break the immunologic quarantine of a host's globulin molecular structure. Newly exposed antigenic determinants would appear as foreign and could induce antibody formation directed against the modified globulin molecule. Anti-antibody formation would result against autologous globulins.

Milgrom and Dubiski (139) have applied this concept to an autologous system resulting in hemolytic anemia. The sequence of events is diagrammatically represented in Figure 23. Foreign materials enter the living organism. Such substances are adsorbed onto the erythrocyte surface which functions as an innocent bystander. Concomitantly, antibody formation is initiated with specificity directed against the foreign substance. Antibody-antigen interaction on the erythrocyte surface may then occur. During this process a change in molecular conformation of the antibody leads to breaking of the immunologic quarantine. Antibody formation directed against the modified autologous antibody occurs. Reaction of this anti-antibody with the original antibody may then occur. The original antibody is fixed to the antigen, which in turn is adsorbed to the erythrocyte surface. During this second immunologic interaction, damage and premature death of erythrocytes develop. A self-perpetuating chain of events can be visualized with continual modification of autologous antibody and production of anti-antibody against modified globulin. The presence of anti-antibody on the erythrocyte surface will lead to a positive antiglobulin reaction. Without identifying the original foreign substance or its specific antibody, the anti-antibody may be erroneously considered to be an erythrocyte autoantibody.

Some experimental data have been presented to support this hypothesis. Milgrom and associates (140) in 1956 described a human anti-antibody with the ability to agglutinate human erythrocytes coated with anti-Rh_o(D). A similar serum was described in 1958 by Lille-Szyszkowicz and Gulmantowicz (141). Milgrom (142) in 1962 reported an identical observation with rabbit serum. Transformation of autologous antibody molecules in the course of immunologic interactions may result after combination with various antigens. Anti-antibody formation directed against autologous rabbit globulin has followed prolonged immunization with guinea pig leukocytes, streptococci, coliform organisms and ferritin (137).

Fudenberg and associates (143) defined many of the characteristics of anti-antibodies. They appear as IgM immunoglobulins and combine with IgG antibody. The molecular transformation detected by anti-antibody takes place on the Fab fragment of the IgG molecule. Reaction of antibody with a precipitating antigen is necessary in order for molecular transformation to occur. Univalent or bivalent hapten does not bring about changes detectable by anti-antibody.

Summary

All of the mechanisms derived above can initiate hemolytic anemia characterized by

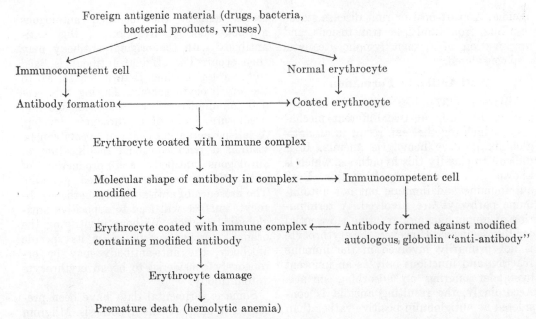

FIGURE 23. The development of hemolytic anemia through anti-antibody formation.

fixation of host antibody to host erythrocytes. A loss of erythrocyte self-recognition is not involved in antibody formation or the antibody itself is not primarily directed against the erythrocyte. True autoimmunization therefore does not occur, and the term antiglobulin positive hemolytic anemia has been applied to this group. Many of the proposed mechanisms are only theoretical speculations at this time. The true significance and incidence of such antiglobulin positive hemolytic anemias are still to be determined.

BIBLIOGRAPHY

1. Roth, K. L.: Interaction of heparin with auto-agglutinins in idiopathic acquired hemolytic anemia. Proc. Soc. Exp. Biol. Med. **86:** 352, 1954.
2. Roth, K. L., and Frumin, A. M.: In vitro differentiation between auto- and iso-immune antibodies by protamine and trypsin. Science **120:** 945, 1954.
3. Pirofsky, B.: Immunologic differences between iso-antibodies and auto-antibodies. Amer. J. Clin. Path. **29:** 120, 1958.
4. Witebsky, E.: Historical roots of present concepts of immunopathology. In *Immunopathology, First International Symposium,* edited by P. Graber and P. Miescher. Schwabe and Company, Basel, 1958.
5. Boyd, W. C.: *Introduction to Immunochemical Specificity.* Interscience Publishers, Inc., New York, 1962.
6. Watkins, W. M., and Morgan, W. T. J.: Neutralization of the anti-H agglutinin in eel serum by simple sugars. Nature (London) **169:** 828, 1952.
7. Boyd, W. C., Brown, R., and Boyd, L. G.: Agglutinins for human erythrocytes in mollusks. J. Immun. **96:** 301, 1966.
8. August, A., and Pirofsky, B.: Interaction of basic polyelectrolytes and human blood: the effect of antiheparin agents. Transfusion **6:** 74, 1966.
9. Sutherland, D. A., and Eisentraut, A. M.: The direct Coombs test in lead poisoning. Blood **11:** 1024, 1956.
10. Watanabe, K.: Immunological study on experimental hemolytic anemia induced by lead acetate. Jap. Arch. Intern. Med. **8:** 469, 568, 1961.
11. Jandl, J. H., and Simmons, R. L.: The agglutination and sensitization of red cells by metallic cations: interactions between multivalent metals and the red cell membrane. Brit. J. Haemat. **3:** 19, 1957.
12. Brown, D. V., Boehni, E. M., and Norlind, L. M.: Anemia with positive direct Coombs test induced by trypan blue. Blood **18:** 543, 1961.
13. Norlind, L. M., Boehni, E. M., and Brown, D. V.: Positive direct Coombs test induced by various azo dyes. Proc. Soc. Exp. Biol. Med. **119:** 970, 1965.
14. Muirhead, E. E., Groves, M., and Bryan, S.: Positive direct Coombs test induced by

phenylhydrazine. J. Clin. Invest. **33**: 1700, 1954.

15. Muirhead, E. E., and Groves, M.: Positive antiglobulin (Coombs) test of canine erythrocytes induced by lipid solvents in vitro. Amer. J. Clin. Path. **26**: 844, 1956.

16. Gralnick, H. R., Wright, L. D., and McGinniss, M. H.: Coombs positive reactions associated with sodium cephalothin therapy. J. A. M. A. **199**: 135, 1967.

17. Molthan, J., Reidenberg, M. M., and Eichman, M. F.: Positive direct Coombs tests due to cephalothin. New Eng. J. Med. **277**: 123, 1967.

18. Brody, J. I., and Finch, J. C.: Serum factors of acquired hemolytic anemia in leukemia and lymphoma. J. Clin. Invest. **40**: 181, 1961.

19. Osgood, E. E.: Antiglobulin-positive hemolytic anemias. Arch. Intern. Med. (Chicago) **107**: 313, 1961.

20. Hinz, C. F., and Boyer, J. T.: Dysgammaglobulinemia in the adult manifested as autoimmune hemolytic anemia. New Eng. J. Med. **269**: 1329, 1963.

21. Schapiro, M.: Familial autohemolytic anemia and runting syndrome with Rh₀ specific autoantibody. Transfusion **7**: 281, 1967.

22. Fialkow, P. J., Fudenberg, H., and Epstein, W. V.: "Acquired" antibody hemolytic anemia and familial aberrations in gamma globulins. Amer. J. Med. **36**: 188, 1964.

23. Pirofsky, B.: Hereditary aspects of autoimmune hemolytic anemia; a retrospective analysis. Vox Sang. **14**: 334, 1968.

24. Campbell, D. H.: Some speculations on the significance of formation and persistence of antigen fragments in tissues of immunized animals. Blood **12**: 589, 1957.

25. Dubert, J. M.: La tolérance immunitaire. Rev. Franc. Etud. Clin. Biol. **2**: 889, 1957.

26. Gear, J.: Autoantibodies and the hyperreactive state in the pathogenesis of disease. Acta Med. Scand. **152**: Suppl. 306, 39, 1955.

27. Stats, D., and Wasserman, L. R.: A critique on our knowledge of the etiology of hemolytic anemia. Trans. N. Y. Acad. Sci. **14**: 238, 1952.

28. Hamamoto, Y., and Yoshikawa, S.: Experimental auto-immune hemolytic anemia. Hematological observation. Acta Haemat. Jap. **26**: 650, 1963.

29. Pirofsky, B., and Vaughn, M.: Addisonian pernicious anemia with positive antiglobulin tests; a multiple autoimmune disease syndrome. Amer. J. Clin. Path. **50**: 459, 1968.

30. Singer, K., and Motulsky, A. G.: The developing (Coombs) test in spherocytic hemolytic anemias. J. Lab. Clin. Med. **34**: 768, 1949.

31. Young, L. E., and Miller, G.: Differentiation between congenital and acquired forms of

hemolytic anemia. Amer. J. Med. Sci. **226**: 664, 1953.

32. Alagille, D., Tron, P., Tupin, J. et al.: Erythroblastopénie aiguë avec test de Coombs passagèrement positif chez deux enfants porteurs d'une sphérocytose héréditaire. Arch. Franc. Pediat. **23**: 313, 1966.

33. Dausset, J., and Contu, L.: Drug induced hemolysis. Ann. Rev. Med. **18**: 55, 1967.

34. Dacie, J. V.: *The Haemolytic Anaemias, Part II*, Ed. 2. Grune & Stratton, Inc., New York, 1962.

35. Snapper, I., Marks, D., Schwartz, L., and Hollander, L.: Hemolytic anemia secondary to mesantoin. Ann. Intern. Med. **39**: 619, 1953.

36. Ackroyd, J. F.: The cause of thrombocytopenia in recurrent purpura. Clin. Sci. **7**: 249, 1949.

37. Harris, J. W.: Studies on the mechanism of a drug induced hemolytic anemia. J. Lab. Clin. Med. **47**: 760, 1956.

38. Torregrosa, M. V. V., Rosando, A. L., and Montilla, E.: Hemolytic anemia secondary to stibophen therapy. J.A.M.A. **186**: 182, 1963.

39. deGruchy, G. C.: The diagnosis and management of acquired haemolytic anaemia. Aust. Ann. Med. **3**: 106, 1954.

40. Muirhead, E. E., Halden, E. R., and Groves, M.: Drug dependent Coombs (antiglobulin) test and anemia. Observations on quinine and acetophenetidin (Phenacetin). Arch. Intern. Med. (Chicago) **101**: 87, 1958.

41. MacGibbon, B. H., Loughridge, L. W., Hourihane, D. O'B., and Boyd, D. W.: Autoimmune haemolytic anaemia with acute renal failure due to phenacetin and p-aminosalicylic acid. Lancet **1**: 7, 1960.

42. Dausset, J., and Bergerot-Blondel, Y.: Etude d'un anticorps allergique actif en présence de para-amino-salicylate de soude (PAS) contre les hématies, les leucocytes et les plaquettes humaines. Vox Sang. **6**: 91, 1961.

43. Freedman, A. L., Barr, P. S., and Brody, E. A.: Hemolytic anemia due to quinidine: observations on its mechanism. Amer. J. Med. **20**: 806, 1956.

44. Eyster, M. E.: Melphalan (Alkeran) erythrocyte agglutinin and hemolytic anemia. Ann. Intern. Med. **66**: 573, 1967.

45. Lindberg, L. G., and Norden, A.: Severe hemolytic reaction to chlorpromazine. Acta Med. Scand. **170**: 195, 1961.

46. Muirhead. E. E., Groves, M., Guy, R., Halden, E. R., and Bass, R. K.: Acquired hemolytic anemia, exposures to insecticides and positive Coombs test dependent on insecticide preparations. Vox Sang. **4**: 277, 1959.

47. Miescher, P., Cooper, N. S., and Hurez, D.: The in vitro action of antigen-antibody complexes on thrombocytes and erythrocytes. In *Cellular Aspects of Immunity,*

edited by G. E. W. Wolstenholme and M. O'Connor. Little, Brown and Company, Boston, 1959.

48. Schulman, N. R.: A mechanism of cell destruction in individuals sensitized to foreign antigens and its implications in autoimmunity. Ann. Intern. Med. **60**: 506, 1964.

49. Ley, A. B., Harris, J. P., Brinkley, M., Liles, B., Jack, J. A., and Cahan, A.: Circulating antibody directed against penicillin. Science **127**: 1118, 1958.

50. Penicillin therapy and haemolytic anaemia (lead article). Brit. Med. J. **2**: 658, 1966.

51. Petz, L. D., and Fudenberg, H. H.: Coombs-positive hemolytic anemia caused by penicillin administration. New Eng. J. Med. **274**: 171, 1966.

52. Swanson, M. A., Chaumougan, D., and Schwartz, R. S.: Immunohemolytic anemia due to anti-penicillin antibodies. New Eng. J. Med. **274**: 178, 1966.

53. Theil, J. A., Mitchell, S., and Parker, C. W.: Specificity of hemagglutination reactions in human and experimental penicillin hypersensitivity. J. Allerg. **35**: 399, 1964.

54. Carstairs, K. C., Breckenridge, A., Dollergy, C. T., and Worlledge, S.: Incidence of a positive direct Coombs test on patients on α-methyldopa. Lancet **2**: 133, 1966.

55. Worlledge, S., Carstairs, K. C., and Dacie, J. V.: Autoimmune haemolytic anaemia associated with α-methyldopa therapy. Lancet **2**: 135, 1966.

56. LoBuglio, A. F., and Jandl, J. H.: Nature of the methyldopa red-cell antibody. New Eng. J. Med. **276**: 658, 1967.

57. Wurzel, H. A., and Silverman, J. L.: The effect of alpha-methyl-3,4-dihydroxyl-L-phenylalanine (methyldopa, aldomet) on erythrocytes. Transfusion **8**: 84, 1968.

58. Breckenridge, A., Dollery, C. T., Worlledge, S. M., Holborow, E. J., and Johnson, G. D.: Positive direct Coombs tests and antinuclear factor in patients treated with methyldopa. Lancet **2**: 1265, 1967.

59. Neter, E.: Bacterial hemagglutination and hemolysis. Bact. Rev. **20**: 166, 1956.

60. Keogh, E. V., North, E. A., and Warburton, M. F.: Haemagglutinins of the haemophilus group. Nature (London) **160**: 63, 1947.

61. Ceppellini, R., and DeGregorio, M.: Crisi emolitica in animali batterioimmuni transfusi con sanque omologo sensibilizyata in vitro mediante l'antigene batterico specifico. Boll. Ist. Sieroter. Milan. **32**: 445, 1953.

62. Boyden, S. V.: Fixation of bacterial products by erythrocytes in vivo and by leukocytes. Nature (London) **171**: 402, 1953.

63. DeGregorio, M.: Fizzazione di antigeni sulla superficie cellulare. Boll. Inst. Sieroter. Milan. **34**: 118, 1955.

64. Shumway, C. N., Bokkenheuser, V., Pollock, D., and Neter, E.: Survival in immune and nonimmune rabbits of Cr^{51} labeled erythrocytes modified by bacterial antigen. J. Lab. Clin. Med. **62**: 600, 1963.

65. Suzuki, T., Gorzyuski, E. A., Whang, H. Y., and Neter, E.: Hemolysis in immune rabbits of autologous erythrocytes modified with common enterobacterial antigens. Experienta **20**: 75, 1964.

66. Skillman, R. K., Spurrier, W., Friedman, I. A., and Schwartz, S. O.: Rheumatic fever activity determined by two correlative methods. Arch. Intern. Med. (Chicago) **96**: 51, 1955.

67. Stormont, C., Suzuki, Y., and Miller, W. J.: Bacterially mediated false-positive reactions in lytic blood-typing tests. Nature (London) **186**: 247, 1960.

68. Cohen, I. R., and Norins, L. C.: Natural human antibodies to gram-negative bacteria: Immunoglobulins G, A, and M. Science **152**: 1257, 1966.

69. Boyden, S. V., and Andersen, M. E.: Agglutination of normal erythrocytes in mixtures of antibody and antigen, and haemolysis in the presence of complement. Brit. J. Exp. Path. **36**: 162, 1955.

70. Dameshek, W., and Schwartz, S. O.: The presence of hemolysins in acute hemolytic anemia; preliminary note. New Eng. J. Med. **218**: 75, 1938.

71. Farrar, G. E., Burnett, W. E., and Steigman, A. J.: Hemolysinic anemia and hepatic degeneration cured by splenectomy. Amer. J. Med. Sci. **200**: 164, 1940.

72. Huebener, C.: Untersuchungen über Isoagglutination mit besonderer berücksichtigung scheinbarer Abweichungen vorm Gruppenschena. Z. Immunitaetsforsch. **45**: 223, 1916.

73. Thomsen, O.: Ein vermehrungsfähiges Agens als Veränderer des isoagglutinatorischen Verhaltens der roten Blutkörperchen, eine bisher unbekannte Quelle der Fehlbestimmung. Z. Immunitaetsforsch. **52**: 85, 1927.

74. Friedenreich, V.: *The Thomsen Hemagglutination Phenomenon.* Levin & Munksgaard, Copenhagen, 1930.

75. Chu, C. M.: Enzymic action of viruses and bacterial products on human red cells. Nature (London) **161**: 606, 1948.

76. Poulsen, M. P. E.: Polyagglutinabilitet og t-omdannelse (medical dissertation, Copenhagen, 1961), quoted by Jørgensen (Reference 77).

77. Jørgensen, J. R.: Prenatal t-transformation? A case of polyagglutinable cord blood erythrocytes. Vox Sang. **13**: 225, 1967.

78. Ejby-Poulsen, P.: Hemolytic anemia produced experimentally in the guinea pig by t-transformation of the erythrocytes in vivo with purified concentrated enzyme. Nature (London) **174**: 929, 1954.

79. Freiesleben, E., Jensen, K. G., and Kundsen, E. E.: Permanent mixed field polyagglutinability. In *Proceedings of the Eighth Con-*

gress of the European Society of Hematology. S. Karger, Basel, 1962.

80. Dausset, J., Moullec, J., and Bernard, J.: Acquired hemolytic anemia with polyagglutinin ability of red blood cells due to a new factor present in normal human serum (anti-Tn). Blood 14: 1079, 1959.

81. van der Hart, M., Moes, M., van Loghem, J. J., Enneking, J. H. J., and Leeksin, C. H. W.: A second example of red cell polyagglutinability caused by the Tn antigen. Vox Sang. 6: 358, 1961.

82. Wiener, A. S.: Origin of naturally occurring hemagglutinins and hemolysins: a review. J. Immun. 66: 287, 1951.

83. Stadsbaeder, S.: Discussion critique de l'auto-immunization au cours des anémies hémolytiques acquises. Acta Clin. Belg. 14: 480, 1959.

84. Costea, N., Yakulis, V., and Heller, P.: Experimental production of cold agglutinins in rabbits. Blood 26: 323, 1965.

85. Smith, C. B., McGinniss, M. H., and Schmidt, P. J.: Changes in erythrocyte I agglutinogen and anti-I agglutinins during Mycoplasma pneumoniae infection in man. J. Immun. 99: 333, 1967.

86. Goldstein, I., Halpern, B., and Robert, L.: Immunological relationship between Streptococcus A polysaccharide and the structural glycoprotein of heart valve. Nature (London) 213: 44, 1967.

87. Jochem, E. M.: Rôle des streptocoques dans la panhémagglutination et la polyagglutinabilité. Ann. Inst. Pasteur (Paris) 95: 756, 1958.

88. Evans, R. S., Bingham, M., and Weiser, R. S.: A hemolytic system associated with enteritis in rabbits. I. Nature of the cell change and the serum factors concerned. J. Exp. Med. 117: 647, 1963.

89. Evans, R. S., Bingham, M., and Weiser, R. S.: A hemolytic system associated with enteritis in rabbits. II. Studies on the survival of transfused red cells. J. Lab. Clin. Med. 62: 559, 1963.

90. Brendemoen, O. J.: A cold agglutinin specifically active against stored red cells. Acta Path. Microbiol. Scand. 31: 574, 1952.

91. Hougie, C., Danbridge, J., and Bobbit, O. B.: A new autoagglutinin against stored erythrocytes. In Proceedings of the Seventh Congress of the International Society of Blood Transfusion. S. Karger, Basel, 1958.

92. Stratton, F., Renton, P. H., and Rawlinson, V. I.: Serological difference between old and young cells. Lancet 1: 1388, 1960.

93. Jenkins, W. J., and Marsh, W. L.: Autoimmune haemolytic anaemia. Three cases with antibodies specifically active against stored red cells. Lancet 2: 16, 1961.

94. Boyden, S. V.: The adsorption of proteins on erythrocytes treated with tannic acid and subsequent hemagglutination by antiprotein sera. J. Exp. Med. 93: 107, 1951.

95. Pirofsky, B., August, A., Nelson, H., and Pittenger, R.: Rapid mass anti-D (Rho) typing with bromelin. J. Lab. Clin. Med. 56: 911, 1960.

96. Davidsohn, I., and Toharsky, B.: The production of bacteriogenic hemagglutination. J. Infect. Dis. 67: 25, 1940.

97. Pirofsky, B., Cordova, M. S., and Rigas, D.: The mechanism of streptomycin inhibition of erythrocyte antibodies. Vox Sang. 9: 653, 1964.

98. Gralnick, H. R., and McGinniss, M.: Nature of the Coombs positive reaction with sodium cephalothin (abstract). Paper presented at the Twentieth Annual Meeting, American Association of Blood Banks, New York, 1967.

99. Pirofsky, B., Cordova, M., and Imel, T. L.: The function of proteolytic enzymes and tannic acid in inducing erythrocyte agglutination. J. Immun. 89: 767, 1962.

100. Masouredis, S. P.: Reaction of I^{131} anti-Rho(D) with enzyme treated red cells. Transfusion 2: 363, 1962.

101. Hughes-Jones, N. C., Gardner, B., and Telford, R.: The effect of ficin on the reaction between anti-D and red cells. Vox Sang. 9: 175, 1964.

102. Chang, R. S., Murray, E. S., and Snyder, J. C.: Erythrocyte-sensitizing substances from rickettsiae of the Rocky Mountain spotted fever group. J. Immun. 73: 8, 1954.

103. Muniz, J.: On the value of "conditioned hemolysis" for the diagnosis of American trypanosomiasis. Hospital (Rio) 38: 685, 1950.

104. Kagan, I. G.: Hemagglutination after immunization with schistosome antigens. Science 122: 376, 1955.

105. Vogel, R. A., and Collins, M. E.: Hemagglutination test for detection of Candida albicans antibodies in rabbit antiserum. Proc. Soc. Exp. Biol. Med. 89: 138: 1955.

106. Norden, A.: Agglutination of sheep's erythrocytes sensitized with histoplasmin. Proc. Soc. Exp. Biol. Med. 70: 218, 1949.

107. McEntegart, M. G.: The application of a haemagglutination technique to the study of trichomonas vaginalis infections. J. Clin. Path. 5: 275, 1952.

108. Hirst, G. K.: The agglutination of red cells by allantoic fluid of chick embryos infected with influenza virus. Science 94: 22, 1941.

109. McClelland, L., and Hare, R.: The adsorption of influenza virus by red cells and a new in vitro method of measuring antibodies for influenza virus. Canad. Pub. Health J. 32: 530, 1941.

110. Briody, B. A.: Action of viruses on red blood cells. Trans. N. Y. Acad. Sci. Series II, 14: 231, 1952.

111. Chu, L.-W., and Morgan, H. R.: Studies of the hemolysis of red blood cells by mumps virus. II. The relationship of hemagglutina-

tion, virus elution, and hemolysis. J. Exp. Med. **91**: 403, 1950.

112. Kilham, L.: A Newcastle disease virus (NDV) hemolysin. Proc. Soc. Exp. Biol. Med. **71**: 63, 1949.

113. Springer, G. F., and Ansell, N. J.: Inactivation of human erythrocyte agglutinogens M and N by influenza viruses and receptor-destroying enzyme. Proc. Nat. Acad. Sci. USA **44**: 182, 1958.

114. Burnet, F. M.: Modification of human red cells by virus action. III. A sensitive test for mumps antibody in human serum by the agglutination of human red cells coated with a virus antigen. Brit. J. Exp. Path. **27**: 244, 1946.

115. Stewart, W. B., Petenyi, C. W., and Rose, H. M.: The survival time of canine erythrocytes modified by influenza virus. Blood **10**: 228, 1955.

116. Wright, C. S., and Gardner, E., Jr.: A study of the role of acute infections in precipitating crises in chronic hemolytic states. Ann. Intern. Med. **52**: 530, 1960.

117. Vivell, O.: Ergebnisse virologischer Studien bei Fällen von akuter hämolytischer Anämie (Lederer-Brill). Mschr. Kinderheilk. **102**: 113, 1954.

118. van Loghem, J. J.: Concepts on the origin of autoimmune diseases. The possible role of viral infection in the aetiology of idiopathic autoimmune diseases. Series Haemat. **9**: 1, 1965.

119. Burnet, F. M.: *The Clonal Selection Theory of Acquired Immunity*, pp. 126–129. Vanderbilt University Press, Nashville, 1959.

120. Motulsky, A. G., and Crosby, W. H.: Experimental production of red cell autoimmunization (abstract). Amer. J. Med. **17**: 102, 1954.

121. Moolten, S. E., and Clark, E.: Viremia in acute hemolytic anemia and in autohemagglutination. Arch. Intern. Med. (Chicago) **89**: 270, 1952.

122. Moolten, S. E., and Clark, E.: The red blood cell as a vehicle of virus transport. II. Role of blood-borne viruses in autohemagglutination and in hemolytic anemia. Trans. N. Y. Acad. Sci. **14**: 235, 1952.

123. Moolten, S. E., Clark, E., Glasser, M. F., Katz, E., and Miller, B. S.: Blood stream invasion by Newcastle disease virus associated with hemolytic anemia and encephalopathy. Report of three cases. Amer. J. Med. **14**: 294, 1953.

124. Morgan, H. R.: Acquired hemolytic anemia and viremia. J. Lab. Clin. Med. **40**: 924, 1952.

125. Morgan, H. R.: Acquired hemolytic anemia and viremia. J. Lab. Clin. Med. **46**: 580, 1955.

126. Eyquem, A., and Dausset, J.: Recherche des propriétés inhibitrices de l'agglutination par le virus de la maladie de Newcastle dans les sérums de malades atteints d'anémie hemolytique acquise. Ann. Inst. Pasteur (Paris) **83**: 407, 1952.

127. Cappell, D. F., and McFarlane, M. N.: Inclusion bodies (protozoan-like cells) in the organs of infants. J. Path. Bact. **59**: 385, 1947.

128. Wyatt, J. P., Saxton, J., Lee, R. S., and Pinkerton, H.: Generalized cytomegalic inclusion disease. J. Pediat. **36**: 271, 1950.

129. Zuelzer, W. W., Stulberg, C. S., Page, R. H., Teruya, J., and Brough, A. J.: The etiology and pathogenesis of acquired hemolytic anemia. Transfusion **6**: 438, 1966.

130. Cajano, A., Miller, A., Finch, S. C., and Ross, J. F.: Autoimmunization to blood cells. Sang **26**: 141, 1955.

131. Stadsbaeder, S.: Différences des auto-anticorps au cours des anémies hémolytiques. Acta Clin. Belg. **11**: 78, 1956.

132. Liu, C. K., and Evans, R. S.: Production of positive antiglobulin serum test in rabbits by intraperitoneal injection of homologous blood. Proc. Soc. Exp. Biol. Med. **79**: 194, 1952.

133. Eng, L.-I. L., and Suinadurai, C.: Syndrome of erythremia di Guglielmo after lightning injury with autoimmune antibodies and terminating in acute monocytic leukemia. Blood **25**:845, 1965.

134. Pirofsky, B., Sutherland, D. W., Starr, A., and Griswold, H. E.: Hemolytic anemia complicating aortic-valve surgery. New Eng. J. Med. **272**: 235, 1965.

135. Lustumbo, M. M., Holland, P. V., and Schmidt, P. J.: Isoimmunization after multiple transfusions. New Eng. J. Med. **275**: 141, 1966.

136. Polesky, H. F., Smith, R., and Weirich, F.: Positive direct anti-human globulin tests in cardiac surgery patients (abstract). Paper presented at the Twentieth Annual Meeting of the American Association of Blood Banks, New York, 1967.

137. Milgrom, F.: Antibodies to denatured autologous antigens. Ann. N. Y. Acad. Sci. **124**: 118, 1965.

138. Najjar, V. A., and Fisher, J.: Mechanism of antibody-antigen reaction. Science **122**: 1272, 1955.

139. Milgrom, F., and Dubiski, S.: Mécanisme de l'auto-immunisation au cours des anémies hémolytiques. Sang **28**: 11, 1957.

140. Milgrom, F., Dubiski, S., and Woźnickzo, G.: Human sera with "anti-antibody." Vox Sang. **1**: 172, 1956.

141. Lille-Szyszkowicz, J., and Gulmantowicz, A.: A further case of a human serum containing "anti-antibodies." Vox Sang. **3**: 100, 1958.

142. Milgrom, F.: Rabbit sera with "anti-antibody." Vox Sang. **7**: 545, 1962.

143. Fudenberg, H. H., Goodman, J. W., and Milgrom, F.: Immunochemical studies on rabbit anti-antibody. J. Immun. **92**: 227, 1964.

Chapter 15

The Autoimmune Hemolytic Anemias

Autoimmune hemolytic anemia occupies a central position in any study of autoimmunization. Self-recognition and "horror autotoxicus" were originally demonstrated in red cell test systems. The first description of an autoantibody was the hemolysin in paroxysmal cold hemoglobinuria. The pathophysiologic implications of autoimmunization in human disease were initially applied in autoimmune hemolytic anemia. In fact, "autoimmune" was coined specifically to describe acquired hemolytic anemia characterized by fixation of immunoglobulins to the erythrocyte surface.

There are several advantages in employing autoimmune hemolytic anemia as a model system of autoimmunization. The disease is common and red cells and erythrocyte antibodies are easily obtained in relatively pure forms. Precise immunohematologic procedures have been developed for a parallel system of isoantibodies. Methods to measure the life span of the erythrocyte are available and may be used to quantitate, locate and monitor in vivo immune interactions. Extensive physiologic, biochemical, genetic and immunologic studies have made available a cellular pattern unique for human tissues.

On a theoretical basis autoimmune hemolytic anemia is an excellent prototype for the entire field of autoimmunization. Erythrocytes freely circulate and are in continual contact with the host's immune apparatus. These cells with prominent and well documented surface antigens must exist in a state of natural immune tolerance. Immunologic quarantine does not exist. If it can be shown that self-recognition of erythrocytes can be disrupted, with the production of autoantibodies and autoimmune anemia, then a similar process involving any host tissue may be anticipated.

Most investigators have dismissed a non-immunologic pathogenesis in the development of immunohemolytic anemia. This concept is limited to a relatively uncommon set of clinical conditions. Antiglobulin positive hemolytic anemia due to immunologic but not autoimmune mechanisms is more common. However, a relatively small number of the total cases may be unequivocally classified as this type. Although future studies may greatly expand this group, the vast majority of cases appear to require other mechanisms to explain clinical observations. The theories of autoimmunization supply the necessary pathologic and physiologic pathways. Until definitive evidence proves otherwise, most examples of immunohemolytic anemia are best considered to result from autoimmunization. At least six mechanisms may be suggested to explain formation of erythrocyte autoantibodies directed against unmodified host erythrocyte antigens.

A Violation of Immunologic Quarantine

The violation of immunologic quarantine is involved in the majority of accepted human autoimmune diseases (1). These include thyroiditis, allergic encephalomyelitis and autoantibody production directed against the testes, the lens of the eye, the adrenal gland, etc. Autoimmune hemolytic anemia differs from these syndromes. The erythrocyte is a host constituent in early, continuous and intimate contact with the immune apparatus. In addition, antigenic determinants are prominent surface characteristics. Accordingly, there is little if any evidence suggesting that autoimmune hemolytic anemia may reflect the availability of previously inaccessible erythrocyte antigens. This postulate has been suggested in di Guglielmo's syndrome, for which multiple immunologic aberrations have been described (2). The proliferation of neoplastic bone marrow elements presumably exposes previously inaccessible constituents. A break in immunologic quarantine is also necessary to explain anti-antibody formation in immunohemolytic anemia. Immunoglobulins are modified in this mechanism and the erythrocyte functions only an an innocent bystander.

The exposure of hidden erythrocyte antigenic determinants is assumed as an explanation for the rare examples of erythrocyte polyagglutinability. Antigenic determinants with T and Tn specificity are made accessible after bacterial enzymes act on erythrocytes (Chapter 14). This postulate can be challenged. The presence of anti-T and anti-Tn in normal human sera suggests that the host antigen is not inaccessible. In addition there is little proof that enzyme action exposes surface antigens.

Enhanced Sensitivity of Antibody Forming Tissue

The assumption that certain individuals have an enhanced ability to form antibodies has been utilized to explain autoimmune hemolytic anemia. Unfortunately this concept has been ill stated and poorly documented. It is well known that the human system varies tremendously in the ability to form antibodies. After immunization with a potent antigen such as $Rh_o(D)$, only 90 per cent of $Rh_o(D)$ negative individuals produce demonstrable antibody. The reverse is equally true. Other individuals may respond in an excessive fashion to minimal antigenic exposure and produce potent high titer antibodies.

Investigators concerned with transfusion therapy have frequently encountered individuals of this latter type. They suffer from frequent transfusion reactions and form post-transfusion erythrocyte isoantibodies with remarkable ease. A high percentage of such patients have suffered from autoimmune disease, particularly systemic lupus erythematosus and autoimmune hemolytic anemia (3–5).

This observation has been employed in deriving an etiologic concept for autoimmune hemolytic anemia. Hennemann (6) reported a patient whose serum contained anti-C+D. Autoimmune hemolytic anemia occurred. A tremendous rise in isoantibody titer was noted concomitant with the production of erythrocyte autoantibodies. Gear (7) suggested that excessive reactions to infection or intoxication were important factors in the development of autoimmune disorders. Kissmeyer-Nielsen (8) presented a similar hypothesis. He suggested an increased ability of the reticuloendothelium to produce antibodies as the primary abnormality in autoimmune hemolytic anemia. Erythrocyte autoantibody formation was a reflection of this propensity to form antibodies.

How an increased antibody producing capacity initiates erythrocyte autoantibody formation is not clearly stated. Two restrictions are pertinent. First, there is little to suggest that the enhanced ability to form antibodies is sufficient in itself to initiate autoantibody formation. The presumed sensitivity for antibody production must be combined with a supply of antigenic determinants foreign to the immune apparatus. Glynn and Holborow (9) have emphasized that "the crucial point in any theory of autoantibody production is the ability of the antibody-forming tissue to regard as foreign the autologous antigens that come within its range of action." Studies on immunoconglutination (10) and anti-antibody formation (11) suggest that autologous proteins may become antigenic through normal metabolic modifications. The capacity of the reticuloendothelial system to initiate antibody formation depends on the ability to recognize such changes as foreign. It is logical to expect variations in individual capacity to distinguish slight changes in antigenic patterns of modified host antigens. In the vast majority, changes in antigenic patterns are insufficient to provoke recognition as foreign and antibody production does not occur. An enhanced sensitivity of the reticuloendothelium in a limited number of subjects permits recognition of these modifications as foreign, leading to autoantibody formation.

The above hypothesis is not entirely satisfactory. No statement has been made as to what produces or controls the postulated increased sensitivity. Such an enhanced ability to form antibody may constitute the functional abnormality of the lymphoid apparatus crucial to Burnet's postulate of forbidden clones (12). Accordingly, the variations encountered in humans may be genetically determined. This appears to be compatible with the tendency of many autoimmune diseases to exhibit multiple autoantibody formation against various host constituents. It is also compatible with the familial predisposition to develop autoimmune diseases such as lupus erythematosus (13), thyroiditis (14, 15), pernicious anemia (15) and autoimmune hemolytic anemia (16). Figure 24 illustrates this mechanism diagrammatically.

No firm statement can currently be made of the role of an unusual propensity to form antibodies in autoimmune hemolytic anemia. Although variations exist in the ability of living organisms to respond to antigenic stimuli, it is not known whether such variations are significant.

A Foreign Clone of Cells

The majority of mechanisms previously described have involved an abnormality or modification of the target antigen. Dameshek and Schwartz (17) have reversed this approach. They suggest that autoimmunization involving the erythrocyte may reflect an abnormality of the antibody producing cell.

On clinical grounds this assumption has merit. Massive production of a single

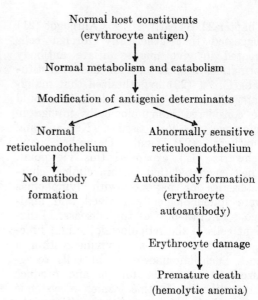

FIGURE 24. Autoimmune hemolytic anemia. An enhanced, abnormal sensitivity of the immunologic apparatus leads to erythrocyte autoantibody formation.

immunoglobulin as seen in plasma cell myeloma does not necessarily lead to an immunologic event. The isolated production of a single circulating antibody in itself does not usually result in a disease state. This is evident with thyroid autoantibodies, lupus erythematosus cell production, rheumatoid factors and even erythrocyte autoantibodies. In contrast, most autoimmune diseases manifest multisystem involvement associated with lymphoid hyperplasia. Dameshek and associates (17–19) suggested that autoimmune hemolytic anemia may appear as one part of such a multisystem immunologic abnormality resembling experimental graft-host disease (GVH disease, runt disease, homologous disease, wasting disease, secondary disease).

Theoretical Concepts

Graft-host disease has been shown to result from immunologic mechanisms (20). The survival and replication of foreign lymphocytes in a host is a necessary prerequisite. The theoretical and experimental studies relating graft-host disease to autoimmune hemolytic anemia are reviewed in

Chapter 22. As early as 1953 Ahrengot (21) suggested that genetically foreign cells created in vivo might initiate antibody formation against normal host constituents. Green (22) hypothesized that malignant cells of the reticuloendothelium could be considered immunologically foreign in reference to host tissues. Kaplan and Smithers (23) and Dameshek and Schwartz (17) expanded this viewpoint. They suggested that certain clinical characteristics of patients with lymphomas were immunologically derived and analogous to graft-host or runt disease. Malignant cells of the reticuloendothelium function as foreign cells surviving within a host. Such immunocompetent cells recognize host tissues as foreign and produce autoantibodies. In this fashion a systemic immunologic disease with multiple abnormalities would occur. Autoimmune hemolytic anemia would represent one part of a systemic syndrome similar to graft-host disease. This hypothesis could be expanded to include nonmalignant lymphoproliferative diseases. Billingham (24) suggested that maternal lymphoid cells may cross the placenta, implant in the fetus and survive. Proliferation of such cells after birth could produce a foreign clone with the capacity to form antibodies against host constituents.

Somatic mutations arising spontaneously or from the action of viruses, chemicals or radiation may lead to gene deletion and to a similar foreign clone of cells surviving in the host. If such cells are immunocompetent and sufficiently modified so as not to recognize host constituents, antibodies may be produced. Fudenberg and Solomon (25) suggested a graft-host disease etiology to explain the development of some forms of autoimmune hemolytic anemia. Two patients with acquired agammaglobulinemia had an associated autoimmune hemolytic anemia. Since this observation, other investigators have postulated a graft-host disease syndrome in patients with multiple immunologic defects. Pirofsky and associates (26) employed the graft-host disease concept to explain a transient antiglobulin positive hemolytic anemia seen in cardiac surgery.

The foreign immunocompetent lymphocytes were presumably supplied by massive transfusion therapy. Development of a febrile lymphocytic splenomegaly syndrome in four of seven cases supports this postulate. Modified lymphocytes can be identified and may possibly be etiologically involved in both hemolysis and the febrile syndrome. The transient nature of the syndrome is assumed to result from the eventual rejection of the transfused lymphocytes.

Application of these concepts to autoimmune hemolytic anemia requires an immunocompetent precursor cell with the potential for rapid proliferation. This cell, termed the immunoblast or immunocyte (27), is acted upon by environmental factors. Malignant changes and virus interactions appear to be particularly important. Either these abnormal immunocytes are not sufficiently modified to be recognized as foreign and rejected, or else an aberrant immune apparatus of the host prevents rejection. Such abnormal cells may have a growth potential sufficient to overcome the body's ability to reject them. The persisting abnormal immunocyte proliferates, creating a clone of cells with the same abnormality. Such cells may preserve their antibody producing capacity, although the ability to recognize self-constituents is lost. The immunologic situation that results is identical with that created in experimental graft-host disease. The autologous modified cells may mature to large lymphocytes, small lymphocytes and plasma cells. With the loss of self-recognition, antibody formation against multiple host antigens can occur, leading to a systemic immunologic disease. The erythrocyte may be one of several host tissues involved in this process. This will be clinically identified as autoimmune hemolytic anemia. Figure 25 diagrammatically presents the proposed sequence of events.

Clinical Application of the Foreign Clone Theory

This concept is particularly well suited for application in reticuloendothelial neoplasia. The peculiar predilection of pa-

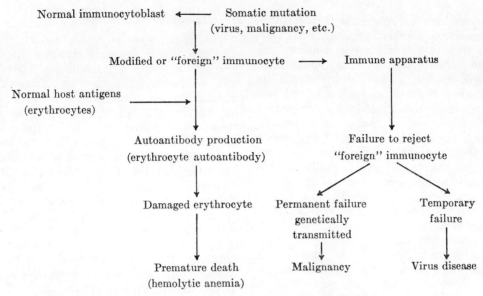

FIGURE 25. Autoimmune hemolytic anemia. The formation of a foreign clone of cells. If such cells are immunocompetent, erythrocyte autoantibodies may be produced.

tients with chronic lymphocytic leukemia to develop autoimmune hemolytic anemia is well known; such a complication occurs in approximately 25 per cent of cases. In chronic lymphocytic leukemia a somatic mutation of the lymphocyte results in a clone of malignant immunocompetent cells. Self-recognition for host antigens may be lost while the potential to produce antibodies is preserved. Involvement of the erythrocyte in this process leads to autoimmune hemolytic anemia.

In addition to autoimmune hemolytic anemia, other confusing aspects of chronic lymphocytic leukemia are compatible with this hypothesis. Many symptoms and signs characteristic of the leukemic state, e.g., fever, wasting and malaise, may be related to a graft-host symptom complex (17, 23). The clinical picture suggests a widespread multisystem immune reaction. Lewis and associates (28) reported that patients with lymphoma or chronic lymphocytic leukemia may manifest accelerated or initial immunologic activity directly after radiation or chemotherapy. It may be postulated that immunologic homeostasis is established between host constituents and antibody production directed against host constituents. Therapy

which reduces the growth rate of host cells may adversely disturb the homeostatic state, leading to more overt evidence of immunologic activity. This could reflect a state of partial immune tolerance between host constituents and immunocompetent cells which is disturbed through therapy, thereby precipitating immunologic activity.

Although autoimmune hemolytic anemia in chronic lymphocytic leukemia is common, such a complication is rare in acute lymphocytic leukemia. This discrepancy is also explainable with the proposed abnormal clone of immunocompetent cells. In chronic lymphocytic leukemia, large numbers of abnormal cells mature to a stage compatible with antibody production. In the acute stage, cell death generally occurs early and the abnormal cells remain primarily in the immunoblast stage. A population of potential antibody producing cells exists. Such cells, however, do not mature sufficiently to produce antibody actively.

Autoimmune hemolytic anemia is frequently considered to be a result of increased antibody production. This is difficult to reconcile with the observation that patients with malignancies of the reticuloendothelium are particularly susceptible to recurrent infectious disease. Such subjects seem unable to marshal a normal immune response (29, 30). The foreign clone theory supplies a working hypothesis for this state. Survival of such modified cells implies a greater capacity for replication, with more efficient metabolic pathways, than is the case with normal lymphocytes. Metabolic competition between abnormal and normal immunocytes results in the gradual replacement of normal cells by malignant cells. The reduction in the number of normal immunocytes is reflected in a loss of ability to produce immunoglobulins directed against foreign antigens. Simultaneously there is an increase in malignant cells with the capacity to produce autoantibodies. The production of large amounts of a single immunoglobulin in plasma cell myeloma illustrates this process.

Infectious mononucleosis is a nonmalignant lymphoproliferative syndrome which suggests a similar foreign clone state (31). Modification of an immunocompetent cell occurs secondarily to virus infection. Proliferation of such modified cells may create a lymphocyte population recognizing host constituents as foreign. Characteristic findings in this disease could then be interpreted as the result of immunologic activity. These would include lymphocytic proliferation, liver damage, the production of heterophile agglutinins, a false positive serologic test for syphilis, cold hemaglutinins, anti-i antibodies and, rarely, autoimmune hemolytic anemia and autoimmune idiopathic thrombocytopenic purpura. Dameshek has projected this concept further (31). He speculates that infectious mononucleosis may represent "a highly atypical self limited form of lymphocytic leukemia." The ability of the foreign clone of cells to persist is crucial. Continued replication of modified cells will result in chronic lymphocytic leukemia and a chronic immunologic problem. Rejection of modified cells by immune homeostasis creates the transient picture of infectious mononucleosis. Complicating heteroimmune and autoimmune states would also disappear.

The Role of the Immunocyte

The immunocyte is critical to the concept of a foreign clone and deserves amplification (27, 32). A fundamental characteristic distinguishes this cell from the immunocompetent cell concept developed by Burnet (33) in the clonal selection theory. With clonal selection the immunocompetent cell has the potential to produce only one or two predetermined antibody molecular structures. In contrast, the immunocyte is considered to be a precursor cell with an unlimited capacity for the production of various antibody molecular structures. Immature immunocompetent cells (immunoblasts) undergo transformation from the large lymphocytes to small lymphocytes or plasma cells. On the basis of phytohemagglutinin studies, as well as other evidence, it appears that small lymphocytes have the capcity to revert to the immature large lymphocyte state and to recycle again to active antibody production. The potential ability of the plasma cell to recycle is still an open question. The theoretical implications of this distinction in relation to autoimmune hemolytic anemia are discussed in Chapter 13. Pertinent reviews delineating the role of the immunocyte have been presented by Dameshek (27) and Berman (32). Silverstine and Prendergast have reviewed this problem and emphasize that precursors of antibody producing cells do not appear to be unique (34). Gorman and Chandler (35) suggest that there may be immunologically incompetent cells with the capacity to replicate under the influence of antigen but not to produce antibody.

Experimental Support for the Foreign Clone Theory

Clinical observations support the concept of a foreign clone of cells involved in autoimmune hemolytic anemia. The relationship is most apparent with lymphoproliferative states such as chronic lymphocytic leukemia and the lymphomas (17, 30, 36). Several experimental studies have examined the role of abnormal lymphocytes in the production of erythrocyte autoantibodies. Pirofsky (37) was unable to demonstrate antigenic material related to erythrocyte autoantibodies in extracts of lymphocytes obtained from cases of chronic lymphocytic leukemia. Potent hemolysins and agglutinins acting against trypsinized erythrocytes were found. This was confirmed by Ponder (38). These agglutinins and hemolysins differed from erythrocyte autoantibodies. Direct production of erythrocyte autoantibodies by abnormal lymphocytes could not be demonstrated. Brody and Beizer (39) showed that abnormal lymphocytes were coated with erythrocyte autoantibodies. This suggests a common antigen on erythrocytes and lymphocytes. Excellent experimental data have documented autoimmune hemolytic anemia and a positive antiglobulin test as part of a graft-host disease syndrome (18, 40–45). Pertinent discussions of the immunologic capacity of lymphocytes related to autoimmunization and graft-host disease have been presented (27, 35, 46–49).

Oliner and associates (18) in 1961 studied graft-host disease in mice and emphasized the hematologic and immunologic consequences. The following observations were made: (1) positive antiglobulin test, (2) anemia with a shortened erythrocyte survival time, (3) the antibody coating erythrocytes were derived from grafted spleen cells, (4) leukopenia, (5) thrombocytopenia, (6) wasting, (7) hypothermia, (8) irregular alopecia, (9) splenomegaly, and (10) hyperglobulinemia. The similarity of experimental graft-host disease and autoimmune hemolytic anemia complicating reticuloendothelial neoplasia is striking. Table 83 summarizes the contrasting observations in these two syndromes. The significance of these studies is further discussed in Chapter 22.

The Development of "Forbidden Clones"

Burnet has suggested an explanation for autoimmunization within the framework of clonal selection (33). The persistence

TABLE 83. *Similarities and dissimilarities between graft-host (runt) disease and secondary forms of autoimmune hemolytic anemia*

	Graft-host Disease	Autoimmune Hemolytic Anemia
General findings		
Growth	Runting	Wasting
Temperature	Hypothermia	Hyperthermia
Alopecia	Yes	Yes
Malaise	?	Yes
Protein abnormalities		
Hypergammaglobulinemia	Yes	Yes
Positive antiglobulin tests	Yes	Yes
Source of erythrocyte antibody	Transplanted cells	Host cells
Hematologic changes		
Anemia	Yes	Yes
Shortened Cr^{51} half-life	Yes	Yes
Leukopenia	Yes	Yes
Thrombocytopenia	Yes	Yes
Splenomegaly	Yes	Yes
Foreign lymphocytes	Yes (transplant)	Yes (malignancy, virus)
Other autoimmune phenomena	Yes	Yes
Death	Yes	Yes

and proliferation of "forbidden clones" are necessary (12). Burnet conceived of immunocompetent cells as having the capacity to respond to a specific antigenic determinant by replication. A clone of cells would develop capable of producing a specific globulin structure complementary to the antigenic determinant. Self-recognition occurs through destruction or inhibition of cells able to respond to self-antigenic materials. MacKay and Burnet (50) hypothesize that the simplest and most direct explanation for autoimmunization is the survival of such immunocompetent cells. Proliferation of such cells would result in a clone able to produce antibodies directed against host constituents. This postulated collection of cells has been termed the "forbidden clone."

Theoretical Concepts

The following sequence of events may be suggested to explain autoimmune hemolytic anemia within this framework. It is necessary to postulate the failure of homeostatic mechanisms which normally inhibit immunocompetent cells able to produce antibodies against host erythrocytes. Inhibition presumably occurs during fetal life. The process occurs in the thymus gland before seeding of lymphocytes populates the reticuloendothelium. MacKay and Burnet (50) state that "perhaps all that can be said about the nature of the homeostatic mechanisms is that they depend principally on the relatively high concentration and persistence of the self components concerned."

If the immunocompetent cell able to produce antibodies against host erythrocytes escapes destruction, a forbidden clone exists. This establishes the potential for the development of a self-perpetuating disease. Two possible mechanisms may be involved in establishing a forbidden clone. The immunocompetent cell simply may be sequestered and may escape destruction because of an aberrant immune homeostatic system. Alternatively, inhibition may be avoided through somatic mutation and creation of a functional abnormality of the lymphoid tissue. Viruses

may function by increasing the rate of somatic mutation, thereby creating foreign cells containing the forbidden pattern. They may also induce the functional modification of the lymphoid tissue postulated above as necessary to prevent the elimination of the cell through immune homeostasis. It is conceivable that persistence of forbidden clones and their ability to escape destruction may be genetically mediated. The fundamental defect in autoimmune hemolytic anemia would then be the genetic tendency to develop cells with the capacity to react with host constituents and not be eliminated during fetal life.

The forbidden clone may therefore be considered as a group of sequestered immunocompetent cells left from fetal life. They also may be thought of as immunocompetent cells modified by somatic mutations through virus action. Such cells have the capacity to initiate antibody formation against host antigens. The simple survival of a forbidden clone, however, is insufficient to explain the production of erythrocyte autoantibodies. Current theories indicate that such immunocompetent cells always exist. What is needed is an explanation for active proliferation. MacKay and Burnet (50) suggested that forbidden clones are sequestered and that proliferation occurs only upon dispersal of these cells from the thymus gland. The initiating factors of this phase of the reaction are unknown. It is possible that the endocrine glands, particularly the gonads and adrenals, are involved. Proliferation of the forbidden clone results in anti-erythrocyte autoantibody formation with autoimmune hemolytic anemia. A diagrammatic representation of the forbidden clone concept is presented in Figure 26.

Experimental Support for the Forbidden Clone Theory

Several experimental studies offer support for this concept. A familial predisposition has been described in various autoimmune syndromes (13–16). This reinforces Burnet's contention that the abnormality preventing inhibition of the immunocompetent cell is genetically determined. Additional support is supplied by recent evidence of chromosomal aberrations associated with autoantibody formation (51, 52). A high incidence of thyroid disease and of thyroid autoantibodies in the mothers of patients with Down's syndrome has been documented (51). Burch and associates (52) expanded this observation and postulated that diabetes mellitus is a spontaneous disturbed tolerance autoimmune disorder. Diabetes is conceived of as a genetically dependent disease initiated by five dependent type random events. Predisposition for diabetes is polygenic, involving an X-linked allele together with an autosomal factor or factors. Burch and coworkers (52) postulate that the intrinsic molecular instability of genetic material makes it inevitable that there be at least one disturbed tolerance autoimmune disorder associated with every distinctive target tissue in the body. Childs (53) suggests that somatic mutations at an X-linked locus, which has control over the structure of immunoglobulins, might explain the excess of affected females and the earlier onset in females of autoimmune diseases.

Development of the NZB strain of mice by Bielschowsky and associates (54) offers more direct evidence of genetic influences in autoimmune syndromes. These animals, developed purely on the basis of inbreeding, manifest spontaneous autoimmune hemolytic anemia. Positive antiglobulin tests are first noted at 6 months of age. Subsequent inbreeding studies have developed additional strains with a high incidence of renal disease resembling human lupus nephritis (see Chapter 22). Recent data may nullify the genetic influences. Mellors and Huang (55) suggest that vertical transmission of a virus may be involved.

The important role of the thymus gland in this genetic concept of forbidden clones has also received experimental support. Burnet (56) has suggested that the thymus gland plays a key role in immunologic homeostasis. This organ normally does not have germinal follicles in the adult mouse. In the NZB mice germinal centers are found in the thymus gland (57).

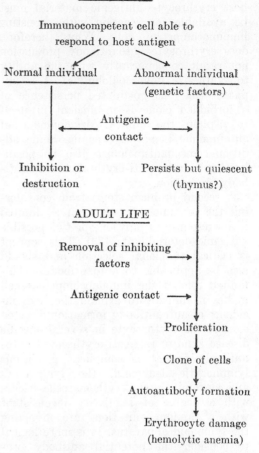

FIGURE 26. Autoimmune hemolytic anemia. The proliferation of a "forbidden clone," leading to erythrocyte autoantibody formation.

Persistence of germinal centers in the thymus gland has also been reported in various human autoimmune syndromes (58). The role of the thymus gland in autoimmune diseases is discussed in Chapter 22.

Clinical Implications of the Forbidden Clone Theory

In spite of excellent theoretical and experimental support of a forbidden clone etiology in autoimmune hemolytic anemia, several clinical observations are difficult to explain. With this hypothesis we must assume the persistence of immunocompetent cells able to produce antibodies against host erythrocytes long after the embryonic period. Simultaneously a large amount of host erythrocyte antigenic material must be available for reaction with persisting immunocompetent cells. Why, therefore, does erythrocyte autoantibody production not result concomitantly with the ability to synthesize immunoglobulins? It is apparent that the postulated persistence of a forbidden clone is insufficient in itself to explain the clinical development of autoimmune hemolytic anemia. Some additional mechanism must also be postulated to initiate anti-erythrocyte autoantibody production.

A second problem stems from considering the immunocompetent cell as limited in its response to only one or two possible antigenic determinants (33). This concept is critical to clonal selection and should also be applicable to autoantibodies. This limited role of the immunocompetent cell makes it difficult to explain the high incidence of autoantibody formation directed against the erythrocyte in several specific disease syndromes. Anti-erythrocyte autoantibody formation complicating chronic lymphocytic leukemia, the lymphomas and systemic lupus erythematosus occurs with a degree of regularity inconsistent with a random mutation rate involving the lymphoid apparatus. It is more logical to consider the potential antibody producing cell as an immunoblast with the capacity to form any one of or even several different antibody molecular structures (27).

An extension of this problem introduces another difficulty in reconciling the forbidden clone concept with clinical observations in autoimmune disease. The autoimmune diseases are more complex than was originally thought. Theories of antibody formation must now contain an explanation for the ability to produce antibodies directed against multiple and apparently unrelated host constituents. For example, there is a high incidence of thyroid autoantibodies in patients with pernicious anemia (15). The reverse is also seen. Multiple autoantibody formation is commonly found in systemic lupus erythematosus (13). In the clinical section of this volume the frequent association of autoimmune hemolytic anemia with other autoimmune syndromes is emphasized. Multiple autoantibody formation appears to be typical of autoimmunization (30). This viewpoint magnifies the difficulty of correlating random mutations with the concept of an immunocompetent cell able to produce only a single specific antibody. It is now necessary to formulate a hypothesis which will account for the production or maintenance of multiple specific immunocompetent cells, on a random basis, in order to explain clinical syndromes which occur with disastrous regularity.

The objections discussed above suggest that the concept of a forbidden clone is insufficient to account for the clinical characteristics of autoimmune hemolytic anemia. However, the postulate suggests experimental approaches which may clarify this difficulty. A delineation of the role of the thymus gland is crucial. Possibly the most productive approach will lie in an understanding of the genetic mechanisms involved. Are the defects encountered truly genetic (16)? Is it possible that specific chromosomal regions will be involved, as was suggested in the study of diabetes and Down's syndrome (51, 52)? Can several of the confusing associations be explained by involvement of the same chromosome, in a fashion analogous to the Philadelphia chromosome? Are there genetically related antigenic characteristics similar to the histocompatibility loci? The experimental development of these problems is essential to evaluate the role of forbidden clones in autoimmune diseases.

The Immunodeficient Individual

The concepts of foreign and forbidden clones supply an excellent theoretical matrix for the analysis of autoimmune hemolytic anemia. Individually, however, they have limited applicability to all forms of autoimmune hemolytic anemia. In addition, several theoretical contradictions are apparent which prevent their universal application. Many of these problems can be resolved by combining elements of both postulates into a unified system. The hypothesis of an immunodeficient individual offers such a framework.

Theoretical Considerations

There is excellent evidence that individuals may have a deficient immune apparatus (59). Congenital and acquired agammaglobulinemia and the lymphopenic syndromes classified under the term "Swiss type" are well known. This limited group has been expanded by the inclusion of other clinical syndromes characterized by various degrees and types of immunodeficiency. These include abnormalities of the thymus gland, reticuloendothelial neoplasia, sarcoidosis, mycosis fungoides, exfoliative erythroderma and pernicious anemia. Autoimmune disease has a close relationship to many of these syndromes.

It may be postulated that individuals have either congenital or acquired abnormalities of their immune apparatus which prevent normal immunologic activity (30). Immunologic homeostatic mechanisms are defective in such individuals. An overt manifestation of this deficiency would be an increased susceptibility to bacterial and virus infections. This reflects the inability to synthesize normal amounts and types of immunoglobulins. If the deficiency should involve cellular immune reactivity, delayed hypersensitivity would also be inadequate.

Actively metabolizing cells are susceptible to somatic mutations and modifications resulting from environmental factors. If such changes are lethal or if they create cells unable to compete with normal cellular elements, replication of the modified structures will not occur. If such modifications establish more efficient cells, survival may be anticipated. Antigenic determinants establishing tolerance may be eliminated. Alternatively, new antigenic determinants may be present for which tolerance has not been established. The immune homeostatic mechanism should recognize these changes and initiate immunologic activity resulting in rejection of the immunologically foreign host tissue.

An immunodeficient individual may not have the immunologic capacity to activate an adequate homeostatic response leading to rejection. A persisting permanent somatic mutation creates malignancy. If temporary modifications are present, such as those induced by viruses, a chronic or transient persistence of modified cells will occur. Tissues with a rapid growth and turnover rate will be particularly susceptible to this condition on chance alone. These include the reticuloendothelium, the basal epithelium and the lining of the gastrointestinal tract. If cells of the reticuloendothelium are involved, additional complications may be anticipated. Such cells are immunologically competent and have the capacity to initiate immune reactions. The acquired modification may not destroy this immunologic capacity. However, the induced change can alter the ability of such immunocompetent cells to recognize normal host antigens. Autoantibody formation may be anticipated. A situation identical to experimental graft-host disease will have occurred.

Theoretically a malignancy of the reticuloendothelium may produce only a single autoantibody. However, the malignant process may "unlock" the immunoglobulin synthesizing capacity of such cells, leading to multiple clones producing different immunoglobuins. A more likely pattern would involve the sequential formation of multiple, nonmalignant, modified immunocompetent cells which would develop and persist throughout the natural history of the immunodeficient state. This would eventually lead to complex and variable clinical syndromes characterized by multisystem immunologic involvement (30). Figure 27 diagrammatically depicts this sequence of events.

This hypothesis is dependent on the foreign clone concept of a graft-host disease syndrome as outlined by Dameshek and associates (17–19, 27, 31, 36). It also requires a multipotential cell such as the immunoblast postulated by Dameshek (27). However, it suggests that the fundamental abnormality is immunologic incompetence with a deficient immune homeostatic mechanism. Burnet's hypothesis of a functional abnormality of the lymphoid apparatus appears to be pertinent (12, 50). The postulated immune aberration may be genetically mediated as suggested by Ziff (60), Leonhardt (13), Fialkow and associates (61), Fudenberg (62) and Pirofsky (16).

The concept of an immunodeficient state leading to autoimmunization is rapidly being developed. Several excellent reviews of various aspects of this postulate are available. The most extensive has been presented by Good and associates (59). Bridges and Good (63) summarized 27 cases of agammaglobulinemia and noted that nine developed various collagen diseases. Gorman and Chandler (35) suggested the presence of an immunologically incompetent lymphocyte. Pirofsky and associates related this pathogenesis to autoimmune hemolytic anemia associated with reticuloendothelial neoplasia (30), pernicious anemia (64), ulcerative colitis (65) and a familial predisposition (16). Clark and associates (66) and Conn and colleagues (67) suggested that pernicious anemia may develop within the framework of immune deficiency. Bierman (68) extensively reviewed this problem in terms of the lymphomas and dermatologic manifestations.

Clinical Applications

Immunodeficiency resulting in a graft-host syndrome is a powerful theoretical tool for application to human disease. Many confusing clinical observations are clarified with this concept. These include (a) the tendency for agammaglobulinemia patients to develop lymphomas, leukemia and collagen diseases, (b) the frequency of hypogammaglobulinemia and/or autoimmune hemolytic anemia in patients with chronic lymphocytic leukemia, (c) the paradox of patients unable to resist bac-

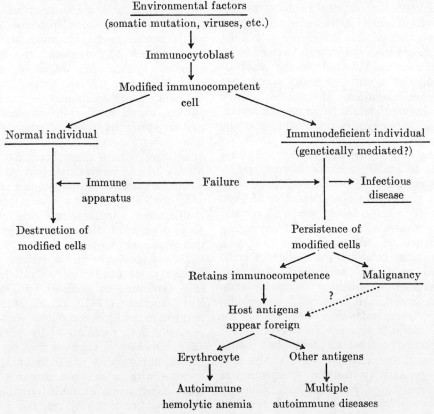

FIGURE 27. Autoimmune hemolytic anemia. The development and persistence of modified immunocompetent cells in an immunodeficient subject. Complex multisystem disease may develop, characterized by autoimmune hemolytic anemia, other autoimmune syndromes, malignancies and infectious disease.

terial and viral infections while appearing to be hyperantibody producers with autoimmune hemolytic anemia, (d) the relationship of thymus gland abnormalities to multiple immunologic deficiences, (e) the predilection of patients with reticuloendothelial neoplasia to develop autoimmune hemolytic anemia, and (f) the sequential or simultaneous development of more than one autoimmune syndrome in the same patient.

These concepts have excellent clinical support. The complications of agammaglobulinemia have already been alluded to (63, 69). Hathaway and associates (70) described the association of aplastic anemia, alymphocytosis and hypogammaglobulinemia in a probable graft-host disease. Thompson and Johnson (71) reported hemolytic anemia, and Clark and associates (66) and Conn and associates (67) reported pernicious anemia with hypogammaglobulinemia. The Swiss type of agammaglobulinemia resulting in an immunodeficiency syndrome has been reported by Hitzig and associates (72), Tobler and Cottier (73) and Rosen and associates (74). Thymic abnormalities are frequently related to immunologic deficiencies, and the association of thymomas with autoimmune hemolytic anemia has been recorded (see Chapter 6 and Cases 6, 20 and 36). The relationship of reticuloendothelial neoplasia, immunodeficiency and hemolytic anemia has been reviewed by Hoffbrand (75) and Pirofsky (30).

Most etiologic theories for autoimmune hemolytic anemia are inadequate to explain clinical observations. In general these theories supply the mechanism for the production of a single set of autoantibodies directed against erythrocytes. The clinical section of the current volume has emphasized that autoimmune hemolytic anemia infrequently appears as an isolated abnormality related to anti-erythrocyte autoantibody production. Most often autoimmune hemolytic anemia is one part of a complex multisystem disease. Pirofsky (16) has suggested that the idiopathic appearance may be illusory and may represent only a small diagnosable part of a systemic aberration. The immunodeficient hypothesis presents an etiologic mechanism which is compatible with the clinical appearance of a variable, complex, multisystem immunologic abnormality. The value of this hypothesis may be seen by reviewing the clinical data presented earlier. The immunodeficiency postulate was employed as an etiologic mechanism for autoimmune hemolytic anemia associated with reticuloendothelial neoplasia, infections, collagen diseases, ulcerative colitis, pernicious anemia, thyroid disease, malignancies and even ovarian cysts.

The Termination of Normal Immune Tolerance

A major flaw in several of the proposed etiologic mechanisms for autoimmune hemolytic anemia is their limited applicability. The foreign clone concept developed by Dameshek (17–19, 27, 31, 36) is an excellent model to explain autoimmune hemolytic anemia complicating chronic lymphocytic leukemia or lymphosarcoma. However, an etiologic mechanism to explain autoimmune hemolytic anemia in the absence of lymphocytic proliferation is also necessary. In one published report, 35 per cent of 137 cases of autoimmune hemolytic anemia did not appear to have an abnormality of lymphocytes (76). The concept of persisting forbidden clones as presented by Burnet (12, 50, 56) offers great promise in understanding autoimmunization characterized by a familial incidence. However, a familial occurrence of autoimmune hemolytic anemia is rare. The limited applicability of this concept to multisystem immunologically mediated diseases is a major handicap.

What is necessary is a general postulate compatible with the diverse clinical picture typical of autoimmune hemolytic anemia. An immunodeficiency state has been suggested in this regard. A mechanism involving termination of natural immune tolerance also appears to be ideally suited for this purpose. A combination of antigenic modification with termination of tolerance offers the versatility required.

TABLE 84. *Termination of tolerance to bovine serum albumin (BSA) in rabbits when animals were immunized with other sources of serum albumin*[*]

Source of Albumin Immunization	Cross Reaction with Anti-BSA	Rabbits Tolerant to BSA Immunized with Other Albumin	
		Producing anti-BSA (termination of tolerance)	Producing antibody to other albumin
	%	%	
Bovine (control)	100	0	
Sheep	75	0	0
Pig	22	33.3	33.3
Human	15	86.6	100
Horse	15	88.9	100

* After Weigle (77, 78).

Theoretical Concepts

Artificial immune tolerance produced for soluble antigens appears to be similar to the normal immune tolerance which characterizes self-recognition. Accordingly, mechanisms shown to terminate experimental immune tolerance may have a counterpart in termination of normal immune tolerance, i.e., autoimmunization. Weigle (77, 78) has documented the following characteristics of loss of tolerance for bovine serum albumin and bovine gamma-globulin in rabbits. (a) Tolerance may be terminated by injecting an antigen that is serologically related to the original tolerance inducing antigen. With the various serum albumins, the more distantly related they appear serologically, the more effective they are in terminating tolerance. Table 84 summarizes Weigle's data in this respect. (b) Incorporation of the tolerance inducing antigen (bovine gamma-globulin) in Freund's adjuvant is effective in terminating tolerance. (c) Chemical modification of the tolerance inducing antigen may terminate tolerance. Coupling of the diazonium derivatives of both arsanilic and sulfanilic acid to bovine serum albumin appeared most effective in terminating artificially induced tolerance to bovine serum albumin (BSA). (d) Modification of the tolerance inducing antigen by pepsin digestion, by heat denaturation and by combination with specific antisera (anti-BSA) was unsuccessful in terminating tolerance. (e) Readministration of the antigen inducing tolerance, after tolerance has been terminated, initially results in antibody production. Repeated administration of the antigen, however, reestablishes the tolerant state. Once tolerance is restored it can again be terminated by reinjection of serologically related antigens. (f) The termination of tolerance following the injection of serologically related antigens could be prevented by simultaneously administering the tolerance inducing antigen. (g) Thymectomy did not prevent the termination of bovine serum albumin tolerance induced by injecting arsanil-sulfanil-BSA.

Against this background the following sequence of events may be postulated to explain the development of autoimmune hemolytic anemia. Environmental factors act on the erythrocyte surface, resulting in either modification or denaturation of normal antigens. Chemical haptens of normal erythrocyte antigens may also play a significant role. The environmental factors to be particularly considered are drugs, bacteria, bacterial products, viruses, physical factors and various diseases previously discussed. If modification of erythrocyte surface antigens is sufficiently marked, a foreign but serologically related erythrocyte antigen may be created. When the induced change is significant, antibody formation directed against the modified antigen can result. This process is not true autoimmunization. There is little to suggest that such anti-erythrocyte antibody production is either self-perpetuating or directly related to the hemolytic stage. At this point Weigle's experimental data have special significance (77, 78). The unmodified erythrocyte antigen is in a state of normal immune tolerance to the host's immune capacity. However, antibody formation directed against modified but serologically related antigens can terminate the tolerant state for unmodified erythrocyte antigens. Autoantibody formation directed against normal erythrocytes may develop with autoimmune hemolytic anemia. Figure 28 diagrammatically depicts this sequence of events.

Several unanswered problems must be considered before accepting a termination of tolerance as a major etiologic mechanism in autoimmune hemolytic anemia. The method by which modified antigenic material terminates tolerance has not been elicited. Exactly what constitutes the normal state of immune tolerance has as yet to be determined. This concept is dependent on the assumption that similar mechanisms are involved in the establishment of both artificial and natural states of immune tolerance.

Clinical Application of the Termination of Tolerance Theory

The termination of tolerance hypothesis is particularly valuable in explaining the diversity of underlying disease processes associated with autoimmune hemolytic anemia. Modification of the erythrocyte surface can occur through various disease processes, drugs, bacteria, bacterial products, viruses and physical interactions. Each of these pathways will contribute to the clinical pattern of the immunohemolytic anemia.

The hypothesis offers an excellent explanation for the varied clinical courses characterized by remissions and exacerbations. Weigle's data (77, 78) suggest that continual modification of the erythrocyte surface by environmental influences will result in chronic, unremitting autoimmune hemolytic anemia. A transient, environmentally induced erythrocyte modification would permit eventual reestablishment of the immune tolerant state. This would reflect the disappearance of the modified erythrocytes. Clinically this may represent the spontaneous remissions not uncommonly seen in autoimmune hemolytic anemia. Reactivation of the mechanism leading to erythrocyte surface modification would again create modified erythrocyte antigens and terminate the immune tolerant state. Clinically this would ap-

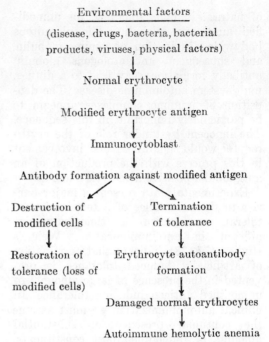

FIGURE 28. Autoimmune hemolytic anemia. The termination of tolerance. Modification of normal antigens by environmental factors leads to cross antibody formation. During the process tolerance for the unmodified antigen is terminated. Destruction of modified cells restores tolerance. Autoantibodies may further damage the cells, creating a self-perpetuating syndrome.

pear as an exacerbation of the autoimmune hemolytic anemia.

An expansion of the termination of tolerance concept permits an innocent bystander role of the erythrocyte to assume autoimmune significance. An identical sequence of events may occur, as proposed by Milgrom and associates (79), in the formation of anti-antibody. Introduction of a foreign substance into a host will result in normal antibody formation. The foreign substance could be a drug, bacteria, bacterial products or viruses. During antibody-antigen union denaturation of autologous antibody results in the exposure of previously inaccessible antigenic determinants. This break of immunologic quarantine leads to formation of anti-antibody. The production of such a serologically related but modified autologous globulin may also lead to termination of natural immune tolerance for unmodified autologous globulin. The ubiquitous bodywide distribution of gamma-globulin, and subsequent antiautologous globulin antibody formation, may lead to a diffuse, multisystem autoimmune disease. The deposition of immune complexes appears to be particularly important in this sequence. The innocent bystander role of the erythrocyte would guarantee its involvement in this process with the production of an antiglobulin positive hemolytic anemia.

Experimental data present a major barrier to the acceptance of a termination of tolerance mechanism as etiologically significant in autoimmunization. Weigle's studies (77, 78) indicate that termination of artificially induced tolerance is prevented in the presence of large amounts of unmodified antigen inducing tolerance. In clinical autoimmunization we must assume the continual presence of substantial amounts of unmodified host constituents. This is particularly apparent in autoimmune hemolytic anemia, in which large numbers of erythrocytes exist with prominent surface antigens. A substantial number of erythrocytes must be modified to allow this mechanism to act. Diseases such as pernicious anemia may be particularly susceptible to this action (64). The proposed anti-antibody mechanism with autoantibodies formed against autologous globulins is especially hard to defend. It is difficult to envision antiautologous globulin antibody formation while the host exists in a veritable sea of unmodified normal globulin.

Experimental Support for the Termination of Tolerance Theory

In spite of these theoretical objections there is excellent experimental evidence that a termination of tolerance can occur. The role of the lymphocyte in this process has been discussed by Bussard and Hannoun (80) and Denman and associates (81). Weigle (78) has presented an excellent series of studies indicating the role of this mechanism with modified thyroglobulin. Dowden and Sercarz (82) have

suggested a sequence in which spontaneous escape from tolerance involves paralysis, generation of memory cells and contact with endogenous retained antigen.

Many heterologous systems have been utilized in studying termination of tolerance. Such studies have generally employed the introduction of antigens from one species into a second species. The anticipated antibody production against the foreign antigen results. In addition, antibody formation against the host's own serologically related constituents also may occur, leading to autoimmunization. The systems which have been reported include human liver nucleoprotein into rabbits (83), rabbit or rat liver ribosomes into rabbits (84), rat liver into rabbits (85), rabbit connective tissue into guinea pigs (86), various heterologous heart antigens into rabbits (87), glomerular basement membrane of heterologous kidney into sheep (88), homologous or heterologous kidney into rats (89, 90), homologous or heterologous muscle incorporated into complete Freund's adjuvant into rabbits and guinea pigs (91) and rat bowel antigens into rabbits (92). In several of these studies tissue damage and disease resulted, as well as antibodies directed against the heterologous and autologous antigens. Autologous infarcted renal tissue has been shown to induce hypertension and autoantibody formation when rats are immunized with this tissue (93). Homologous or stored autologous leukocytes employed to immunize rabbits can also lead to autoantibody formation and granulocytopenia (94).

There is even experimental evidence supporting a termination of tolerance for autologous gamma-globulin. Milgrom and Witebsky (95) reported rabbit antirabbit antibody following immunization with autologous globulin prepared by ammonium sulfate fractionation. Circulating antibody directed against autologous rabbit globulin has been noted in rabbits immunized with protein antigens (96), bacteria (97–99), guinea pig leukocytes (100) and ferritin (96). Two possible examples exist for human disease. Williams and Kunkel (101) reported rheumatoid factor in approximately 50 per cent of untreated cases of subacute bacterial endocarditis. Treatment of endocarditis resulted in a titer drop of rheumatoid factor. Rheumatoid factors probably represents antiglobulin antibody. The diminution in titer of such antibody following therapy for subacute bacterial endocarditis suggests restoration of the normal immune tolerant state by removal of the underlying pathology leading to modification of autologous globulin. Loghem-Langereis and associates (102) have reported a patient with hypogammaglobulinemia and hemolytic anemia. They were able to demonstrate the occurrence of gamma-globulin/anti-gamma-globulin complexes in this case.

Four studies are available which suggest that erythrocytes may be involved in the termination of the tolerance mechanism, resulting in erythrocyte autoantibodies. Ovary and Speigleman (103) employed a rabbit test system. They documented the formation of iso- and auto-panhemagglutinins directed against both donor and recipient erythrocytes when a rabbit was immunized with donor erythrocytes. The isoantibodies produced were a mixture of IgG and IgM molecules; the autopanhemagglutinin was an IgM antibody reactive only at 4°C.

Zmijewski (104) studied a primate system with chimpanzees immunized with human erythrocytes. A circulating antibody directed against human erythrocytes was found. In addition, autoantibody directed against chimpanzee erythrocytes could be demonstrated. Increased erythrocyte destruction did not occur, but complement binding could be shown.

In 1961 Bowman and associates (105) employed a human test system. They transfused plasma containing potent anti-CD antibodies into a C^wDe/C_e (R^wR_1) volunteer recipient. An acute isoimmune hemolytic anemia resulted. Possible erythrocyte autoantibody formation wes noted 105 to 140 days after transfusion. Mohn and associates (106) expanded this study.

Plasma containing potent anti-CD antibodies was transfused into two recipients of blood group CDe/c_E (R_1R_2) and one recipient of blood group cDE/c_E (R_2R_2). All three recipients developed acute anemia, spherocytosis, hemoglobinemia, hypohaptoglobinemia, bilirubinemia and reticulocytosis. One recipient of blood group Cde/c_E developed an erythrocyte auto-antibody with specificity of anti-E. The authors postulate that the autoantibody developed in response to alterations at the rhesus site. Damage to or alteration of this site was produced by action of the anti-CD antibody.

Pirofsky and associates (26) in 1965 reported seven cases of transient acute hemolytic anemia with positive antiglobulin tests following aortic valve surgery. The authors speculate that mechanical damage to the erythrocyte surface resulted from hemodynamic factors involved in aortic stenosis and valve implantation. This was presumed to modify or denature erythrocyte surface antigens. Antibody formation directed against modified surface antigens may occur and with it, termination of tolerance for normal erythrocytes. Anti-erythrocyte autoantibodies are accordingly formed. The spontaneous correction of autoimmune hemolytic anemia presumably occurs with reestablishment of the tolerant state. This in turn results from the disappearance of modified erythrocytes from the circulation.

A termination of natural tolerance appears to be the most versatile mechanism for application to human autoimmunization. It is compatible with the diverse clinical patterns which may be associated with autoimmune hemolytic anemia. It combines the advantages of systems dependent on modification of antigens as well as abnormalities of the antibody producing apparatus. Different mechanisms which are experimentally supported may be incorporated into a workable system leading to autoantibody formation. The confusing spectrum of chronic hemolytic anemia contrasted with spontaneous remission and exacerbation is clarified with this concept.

Summary of Autoimmune Mechanisms

Etiologic discussions of autoimmune hemolytic anemia have frequently created misunderstandings and confusion among investigators. Three major reasons exist for such difficulties.

First, it is erroneous to search for *the etiology* of autoimmune hemolytic anemia. This syndrome is best considered as an end stage phenomenon resulting from loss of self-recognition and concomitant production of erythrocyte autoantibodies. This does not imply that there is only one way in which self-recognition may be abrogated. Data now available suggest that many different mechanisms may create this state, although the end stage evidence of autoimmunization is similar. The investigator should therefore document and champion a specific pathway only for a specific example of autoimmunization. Caution should be exercised before generalities are drawn. This simply requires the acceptance of experimental data as applied to a specific study. Delineation of one etiologic mechanism does not invalidate an entirely different concept based on different data in other systems. A prerequisite of this view is the realization that autoimmune hemolytic anemia is a symptom complex resulting from different pathophysiologic processes.

There is no reason to assume that a specific mechanism exists independently of other mechanisms. Thirteen different mechanisms are presented in this volume, each with experimental support for an etiologic relationship to immunohemolytic anemia and positive serologic tests. Many of these mechanisms by themselves contain unsolved problems and contradictions which prevent any one of them from standing alone as a satisfactory hypothesis. However, a combination of several of these mechanisms creates a composite picture answering individual objections. The innocent bystander concept, combined with a break in immunologic quarantine, permits the action of anti-antibody. Modification of antigenic structures appears to be insufficient to explain autoimmune

hemolytic anemia. When combined with a termination of tolerance, both mechanisms assume great potential.

The last and most difficult area to resolve is terminology. Much of the controversy characterizing etiologic discussions of autoimmune hemolytic anemia has resulted from lack of agreement as to what constitutes an autoantibody and autoimmunity. Although semantics plays a part in this difficulty, certain fundamental immunologic concepts are involved. A universally acceptable definition of antibody is still not available. It is necessary to resolve the conflict of "instruction" versus "selection" theories of antibody formation. The self-recognition phenomenon must be understood. The initiation, maintenance and termination of immune tolerance must be clarified. Only when this is accomplished will autoantibody formation and autoimmunity be placed on a firm semantic base.

In the current discussion autoimmunization is assumed only when a loss of self-recognition of normal host antigens occurs in relationship to the immune apparatus. The involvement of an erythrocyte as an innocent bystander offering an adsorption surface for an unrelated immunologic event does not satisfy this criteria. This is not considered to be autoimmunization. Dameshek (31) has also stated this point of view. Petz and Fudenberg (107) have strongly reiterated this concept in discussing the antiglobulin positive hemolytic anemia complicating penicillin therapy.

A more controversial area involves the modification of erythrocyte antigens by various environmental effects. The point of view has been taken that such antigen modifications result in a serologically foreign substance which initiates a normal immune response. Self-recognition and immune tolerance have not been abrogated. Antibody formation results from recognition of the foreign state and activation of normal immune homeostatic mechanisms. This state is not termed autoimmunization and the resulting hemolytic anemia has been classified as antiglobulin positive hemolytic anemia. On both clinical and theoretical grounds it is important to distinguish between these different pathogeneses.

Dacie (108) has examined the same problem. He presents two alternate definitions of autoimmunization in relation to erythrocytes. A narrow definition requires an erythrocyte autoantibody to be formed by normal antibody forming cells, with the subject's own normal erythrocytes acting as an antigen. A broader definition would classify an erythrocyte autoantibody as one capable of being adsorbed by autologous cells, without specifying that the erythrocytes themselves or the antibody forming mechanisms are normal. Dacie (108) is inclined to this latter interpretation.

Final agreement as to what constitutes an autoantibody and autoimmune hemolytic anemia will depend on the eventual delineation of the basic immunologic concepts. Until this occurs, needless misinterpretations can be avoided by a clear statement of definitions by the reporting investigator.

BIBLIOGRAPHY

1. Waksman, B. H.: Experimental Allergic Encephalomyelitis and the "Auto-allergic" Diseases. S. Karger, Basel, 1959.
2. Finkel, H. E., Brauer, M. J., Taub, R. N., and Dameshek, W.: Immunologic aberrations in the di Guglielmo syndrome. Blood 23: 634, 1966.
3. Callender, S., Race, R. R., and Pazkoc, Z. V.: Hypersensitivity to transfused blood. Brit. Med. J. 2: 83, 1945.
4. Waller, R. K., and Race, R. R.: Six blood group antibodies in the serum of a transfused patient. Brit. Med. J. 1: 225, 1951.
5. Clinicopathologic Conference, Washington University School of Medicine: Lupus erythematosus with severe anemia, selective erythroid hypoplasia and multiple red blood cell isoantibodies. Amer. J. Med. 44: 590, 1968.
6. Hennemann, H. H.: La formation d'anticorps multiples au cours d'anémies hémolytiques acquises. Rev. Belge. Path. 24: 479, 1955.
7. Gear, J.: Autoantibodies and the hyper-reactive state in the pathogenesis of disease. Acta Med. Scand. 152: Suppl. 306, 39, 1955.
8. Kissmeyer-Nielsen, F.: Specific auto-antibodies in immunohaemolytic anaemia. With a note on the pathogenesis of autoimmunization. In P. H. Andresen: Papers in Dedication of his Sixtieth Birthday. Einar Munksgaard Forlag, Copenhagen, 1957.
9. Glynn, L. E., and Holborow, E. J.: Autoimmunity and Disease. F. A. Davis Company, Philadelphia, 1965.
10. Coombs, R. R. H., Coombs, A. M., and Ingram, D. G.: The Serology of Conglutination and its Relation to Disease. Blackwell Scientific Publications Ltd., Oxford, 1961.
11. Najjar, V. A.: Some aspects of antibody-antigen reactions and theoretical considerations of the immunologic response. Physiol. Rev. 43: 243, 1963.
12. Burnet, F. M.: Autoimmune disease. II. Pathology of the immune response. Brit. Med. J. 2: 720, 1959.
13. Leonhardt, T.: Familial studies in systemic lupus erythematosus. Acta Med. Scand. 176: (suppl.) 416, 1964.
14. Hall, R., Owen, S. G., and Smart, G. A.: Evidence for genetic predisposition to formation of thyroid autoantibodies. Lancet 2: 187, 1960.
15. Doniach, D., Roitt, I. M., and Taylor, K. B.: Autoimmunity in pernicious anemia and thyroiditis: a family study. Ann. N. Y. Acad. Sci. 124: 605, 1965.
16. Pirofsky, B.: Hereditary aspects of autoimmune hemolytic anemia; a retrospective analysis. Vox Sang. 14: 334, 1968.
17. Dameshek, W., and Schwartz, R. S.: Leukemia and auto-immunization—some possible relationships. Blood 14: 1151, 1959.
18. Oliner, H., Schwartz, R., and Dameshek, W.: Studies in experimental autoimmune disorders. I. Clinical and laboratory features of autoimmunization (runt disease) in the mouse. Blood 17: 20, 1961.
19. Dameshek, W.: Theories of autoimmunity. In Conceptual Advances in Immunology and Oncology. Hoeber Medical Division, Harper & Row, Publishers, New York, 1963.
20. Simonsen, M.: The impact on the developing embryo and newborn animal of adult homologous cells. Acta Path. Microbiol. Scand. 40: 480, 1957.
21. Ahrengot, V.: De serologiske forhold hos en patient med immunologtisk haemolyisk anaemi og en antistofholdig abdominalcyste. Nord. Med. 50: 1570, 1953.
22. Green, H. N.: An immunological concept of cancer: A preliminary report. Brit. Med. J. 2: 1374, 1954.
23. Kaplan, H. S., and Smithers, D. W.: Autoimmunity in man and homologous disease in mice in relation to the malignant lymphomas. Lancet 2: 1, 1959.
24. Billingham, R. E.: Immune tolerance and autoimmune disease. Paper presented at the Second Annual Meeting of the American Society of Hematology, St. Louis, November 23, 1959.

25. Fudenberg, H., and Solomon, A.: "Acquired agammaglobulinemia" with autoimmune hemolytic disease: graft-versus-host reaction? Vox Sang. **6**: 68, 1961.

26. Pirofsky, B., Sutherland, D. W., Starr, A., and Griswold, H. E.: Hemolytic anemia complicating aortic-valve surgery. New Eng. J. Med. **272**: 235, 1965.

27. Dameshek, W.: "Immunoblasts" and "immunocytes"—an attempt at a functional nomenclature. Blood **21**: 243, 1963.

28. Lewis, F. B., Schwartz, R. S., and Dameshek, W.: X-radiation and alkylating agents as possible "trigger" mechanisms in the autoimmune complications of malignant lymphoproliferative disease. Clin. Exp. Immun. **1**: 1, 1966.

29. Aisenberg, A. C.: Studies on delayed hypersensitivity in Hodgkin's disease. J. Clin. Invest. **41**: 1964, 1962.

30. Pirofsky, B.: Autoimmune hemolytic anemia and neoplasia of the reticuloendothelium. With a hypothesis concerning etiologic relationships. Ann. Intern. Med. **68**: 109, 1968.

31. Dameshek, W.: Autoimmunity: theoretical aspects. Ann. N. Y. Acad. Sci. **124**: 6, 1965.

32. Berman, L.: The immunologically competent cell (immunocyte) system—an attempt at a delineation of cellular relationships. Blood **21**: 246, 1963.

33. Burnet, F. M.: *The Clonal Selection Theory of Acquired Immunity*. Vanderbilt University Press, Nashville, 1959.

34. Silverstein, A., and Prendergast, R. A.: What is immunologic competence? An attempt to define the attributes of the immunologically functioning cell. Blood **22**: 770, 1963.

35. Gorman, J. G., and Chandler, J. G.: Is there an immunologically incompetent lymphocyte? Blood **23**: 117, 1964.

36. Dameshek, W.: Chronic lymphocytic leukemia—An accumulative disease of immunologically incompetent lymphocytes. Blood **29**: 566, 1967.

37. Pirofsky, B.: Studies on leukemic leukocyte extracts. I. Lack of antigenic relationship in acquired hemolytic anemia. II. The demonstration of a hemolysin and agglutinin. J. Lab. Clin. Med. **48**: 745, 1956.

38. Ponder, E.: Hemolysins of tissues and tumors: recent advances with special reference to electrophoretic properties. In *Cell Electrophoresis*, edited by E. J. Ambrose. Little, Brown and Company, Boston, 1965.

39. Brody, J. I., and Beizer, L. H.: Globulin coating of neoplastic lymphocytes in chronic lymphocytic leukemia. Blood **22**: 139, 1963.

40. Cock, A. G., and Simonsen, M.: Immunological attack on newborn chickens by injecting adult cells. Immunology **1**: 103, 1958.

41. Simonsen, M., and Jensen, E.: The graft versus host assay in transplantation chimeras. In *Biological Problems of Grafting*, edited by F. Albert and P. B. Medawar. Blackwell Scientific Publications Ltd., Oxford, 1959.

42. Meier, H., and Brown, B.: The "runt disease" syndrome associated with immune hemolytic anemia and splenomegaly. Sang **30**: 776, 1959.

43. Piomelli, S., and Brooke, M. S.: An immune hemolytic anemia as a component of secondary disease in rabbit radiation chimeras. Transplant. Bull. **7**: 428, 1960.

44. Rask-Nielsen, R.: Coombs-positive hemolytic anemia and generalized amyloidosis in mice following transmission of subcellular leukemic material. Proc. Soc. Exp. Biol. Med. **116**: 1154, 1964.

45. Goldman, A. S., Haggard, M. E., McFadden, J., Ritzmann, S. E., Houston, E. W., Bratcher, R. L., Weiss, K. G., Box, E. M., and Szekrenyes, J. W.: Thymic alymphoplasia, lymphoma and dysgammaglobulinemia, hyper gamma A, normo gamma M, hypo gamma G, agamma D, and gamma E globulinemia, plasmacytosis, normal delayed hypersensitivity, severe allergic reactions, and Coombs positive anemia. Pediatrics **39**: 348, 1967.

46. Mackiewicz, S., and Burchardt, K.: Ostra choroba autoimmunizacyjna w przebiegu nietypowego rozplemu komórek immunologicznie wlasciwyck. Pol. Arch. Med. Wewnet. **35**: 723, 1965.

47. Cajano, A.: Auto-immunization and physiological cell auto-incompatibility patterns of auto-immunization in hematology. Bibl. Haemat. **23**: 66, 1965.

48. McBride, R. A.: Graft versus host reaction in lymphoid proliferation. Cancer Res. **26**: 1135, 1966.

49. Holborow, E. J.: An ABC of modern immunology. V. The immunological capability of small lymphocytes. Lancet **1**: 1049, 1967.

50. MacKay, I. R., and Burnet, F. M.: *Autoimmune Diseases*. Charles C Thomas, Publisher, Springfield, Ill., 1963.

51. Fialkow, P. J., Hecht, F., Uchida, I. A., and Motulsky, A. G.: Increased frequency of thyroid autoantibodies in mothers of patients with Down's syndrome. Lancet **2**: 868, 1965.

52. Burch, P. R. J., Rowell, N. R., and Burwell, R. G.: Autoimmunity and chromosomal aberrations. Lancet **2**: 170, 1966.

53. Childs, B.: Genetic origin of some sex differences among human beings. Pediatrics **35**: 798, 1965.

54. Bielschowsky, M., Helyer, B. J., and Howie, J. B.: Spontaneous hemolytic anemia in mice of the NZB/Bl strain. Proc. Univ. Otago Med. Sch. **37**: 9, 1959.

55. Mellors, R. C., and Huang, C. Y.: Immunopathology of NZB/Bl mice. VI. Virus separable from spleen and pathogenic for Swiss mice. J. Exp. Med. **126**: 53, 1967.

56. Burnet, F. M.: The immunological function

of the thymus. Aust. Ann. Med. **11**: 79, 1962.

57. Holmes, M. C., and Burnet, F. M.: The natural history of autoimmune disease in NZB mice. Ann. Intern. Med. **59**: 265, 1963.

58. Burnet, F. M., and MacKay, I. R.: Lympho-epithelial structures and auto-immune disease. Lancet **2**: 1030, 1962.

59. Good, R. A., Kelly, W. D., Rotstein, J., and Varco, R. L.: Immune deficiency diseases. Progr. Allerg. **6**: 187, 1962.

60. Ziff, M.: Genetics, hypersensitivity and the connective tissue diseases. Amer. J. Med. **30**: 1, 1961.

61. Fialkow, P. J., Fudenberg, H., and Epstein, W. V.: "Acquired" antibody hemolytic anemia and familial aberrations in gamma globulins. Amer. J. Med. **36**: 188, 1964.

62. Fudenberg, H.: Immunology deficiency, autoimmune disease, and lymphoma: observations, implications and speculations. Arthritis Rheum. **9**: 464, 1966.

63. Bridges, R. A., and Good, R. A.: Connective tissue diseases and certain serum protein components in patients with agammaglobulinemia. Ann. N. Y. Acad. Sci. **86**: 1089, 1960.

64. Pirofsky, B., and Vaughn, M.: Addisonian pernicious anemia with positive antiglobulin tests; a multiple autoimmune disease syndrome. Amer. J. Clin. Path. **50**: 459, 1968.

65. Bardana, E. J., and Pirofsky, B.: Autoimmune hemolytic anemia and ulcerative colitis; a multisystem immunodeficiency disease?, to be published.

66. Clark, R., Tornyos, K., Herbert, V., and Twomey, J. J.: Studies on two patients with concomitant pernicious anemia and immunoglobulin deficiency. Ann. Intern. Med. **67**: 404, 1967.

67. Conn, H. O., Binder, H., and Burns, B.: Pernicious anemia and immunologic deficiency. Ann. Intern. Med. **68**: 603, 1968.

68. Bierman, S. M.: Speculation on the role of immunologic aberrations in the pathogenesis of lymphoma with particular reference to mycosis fungoides and exfoliative erythroderma. Arch. Derm. (Chicago), **97**: 699, 1968.

69. Page, A. R., Hansen, A. E., and Good, R. A.: Occurrence of leukemia and lymphoma in patients with agammaglobulinemia. Blood **21**: 197, 1963.

70. Hathaway, W. E., Brangle, R. W., Nelson, T. L., and Roeckel, I. E.: Aplastic anemia and alymphocytosis in an infant with hypogammaglobulinemia. Graft versus host reaction? J. Pediat. **68**: 713, 1966.

71. Thompson, E. N., and Johnson, R. S.: A case of primary idiopathic hypogammaglobulinemia associated with haemolytic anaemia. Postgrad. Med. J. **38**: 292, 1962.

72. Hitzig, W. H., Biro, Z., Bosch, H., and Huser, H. J.: Agammaglobulinämie und Alymphocytose mit Schwund des lymphatischen Gewebes. Helv. Paediat. Acta **13**: 551, 1958.

73. Tobler, R., and Cottier, H.: Familiäre Lymphopenie mit Agamma-globulinämie und schwerer Moniliasis: die "essentielle Lymphocytophthise" als besondere Form der frühkindlichen Agammaglobulinämie. Helv. Paediat. Acta **13**: 313, 1958.

74. Rosen, F. S., Gitlin, D., and Janeway, C. A.: Alymphocytosis, agammaglobulinemia, homografts and delayed hypersensitivity: study of a case. Lancet **2**: 380, 1962.

75. Hoffbrand, B. I.: Haemolytic anaemia in Hodgkin's disease associated with immunoglobulin deficiencies. Brit. J. Cancer **18**: 98, 1964.

76. Pirofsky, B.: Serologic and clinical findings in autoimmune hemolytic anemia. Series Haemat. **9**: 47, 1965.

77. Weigle, W. O.: The antibody response in rabbits to previously tolerated antigens. Ann. N. Y. Acad. Sci. **124**: 133, 1965.

78. Weigle, W. O: *Natural and Acquired Immunologic Unresponsiveness.* World Publishing Company, Cleveland, 1967.

79. Milgrom, F., Dubiski, S., and Wozniczko, G.: Human sera with "anti-antibody." Vox Sang. **1**: 172, 1956.

80. Bussard, A., and Hannoun, C.: In vitro synthesis of autoantibodies by rabbit lymph node cells following cross immunization in vivo. Nature (London) **194**: 881, 1962.

81. Denman, A M., Vischer, T. L., and Stastny, P.: Termination of acquired tolerance by administration of small lymphocytes. J. Immun. **98**: 442, 1967.

82. Dowden, S. J., and Sercarz, E. E.: The X-Y-Z scheme of immunocyte maturation. II. The effect of antigen on spontaneous escape from immune paralysis. J. Immun. **98**: 827, 1967.

83. Goodman, H. C.: Antibodies to nucleoprotein extracts in patients with lupus erythematosus and rabbits immunized with nucleoprotein extracts. Clin. Res. **7**: 264, 1959.

84. Dodd, M. C., Bigley, N. J., Geyer, V. B., McCoy, F. W., and Wilson, H. E.: Autoimmune response in rabbits injected with rat and rabbit ribosomes. Science **137**: 688, 1962.

85. Asherson, G. L., and Dumonde, D. C.: Characterization of autoantibodies produced in the rabbit by the injection of rat liver. Brit. J. Exp. Path. **43**: 12, 1962.

86. Heller, P., and Yakulis, V. J.: Antigenicity of connective tissue extracts. II. Stimulation of auto- and iso-antibodies by heterologous antigen. Proc. Soc. Exp. Biol. Med. **104**: 590, 1960.

87. Kaplan, M. H., and Graig, J. M.: Immunologic studies of heart tissue. VI. Cardiac

lesions in rabbits associated with autoantibodies to heart induced by immunization with heterologous heart. J. Immun. **90**: 725, 1963.

88. Steblay, R. W.: Glomerulonephritis induced in sheep by injections of heterologous glomerular basement membrane and Freund's adjuvant. J. Exp. Med. **116**: 253, 1962.

89. Heymann, W., Kmetec, E. P., Wilson, S. G. F., Hunter, J. L. P., Hackel, D. B., and Cuppage, F.: Experimental autoimmune renal disease in rats. In *Immunopathology, Third International Symposium,* edited by P. Grabor and P. Miescher. Schwabe and Company, Basel, 1963.

90. Unanue, E. R., and Dixon, F. J.: Experimental allergic glomerulonephritis induced in the rabbit with heterologous renal antigens. J. Exp. Med. **125**: 149, 1967.

91. Tal, C., and Libau, E.: Experimental production of muscular dystrophy-like lesions in rabbits and guinea pigs by an autoimmune process. Brit. J. Exp. Path. **43**: 525, 1962.

92. Holborow, E. J., Asherson, G. L., and Wigley, R. D.: Autoantibody production in rabbits. VI. The production of autoantibodies against rabbit gastric, ileal and colonic mucosa. Immunology **6**: 551, 1963.

93. White, F. N., and Grollman, A.: Autoimmune factors associated with infarction of the kidney. Nephron **1**: 93, 1964.

94. Okubo, H.: Experimental studies on homologous or auto-leukocyte immunization. Bibl. Haemat. **23**: 62, 1965.

95. Milgrom, F., and Witebsky, E.: The rheumatoid factor and its possible pathogenic role. In *The Mechanism of Cell and Tissue Damage Produced by Immune Reactions,* Second International Symposium on Immunopathology, edited by P. Grabar and P. Miescher. Schwabe and Company, Basel, 1961.

96. Williams, R. C., and Kunkel, H. G.: Antibodies to rabbit γ-globulin after immunization with various preparations of autologous γ-globulin. Proc. Soc. Exp. Biol. Med. **112**: 554, 1963.

97. Eyquem, A., Guyot-Jeannin, N., and Podliachouk, L.: Présence dans les immusérums anti-bactérienes de facteurs antiglobu-

liniques analogues à ceux de la polyarthrite chronique évolutive. Ann. Inst. Pasteur (Paris) **96**: 295, 1959.

98. Milgrom, F., and Witebsky, E.: Rabbit antibodies against gamma globulins resembling the rheumatoid factor. Fed. Proc. **19**: 197, 1960.

99. Christian, C. L.: Rheumatoid factor properties of hyperimmune rabbit sera. J. Exp. Med. **118**: 827, 1963.

100. Milgrom, F., and Dubiski, S.: Antigenicity of antibodies of the same species. Nature (London) **179**: 1351, 1957.

101. Williams, R. C., and Kunkel, H. G.: Rheumatoid factor, complement, and conglutinin aberrations in patients with subacute bacterial endocarditis. J. Clin. Invest. **41**: 666, 1962.

102. Loghem-Langereis, E., Peetoom, F., and van der Hart, M.: The occurrence of gamma globulin/anti-gamma globulin complexes in a patient suffering from hypogammaglobulinemia and haemolytic anaemia. Bibl. Haemat. **23**: 55, 1965.

103. Ovary, Z., and Spiegelman, J.: The production of cold "autohemagglutinins" in the rabbit as a consequence of immunization with isologous erythrocytes. Ann. N. Y. Acad. Sci. **124**: 147, 1965.

104. Zmijewski, C. M.: The production of erythrocyte autoantibodies in chimpanzees. J. Exp. Med. **121**: 657, 1965.

105. Bowman, H. S., Brason, F. W., Mohn, J. F., and Lambert, R. M.: Experimental transfusion of donor plasma containing bloodgroup antibodies into incompatible normal human recipients. II. Induction of isoimmune hemolytic anemia by a transfusion of plasma containing exceptional anti-CD antibodies. Brit. J. Haemat. **7**: 130, 1961.

106. Mohn, J. F., Lambert, R. M., Bowman, H. S., and Brason, F. W.: Experimental production in man of autoantibodies with Rh specificity. Ann. N. Y. Acad. Sci. **124**: 477, 1965.

107. Petz, L. D., and Fudenberg, H. H.: Coombs-positive hemolytic anemia caused by penicillin administration. New Eng. J. Med. **274**: 171, 1966.

108. Dacie, J. V.: *The Haemolytic Anaemias, Part II,* Ed. 2. Grune & Stratton, Inc., New York, 1962.

Chapter 16

The Antibody in the Autoimmune Hemolytic Anemias

The starting point for any clinical or laboratory investigation of autoimmune hemolytic anemia is the autoantibody. A definitive diagnosis of the syndrome can be made only by identifying this substance. Therapy and prognosis are closely bound to the type of immunologic reactivity manifested by such antibodies. These materials have distinctive qualities which must be understood for a comprehensive view of autoimmune hemolytic anemia. It is therefore not surprising that a great deal of serologic and theoretical information has accumulated. The volume of technical material to be mastered is swelled by information obtained from analysis of erythrocyte isoantibodies. A close similarity exists between erythrocyte iso- and autoantibodies. Serologic data obtained from one system are pertinent to the other.

In the past two decades major advances have been made in understanding the structure, function and formation of antibodies. Serologic reactivity is dependent on antibody structure. An evaluation of erythrocyte autoantibodies therefore requires a correlation of their molecular structure with laboratory observations. In order to approach this problem it is necessary to summarize current concepts of antibody structure and function. No attempt is made to record all of the pertinent publications in this rapidly expanding field. Rather, the summary presented below is designed expressly for the clinician in order to introduce the necessary terminology and con-

cepts for application in human disease. Many excellent reviews of this subject are available and should be consulted (1–19).

Tiselius (20) in 1937 applied the moving boundary electrophoresis technique to the study of serum proteins. At pH 7.5 to 9.0, serum proteins were found to migrate into five distinct fractions under the influence of an electrical field. These fractions, cited in order of decreasing mobility, have been termed albumin, alpha 1, alpha 2, beta- and gamma-globulins. Antibody activity was first localized to the globulin zone. Subsequently they were more specifically described in the gamma- and beta-globulin fractions. Figure 29 presents a typical electrophoretic pattern of human serum identifying the various protein fractions. The regions manifesting antibody activity are indicated and the serum proteins are termed immunoglobulins.

The Immunoglobulins

Proteins may be classified on the basis of physical, chemical or biologic characteristics. The terminology subdividing globulins into alpha, beta and gamma fractions is dependent on the rate of migration in an electrical field. Each of the globulin fractions, even when represented by a symmetrical electrophoretic or ultracentrifugal peak, consists of a heterogeneous population of molecules differing in regard to molecular weight, electrical charge and antigenic determinants. The complexity of such crude

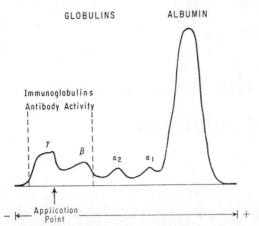

FIGURE 29. Electrophoretic pattern of human serum, indicating the zone containing antibody activity, i.e., the immunoglobulins.

TABLE 85. *Recommended terminology for the immunoglobulins*

Immunoglobulin Terminology		
Recommended	Alternative	Past synonyms
Gamma G	IgG	7S, γ_2, γ_2S, γ_{ss}, 6.8S
Gamma A	IgA	γ_1A, β_2A
Gamma M	IgM	19S, β_2M, γ_1M
Gamma D	IgD	
Gamma E	IgE	

serum components is apparent. For example, immunoelectrophoresis defines a protein molecule in terms of electrophoretic mobility and immunochemical specificity. With this procedure as many as 30 different antigenic components of serum can be identified. By adding another parameter to electrical charge, e.g., biologic activity as an antibody, the group of globulins can be further subdivided and classified as immunoglobulins.

A confusing jargon of terminology developed in an attempt to incorporate electrophoretic mobility, immunochemical specificity and physical characteristics in naming the various serum components involved in immunologic activity. This problem has been resolved (1–3), and Table 85 lists the recommended terminology and synonyms employed for the immunoglobulins. Detailed chemical, physical, metabolic, immunologic and genetic studies have been performed with these serum fractions. The pertinent studies are discussed below and summarized in Tables 86 to 88. Five classes of immunoglobulins are currently recognized: gamma G (IgG), gamma A (IgA), gamma M (IgM), gamma D (IgD) and gamma E (IgE). An additional class of immunoglobulins has been postulated. This has been tentatively termed gamma ND (IgND) and it appears to be identical to gamma E.

Gamma G Immunoglobulins

The gamma G immunoglobulins have previously been termed 7S, gamma 2, gamma 2-S and gamma ss. They are found in the gamma portion of serum after electrophoresis. Their molecular weight is approximately 140,000 to 160,000 and they sediment in the ultracentrifuge in a single symmetrical 7S or 6.8S peak. In normal human serum they constitute about 70 per cent of the gamma-globulins, representing a serum concentration of 1.2 gm. per cent. The majority of acquired antibodies are IgG molecules, as is the lupus erythematosus cell factor. Treatment of such antibodies with reducing agents does not inactivate immunologic reactivity. In fact, incomplete IgG erythrocyte antibodies may function as complete saline agglutinating antibodies after such treatment. IgG molecules have a low carbohydrate content (approximately 2.5 per cent) in contrast with IgA and IgM globulins. The abnormal serum proteins which may be seen in the sera of patients with plasma cell myeloma are frequently of an IgG class (70 per cent). During fetal life maternal IgG molecules are actively transported across the placenta. Antigenic stimulation initially leads to the production of IgM antibodies and is subsequently followed by the appearance of IgG antibodies. The production of IgG antibody is accompanied by marked reduction in the rate of synthesis of IgM antibody. Accordingly, IgG antibodies form the major portion of the secondary immunologic response. The appearance of gamma G

TABLE 86. *Physical, chemical and genetic properties of the immunoglobulins*

	Gamma G	Gamma A	Gamma M	Gamma D
Electrophoretic zone	γ	Slow β	γ-B	γ-B
Sedimentation rate	7S (6.8)	7S (9S, 11S, 13S)	19S	7S
Molecular weight	140,000	160,000	890,000	?
Carbohydrate (%)	2.5	10	10	?
Polymerization	No	Yes	Yes	?
Gm typing	+	−	−	−
InV typing	+	+	+	+
Paraprotein	Gamma-G myeloma protein	Gamma-A myeloma protein	Macroglobulin	Gamma-D myeloma protein
Disease with paraprotein	Myeloma	Myeloma	Macroglobulinemia	Myeloma

TABLE 87. *Antibody characteristics of the immunoglobulins*

	Gamma G	Gamma A	Gamma M	Gamma D
Antigenic specificity	γ	α	μ	δ
Effects of reducing agents	No loss of activity	?	Loss of activity	?
Primary antibody response, human	No	No	Yes	?
Bulk of secondary antibody response, human	Yes	No	No	?
Occurrence in phylogeny	Late	?	Early	?
Production in immature, human	No	?	Yes	?
Production in adult, human	Yes	Yes	Yes	Yes
Ability to traverse placenta, human	Yes	No	No	No
Example of antibody type	Incomplete warm acting autoantibody; anti-Rh₀(D)	?	Complete cold acting autoantibody; anti-A, anti-B	?

immunoglobulins reflects the response of the host to its environment with the bacterial flora playing a crucial role. In germ free animals the synthesis of IgG molecules may be reduced to only 5 per cent of normal. Approximately 40 per cent of IgG molecules are distributed in the intravascular pool and they are catabolized at an approximate daily rate of 3 per cent. This indicates a half-life survival time of about 23 days. The normal rate of synthesis is approximately 2.3 gm. daily. The rate of IgG catabolism is partially dependent on the serum level of IgG.

Gamma A Immunoglobulins

The gamma A immunoglobulins were first discovered by immunoelectrophoresis of normal serum and serum obtained from patients with plasma cell myeloma. They have been variously called gamma 1-A or beta 2-A globulins. On electrophoresis they migrate either as fast gamma or slow beta serum components. These proteins constitute about 20 to 25 per cent of the normal serum gamma-globulin and have a concentration of approximately 350 mg. per cent. About 30 per cent of human myeloma sera, and a significantly higher number of sera from mice with experimentally induced plasma cell tumors, have an abnormal amount of IgA immunoglobulins. IgA molecules have a monomeric molecular weight of approximately 160,000. They have a tendency to polymerize which appears to be related to their 10 per cent carbohydrate

TABLE 88. *Metabolic characteristics of the immunoglobulins**

	Gamma G	Gamma A	Gamma M	Gamma D
Serum levels (gm. %)	1.24	0.39	0.12	0.003
Immunoglobulins (%)	70	20–25	7	0.02
Present intravascularly (%)	40	40	80	?
Half-life survival (days)	23	6	5	?
Catabolized daily (%)	3	12	14	?
Synthesis (gm./day)	2.3	2.7	0.4	?

* After Fahey (10).

content. Accordingly, their ultracentrifugal sedimentation peaks are frequently asymmetrical and skewed. This tendency to polymerize results in a family of different sedimentation coefficient peaks with values of 7S, 9S, 11S and 13S after ultracentrifugation. The polymers can be dissociated into 7S monomers by breaking disulfide bonds with reducing agents. Diptheria and tetanus toxoid antibodies and typhoid O and paratyphoid B antibodies have been described in partially purified IgA fractions; however, contamination with IgG molecules cannot be excluded. Antibody activity directed against insulin and thyroglobulin have been detected in the IgA class of molecules. Antibodies against these components were also found in the IgG and IgM groups. It has been suggested that reaginic antibodies responsible for allergic disease are IgA immunoglobulins. Recent studies based on ragweed reagins have not confirmed this observation. A special form of gamma A immunoglobulin is present in saliva, colostrum and parotid gland secretions. Tomasi and associates (21) have presented evidence that IgA is synthesized as well as secreted by the parotid gland. Such secretory forms of IgA are unique in possessing an additional structural fragment or piece which stabilizes the molecule (22). A selected deficiency in gamma A immunoglobulins has been reported in normal individuals and in patients with ataxia telangiectasia. The significance of this type of agammaglobulinemia is unknown, but it may be related to respiratory and gastro-intestinal tract infectious problems. Approximately 40 per cent of the IgA molecules are distributed in the intravascular pool. A very rapid catabolism approximating 12 per cent daily results in half-life survivals of only 6 days. The normal rate of synthesis is similar to IgG and approximates 2.7 gm. daily.

Gamma M Immunoglobulins

The gamma M immunoglobulins are large macromolecules with a molecular weight of plus or minus one million (890,000). They have previously been termed 19S, beta 2-M and gamma 1-M macromolecules, and they migrate electrophoretically between gamma- and beta-globulin peaks. They appear as a minor component of normal serum comprising approximately 7 per cent of total gamma-globulin. Their serum concentration is about 100 mg. per cent. IgM immunoglobulins, similar to IgA immunoglobulins, have a 10 per cent concentration of carbohydrates and exhibit the same tendency to polymerize and combine with other serum components. Sedimentation coefficients of 19S are obtained with minor peaks of 24S and 32S after ultracentrifugation. Reducing agents splitting disulfide bonds will dissociate IgM molecules into five or six component parts with sedimentation coefficients of about 7S and molecular weights approximating 160,000 to 180,000. Fractions obtained by reduction are not true IgA or IgG molecules and are immunologically distinct. In contrast with IgG antibodies, reduction of IgM antibodies by 2-mercaptoethanol or Cleland's reagent destroys immunologic activity. IgM immunoglobulins are synthesized at an earlier evolutionary stage than are IgG molecules. Ontogony recapitulates phylogeny in formation of the immunoglobulins. IgM molecules can be synthesized by the human fetus and may be present by the 6th gestational month. In contrast, IgG immunoglobulins are not synthesized until approximately 3 months after birth and do not reach normal levels until several years of age. IgM immunoglobulins will not pass the placental barrier. The small quantities present at birth represent fetal and newborn synthesis. Accordingly, the initial antibody forming capacity of the human is essentially limited to the production of IgM molecules. This pattern is carried into adult life. Exposure of the human to an antigenic stimulus initially results in the formation of IgM antibody. Production of IgG antibody can subsequently be demonstrated and is accompanied by marked reduction in synthesis of IgM antibodies. The abnormal proteins found in Waldenström's macroglobulinemia and in cold hemagglutinin disease are IgM immunoglobulins. The saline acting complete isohemagglutinins (anti-A, anti-B, anti-Rh$_0$(D), etc.), the cold hemagglutinins, rheumatoid factor, antibodies against somatic "O" antigens of gram negative bacteria and many heterophile antibodies are IgM immunoglobulins. The IgM molecules are largely (80 per cent) distributed in the intravascular pool. They are rapidly catabolized (14 per cent daily) with a half-life of only 5 days. The rate of synthesis is only ⅙ the rate of IgG molecules, with 0.4 gm. produced daily.

Gamma D Immunoglobulins

The IgD class of immunoglobulins was described by Rowe and Fahey in 1965 (23). An immunologic study was performed on sera obtained from patients with plasma cell myeloma. It was noted that the abnormal protein present in certain pathologic sera did not react with antisera specific for IgG, IgA or IgM immunoglobulins. A new immunoglobulin class was postulated and termed gamma D (IgD). Antiserum produced against this protein demonstrated antigenic specificity which could distinguish it from other immunoglobulins. Many characteristics of this class are still to be determined. By electrophoresis IgD immunoglobulins are found in the range between gamma- and beta-globulins. Their sedimentation coefficient in the ultracentrifuge is similar to that of IgG, appearing as a 7S peak. They do not cross the placental barrier. The normal serum level varies widely, with a median value of 0.003 gm. per cent reported by Rowe and Fahey (23). This represents a trace concentration of 0.2 per cent of the total serum immunoglobulins. Hobbs and associates (24) found an in-

cidence of 3 per cent of an IgD type of plasma cell myeloma in 204 patients studied with this disease. In pathologic sera IgD concentrations averaged 0.7 gm. per cent and had a half-life of 2 to 4 days. It is interesting to note that all six IgD proteins described had a type L light chain. Rowe and Fahey (23) had previously studied 17 cases of an IgD type of myeloma and 15 had a type L and only two had a type K light chain.

Gamma E Immunoglobulins

It was originally suggested that reaginic antibody activity was located in the IgA group of immunoglobulins. However, many investigators demonstrated that reaginic activity was obtained from serum protein components free of IgA immunoglobulins. Goodfriend and associates (25) studied reaginic fractions obtained chromatographically from the sera of six ragweed allergic patients. Immunoadsorption with anti-IgG and anti-IgA did not reduce reaginic activity. The authors concluded that ragweed reagins belong to an as yet uncharacterized immunoglobulin class. Ishizaka and associates (26) obtained similar data. Antiserum was produced which removed the reagin rich fraction from the sera of atopic patients and which would not react with IgG, IgA, IgM or IgD globulins. These workers named the immunoglobulin class gamma E or IgE and suggested that reaginic antibody is of this globulin type. Little is known about this immunoglobulin class. Several physical characteristics have been documented by Ishizaka and associates (26). The electrophoretic mobility in agarose gel is that of a gamma 1 protein. Chromatographic fractions obtained from DEAE cellulose columns indicate a different separation from that of IgG, IgA and IgM, but it appears similar to that of IgD. IgE immunoglobulin elutes faster through a Sephadex G-200 column and sediments faster in sucrose density gradient ultracentrifugation. In the analytic ultracentrifuge a sedimentation coefficient of approximately 8S is obtained. The protein is present only in trace amounts in most sera and appears at a lower concentration than do IgD immunoglobulins.

The relationship of gamma E immuno-globulins to reaginic antibody is still un-clear. Studies by Johansson and associa'es suggest that reaginic activity may be found in an immunoglobulin class which they have termed *gamma ND* or *IgND*. Johans-son and Bennich (27) identified this globu-lin as a myeloma serum component. The protein migrates in the fast gamma range on electrophoresis, has an 8S sedimentation constant and elutes from a Sephadex G-200 column as IgA does. The molecular weight is approximately 200,000 with a carbohy-drate content of 10.7 per cent. Antisera specific to determinants of the heavy chain do not react with IgG, IgA, IgM or IgD. Recent studies suggest that gamma E and gamma ND are identical immunoglobulin classes.

The Structure of Antibodies

The structure, composition and genetics of the immunoglobulins have been inten-sively studied. The information obtained is of extraordinary interest and is funda-mental to the understanding of antibody formation and function. Antibodies present a wide diversity of biologic activity in molecules of very similar structure. Porter (6) points out that only a detailed knowl-edge of the full structure of the antibody molecule, with localization of biologic activ-ity to different parts, can permit under-standing of the chemical basis of antibody function and specificity.

Papain Digestion Studies

Porter (4–6) approached this problem by splitting the rabbit 7S IgG molecule by means of the enzymatic action of papain. Three fractions were chromatographically obtained, which accounted for over 90 per cent of the original molecular weight. Frac-tions I and II appeared almost identical, with a molecular weight each of 45,000; each fraction contained a single antibody combining site. In specificity and combin-ing power the antibody combining site seemed unchanged from what it had been in the intact molecule. The third piece of the rabbit IgG molecule was called fraction III. It is a heavier fraction with a molecu-lar weight of 55,000 and was easily crystal-lized. The fractions obtained by papain digestion were subjected to electrophoretic studies. Fractions I and II were termed S or slow fragments and fraction III was designated the F or fast fragment. Expan-sion of these studies employing immunoglob-ulins obtained from other animal species and from the human being gave essentially identical results. Three fractions were simi-larly obtained, although the mobility and ease of separation varied.

The recommended terminology describ-ing the fragments of the IgG immunoglobu-lins obtained after papain digestion are listed in Table 89 with their synonyms. Fab is employed to describe Porter's frac-tions I and II and the S or slow fragments. Fc refers to Porter fraction III, the F or fast fragment. A portion of the Fab frag-ment is derived from the H chain, contains part of the antibody combining site and is termed the Fd fragment.

Reduction Studies

In 1961 Edelman and Pulik (28) split the globulin molecule by reduction, employ-ing 2-mercaptoethanol in a strong urea solution. When the products of reduction were examined by starch gel electrophoresis, two major components were recognized and isolated. Terminology at this point became a bit sticky. The two fragments obtained by disulfide reduction had different molec-ular weights. The heavy fragment was termed the H fragment and the lighter frag-ment was termed the L fragment. On the basis of his reduction studies, Porter termed the heavy (H) fragment the A component and the lighter (L) fragment the B com-ponent. Comprehensive physicochemical and immunochemical studies of the various gamma-globulin fragments were performed. The papain digested electrophoretic S frag-ment was shown to be closely related to the chemically produced L or B fragment, and the papain digested electrophoretic F frag-ment was shown to be similar to the H or A fragment. Antisera specific for papain fraction Fab and papain fraction Fc were produced and tested against the L (B) and H (A) fragments obtained by reduction.

TABLE 89. *Breakdown products obtained after disrupting the rabbit IgG molecule*

Procedure	Analysis	Author	Components	
Papain digestion	Chromotographic	Porter (4–6)	Fractions I and II	Fraction III
		Franklin (12)	Fractions A and C	Fraction B
	Electrophoresis	Fahey (10)	S (slow)	F (fast)
			Fab*	**Fc**
Reduction with 2-mer-captoethanol	Molecular weight	Porter (4–6)	B	A
		Edelman and Poulik (28)	L (light)	H (heavy)
			L (light)	**H (heavy)**
Chains of IgG molecule		Porter (4–6)	B	A
		Edelman and Poulik (28)	L	H
			L	H

* **Boldface** designates recommended terminology: Fab, L chain + part of H chain; Fc, remainder of H chain; Fd, H chain part of Fab fragment.

Antiserum against fraction Fab reacted with both the L (B) and the H (A) fragments, whereas antiserum against fraction Fc reacted only with the H (A) fragment. Fraction Fab obtained by papain digestion therefore contained the L (B) chain of the globulin molecule and part of the H (A) chain. Fraction Fc obtained by papain digestion contained only the remainder of the globulin molecule (H chain). The L and H terminology is now recommended and is employed for the rest of this discussion. The various terminologies that have been developed are listed in Table **89**.

Structure of the Globulin Molecule

The above observations have led to a postulated four-chain structure for normal IgG immunoglobulins. Figure 30 illustrates a schematic representation of the assumed structure, the source of fragments Fab, Fc and Fd and the theorized relationship of the L and H chains. This schematic molecule is composed of two L polypeptide chains linked by disulfide bonds and non-covalent bonds to two H polypeptide chains. Detailed physical, chemical, genetic and immunologic studies of these two chains and of the related papain digest fractions have been carried out. Terminal amino acids of the L chains originally appeared to be alanine and aspartic acid. Since then other

amino acids have been found. The carbohydrate moiety is bound to the H chains. There is general agreement that the fundamental IgA and the IgM immunoglobulin subunits are similarly composed of two L chains bound by interchain disulfide bonds to two H chains. The specific characteristics of L chains and H chains are listed in Table 90 and are discussed below.

Characteristics of Light (L) Chains

There are two L chains in each divalent IgG antibody molecule. Considerable evidence has accumulated indicating that two antigenic types of L chains exist. These have been termed type kappa or K (I) and type lambda or L (II) and correspond to the two major antigenic types found for Bence-Jones protein. The two L chain types differ from each other in amino acid composition and in antigenic determinants. Normally both types of L chains are present in human sera. However, a single immunoglobulin molecule contains only one type of L chain. In normal human serum the lambda type of L chain comprises approximately 30 per cent, whereas the kappa type comprises 60 per cent of the total L chains. The remaining 10 per cent of L chains are not as yet classified. The C terminal amino acid has been determined in both types of L chains. In the kappa type it is cysteine and in the lambda type it is serine preceded

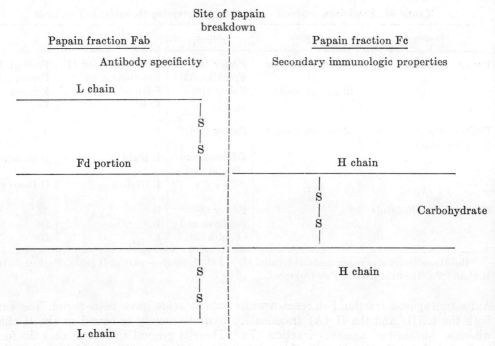

FIGURE 30. Schematic representation of rabbit gamma G (IgG) immunoglobulin. (After Porter (4–6).)

TABLE 90. *Characteristics of the immunoglobulin light and heavy chains*

	Light Chain	Heavy Chain
Synonyms	L chain	H chain
	B chain	A chain
Molecular weight	25,000	55,000
Electrophoresis	Slow	Fast
	Heterogeneous	Heterogeneous
Types	Kappa or K (κ) (I)	γ, α
	Lambda or L (λ) (II)	μ, δ, ϵ
Genetic factors	InV	Gm
Carbohydrates	–	+
Allotypic antigen	+	–
Isotypic antigen	–	+
Antibody specificity	–	+
Full antibody activity	+	+
Placental passage	–	+
Regulation of catabolism	–	+
Complement binding	–	+
Skin fixation	–	+
Reaction with rheumatoid factor	?	+
Production in disease	Bence-Jones protein, "light chain" disease	H chain disease

by cysteine. The cysteine is critical to the immunoglobulin structure as it provides the S—S bond between the L and H chains.

The L chains of all immunoglobulin classes appear to be similar and are immunologically identical. Antiserum prepared against L chains obtained from IgG molecules will accordingly react with IgA,

IgD and IgM immunoglobulins. The allotypic antigenic sites of immunoglobulins are therefore incorporated in the L chain. The L chains migrate slower in electrophoresis than do the H chains and they form a heterogeneous pattern. They have a molecular weight of about 25,000 and are devoid of conjugated carbohydrate. The similarity of L chains to Bence-Jones protein is striking. This similarity is reinforced by the observation that L chains have the characteristic solubility and thermal properties of Bence-Jones protein. L chains do not carry antibody specificity of the intact IgG antibody molecule. However, it appears that the L chains must be combined with H polypeptide chains for full antibody activity. One H chain and one L chain are associated with each antigenic binding site.

There is excellent evidence that the L and H chains are under separate genetic control. The InV genotype marker is a function of the L chains. Accordingly, InV activity is associated not only with IgG globulins but also with IgA, IgM, IgD and Bence-Jones protein.

Studies performed on the sera of patients with plasma cell myeloma suggest that the synthesis of L chains proceeds independently from that of the intact myeloma protein. The production of Bence-Jones protein may therefore reflect the malignant process with an abortive synthesis of the entire IgG, IgD or IgA immunoglobulin. L chain or Bence-Jones protein may now exist freely in the serum. Such Bence-Jones proteins (L chains) are predominantly of one type, i.e., kappa or lambda, and illustrate the monoclonal etiology of the synthesized protein. Williams and associates (29) have described a variant of plasma cell myeloma characterized by hypogammaglobulinemia (gamma-globulin of less than 0.7 gm. per cent) and an elevation of free serum L chains or Bence-Jones protein. The authors have termed this syndrome light chain disease.

Attempts have been made to characterize light chains more specifically. The sera of mice and of humans suffering from plasma cell myeloma have been extensively utilized in this regard. Light chains have been shown to be simple polypeptide chains containing somewhat more than 200 amino acid residues. Each polypeptide chain is divided near the midpoint of its amino acid sequence into a variable region, which differs for each light chain, and an invariable or common region, which is similar for all light chains of a given class. Hood and associates (30) have summarized these studies as follows. (a) Light chains are single polypeptide chains. (b) Light chains derived from the sera of mice with different plasma cell myeloma tumors have different amino acid sequences in the variable region. (c) The amino terminal portion of the L chain has remarkably similar amino acid sequences. (d) The differences at any one position in the sequence are limited to a small number of amino acids. (e) Variation in the amino acid sequence occurs from positions 1 through 105 in the amino terminal portion of the light chain. (f) In mouse light chains a variation in amino acid sequence does not occur in the entire carboxyl terminal portion. This includes amino acid positions 106 through 212. (g) There are small changes in amino acid sequences in the carboxyl terminal region of human light chains. These changes probably represent genetic heterogeneity in the human population. (h) It appears that some portion of the light chains, presumably the carboxyl terminal half, is coded by a single gene. There is significant variation of amino acid sequences between mouse kappa and mouse lambda light chains. Hood and associates suggest that the most reasonable theory of light chain formation involves the coding of the amino terminal half of the molecule by many genes. The studies of Hilschmann and Craig (31) suggest that the allotypic antigenic determinants (InV) are on the invariable or carboxyl terminal half of the L chain.

Milstein (32) investigated the differences between kappa and lambda type L chains. Comparison of the carboxyl terminal halves suggests an evolutionary relationship between the common regions of these two polypeptide types. Hood and associates (33) studied the amino terminal sequence of four human lambda light chains. They noted a strong analogy between kappa and lambda types in the first 20 residues if deletion was assumed to have occurred between positions 9 and 10 in the L chain. These studies strongly suggest that the genes coding for both the variable and invariable regions of the kappa and lambda chains have evolved from a common ancestor. Figure 31 diagrammatically represents the structural concepts of the L chain.

Characteristics of Heavy (H) Chains

The largest portion of an immunoglobulin molecule is the two H or heavy chains. In contrast to L chains, H chains are structurally different in each immunoglobulin class and are responsible for antigenic specificity of the class. Five types of H or

Single polypeptide chain	
212 Amino acids	
Common gene ancestry ?	
Multiple gene control ?	Single gene control ?
	InV site
Variable zone	Invariable zone
Amino acids 1–105	Amino acids 106–212
Amino region	Carboxyl region

FIGURE 31. Schematic representation of the amino acid structure of the immunoglobulin light (L) chain.

heavy chains are known, one type for each class of immunoglobulin. The H chain of the IgG immunoglobulins is called the gamma (γ) chain. In a similar fashion, alpha (α), mu (μ), delta (δ) and epsilon (ϵ) chains have been designated to describe the H chains of IgA, IgM, IgD and IgE immunoglobulins, respectively. When these are taken in conjunction with the two types of L chains, it is apparent that 10 basic immunoglobulin structures are present. A simple notation is available to describe an immunoglobulin molecule composed of two heavy and two light chains. IgG immunoglobulins are composed of $\gamma_2\kappa_2$ and $\gamma_2\lambda_2$ molecules. IgA immunoglobulins are described as $\alpha_2\kappa_2$ and $\alpha_2\lambda_2$ molecules. Polymerization of the individual molecules may be indicated by $(\alpha_2\kappa_2)n$. IgM immunoglobulins are polymers consisting of five or six units; they may accordingly be designated as $(\mu_2\kappa_2)_5$ or $(\mu_2\lambda_2)_5$. Table 91 lists this type of classification.

The information presented in the following discussion and summarized in Table 90 has been obtained primarily from studies of IgG immunoglobulin H chains. H chains electrophoretically migrate more rapidly than do L chains, and they appear to be heterogeneous. They are larger than L chains and have a molecular weight of 55,000. The carbohydrate moiety is bound to the H chain and may play a role in establishing different antigenic specificities of the five types. Antibody specificity of the

TABLE 91. *Classification and terminology of immunoglobulin types**

	Gamma G	Gamma A	Gamma M	Gamma D	Gamma E
L chains	Type K	Type K	Type K	Type K	Type K
	Type L	Type L	Type L	Type L	Type L
H chains	Gamma (γ)	Alpha (α)	Mu (μ)	Delta (δ)	Epsilon (ϵ)
Structure	$\gamma_2\kappa_2$	$\alpha_2\kappa_2$	$\mu_2\kappa_2$	$\delta_2\kappa_2$	$\epsilon_2\kappa_2$
	$\gamma_2\lambda_2$	$\alpha_2\lambda_2$	$\mu_2\lambda_2$	$\delta_2\lambda_2$	$\epsilon_2\lambda_2$
		$(\alpha_2\kappa_2)n$	$(\mu_2\kappa_2)_5$		
		$(\alpha_2\kappa_2)n$	$(\mu_2\lambda_2)_5$		

* Terminology:

L chains: Type Kappa = Type K = Type κ = Type I

Type Lambda = Type L = Type λ = Type II

H chains: gamma or γ; alpha or α; Mu or μ; delta or δ; epsilon or ϵ.

globulin molecule resides in the sections of the H chain in close proximity to the L chain. Antibody activity of the isolated H chain is limited unless the latter is combined with L polypeptide chains. Fraction Fab of the papain digest contains this combination of L chains and fragments of H chains. The portion of the H chain included is termed the Fd fraction. Other biologic features of the immunoglobulin reside in a different part of the H chain. This corresponds to the fraction Fc of the papain digest. These include the placental transport mechanism, regulation of catabolism, complement binding capacity, skin fixation and sensitization and reaction with rheumatoid factor. An overproduction of L chains in proportion to H chains may occur in various diseases, resulting in Bence-Jones protein. In a similar fashion disease states may lead to a proportional overproduction of Fc fractions of the H chain. Such a clinical syndrome was originally described by Franklin and associates (34) and confirmed by Osserman and Takatsuki (35) under the term H or heavy chain disease.

As each immunoglobulin class has a different H chain structure, it is probable that different H chains reflect different genetic control. InV activity is absent with H chains. Gm activity is present with IgG immunoglobulins but absent in IgA, IgD and IgM immunoglobulins. Accordingly, the Gm genotype marker is specific for the H chains of IgG immunoglobulins (γ-chain). We may assume that additional specific protein isotypic groups will eventually be

found to characterize the H chains of the IgA, IgM, IgD and IgE classes.

By combining genetic studies with immunologic procedures the complexity of H chains becomes apparent. This may be illustrated in the IgG class of human immunoglobulins. On the basis of immunologic analysis the heavy chains of human IgG immunoglobulins have been divided into four different subgroups. Three of these four subgroups possess one or more genetic factors which appear to be confined to a single class of heavy chain. Table 92 summarizes these data. Kunkel and associates (36) have therefore suggested that there are four closely linked heavy chain genetic loci for IgG immunoglobulins; one locus directs the synthesis of each type of chain.

Litwin and Kunkel (37) have studied in detail the two major genetic antigens associated with the IgG_1 subclass of gamma heavy chains, Gm (1) and Gm (4). They demonstrated that two new genetic antigens, Gm (17) and Gm (22) occurred in association with Gm (1) and Gm (4), respectively. Using enzymatic splitting and recombination between light and heavy chains, they found that the Fc fragment was Gm (1+) and Gm (17−) and that the Fab fragment was Gm (17+) and Gm (1−); Gm (17) was localized to the Fd piece of the heavy chain. In a similar fashion Gm (22) was localized to the Fc fragment and Gm (4) to the Fd piece. These studies indicate that the genetic factors on the Fc fragment and those on the portion of the Fd fragment containing Gm (17) and Gm (4) are under the same

TABLE 92. *Recommended terminology and classification of the subclasses of IgG heavy chains*

	Serum Proteins				Genetic Factors
Class: Chain:	Gamma G immunoglobulin; IgG Heavy gamma (γ) chain				InV, Gm Gm
	Immunoglobulin	Heavy chain	Synonyms	Incidence	GM types
Subclass:	IgG_1 ; γG_1	γ_1	We; γ_2b; C	% 70–80	1(a); 2(x); 4(f); 17(z); 22(y)
	IgG_2 ; γG_2	γ_2	Ne; γ_2a	13–18	M
	IgG_3 ; γG_3	γ_3	Vi; γ_2c; Z	6–8	5(b_1); 13(b_3); 14(b_4); 6(c); 15(s)
	IgG_4 ; γG_4	γ_4	Ge; γ_2d	3	?

genetic control. Unfortunately, the exact relationship of these genetic factors to the variable and constant parts of the H chain is not as yet known.

H chains resemble L chains in also presenting variable and invariable portions. The N terminal amino acid portion, which corresponds to the Fd fragment, may be roughly divided in half. The N terminal amino acid part is highly variable and takes part in forming antibody specificity. The remaining portion of the Fd fraction of the H chain appears to be invariable.

Edelman and Gally (16) have presented a model of the IgG antibody molecule which aids greatly in visualizing the interrelationship between H and L chains. This is diagrammatically shown in Figure 32, modified from their publication. The Fab, Fd and Fc fractions are illustrated.

A more recent model has been proposed by Singer and Thorpe (38). Using affinity labeling, the variable region of both light

and heavy chains was found to be related to antibody activity. The functional area was localized to segments about tyrosine, in position 86. Invariable regions of both light and heavy chains are visualized in close proximity, thereby stabilizing the molecule.

Studies relating structure, genetic control and function of antibodies have introduced a new era in our understanding of immune reactivity. Experimental work in this area is expanding rapidly. The reader is encouraged to master these basic new concepts quickly in anticipation of further major advances.

The Nature of Erythrocyte Autoantibodies

The erythrocyte coating material characteristic of autoimmune hemolytic anemia has been the object of many investigations. Initial studies were primarily concerned with proving the antibody nature of such

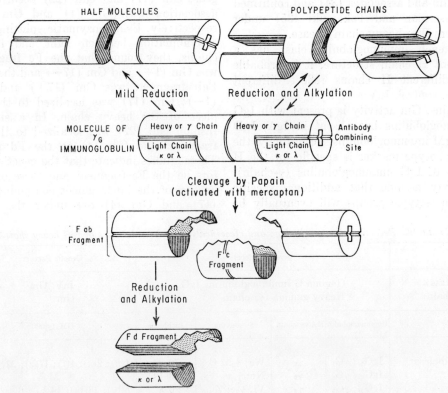

FIGURE 32. Proposed model of a gamma G immunoglobulin. The production of the Fab, Fc and Fd fragments is shown. (Modified from Edelman and Gally (16).)

substances. These studies emphasized the serologic reactivity of erythrocyte auto-antibodies. More recently, a limited but productive area of investigation has documented and correlated the structure and function of erythrocyte iso- and auto-antibodies.

Historical Background

Several of the most famous investigators in immunology made the initial observation that antibodies present in a patient's serum might interact with his own erythrocytes. In 1899 Ehrlich and Morganroth (39) speculated as to the nature of the lytic properties of normal serum. They theorized that certain forms of hemoglobinuria could originate through the development of autologous hemolysins. These investigators also suggested that paroxysmal cold hemoglobinuria might result from the action of amboceptor-alexin lysis. In 1903 Landsteiner (40) noted that chilling the blood of various mammals would lead to agglutination of the erythrocytes. This was followed by the classic paper of Donath and Landsteiner (41) reporting studies performed in three patients suffering from paroxysmal cold hemoglobinuria. They presented the first description of erythrocyte autoantibodies. It was demonstrated that fixation of an autolysin present in the patient's serum to his own erythrocytes, in the cold, was subsequently followed by lysis of erythrocytes caused by the action of labile serum factors (alexin or complement) on the warmed sensitized cells.

Soon after these initial studies on "cold acting" erythrocyte autoantibodies, the French school of investigators described "warm acting" serum components in diseases they termed acquired hemolytic anemia. Reports of Widal and associates (42) and Chauffard and Troisier (43) documented the presence of substances in the patient's blood which could agglutinate and hemolyze his own erythrocytes. They suggested a relationship between such hemolysins and hemagglutinins and the development of rapid in vivo hemolysis.

A major advance was made with the development of the antiglobulin test by Coombs and associates (44). This test was applied to cases of idiopathic hemolytic anemia by Boorman and associates (45) and Loutit and Mollison (46). Positive reactions established the presence of a serum globulin coating the erythrocyte surface. Documentation of an erythrocyte coated with a serum globulin soon became a necessary prerequisite for the diagnosis of autoimmune hemolytic anemia.

These important initial observations introduced two major concepts. First, an antibody produced by an individual had the capacity to react with his own erythrocytes, leading to premature death of the cell and hemolytic anemia. Second, two distinct types of antibodies, one cold acting and the other warm acting, could be involved in the process. Although this division of erythrocyte autoantibodies into cold acting and warm acting varieties is artificial, there is an advantage in discussing and treating them separately. The hemolytic anemia associated with these erythrocyte autoantibody types differs in clinical manifestations, etiology, prognosis and therapeutic approaches.

Chance alone was not responsible for the original description of erythrocyte autoantibodies as cold acting materials. Although a complex serologic test system was involved, the laboratory procedure required a simple cooling of blood and examination for hemagglutination or hemolysis of the cooled or warmed specimens. The basis for this test system was simultaneously established for the erythrocyte isoantibodies now known as natural anti-A and anti-B.

In contrast with cold acting antibodies, it was necessary to await the development of entirely new test systems before warm acting erythrocyte autoantibodies could be accurately and consistently demonstrated. Such test systems were intimately concerned with warm acting erythrocyte isoantibodies, particularly the anti-rhesus antibody. In 1944 Wiener (47) and Race (48) independently demonstrated that anti-rhesus antibodies existed in two forms. In addition to the previously documented cold acting antibody which agglutinated saline suspended erythrocytes, another type of anti-rhesus antibody was described. This antibody did not agglutinate saline suspended erythrocytes. Race (48) conceived of hemagglutination as resulting from a two-step process similar to a lattice formation in precipitin reactions. The first phase of hemagglutination involved coating of the erythrocyte surface by the antibody fixing to its antigen. The second phase of hemagglutination required interaction of antibody coated erythrocytes until aggregates of erythrocytes were visible as hemagglutination. Cold acting antibodies which produced agglutination of saline suspended erythrocytes were considered to be "complete" antibodies, inducing phases 1 and 2 of the hemagglutination reaction. The second type of antibody was classified as an "incomplete" antibody. It was suggested that phase 1 of the hemagglutination reaction occurred, resulting in an antibody coated erythrocyte. Phase 2, however, did not occur and agglutination of saline suspended erythrocytes did not result.

Wiener (47) simultaneously arrived at the same conclusion. He demonstrated that antibodies which did not induce agglutination of saline suspended erythrocytes possessed the ability to fix to the erythrocyte. Such antibodies saturated the antigenic sites of the cell and blocked the subsequent action of saline agglutinating antibodies. Wiener termed these nonagglutinating antibodies "blocking" antibodies. In order to explain the different actions of these two types of antibodies, it was postulated that the saline agglutinating cold acting antibody (complete antibody) possessed two antibody combining sites and was bivalent. The newly discovered antibody which did not induce agglutination of appropriate erythrocytes (incomplete antibody) was considered to be univalent with one antibody site able to combine with antigen. This could saturate antigenic sites without inducing agglutination. The univalent concept is no longer acceptable (see Chapter 17), but this important postulate led to the development of diagnostic procedures such as the antiglobulin test (44). Figure 33 diagrammatically represents these two types of antibodies reacting with appropriate erythrocytes.

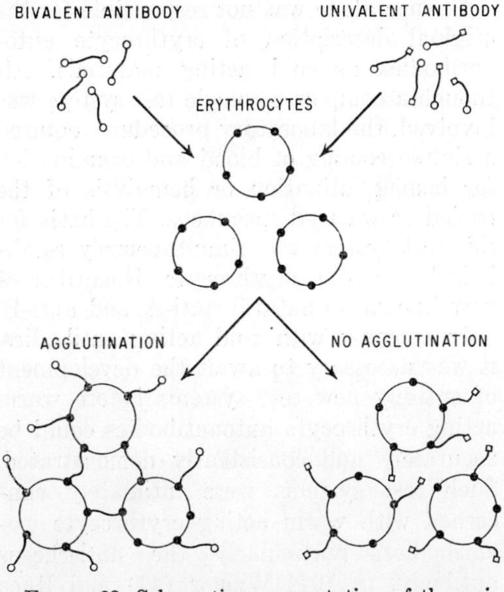

Terminology

Various terms have been employed to describe the two forms of erythrocyte antibodies. As a general but not absolute rule, warm acting antibodies have appeared as incomplete antibodies, in contrast to the saline agglutinating action of cold acting complete antibodies. As indicated above, such incomplete antibodies have been termed "blocking" antibodies by Wiener (47). The role of incomplete antibodies in hemagglutination led to the descriptive term "coating" antibody. It was noted that suspending erythrocytes coated with incomplete antibodies in serum would occasionally induce hemagglutination. Incomplete antibodies have therefore been termed "serum" antibodies, in contrast with the use of "saline" antibodies as a descriptive phrase for complete antibodies. The agglutination potentiating effect of serum on incomplete antibodies resulted in the addition of bovine serum albumin to the test system (49). Incomplete antibodies which

FIGURE 33. Schematic representation of the univalent and bivalent concept of erythrocyte antibodies. Bivalent antibodies bridge between two erythrocytes, inducing agglutination. Univalent antibodies "coat" the erythrocyte and by saturating the antigen sites create a "blocking" effect. (After Wiener (47).)

agglutinated erythrocytes suspended in such media were called "albuminoid" antibodies.

Further study of complete and incomplete erythrocyte antibodies revealed another general although not universal rule. Many cold acting complete antibodies were found in subjects without evidence of prior immunization. In contrast, warm acting or incomplete antibodies generally were produced in individuals with well documented episodes of sensitization. The term "naturally" occurring antibody was employed for such complete antibodies and the term "immune" antibody was used to describe the incomplete variety.

Fudenberg and Kunkel (50) documented specific physical differences between the two forms of antibody by applying density gradient and analytic ultracentrifugation techniques. Again a general although not universal pattern appeared. The cold acting complete antibodies were shown to be macromolecules and were termed 19S and, more recently, IgM antibodies. The warm acting incomplete antibodies appeared as 7S or IgG immunoglobulins. Table 93 lists the various synonyms which have been employed in discussing the two forms of erythrocyte iso- and autoantibodies.

It should be emphasized that all terms used are descriptive. The characteristics implied in such classifications do not necessarily carry over into all groups. A blending of various features typifying either cold acting or warm acting antibodies is not uncommon for a specific antibody. Accordingly, cold acting incomplete autoantibodies can be found. The immunologic reactivity of cold acting antibodies may be increased by applying techniques usually employed to demonstrate warm acting autoantibodies. In other cases such techniques will inhibit the action of cold acting complete antibodies. Immunization will frequently result in the production of immune warm acting antibodies and an increase in titer of natural cold acting antibodies.

Two conclusions have developed from many detailed studies of erythrocyte iso- and autoantibodies. A serum containing an erythrocyte antibody seldom if ever contains only one form of antibody. A mixture of cold acting and warm acting antibodies almost always occurs. The serologic characteristics of the serum are dependent on the amount and avidity of the individual components. This observation of a variation of erythrocyte antibody characteristics must be further extended. A marked heterogeneity exists among erythrocyte iso- and autoantibodies. A study by van der Giessen and associates (51) using various anti-$Rh_o(D)$ antisera illustrates this point. Fractionation of these sera revealed the presence of both 7S and 19S anti-$Rh_o(D)$. When these two groups were further tested in saline, antiglobulin and bromelin proteolytic enzyme test procedures, five different serologic patterns were apparent. Constantoulakis and associates (52) similarly encountered marked heterogeneity of erythrocyte iso- and autoantibodies. The degree of heterogeneity explains to some extent the serologic and biologic variations seen in any extensive study of anti-erythrocyte antibody activity. Yamada (53) has emphasized the heterogeneity seen with warm acting erythrocyte autoantibodies. Yokoyama and Fudenberg (54) have described the heterogeneity of immune anti-A in relation to the Forssman antigen. Such heterogeneity is not an exclusive characteristic of erythrocyte autoantibodies. It appears as a fundamental part of any immune response (55, 56). The variations introduced by antibody heterogeneity should be con-

TABLE 93. *Various descriptive synonyms employed for erythrocyte antibodies*

Erythrocyte Antibodies	
Warm acting type	Cold acting type
Incomplete	Complete
Univalent	Bivalent
Serum	Saline
Immune	Natural
Blocking	Hemagglutinating
Atypical	Typical
7S type	19S type
IgG type	IgM type
Albuminoid	Macroantibody
Coating	Hemagglutinating

sidered in the detailed discussions of warm
and cold acting erythrocyte antibodies presented in subsequent chapters.

BIBLIOGRAPHY

1. Nomenclature of human immunoglobulins. Bull. WHO **30**: 447, 1964.
2. Notation for genetic factors of human immunoglobulins. Bull. WHO **33**: 721, 1965.
3. Notation for human immunoglobulin subclasses. Bull. WHO **35**: 953, 1966.
4. Porter, R. R.: Structure of gamma-globulin and antibodies. In *Basic Problems in Neoplastic Disease,* edited by A. Gellhorn and E. Hirschberg. Columbia University Press, New York, 1962.
5. Porter, R. R., and Press, E. M.: Immunochemistry. Ann. Rev. Biochem. **31**: 625, 1962.
6. Porter, R. R.: Chemical structure of γ-globulin and antibodies. Brit. Med. Bull. **19**: 197, 1963.
7. Cohen, S., and Milstein, C.: Structure and biological properties of immunoglobulins. Advances Immun. **7**: 1, 1967.
8. Cohen, S.: The structure of antibody. In *Immunological Diseases,* edited by M. Samter. Little, Brown and Company, Boston, 1965.
9. Gitlin, D.: Current aspects of the structure, function, and genetics of the immunoglobulins. Ann. Rev. Med. **17**: 1, 1966.
10. Fahey, J. L.: Antibodies and immunoglobulins. I. Structure and function. II. Normal development and changes in disease. J. A. M. A. **194**: 72, 255, 1965.
11. Fudenberg, H. H.: The immune globulins. Ann. Rev. Microbiol. **19**: 301, 1965.
12. Franklin, E. C.: Immune globulins: their structure and function and some techniques for their isolation. Progr. Allerg. **8**: 58, 1964.
13. Osserman, E. F., and Takatsuki, K.: Plasma cell myeloma: gamma globulin synthesis and structure. Medicine (Balt.) **42**: 357, 1963.
14. Nisonoff, A., and Thorbecke, G. J.: Immunochemistry. Ann. Rev. Biochem. **33**: 355, 1964.
15. Nisonoff, A.: Molecules of immunity. Hosp. Pract. **2**: 19, 1967.
16. Edelman, G. M., and Gally, J. A.: Model for 7S antibody molecule. Proc. Nat. Acad. Sci. USA **51**: 846, 1964.
17. Antibodies. Cold Spring Harbor Symposia on Quantitative Biology, **32**: 1967.
18. Lennox, E. S., and Cohn, M.: Immunoglobulins. Ann. Rev. Biochem. **36**: 365, 1967.
19. Killander, J., editor: *Gamma Globulins.* Interscience Publishers, Inc., New York, 1967.
20. Tiselius, A.: Electrophoresis of serum globulin. II. Electrophoretic analysis of normal and immune sera. Biochem. J. **31**: 1464, 1937.
21. Tomasi, T. B., Jr., Tan, E. M., Solomon, A.,
and Prendergast, R. A.: Characteristics of immune system common to certain external secretions. J. Exp. Med. **121**: 101, 1965.
22. Tomasi, T. B.: The gamma A globulins: first line of defense. Hosp. Pract. **2**: 26, 1967.
23. Rowe, D. S., and Fahey, J. L.: New class of human immunoglobulin. I and II. J. Exp. Med. **121**: 171, 184, 1965.
24. Hobbs, J. R., Slot, G. M. J., Campbell, C. H., Clein, G. P., Scott, J. T., Crowther, D., and Swan, H. T.: Six cases of gamma D-myelomatosis. Lancet **2**: 614, 1966.
25. Goodfriend, L., Perelmutter, L., and Rose, B.: Relationship between ragweed-reagins and serum immunoglobulins. Int. Arch. Allerg. **30**: 542, 1966.
26. Ishizaka, K., Ishizaka, T., and Hornbrook, M. M.: Physico-chemical properties of human reaginic antibody. IV. Presence of a unique immunoglobulin as a carrier of reaginic activity. J. Immun. **97**: 75, 1966.
27. Johansson, S. G. O., and Bennich, H.: Immunological studies of an atypical (myeloma) immunoglobulin. Immunology **13**: 381, 1967.
28. Edelman, G. M., and Poulik, M. D.: Studies on structural units of the γ-globulins. J. Exp. Med. **113**: 861, 1961.
29. Williams, R. C., Brunning, R. D., and Wollheim, F. A.: Light-chain disease. An abortive variant of multiple myeloma. Ann. Intern. Med. **65**: 471, 1966.
30. Hood, L. E., Gray, W. R., and Dreyer, W. J.: On the mechanism of antibody synthesis: a species comparison of L-chains. Proc. Nat. Acad. Sci. USA **55**: 826, 1966.
31. Hilschmann, N., and Craig, L. C.: Amino acid sequence studies with Bence-Jones proteins. Proc. Nat. Acad. Sci. USA **53**: 1403, 1965.
32. Milstein, C.: Variation in amino acid sequence near the disulfide bridges of Bence-Jones proteins. Nature (London) **209**: 370, 1966.
33. Hood, L., Gray, W., and Dreyer, W.: On the evolution of antibody light chains. J. Molec. Biol. **22**: 179, 1966.
34. Franklin, E. C., Lowenstein, J., Bigelow, B., and Meltzer, M.: Heavy chain disease—a new disorder of serum γ-globulins. Amer. J. Med. **37**: 332, 1964.
35. Osserman, E. F., and Takatsuki, K.: Clinical and immunochemical studies of four cases of heavy (H) chain disease. Amer. J. Med. **37**: 351, 1964.
36. Kunkel, H. G., Allen, J. C., Grey, H. M., Mårtensson, L., and Grubb, R.: A relationship between the H chain groups of 7S gamma-globulin and the Gm system. Nature (London) **203**: 413, 1964.
37. Litwin, S. D., and Kunkel, H. G.: The genetic control of γ-globulin heavy chains. J. Exp. Med. **125**: 847, 1967.
38. Singer, S. J., and Thorpe, N. O.: On the location and structure of the active sites of anti-

body molecules. Proc. Nat. Acad. Sci. U.S.A. **60:** 1371, 1968.

39. Ehrlich, P., and Morganroth, J.: Ueber Häemolysine. Zweite Mittheilung. Berlin Klin. Wschr. **36:** 481, 1899.

40. Landsteiner, K.: Ueber Beziehungen zwischen dem Blutserum und den Körperzellen. Munchen. Med. Wschr. **50:** 1812, 1903.

41. Donath, J., and Landsteiner, K.: Ueber paroxysmalen Hämeglobinurie. Munchen. Med. Wschr. **51:** 1590, 1904.

42. Widal, F., Abrami, P., and Brulé, M.: Auto-agglutination des hématies dans l'ictère hémolytique. C. R. Soc. Biol. (Paris) **64:** 655, 1908.

43. Chauffard, M. A., and Troisier, J.: Anémie grave avec hémolysine dans le sérum; ictère hémolysinique. Sem. Med. **28:** 345, 1908.

44. Coombs, R. R. A., Mourant, A. E., and Race, R. R.: A new test for the detection of weak and "incomplete" Rh agglutinins. Brit. J. Exp. Path. **26:** 255, 1945.

45. Boorman, K. E., Dodd, B. E., and Loutit, J. F.: Haemolytic icterus (acholuric jaundice) congenital and acquired. Lancet **1:** 812, 1946.

46. Loutit, J. F., and Mollison, P. L.: Haemolytic icterus (acholuric jaundice) congenital and acquired. J. Path. Bact. **58:** 711, 1946.

47. Wiener, A. S.: A new test (blocking test) for Rh sensitization. Proc. Soc. Exp. Biol. Med. **56:** 173, 1944.

48. Race, R. R.: An "incomplete" antibody in human serum. Nature (London) **153:** 771, 1944.

49. Wiener, A. S.: Conglutination test for Rh sensitization. J. Lab. Clin. Med. **30:** 662, 1945.

50. Fudenberg, H. H., and Kunkel, H. G.: Physical properties of red cell agglutinins in acquired hemolytic anemia. J. Exp. Med. **106:** 689, 1957.

51. van der Giessen, M., van der Hart, M., and van der Weerdt, C. M.: Fractionation of sera containing antibodies against red cells or platelets with special reference to anti-D sera. Vox Sang. **9:** 25, 1964.

52. Constantoulakis, M., Costea, N., Schwartz, R. S., and Dameshek, W.: Quantitative studies of the effect of red-blood-cell sensitization on in vivo hemolysis. J. Clin. Invest. **42:** 1790, 1963.

53. Yamada, A.: Iinvestigations on clinical observations of autoimmune hemolytic anemia and characteristics of the warm autoantibody obtained from patients red cells. Acta Haemat. Jap. **27:** 19, 1964.

54. Yokoyama, M., and Fudenberg, H. H.: Heterogeneity of immune anti-A antibody in relation to Forssman antigen. J. Immun. **96:** 304, 1966.

55. Uhr, J. W.: The heterogeneity of the immune response. Science **145:** 457, 1964.

56. Pike, R. M.: Antibody heterogeneity and serological reactions. Bact. Rev. **31:** 157, 1967.

Chapter 17

Warm Acting Erythrocyte Autoantibodies

The warm acting erythrocyte autoantibodies have two outstanding characteristics. They are maximally reactive with erythrocytes at 37°C. Generally they appear as incomplete erythrocyte antibodies and they do not induce hemagglutination of red cells suspended in saline. Demonstration of the erythrocyte-antibody reaction is frequently dependent on an additional test system. Such systems are discussed in Chapter 18.

Warm acting erythrocyte autoantibodies have profound clinical significance. They are the most common variety of erythrocyte autoantibody encountered in autoimmune hemolytic anemia. Of Dacie's 175 cases of autoimmune hemolytic anemia, 74 per cent were of the warm acting variety (1). Worledge (2) expanded this group to 198 cases with 72 per cent appearing warm acting. Similar frequencies have been reported by other investigators with large series. In the series of van Loghem and associates (3), 74 per cent were of the warm acting variety. Dausset and Colombani (4) noted an 85 per cent incidence of warm acting erythrocyte antibodies in autoimmune hemolytic anemia.

Physical and Immunochemical Characteristics

A complete understanding of warm acting erythrocyte autoantibodies requires an accurate physical and immunochemical documentation of the molecular characteristics. Unfortunately this type of critical information is available only in an incomplete form. Future studies may be expected to expand this knowledge.

The Protein Nature of the Erythrocyte Coating Material

Initial studies of the erythrocyte coating material in autoimmune hemolytic anemia were directed toward their protein and immunoglobulin nature. Electrophoretic serum protein analysis in cases of warm acting autoimmune hemolytic anemia was not considered to be diagnostic (1). It was generally assumed, however, that an immunologic event was occurring and that the erythrocyte coating material was an antibody. In 1947 Coombs and Mourant (5) suggested that such coating substances were gamma-globulin. Neutralization of antiglobulin serum with gamma-globulin prevented the reagent from agglutinating erythrocytes coated with anti-Rh_o(D) antibody. Wiener and associates (6) utilized the same procedure to quantitate the presence of human serum globulin. Hackett (7) demonstrated a similarity between warm acting erythrocyte autoantibodies and the isoantibody anti-Rh_o(D). Adsorption experiments indicated that these two types of antibodies had similar components which reacted with antiglobulin serum.

Gamma-globulin Neutralization Test

Dacie (1) expanded these observations and developed the gamma-globulin neutralization test. He noted that the addition of gamma-globulin to antiglobulin serum led to variable reactions when the modified reagent was used to agglutinate erythrocytes sensitized with erythrocyte autoantibodies. Some but not all warm acting erythrocyte autoantibodies were similar to incomplete anti-Rh_o(D); small amounts of gamma-globulin added to antiglobulin serum prevented the agglutination reaction. These antibodies were called gamma type antibodies. In contrast, large amounts of gamma-globulin had to be added to neutralize antiglobulin serum subsequently used with cold acting erythrocyte autoantibodies. These were considered to be a non-gamma type of antibody. Two suggestions were made to explain this variation of results. Either cold acting erythrocyte autoantibodies appeared not to be gamma-globulin, or else antiglobulin serum reacted with a non-gamma-globulin component of fresh serum adsorbed onto the erythrocyte. Warm acting erythrocyte autoantibodies with a pattern of reaction between these two extremes were also documented. Dacie analyzed 73 cases of warm acting autoimmune hemolytic anemia with this test system. Thirty-two were of the gamma type, 13 were of the non-gamma type and 28 were of the intermediate type. He concluded that warm acting autoantibodies were gamma-globulins.

Similar findings were noted by Vaughan (8) employing anti-gamma and anti-non-gamma antiglobulin serum. Erythrocytes obtained from 16 patients with autoimmune hemolytic anemia were analyzed. In nine the erythrocytes reacted with the anti-non-gamma-globulin serum, in two they reacted with the anti-gamma-globulin serum and in the remaining five they reacted with both reagents. Vaughan concluded that three types of antibodies were involved, i.e., gamma-globulin and warm and cold non-gamma-globulin antibody types. The serologic pattern with modified antiglobulin serum was not necessarily constant. Dacie (9), Wuilleret (10) and Konda and Yamada (11) all reported a change in the type of antibody during various stages of a patient's illness.

Dacie (1) expanded these observations, using two specific types of anti-globulin sera. The first reagent was a pure anti-IgG gamma-globulin and the second was a broad spectrum reagent which was adsorbed with purified IgG gamma-globulin and which was called anti-non-gamma-globulin antiserum. Parallel studies were carried out with an anti-beta 1 globulin antiserum which reacted with components of complement (2). The reactions with anti-non-gamma-globulin serum and anti-beta 1 antiserum were identical, suggesting that the former was directed against complement components. One hundred forty-three examples of warm acting erythrocyte autoantibodies were tested with these antisera (2). Seventy were found to react with the anti-IgG gamma serum, 26 with the anti-non-gamma serum and 47 with both. Accordingly, 82 per cent reacted with the anti-IgG gamma anti-serum. Analysis of these reactions as to primary and secondary types of autoimmune hemolytic anemia and varieties of secondary diseases did not reveal significant differences.

Eyster and associates (12) performed similar studies with 18 cases of warm acting autoimmune hemolytic anemia. The erythrocyte coating substance was gamma G globulin alone in five patients, gamma G globulin in combination with complement in nine patients and complement alone in four patients. Jeannet's experience illustrates the frequency of complement binding in autoimmune hemolytic anemia as discovered by modified antiglobulin serum testing. Thirty patients were studied and only one had an anti-gamma reaction. Three patients had both gamma-globulin and complement on the erythrocyte surface. In 26 patients only complement was present.

Physical Characterization

The most definitive study characterizing the immunoglobulin status of warm acting autoantibodies was performed by Fudenberg and Kunkel (14). They applied density gradient and ultracentrifugation techniques to erythrocyte autoantibodies. The warm acting autoantibodies were found to be 7S globulin molecules and the cold acting autoantibodies were found to be 19S macromolecules. This observation has been repeatedly confirmed. Further studies demonstrated that treatment of warm acting autoantibodies with the reducing agent 2-mercaptoethanol did not affect immunologic reactivity. In contrast, 2-mercapto-

ethanol treatment of cold acting autoantibodies led to a marked or complete loss of
immunologic activity. Unpublished studies
in our laboratories using Cleland's reagent
(dithiothreitol) have revealed essentially
identical results. Cleland's reagent has some
advantage in this test procedure. Less than
one-tenth of the molecular concentration
of 2-mercaptoethanol is required and this
reagent is free from the obnoxious smell and
taste of 2-mercaptoethanol.

Eluate Studies

Warm acting erythrocyte autoantibodies
have been eluted from erythrocytes and used
as an antigen to prepare antiglobulin serum.
Komninos and Aksoy (15) and Komninos
and Désy (16) demonstrated that antiglobulin serum produced in this fashion
is not specific and that it cross reacts with
anti-rhesus antibodies. Fudenberg and associates (17) produced antisera using antigenic eluates obtained from erythrocytes of
patients with idiopathic and secondary
types of autoimmune hemolytic anemia. A
nonspecific antiglobulin serum was obtained which reacted with both primary and
secondary types of autoimmune hemolytic
anemia. The authors noted that the eluates
contained gamma-globulin. However, only
a small portion of eluate nitrogen reacted
with antiglobulin serum. Unpublished studies in our laboratories suggest an explanation of this phenomenon. Eluates prepared
from erythrocytes of patients with warm
acting autoimmune hemolytic anemia contain all globulin fractions and a substantial
amount of albumin. Warm acting antibody
activity is localized to the gamma-globulin
fraction. Similar studies have been reported
by Auerswald and associates (18) employing sera from patients with idiopathic granulocytopenia and thrombocytopenia purpurae. Cassell and Chaplin (19) carried out
an extensive study using antiglobulin reagents prepared from normal sera, from
eluates obtained from erythrocytes coated
with rhesus antibodies and from eluates
obtained from erythrocytes coated with
warm acting erythrocyte autoantibodies.
The antiglobulin sera produced were "nonspecific" and cross reacted with autoantibodies and isoantibodies. A marked hetero-

geneity of autoantibodies was found. The
authors also noted that eluates prepared
from erythrocytes not coated with antibodies produced potent antiglobulin serum.
This finding has been repeatedly confirmed
in our laboratory, and it supports the contention that gamma-globulin normally coats
erythrocytes.

A possible difference in antigenicity of
proteins in autoimmune hemolytic anemia
has been reported by Vulpis (20). Ghost
erythrocytes were prepared and a water
soluble fraction was collected and found to
contain "S" protein. No differences were
noted in S proteins obtained from normal
and hereditary spherocytosis erythrocytes.
However, antiserum prepared against the
S protein from cells having erythrocyte
autoantibodies formed specific precipitins
for autoimmune hemolytic anemia S proteins.

Structural Characteristics

The above studies suggest that the majority of warm acting erythrocyte autoantibodies are gamma G immunoglobulins. Several investigators have studied the light
chains of these antibodies. Franklin and
Fudenberg (21) analyzed three IgG autoantibodies. One antibody contained only
lambda type L chains. The remaining two
autoantibodies were composed of a mixture
of kappa and lambda molecules. Leddy and
Bakemeier (22) investigated eluted IgG
warm acting erythrocyte autoantibodies
obtained from 20 patients with autoimmune
hemolytic anemia. Eight eluates contained
a mixture of kappa and lambda type L
chains. Twelve eluates contained only one
type of L chain; eight of these were of the
kappa type and four were of the lambda
type. Eyster and associates (12) directly
reacted antisera specific for kappa and
lambda L chains with erythrocytes obtained
from nine patients with autoimmune hemolytic anemia. All nine reacted with both
antisera, indicating a mixture of kappa and
lambda L chains. The degree of reaction
suggested a predominance of kappa L
chains in some erythrocyte autoantibodies
and a predominance of lambda L chains in
others. The authors suggest that such a
variation may indicate a complex antigen

with multiple determinants. Khan and Zinneman (23) have studied the amino acid composition of incomplete anti-Rh_0(D). They report that this antibody differed from normal IgG with a higher serine and arginine content and a lower valine and methionine value. This study should be confirmed and expanded to include autoantibodies.

The Bivalence of Incomplete Erythrocyte Antibodies

Wiener (24) originally postulated that incomplete erythrocyte antibodies were univalent molecules. Dausset (25) described incomplete erythrocyte antibodies which reacted in proteolytic enzyme test systems but not with antiglobulin serum. He speculated that such antibodies may have two nonreactive sites, and he suggested the descriptive term "doubly incomplete antibodies."

The univalent concept has been challenged (26). A review of the serologic literature strongly suggests that incomplete erythrocyte antibodies do not act as univalent materials (26). (a) Erythrocytes coated with incomplete antibody spontaneously agglutinate when suspended in solutions containing large numbers of anisometric molecules (27). (b) Erythrocytes pretreated with proteolytic enzymes are directly agglutinated by incomplete antibody (28). (c) Incomplete anti-Rh_0(D) induces saline agglutination of D——/ D—— erythrocytes (29). (d) Group A erythrocytes coated with incomplete anti-A can be prevented from agglutinating by adding A substance (30). (e) Antiglobulin serum induced agglutination of erythrocytes coated with incomplete antibody is not due simply to the supply of nonspecific bivalent links between coating globulin molecules (31). (f) Incomplete erythrocyte antibodies will directly agglutinate erythrocytes at centrifugation speeds above 4430 × gravity (32). (g) Anti-Le^a antibody behaves as a saline or bivalent antibody at 26°C. and may act as an incomplete antibody at 37°C. (33).

On the basis of these studies Pirofsky and Cordova (34, 35) postulated that incomplete erythrocyte autoantibodies were bivalent with one functional antibody combining

site and the other site nonfunctional because of steric interference. It was reasoned that a change in tertiary structure of the antibody molecule might make available the nonfunctioning combining site, converting incomplete antibody into a complete form. In order to test this hypothesis the tertiary structure of incomplete erythrocyte antibodies was modified by exposing them to 2-mercaptoethanol, a reducing agent which disrupts disulfide links. After such reduction treatment, incomplete antibodies were found to induce direct agglutination of saline suspended erythrocytes. The saline activity was only 5 to 10 per cent of antibody activity determined by antiglobulin and proteolytic enzyme testing. Both incomplete anti-Rh antibodies and incomplete erythrocyte autoantibodies gave identical reactions. A similar finding has been noted in our laboratory, using the reducing agent Cleland's reagent. These findings were confirmed by Mandy and associates (36), although the reaction was interpreted differently. They felt that agglutination of saline suspended erythrocytes by reduced incomplete erythrocyte antibodies represented a nonimmunologic phenomenon similar to conglutination with the erythrocyte surface involved in the reaction.

Stolinsky and Fudenberg (37) demonstrated that incomplete erythrocyte antibodies had a polypeptide structure compatible with two antibody combining sites. The bivalent nature of incomplete erythrocyte antibodies was more directly shown by Fudenberg and associates (38). Using pepsin digestion and 2-mercaptoethanol reduction, two univalent fragments of incomplete anti-Rh_0(D) antibody were obtained. Each of these fractions functioned as true univalent antibodies, indicating two antibody combining sites.

Although experimental studies indicate that incomplete warm acting erythrocyte autoantibodies are bivalent, their inability to directly induce agglutination is still not explained. Several hypotheses must be considered.

(a) A nonfunctional antibody combining site due to steric interference. This concept was postulated by Pirofsky and Cordova (34, 35). The antibody mole-

INCOMPLETE ANTIBODY   ERYTHROCYTE

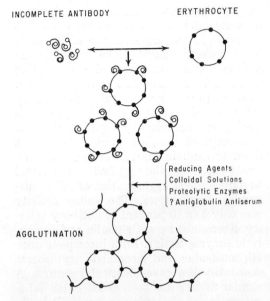

AGGLUTINATION

FIGURE 34. Schematic representation of incomplete erythrocyte antibodies which appear univalent but are potentially bivalent. Agglutination is induced by modifying the molecular conformation, exposing a previously unavailable combining site.

cule is visualized as coiled upon itself, with one antibody combining site exposed and a second site unavailable because of the molecular conformation. It is suggested that macromolecular solutions such as albumin and polyvinylpyrrolidone, proteolytic enzymes, reducing agents and even antiglobulin serum function by changing the steric configuration, exposing the previously hidden reactive group. Figure 34 illustrates this diagrammatically.

(b) The molecular size of the antibody in relation to the antigen combining site. Saline acting complete antibodies are generally macromolecules with a molecular weight approaching one million. These large molecules have a length of about 1000 Å. If the antigenic combining site is depressed into the surface of the erythrocyte, the length of the 19S macromolecule may permit projection of antibody from the surface. This presents a free antibody combining site able to bridge and to combine with an antigen site on a second erythrocyte. In contrast, 7S incomplete antibodies are smaller, with a molecular weight of 140,000

and a length of about 250 Å. Their size may not permit the antibody molecule to project from the erythrocyte surface. Even though an additional antibody site is available and functional, it cannot bridge to a second erythrocyte. Antiglobulin serum functions by supplying bivalent antibody sites able to bridge two erythrocytes through a combination with antigenic determinants of antibodies on different erythrocytes. Figure 35 presents this concept diagrammatically. Enzymes would function by digesting the erythrocyte surface and exposing the depressed antigenic site. This would allow the smaller incomplete antibody to project sufficiently to bridge to a second erythrocyte. The action of macromolecular solutions may be dependent on packing the antigen site sufficiently to project the 7S globulin the distance required to react with an additional erythrocyte.

(c) Surface charge changes. The stud-

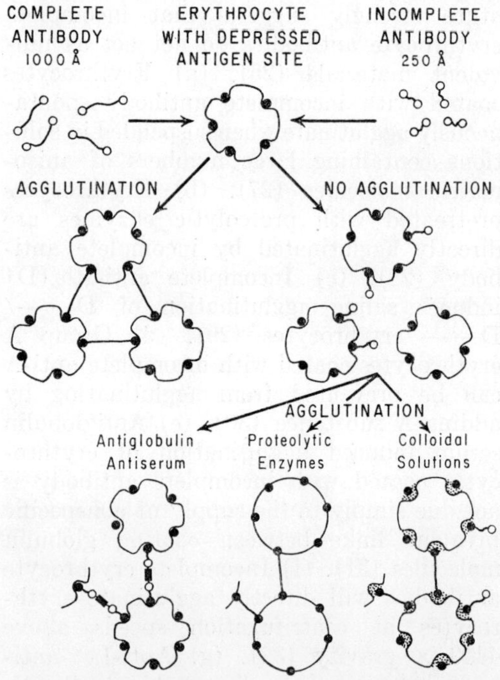

COMPLETE   ERYTHROCYTE   INCOMPLETE
ANTIBODY   WITH DEPRESSED   ANTIBODY
1000 Å   ANTIGEN SITE   250 Å

AGGLUTINATION   NO AGGLUTINATION

AGGLUTINATION

Antiglobulin   Proteolytic   Colloidal
Antiserum   Enzymes   Solutions

FIGURE 35. Schematic representation of the effect of antibody size in creating complete or incomplete antibodies. Agglutination with incomplete antibodies is induced by the bridging effect of antiglobulin serum, by enzymatic digestion of the erythrocyte surface or by "packing" the depressed antigen site.

ies of Seaman and Heard (39) demonstrated that the erythrocyte functions as a polyanion. Proteolytic enzymes release mucoids containing N-acylated neuraminic acids from the red cell and reduce the negativity of the erythrocyte surface (40–42). The magnitude of the change depends on the particular enzyme and on the species from which the erythrocyte was obtained (43). This subject and the use of microscopic electrophoresis have been thoroughly reviewed by Seaman and Cook (44, 45). In addition it has been demonstrated that basically charged molecules will adsorb onto the erythrocyte surface, leading to agglutination (46). Unpublished studies in our laboratory suggest that approximately the same number of molecules are involved in the agglutination induced by incomplete anti-Rh_o(D) and basically charged chemicals such as L-polylysine.

The electrophoretic mobility of erythrocytes is also reduced after treatment with anti-erythrocyte antibody (47–49). It has been suggested that saline acting complete antibodies may function by reducing the zeta potential of erythrocytes. This permits the close proximity of antibody coated erythrocytes, leading to bridging, lattice formation and agglutination. In contrast, incomplete antibodies may not affect the zeta potential sufficiently to overcome the repulsive force of erythrocytes necessary to induce agglutination (50). This tidy system is not confirmed by the detailed experimental studies of Sachtleben (49).

Agglutination is dependent on the balancing of repulsive and attractive forces acting on the erythrocyte surface. The zeta potential seems to be the important factor. Pollack and associates (50) have reported the zeta potential for agglutination of human erythrocytes by complete antibodies as 18 to 20 mv. and 8 to 9 mv. for incomplete antirhesus antibodies. In physiologic saline the zeta potential of human erythrocytes approximates 16 mv. Accordingly, complete antibodies will directly induce agglutination, but a further lowering of the zeta potential is necessary for incomplete antibodies to agglutinate erythrocytes. Proteolytic enzymes, anisometric colloid solutions (albumin, polyvinylpyrrolidone, dextran, etc.) and raising the ionic concentration of NaCl all lower the zeta potential and possibly potentiate agglutination in this manner. The data obtained by Sachtleben (49) cast some doubt on this hypothesis. The latter author noted that complete acting antirhesus antibodies differed from anti-A. Such antibodies induced agglutination without influencing the electrophoretic mobility of erythrocytes.

Other theoretical systems may be constructed to explain the lack of agglutination characteristic of incomplete erythrocyte autoantibodies. Close study of the three theoretical mechanisms described above indicates that they are not mutually contradictory. The possibility should be considered that all or some of the described mechanisms are involved in combination.

Application of These Concepts

The above studies can be interpreted within the framework of our modern concepts of antibody structure. Warm acting erythrocyte autoantibodies are generally bivalent gamma G immunoglobulins. Antisera against such substances cross react with normal gamma-globulin, with incomplete rhesus isoantibody and with warm acting autoantibodies of other patients. This reflects the presence of similar antigenic determinants on the gamma type H chain, on the L chain or on both chains. Eyster and associates (12) noted that antiserum specific for gamma H chains induced agglutination of IgG autoantibody coated erythrocytes in 12 cases. In four additional cases only complement could be demonstrated on the erythrocyte surface and gamma H chain antiserum did not induce agglutination.

The L chains of normal IgG globulins and erythrocyte auto- and isoantibodies have similar antigenic determinants. Franklin and Fudenberg (21), Leddy and Bakemeier (22) and Eyster and associates (12) reported that kappa and lambda type L chain antisera induced agglutination of autoantibody coated erythrocytes. Heterogeneity of the IgG autoantibody population was apparent. Although some monotypic L chain antibodies have been described, a mixture of both kappa and lambda L chains is common. Although the data are incomplete, they suggest that the production of warm acting autoantibody reflects a polyclonal mechanism. It is therefore unlikely that a monoclonal process similar to that seen in plasma cell myeloma, Waldenström's macroglobulinemia and cold hemagglutinin disease is involved. The postulated etiologic mechanisms of monoclonal dysgammaglobulinemia, establishment of a malignant foreign clone and proliferation of a forbidden clone may therefore have only a limited application in warm acting erythrocyte autoantibody production.

The ability of antiglobulin serum to react with normal gamma G globulin and iso- and autoantibodies suggests that the portions of the L and H chains concerned with antibody specificity are not involved in the antiglobulin agglutination reaction. Gamma H chain antiserum generally induces stronger reactions with autoantibodies than do the two L chain antisera. This suggests that antiglobulin serum reactivity primarily involves the Fc portion of the H chain. This assumption may explain a puzzling characteristic of the antiglobulin reaction. Normal human erythrocytes are always coated with large amounts of normal gamma G immunoglobulin (51, 52). Although antiglobulin serum can and does react with such nonimmunologically adsorbed cell bound globulin, agglutination does not occur (31). IgG molecules fixed to the erythrocyte surface in an immunologic linkage may therefore present a different molecular conformation of the Fc portion than nonimmunologic fixed IgG. Immune fixation of globulin to the erythrocyte surface may expose the Fc portion of the H chain. Alternatively, the Fc portion may be bound to the cell. In contrast the nonimmune fixation of globulin to normal erythrocytes probably involves this portion of the H chain in a position offering steric hindrance to its reaction with antiglobulin serum, thereby preventing agglutination. The observation that the Fc portion of the H chain is involved in secondary immunologic properties of the molecule lends support to this view. Gergeley and associates (53) have similarly proposed functional differences in the Fc portion of papain sensitive and papain insensitive immuno-globulins in nonspecific adsorption to the erythrocyte surface.

Serologic Characteristics of Warm Acting Erythrocyte Antibodies

Warm acting erythrocytes autoantibodies have marked serologic heterogeneity. Such variations prevent any simple listing of serologic reactivity as typical, universal or diagnostic. Serologic characterization is further complicated by the frequent admixture of both cold and warm acting types and their variable influences in test procedures. This heterogeneity of warm acting erythrocyte autoantibodies should not surprise the reader and laboratory investigator. Antibody specificity is structurally related to those portions of the H and L chains which interact (Fab fragment). Serologic characteristics, however, are determined by an entirely different portion of the H chain, the Fc fragment. Accordingly, heterogeneity in serologic terms is compatible with antibody specificity. Dacie (1) has presented a detailed review of the serologic characteristics of erythrocyte autoantibodies. The reader is encouraged to consult his volume.

Autohemagglutination and Autohemolysis

It is uncommon for warm acting autoantibodies to induce agglutination or hemolysis of a patient's own erythrocytes. In order to document such a phenomenon, antibody activity must be demonstrated at 37°C. against saline suspended normal and host erythrocytes. The original description of this state by Chauffard and Vincent (54) described hemoglobinuria, a serum isolysin and autolysin present during the acute phase of illness, maximal activity of the lysin at 37°C. and disappearance of the lysin upon recovery. In 1938 Dameshek and Schwartz (55) reported three cases of this phenomenon, and their study reawakened interest in the subject. Hemoglobinuria was present. The autolysin was heat stable and required complement for lysis. Fixation of the antibody occurred without lysis in the absence of heat labile portions of complement. Lysis was prevented by normal human serum. This latter observation was confirmed by

Farrar and associates (56) in 1940. There is a striking similarity between this description and that reported by Boyden and Andersen (57) for bacterial immune complexes adsorbed onto erythrocytes. This may be significant in light of the studies of Moolten and Clark (58), who isolated Newcastle disease virus and herpes simplex virus from the blood of patients with autohemagglutination.

Scattered individual reports have dedescribed various clinical and laboratory characteristics of warm acting autohemagglutinins and hemolysins. Warm acting autohemagglutinins are uncommonly found in autoimmune hemolytic anemia. Evans (59) noted one example in 34 patients studied. van Loghem and associates (3) found five such cases in 122 patients. Dacie (1) specifically looked for this type of antibody in 85 sera containing warm acting autoantibodies. Four patients, or less than 5 per cent, had significant autohemagglutination at 37°C.

Warm acting autohemolysins are even less common. Dausset and Colombani (4) reported four cases in 83 patients investigated. van Loghem and associates (3) found only one warm acting autohemolysin among 122 patients with warm acting erythrocyte autoantibodies; this hemolysin lysed only trypsinized erythrocytes. In Dacie's series (1) of 89 cases of warm acting autoimmune hemolytic anemia, only two examples of autohemolysins active against normal erythrocytes were found. Two other sera had autohemolysin activity with trypsinized erythrocytes or erythrocytes from patients with paroxysmal nocturnal hemoglobinuria.

The Effect of pH

In 1944 David and Minot (60) observed an increased hemolytic activity of a warm acting autohemolysin when the serum pH was lowered. Dacie (1) confirmed this observation. He noted that hemolysis was minimal in unacidified serum but was markedly increased at a serum pH 6.8 to 7.0. Gardner (61) reported that acidification of sera from patients with warm acting autoimmune hemolytic anemia induced agglutination of the patient's own or normal eryth-

rocytes. A pH of 6.5 to 6.7 was optimal. Agglutination was abolished at pH 8.0, although reaction with antiglobulin serum persisted. Gardner and Harris (62) also noted the presence of autohemolysins during acidification. Evans and Weiser (63) studied the effect of serum acidification over a pH range of 6.6 to 8.0 with 29 erythrocyte autoantibody preparations. They were unable to demonstrate spontaneous autohemagglutination throughout this pH range. A pH of 7.4 resulted in significant enhancement of erythrocyte sensitization in only one case. Case 101 illustrates an example of a warm acting autoantibody which induced lysis when the pH was lowered during Cr^{51} labeling of erythrocytes.

Thermal Range of Action

There has been a tendency to ascribe particular significance to the maximal thermal range of activity of erythrocyte antibodies. Cold acting erythrocyte isoantibodies frequently develop without evidence of immunization, and accordingly they have been described as "natural." Warm acting isoantibodies usually follow specific immunization and are termed "immune." Immunization with foreign erythrocytes also reveals a distinction between cold and warm acting antibodies. The cold reacting antibody is seen first, and the warm acting antibody appears as immunization continues. The significance of this sequence was obscure and it was commonly assumed that warm acting erythrocyte antibodies were more significant pathologically. A similar assumption has been made with erythrocyte autoantibodies. This is reinforced by the observation that cold acting erythrocyte autoantibodies are asymptomatically present in almost all normal human sera. In contrast, warm acting erythrocyte autoantibodies are less common and are almost always associated with a pathologic state.

Komninos and Désy (16) studied the activity temperature range of eluted warm acting erythrocyte autoantibodies, and they demonstrated preferential erythrocyte fixation at 37°C. Antibody titers at 3°C. were substantially lower than at 37° C. Evans and Weiser (63) studied eight eluates containing erythrocyte autoantibodies. All eight were active at a temperature range of 5 to 37°C.; five were most active at 37°C. Three eluates were not affected by temperature variations and were found to be nongamma types by gamma-globulin neutralization tests. Schubothe (64) noted similar temperature variations. An optimal reactivity at 40°C. was noted for three sera containing erythrocyte autoantibodies and for anti-Rh₀(D). Two other sera had an optimal thermal range between 10 and 20°C. Heating sera with autoantibodies to 56°C. did not affect their ability to sensitize erythrocytes (65). Schubothe (64) confirmed this observation but noted that a temperature of 60°C. reduced antibody activity.

Filitti-Wurmser and Jacquot-Armand (66) postulated that erythrocyte antibodies were a single molecule type with various antibody groupings sensitive to temperature. Wiener (67) in 1951 suggested that cold acting antibodies resulted from immunization with various cross reacting antigens. A heterogeneous molecular population results. Because such antibodies are cross reacting they have an imperfect fit with human antigenic determinants. This imperfect fit permits increased molecular activity resulting from heat to dissociate antigen-antibody complexes. Schubothe (68) suggests that cold acting hemagglutinins may change their molecular shape under the influence of cold.

Recent physical, chemical and phylogenetic studies give some explanation for these temperature variations. It is clear that two different immunoglobulin types are involved. Fudenberg and Kunkel (14) demonstrated that warm acting autoantibodies are generally IgG molecules and that cold acting erythrocyte autoantibodies are generally IgM molecules. A different set of H chains (gamma H and mu H) are present in these two immunoglobulin types. Secondary immunologic characteristics are a function of the Fc fragment of the H chain. It is therefore not surprising that different temperature requirements characterize these two antibody types. Other secondary immunologic characteristics similarly differ.

This is most apparent with placental transfer (69) and complement fixation. These qualities are also functions of the Fc portion of the H chain. In all probability most immune sera contain a mixture of both types of antibody molecules. The variation and confusion characterizing optimal temperature requirements are therefore understandable.

The production of gamma M immunoglobulins appears as the original immunologic mechanism in lower vertebrates. Gamma G immunoglobulin production is a more recent evolutionary development. In the human, immunization first results in formation of IgM antibodies and is subsequently followed by the formation of IgG antibodies. A particular pathologic significance of "natural" or "immune" antibody becomes meaningless in view of this observation.

It must not be assumed that all warm acting autoantibodies are gamma G immunoglobulins and that all cold acting autoantibodies are gamma M immunoglobulins. The original cold acting autoantibody characteristic of paroxysmal cold hemoglobinuria has been shown by Hinz (70) to be a gamma G antibody rather than the expected IgM type.

The Elution of Warm Acting Autoantibodies

Warm acting erythrocyte autoantibodies are encountered in two forms. They may be fixed to the erythrocyte surface or they may be unbound and circulating freely in the serum. Elution from the cell surface has several real as well as imaginary advantages in the study of erythrocyte autoantibodies. Only by employing eluates can an investigator be sure that documented serologic characteristics actually reflect the antibody fixed to the erythrocyte surface. A positive direct antiglobulin test is frequently found in the presence of a circulating antibody. The assumption may be made that the unbound antibody is identical to that fixed to the patient's own cells. This assumption is unwarranted. An eluate must be made from the antiglobulin positive erythrocytes and tested for specificity. It is not uncommon for two or more erythrocyte antibodies to be present. The eluate may contain an auto-antibody acting as a panhemagglutinin which is unrelated to a circulating erythro-cyte isoantibody.

Negative direct antiglobulin tests can be further investigated by elution of the non-reacting red cells. Such procedures may demonstrate warm acting erythrocyte auto-antibodies. In the present series positive eluates were obtained in 16 instances when the direct antiglobulin test was negative or only trace positive. In five a prozone phe-nomenon was present (see Table 23, Chap-ter 3).

Elution procedures permit the recovery of warm acting erythrocyte autoantibodies in a soluble form. Approximately 50 to 60 per cent of cases of warm acting autoimmune hemolytic anemia have demonstrable anti-body fixed to erythrocytes and unbound in the serum. In the remaining 40 to 50 per cent the antibody is only fixed to erythrocytes. Eluates make available specimens for the study of autoantibody specificity and for physical, chemical and serologic analysis. The ability to elute erythrocyte autoanti-bodies permits the storage of such materials for further study.

There are limitations in the use of elution procedures. Eluates are of dubious value in obtaining pure solutions of warm acting erythrocyte autoantibody. All proteins (globulins and albumin) bound to the erythrocyte surface are released concom-itantly with the autoantibody. Elution tech-niques are of little value in quantitative procedures to evaluate antibody kinetics, number of antibody molecules in relation to antibody titer, etc. Erythrocyte autoanti-bodies are not released by elution in any consistent, quantitative fashion. A careful search will usually reveal washing out of small amounts of autoantibody prior to elution. In addition, substantial amounts of autoantibody remain fixed to the eryth-rocyte or stroma after elution. In our lab-oratory, release of autoantibody may still be demonstrated after more than 10 sep-arate elutions of the same erythrocytes or stroma with the techniques of Landsteiner

and Miller (71), Kidd (72), Greenwalt (73) and Weiner (74).

Many investigators have relied on eluate solutions of autoantibodies for quantitation of physical and serologic characteristics. In retrospect this appears to be a dubious pro-cedure. Elution techniques in terms of pro-tein chemistry are particularly harsh and liable to create denaturation. This is par-ticularly apparent with warm acting eryth-rocyte autoantibodies. Simple warm elution for cold acting erythrocyte autoantibodies appears to be relatively innocuous. It is more desirable to perform analytical analy-sis on unbound warm acting erythrocyte autoantibodies found in sera, rather than to risk modifying physical and serologic char-acteristics through elution.

Elution techniques for obtaining eryth-rocyte autoantibodies have been available for some time. Sturgeon (75) in 1947 dem-onstrated that warm acting erythrocyte au-toantibodies were eluted by incubating sa-line suspensions of erythrocytes at 37° or 56°C. Evans and associates (76) made sim-ilar observations. They found that warm acting erythrocyte autoantibodies could be eluted from saline suspended erythrocytes by heating at 56°C. for 5 minutes. Both of these techniques employed a heat elution procedure originally developed in 1925 by Landsteiner and Miller (71). Many other procedures have since been published. These include the methods of Kidd (72), Green-walt (73), Vos and Kelsall (77), Weiner (74), van Loghem and associates (78) and Kochwa and Rosenfield (79). Jensen (80) in 1959 performed a comparative study of many of these techniques. The best eluates were obtained using the methods of Weiner (74) and van Loghem and associates (78). The Landsteiner-Miller method (71) was the simplest and most rapid procedure and gave adequate eluates. The more recently developed procedure of Kochwa and Rosen-field (79) appears to offer several distinct advantages and can be recommended.

In the current series the Weiner technique (74) has been extensively used, with the procedures of Landsteiner and Miller (71) and Kochwa and Rosenfield (79) occasion-ally employed. Elution was performed in

80 cases. The great majority of such cases were characterized by weak direct antiglobulin tests. Elution was successful in 60 cases or 75 per cent (see Chapter 3).

Caution must be exercised in interpreting elution data. Croucher and associates (81) have pointed out that multiple isoantibodies may be produced (restimulated) after the transfusion of "apparently compatible blood." The presence of such isoantibodies concomitantly with large numbers of transfused erythrocytes containing the pertinent antigens can lead to positive antiglobulin tests and to the simulation of autoimmune hemolytic anemia. Elution may then induce an erroneous assumption of autoantibody specificity.

Fong and Masouredis (82) reported that different elution procedures modify the properties of anti-Rh$_0$(D). Variables are introduced by the composition of the globulin containing fraction, the physical form of the antigen containing cells, the manner of forming stroma and the modality used for elution. Anti-Rh$_0$(D) eluates showed differences in antibody content, rate of association with erythrocytes and zoning in antibody excess. Antigen-antibody complexes are also eluted and increase the ionic charge of the sample.

Ogata and Matuhasi (83, 84) have made a remarkable observation which must be considered whenever elution is performed. The fixation of erythrocyte antibodies to their specific antigens may lead to the nonspecific adsorption of other erythrocyte antibodies in the absence of erythrocyte antigens. This has been termed the *Ogata phenomenon*. Issitt and associates (85) emphasized that the nonspecific binding of antibody is related to erythrocyte-antibody and group specific soluble substance-antibody complexes. Svardal and associates (86) studied a patient whose erythrocytes were characterized as cDE/cDE and were antiglobulin positive. Erythrocyte eluates revealed anti-e, ce, Ce and I. The authors reported that cooling of the blood may permit cold hemagglutinins to fix to the erythrocyte and to simultaneously induce nonspecific adsorption of isoantibodies. This may simulate autoimmune hemolytic anemia, and eluates would give an incorrect appearance of specificity.

Other Characteristics of Warm Acting Erythrocyte Autoantibodies

It is impossible to list all of the individual immunologic variations reported for warm acting erythrocyte autoantibodies. Several important observations, however, should be mentioned.

Placental Transport

Warm acting erythrocyte autoantibodies behave as other IgG molecules and have an active placental transfer mechanism (69). Erythrocyte autoantibodies may therefore traverse the placenta and react with erythrocytes of the fetus. Newborn infants born of mothers with autoimmune hemolytic anemia may have direct and indirect positive antiglobulin tests. Case 2 illustrates such a sequence. This is in contrast with the lack of placental transfer of cold acting IgM erythrocyte autobodies. Such differences appear to be related to the different H chains (Fc portion) comprising the various immunoglobulin classes. The maternal transfer of autoimmune diseases through the placenta is accordingly dependent on passive immunization with IgG immunoglobulins (69).

The Dissociation of Erythrocyte Autoantibodies from the Erythrocyte Surface

Selwin and Hackett (87) in 1949 noted that transfusion of erythrocytes coated with autoantibodies led to positive antiglobulin tests with the recipient's normal erythrocytes. Erythrocyte autoantibodies appeared to dissociate from the original donor erythrocytes and to react with the recipient's cells. Evans and associates (63, 88) demonstrated the same phenomenon in vitro with erythrocyte iso- and autoantibodies. They emphasized that each antibody must have an individual dissociation constant. The concentration of erythrocyte autoantibody and its dissociation constant must influence the presence or absence of unbound erythrocyte autoantibody freely circulating in the serum. Implicit in this concept is the assumption that erythrocyte autoantibody must always be present in the serum, irrespective of the results of antibody testing. Evans and associates (63, 88, 89) suggest that measurement of erythrocyte autoantibody dissociation constants is a more accurate indicator of antibody concentration than is determination of titer. Although the degree of positivity of direct antiglobulin tests might not change, a decrease in the amount of antibody fixed to the erythrocyte surface would result in a decrease of spontaneous dissociation of the antibody.

Hughes-Jones (90) analyzed the dissociation of antibody-antigen complexes containing anti-Rh_o(D) and anti-hr'(c). Dissociation rate constants of the order of 1×10^{-4} to 1×10^{-6} sec.$^{-1}$ were found. Marked heterogeneity was noted and the dissociation half-time ranged from approximately 2 hours to more than 8 days.

Spontaneous erythrocyte autoantibody elution is still not completely understood. It does not appear to be entirely dependent on avidity or other aspects of antibody-antigen union. It has been shown that gamma-globulin fixed to the erythrocyte surface in a nonimmunologic fashion undergoes a similar spontaneous elution (52). At least two populations of globulin molecules are involved. Approximately 30 per cent of the globulin rapidly dissociates, while the remaining molecules gradually leave the cell surface with repeated washings. Dissociation is not complete, with 50 per cent of the globulin remaining bound even after 15 washings (52).

The Effect of Heparin and Protamine

In 1954 Roth (91) reported that heparin inhibited the agglutination of erythrocytes sensitized with autoantibodies and erythrocytes exposed to warm acting erythrocyte autoantibodies. The effect of heparin on the antiglobulin test has been confirmed both in vivo and in vitro. Roth and Frumin (92), McFarland and associates (93), Hartman (94) and Ten Pas and Monto (95) have described the reversal of positive antiglobulin tests after heparin administration.

Heparin's action in the agglutination and lytic reaction is still obscure. In 1929 Ecker and Gross (96) reported that heparin neutralized complement at concentrations of 0.04 to 0.06 mg. of heparin per unit of complement. Heparin appeared to act at the C'3 component. This was confirmed in the studies of Von Falkenhausen (97) and Wising (98). Storti and Vaccari (99) demonstrated that heparin and other anticoagulants could prevent hemolysis in in vitro hemolytic tests systems. Cortisone and Dicumarol were ineffectual in the same system. The active inhibiting materials did not prevent antibody from fixing to erythrocytes. In addition, they were ineffectual in noncomplement dependent hemolytic systems. Storti and Vaccari (99) postulated that the antihemolytic activity of anticoagulants reflected their anticomplementary activity. Ten Pas and Monto (95) demonstrated a reduced complement level during the hemolytic stage in autoimmune hemolytic anemia. After a remission induced by heparin, normal complement levels were found. Rosenfield and associates (100) reported the protective action of heparin on lysis of erythrocytes coated with IgG hemolysins. Inhibition of lysis following a single dose of heparin lasted for less than 4 hours. Lysis was only delayed, indicating that the sensitizing hemolysin remained fixed to the cell. The protective action of heparin appeared to be related to its anticomplementary activity. Highly charged molecules, whether of a positive or negative charge, may be anticomplementary (101). Heparin is a strongly negatively charged compound because of a high degree of esterification with sulfonic acid. This may explain its anticomplementary role.

Roth (102) minimizes the anticomplementary effect of heparin in its antilytic activity. After parenteral administration of heparin, only an insignificant and transient lowering of complement was observed. Roth (91) suggested that the beneficial action of heparin might reflect competition between autoantibodies and heparin. Alternatively, heparin may directly interact with erythrocyte autoantibodies. Incubating erythrocytes coated with antibody with heparin prevented agglutination reactions with antiglobulin serum (102).

Other mechanisms of action may be suggested. Heparin may function through its strong negative charge by interacting with serum globulins, forming heparin-protein complexes. Such complexes may compete for complement with erythrocyte-antibody complexes. Heparin may directly bind to the erythrocyte surface. This would increase the negative charge of the polyanionic erythrocyte, thereby minimizing the lowering of the zeta potential induced by erythrocyte antibodies or by ancillary treatments such as proteolytic enzymes. This would tend to stabilize the repelling forces, preventing the bridging of antibodies and the aggregation of red cells. The formation of a heparin-erythrocyte antibody complex could induce a change in the charge of the antibody molecule. Such an effect might produce a modification of the antibody molecular conformation with steric hindrance of the antibody site. This mechanism has been employed to explain the inhibitory action of basically charged hexosamine antibiotics on erythrocyte antibodies (103). The heparin effect on erythrocyte antibodies deserves detailed investigation. A superficial and unpublished study in our laboratory did not reveal any effect of heparin on crude agglutination titers obtained with anti-rhesus antibodies.

Roth and Frumin (104) in 1954 reported that protamine possessed the ability to agglutinate antibody coated erythrocytes. A difference in the effect of protamine on erythrocyte auto- and isoantibodies was found. The significance of this observation is dubious. Protamine sulfate is a highly basically charged molecule. In view of the discussion above, it may be anticipated that adsorption of such basically charged molecules onto the erythrocyte surface would induce agglutination irrespective of the presence of antibody. Such a nonimmune agglutination of erythrocytes has been reported both with protamine sulfate and with Polybrene (46). August and Pirofsky (46) also noted that serum proteins reacted with these basically charged molecules. Lalezari and associates (105) have applied this observation to sensitize erythrocytes with Polybrene in an attempt to potentiate agglutination. Other basically charged molecules may be expected to induce agglutination in the same manner. Various polymers of L-polylysine, sodium argenate, methylated bovine serum albumin and decamethyldiamine have all been successfully employed in our laboratory. Godal and Norseth (106) noted that TAME (p-tosyl-1-arginine methyl ester, HCl), a basically charged molecule, has a reverse effect on nonantibody induced erythrocyte aggregation. The mechanism of action is obscure.

The Effect of Normal Serum on Erythrocyte Autoantibodies

In 1938 Dameshek and Schwartz (55) noted that normal serum had the ability to block the lytic activity of autohemolysins. This observation was confirmed by Farrar and associates (66). Reports of the influence of serum and serum components on erythrocyte autoantibodies have been infrequent since that time. Martin du Pan (107) reported an autoagglutinin which was inhibited by normal serum. Denys and van den Broucke (108) and Roth and Frumin (104) noted that normal serum decreased the sensitization of erythrocytes exposed to erythrocyte autoantibodies.

Normal human serum and its components may have the reverse effect from that described above. Sera obtained from normal humans may rarely induce agglutination of papain treated erythrocytes. Most human sera contain a substance able to induce the immediate agglutination of trypsinized erythrocytes (109). With continual incubation, agglutination disappears as the serum agglutinin is spontaneously eluted off the erythrocyte. Elution is more rapid in serum than in saline (110).

Various serum components may fix to erythrocytes and occasionally lead to positive reactions typical of warm acting erythrocyte autoantibodies. This phenomenon is well documented but of dubious significance. Janković (111) reported that most human sera incubated at 37°C. will permit the adsorption of serum components to trypsinized erythrocytes. This in turn can produce positive antiglobulin tests. Evans (59) noted that incubating normal erythrocytes at 37°C. with some human sera could create weak positive antiglobulin tests. Delage (112) investigated this phenomenon in detail. He observed that sera obtained from newborns did not have this ability. Sera obtained from infants 14 to 16 months old acquired the reactivity. Anticoagulants and heating the serum to 56°C blocked this reaction.

Weiner and associates (113) reported the capacity of rare sera to induce agglutination of albumin suspended erythrocytes. Agglutination was transient and no thermal preference was noted. No clinical significance could be ascribed to this state. Additional cases of this "albumin autoagglutination" syndrome have been reported (114–119). Marsh and Jenkins (116) found no relationship of this reaction to I or i antigens. Hossaini (119) noted that 30 per cent albumin would induce agglutination but that a 22 per cent concentration was ineffectual. In an investigation of 4580 sera, albumin autoagglutination ability was noted in 11. Nine positive sera were obtained from Negroes out of a total 2216 tested. Two active sera were found in the 2364 sera obtained from Caucasians. The phenomenon appeared to be nonimmunologic and antibodies could not be demonstrated.

The Effect of Hexosamine Antibiotics on Warm Acting Erythrocyte Autoantibodies

In 1955 Kout and Kubickova (120) noted that streptomycin in high concentrations had the ability to prevent agglutination of $Rh_o(D)$ human erythrocytes exposed to anti-$Rh_o(D)$. Boyd and associates (121) simultaneously noted the same phenomenon and attributed it to the N-methyl-L-glucosamine moiety of streptomycin. They postulated that this "unnatural" sugar was closely related to the antigenic structure of $Rh_o(D)$ and that streptomycin may function as an analog of the antigen. These original observations were confirmed by Pirofsky and Cordova (122, 123) who noted that 250 mg. per ml. (0.24 M) solutions of streptomycin were optimal to demonstrate inhibition. Anti-A, anti-B, anti-M and anti-N were not affected by streptomycin. However, warm acting erythrocyte autoantibodies and the anti-rhesus antibodies anti-$Rh_o(D)$, rh'(C), rh"(E), hr'(c) and

hr"(e) were inhibited. Inhibition was not influenced by the IgM or IgG nature of the antibody as determined by 2-mercaptoethanol treatment. Streptomycin inhibited agglutination by preventing antibodies from fixing to the erythrocyte surface (103). Other materials had a similar capacity to inhibit erythrocyte autoantibodies and anti-rhesus antibodies. Nine hexosamine containing antibiotics and their derivatives were documented as possessng the inhibitory capacity. The studies of Pirofsky and associates (103, 122, 123) did not confirm Boyd's assumption (121) that streptomycin functioned as an analog of the antigen. The streptodine portion of the molecule, which was devoid of N-methyl-L-glucosamine, was an active inhibiting agent (123). Evidence was presented that the highly polar basic charge of the streptomycin molecule was critical for inhibition. It was suggested that such a basically charged molecule could adsorb to negatively charged groups of the antibody globulin, resulting in a streptomycin-globulin complex. Such a complex may then present a steric obstruction preventing combination with antigenic determinants (103). The possible therapeutic significance of this reaction has not as yet been explored. The interaction of cephalothin with serum proteins may establish a similar complex which has the capacity to adsorb to the erythrocyte surface, leading to positive antiglobulin tests (124).

BIBLIOGRAPHY

1. Dacie, J. V.: *The Haemolytic Anaemias, Part II*, Ed. 2. Grune & Stratton, Inc., New York, 1962.
2. Worlledge, S. M.: Serologic aspects of the auto-immune haemolytic anaemia. In *Auto-immunity*, edited by R. W. Baldwin and J. H. Humphrey. Blackwell Scientific Publications, Ltd., Oxford, 1965.
3. van Loghem, J. J., van der Hart, M., and Dorfmeier, H.: Serologic studies in acquired hemolytic anemia. In *Proceedings of the Sixth International Congress of the International Society of Hematology*. Grune & Stratton, Inc., New York, 1958.
4. Dausset, J., and Colombani, J.: The serology and the prognosis of 128 cases of autoimmune hemolytic anemia. Blood **14**: 1280, 1959.
5. Coombs, R. R. A., and Mourant, A.: On certain properties of antisera prepared against human serum and its various pro-

tein fractions: their use in the detection of sensitization of human red cells with "incomplete" Rh antibody, and on the nature of this antibody. J. Path. Bact. **59:** 105, 1947.

6. Wiener, A. S., Hyman, M. A., and Handman, L.: A new serologic test (inhibition test) for human serum globulin. Proc. Soc. Exp. Biol. Med. **71:** 96, 1949.

7. Hackett, E.: Coombs test in acute acquired haemolytic anaemia. Lancet **1:** 998, 1950.

8. Vaughan, J. H.: Immunologic features of erythrocyte sensitization. I. Acquired hemolytic disease. Blood **11:** 1085, 1956.

9. Dacie, J. V.: Auto-immune haemolytic anaemias. Acta Haemat. (Basel) **20:** 131, 1958.

10. Wuilleret, B.: L'anémie hémolytique acquise par autoanticorps de l'enfant C. P. étudiée à la lumière des tests immunohématologiques érythrocytaires. Helv. Paediat. Acta **13:** 140, 1958.

11. Konda, S., and Yamada, A.: Characteristics of the autoantibody attached to erythrocytes of the patient with auto-immune hemolytic anemia. Acta Haemat. Jap. **23:** 879, 1960.

12. Eyster, M. E., Nachman, R. L., Christenson, W. N., and Engle, R. L.: Structural characteristics of red cell autoantibodies. J. Immun. **96:** 107, 1966.

13. Jeannet, M.: Specificity of the antiglobulin tests in "auto-immune" hemolytic anemias. Helv. Med. Acta **33:** 151, 1966.

14. Fudenberg, H. H., and Kunkel, H. G.: Physical properties of red cell agglutinins in acquired hemolytic anemia. J. Exp. Med. **106:** 689, 1957.

15. Komninos, Z. D., and Aksoy, M.: Studies on antibodies eluted from erythrocytes in autoimmune hemolytic anemia. J. Clin. Invest. **33:** 949, 1954.

16. Komninos, Z. D., and Désy, L.: Thermal range of activity of antibodies eluted from the red cells in autoimmune hemolytic anemia. J. Lab. Clin. Med. **46:** 74, 1955.

17. Fudenberg, H., Barry, I., and Dameshek, W.: The erythrocyte-coating substance in autoimmune hemolytic disease: its nature and significance. Blood **13:** 201, 1958.

18. Auerswald, W., Doleschel, W., Rosak, M., and Steffen, C.: Physico-chemical characterization of proteins obtained by elution from blood cells incubated with autoantibody containing sera. Vox Sang. **6:** 478, 1961.

19. Cassell, M., and Chaplin, H.: Studies on anti-eluate sera. II. Comparison of a conventional antiglobulin serum with three anti-eluate sera in the study of 70 patients with acquired hemolytic anemia. Vox Sang. **5:** 43, 1960.

20. Vulpis, N.: Studies on the antigens of red cell ghost. Differences in antigenic specificity of human normal adult hereditary sphero-cytosis and autoimmune hemolytic anemia S protein. Acta Haemat. (Basel) **30:** 280, 1963.

21. Franklin, E. C., and Fudenberg, H. H.: Antigenic heterogeneity of human Rh antibodies, rheumatoid factors, and cold agglutinins. Arch. Biochem. **104:** 433, 1964.

22. Leddy, J. P., and Bakemeier, R. F.: Structural aspects of human erythrocyte auto-antibodies. I. L. chain types and electrophoretic dispersion. J. Exp. Med. **121:** 1, 1965.

23. Khan, M. Y., and Zinneman, H. H.: Amino acid composition of anti-D as isolated by immunologic specificity. Amer. J. Clin. Path. **47:** 429, 1967.

24. Wiener, A. S.: A new test (blocking test) for Rh sensitization. Proc. Soc. Exp. Biol. Med. **56:** 173, 1944.

25. Dausset, J.: The agglutination mechanism of trypsin modified red cells. Blood **7:** 816, 1952.

26. Pirofsky, B., Cordova, M., and Imel, T. L.: The function of proteolytic enzymes and tannic acid in inducing erythrocyte agglutination. J. Immun. **89:** 767, 1962.

27. Jandl, J. H., and Castle, W. B.: Agglutination of sensitized red cells by large anisometric molecules. J. Lab. Clin. Med. **47:** 669, 1956.

28. Morton, J. A., and Pickles, M. M.: Use of trypsin in the detection of incomplete anti-Rh antibodies. Nature (London) **159:** 779, 1947.

29. Race, R. R., Sanger, R., and Selwyn, J. G.: A probable deletion in a human Rh chromosome. Nature (London) **166:** 520, 1950.

30. Vos, G. H., and Kirk, R. L.: The "protection" of sensitized A and B cell antigens by water-soluble A and B substances. J. Immun. **80:** 149, 1958.

31. Pirofsky, B., Cordova, M. S., and Imel, T. L.: The mechanism of action of antiglobulin serum. Vox Sang. **7:** 348, 1962.

32. Solomon, J. M.: Behavior of incomplete antibodies in quantitative hemagglutination reactions. Transfusion **4:** 101, 1964.

33. Mollison, P. L.: *Blood Transfusion in Clinical Medicine,* Ed. 3, p. 219. Charles C Thomas, Publisher, Springfield, Ill., 1961.

34. Pirofsky, B., and Cordova, M. S.: Bivalent nature of incomplete anti-D (Rh$_0$). Nature (London) **197:** 392, 1963.

35. Pirofsky, B., and Cordova, M. S.: The nature of incomplete erythrocyte antibodies. Vox Sang. **9:** 17, 1964.

36. Mandy, W. J., Fudenberg, H. H., and Lewis, F. B.: On "incomplete" anti-Rh antibodies: mechanism of direct agglutination induced by mercaptoethanol. J. Clin. Invest. **44:** 1352, 1965.

37. Stolinsky, D., and Fudenberg, H.: On the univalent fragments of human 7S gamma-globulin. Nature (London) **200:** 856, 1963.

38. Fudenberg, H., Mandy, W. J., and Nisonoff, A.: Serologic studies of proteolytic frag-

ments of rabbit agglutinating antibodies. J. Clin. Invest. **41**: 2123, 1962.

39. Seaman, G. V. F., and Heard, D. H.: The surface of the washed human erythrocyte as a polyanion. J. Gen. Physiol. **44**: 251, 1960.

40. Cook, G. M. W., Heard, D. H., and Seaman, G. V. F.: A sialomucopeptide liberated by trypsin from the human erythrocyte. Nature (London) **188**: 1011, 1960.

41. Klenk, E., and Uhlenbruck, G.: On the isolation of mucoids containing neuraminic acid from human erythrocyte stroma, a contribution to the chemistry of agglutinogens. Z. Physiol. Chem. **319**: 151, 1960.

42. Mäkelä, O., Miettinen, T., and Pesola, R.: Release of sialic acid and carbohydrates from human red cells by trypsin treatment. Vox Sang. **5**: 492, 1960.

43. Seaman, G. V. F., and Uhlenbruck, G.: The action of proteolytic enzymes on the red cells of some animal species. Biochim. Biophys. Acta **64**: 570, 1962.

44. Seaman, G. V. F.: Electrophoresis using a cylindrical chamber. In *Cell Electrophoresis,* edited by E. J., Ambrose. Little, Brown and Company, Boston, 1965.

45. Seaman, G. V. F., and Cook, G. M. W.: Modification of the electrophoretic behaviour of the erythrocyte by chemical and enzymatic methods In *Cell Electrophoresis,* edited by E. J. Ambrose. Little, Brown and Company, Boston, 1965.

46. August, A., and Pirofsky, B.: Interaction of basic polyelectrolytes and human blood: the effect of antiheparin agents. Transfusion **6**: 74, 1966.

47. Coulter, C.: The isoelectric point of red blood cells and its relation to agglutination. J. Gen. Physiol. **3**: 309, 1921.

48. Seaman, G. V. F., and Uhlenbruck, G.: Die electrophoretische Beweglichkeit von Erythrocyten nach Behandlung mit verschiedenen Enzymen und Antiserum. Klin. Wschr. **40**: 699, 1962.

49. Sachtleben, P.: The influence of antibodies on the electrophoretic mobility of red blood cells. In *Cell Electrophoresis,* edited by E. J. Ambrose. Little, Brown and Company, Boston, 1965.

50. Pollack, W., Hager, H. J., Reckel, R., Singher, H. O., and Toren, D. A.: A study of the forces involved in the second stage of hemagglutination. Transfusion **5**: 158, 1965.

51. Boursnell, J. C., Coombs, R. R. A., and Rizk, V.: Quantitative studies with antisera marked with iodine[131] isotope and their corresponding red-cell antigens. Biochem. J. **55**: 745, 1953.

52. Pirofsky, B., Cordova, M. S., and Imel, T. L.: The nonimmunologic reaction of globulin molecules with the erythrocyte surface. Vox Sang. **7**: 334, 1962.

53. Gergely, J., Horváth, E., Medgyesi, G. A.,

and Puskas, E.: The papain-sensitivity and nonspecific binding capacity of incomplete anti-Rh₀(D) antibodies. Vox Sang. **14**: 161, 1968.

54. Chauffard, M. A., and Vincent, C.: Hémoglobinurie hémolysinique avec ictère polycholique aigu. Sem. Med. **29**: 601, 1909.

55. Dameshek, W., and Schwartz, S. O.: The presence of hemolysins in acute hemolytic anemia; preliminary note. New Eng. J. Med. **218**: 75, 1938.

56. Farrar, G. E., Burnett, W. E., and Steigman, A. J.: Hemolysinic anemia and hepatic degeneration cured by splenectomy. Amer. J. Med. Sci. **200**: 164, 1940.

57. Boyden, S. V., and Andersen, M. E.: Agglutination of normal erythrocytes in mixtures of antibody and antigen, and haemolysis in the presence of complement. Brit. J. Exp. Path. **36**: 162, 1955.

58. Moolten, S. E., and Clark, E.: The red blood cell as a vehicle of virus transport. II. Role of blood-borne viruses in autohemagglutination and in hemolytic anemia. Trans. N. Y. Acad. Sci. **14**: 235, 1952.

59. Evans, R. S.: Autoantibodies in hematologic disorders. Stanford Med. Bull. **13**: 152, 1955.

60. David, J. K., and Minot, A. S.: Acute hemolytic anemia in infancy. Amer. J. Dis. Child. **68**: 327, 1944.

61. Gardner, F. H.: Transfer to normal red cells of an agglutinin demonstrable in the acidified sera of patients with acquired hemolytic jaundice. J. Clin. Invest. **28**: 783, 1949.

62. Gardner, F. H., and Harris, J. W.: The demonstration of hemolysis in acquired hemolytic anemia. J. Clin. Invest. **29**: 814, 1950.

63. Evans, R. S., and Weiser, R. S.: The serology of autoimmune hemolytic disease. Observations on forty-one patients. Arch. Intern. Med. (Chicago) **100**: 371, 1957.

64. Schubothe, H.: *Serologie und Klinische Bedeutung der Autohämantikörper.* S. Karger, Basel, 1958.

65. Dacie, J. V.: Acquired hemolytic anemia. With special reference to the antiglobulin (Coombs') reaction. Blood **8**: 813, 1953.

66. Filitti-Wurmser, S., and Jacquot-Armand, Y.: Méchanisme de l'effet de la température sur l'isohémagglutination. C. R. Soc. Biol. (Paris) **141**: 577, 1947.

67. Wiener, A. S.: Origin of naturally occurring hemagglutinins and hemolysins: a review. J. Immun. **66**: 287, 1951.

68. Schubothe, H.: Current problems of chronic cold hemagglutinin disease. Ann. N. Y. Acad. Sci. **124**: 484, 1965.

69. Placental transmission of autoimmune diseases (editorial). Brit. Med. J. **1**: 1554, 1966.

70. Hinz, C. F.: Serologic and physico-chemical characterization of Donath-Landsteiner antibodies from six patients. Blood **22**: 600, 1963.

71. Landsteiner, K., and Miller, C. P.: Serologic studies on the blood of the primates. II. The blood groups in anthropoid apes. J. Exp. Med. **42**: 853, 1925.

72. Kidd, P.: Elution of an incomplete type of antibody from the erythrocytes in acquired haemolytic anaemia. J. Clin. Path. **2**: 103, 1949.

73. Greenwalt, T. J.: A method for eluting antibodies from red cell stromata. J. Lab. Clin. Med. **48**: 634, 1956.

74. Weiner, W.: Eluting red-cell antibodies: a method and its application. Brit. J. Haemat. **3**: 276, 1957.

75. Sturgeon, P.: A new antibody in serum of patients with acquired hemolytic anemia. Science **106**: 293, 1947.

76. Evans, R. S., Duane, R. T., and Behrendt, V.: Demonstration of antibodies in acquired hemolytic anemia with anti-human globulin serum. Proc. Soc. Exp. Biol. Med. **64**: 372, 1947.

77. Vos, G. H., and Kelsall, G. A.: A new elution technique for the preparation of specific immune anti-Rh serum. Brit. J. Haemat. **2**: 342, 1956.

78. van Loghem, J. J., Mendes de Leon, D. E., and van der Hart, M.: Recherches sero-logiques dans les anémies hémolytiques acquises. *Congrès Français de Medecine, Trentième Session,* Masson et Compagnie, Editeurs, Paris, 1957.

79. Kochwa, S., and Rosenfield, R. E.: Immuno-chemical studies of the Rh system. I. Isolation and characterization of antibodies. J. Immun. **92**: 682, 1964.

80. Jensen, K. G.: Elution of incomplete antibodies from red cells. A comparison of different methods. Vox Sang. **4**: 230, 1959.

81. Croucher, B. E. E., Crookston, M. C., and Crookston, J. H.: Delayed haemolytic transfusion reactions simulating auto-immune haemolytic anaemia. Vox Sang. **13**: 32, 1967.

82. Fong, S. W., and Masouredis, S. P.: Physico-chemical and immunologic properties of eluates containing I^{125} anti-Rh$_o$(D). J. Immun. **98**: 374, 1967.

83. Ogata, T., and Matuhasi, T.: Problems of specific and cross reactivity of blood group antibodies. In *Proceedings of the Eighth Congress of the International Society of Blood Transfusion.* S. Karger, Basel, 1962.

84. Ogata, T., and Matuhasi, T.: Further observations on the problems of specific and cross reactivity of blood group antibodies. In *Proceedings of the Ninth Congress of the International Society of Blood Transfusion.* S. Karger, Basel, 1964.

85. Issitt, P. D., Allen, F. H., Degnan, T. J., Jackson, V., Reihart, J., and Knowlin, R.: Further observations on the Ogata phenomenon (abstract). Paper presented at the Twentieth Annual Meeting of the American Association of Blood Banks, New York, October 23, 1967.

86. Svardal, J. M., Yarbro, J., and Yunis, E. J.: Ogata phenomenon explaining the unusual specificity in eluates from Coombs positive cells sensitized by autogenous anti-I. Vox Sang. **13**: 472, 1967.

87. Selwyn, J. G., and Hackett, W. E. R.: Acquired haemolytic anaemia: survival of transfused erythrocytes in patients and normal recipients. J. Clin. Path. **2**: 114, 1949.

88. Evans, R. S., Bingham, M., and Boehni, P.: Autoimmune hemolytic disease. Antibody dissociation and activity. Arch. Intern. Med. (Chicago) **108**: 60, 1961.

89. Evans, R. S., Turner, E., and Bingham, M.: Studies of I^{131} tagged Rh antibody of D specificity. Vox Sang. **8**: 153, 1963.

90. Hughes-Jones, N. C.: Nature of the reaction between antigen and antibody. Brit. Med. Bull. **19**: 171, 1963.

91. Roth, K. L.: Interaction of heparin with auto-agglutinins in idiopathic acquired hemolytic anemia. Proc. Soc. Exp. Biol. Med. **86**: 352, 1954.

92. Roth, K. L., and Frumin, A. M.: Effect of intramuscular heparin on antibodies in idiopathic acquired hemolytic anemia. Amer. J. Med. **20**: 968, 1956.

93. McFarland, W., Galbraith, R. G., and Miale, A.: Heparin therapy in autoimmune hemolytic anemia. Blood **15**: 741, 1960.

94. Hartman, M. M.: Reversal of serologic reactions by heparin: therapeutic implications. II. Idiopathic acquired hemolytic anemia (IAHA). Ann. Allerg. **22**: 313, 1964.

95. Ten Pas, A., and Monto, R. W.: The treatment of autoimmune hemolytic anemia with heparin. Amer. J. Med. Sci. **251**: 63, 1966.

96. Ecker, E. E., and Gross, P.: Anticomplementary power of heparin. J. Infect. Dis. **44**: 250, 1929.

97. Von Falkenhausen, M.: Körpereigene (anti-prothrombin bzw. Heparin) und körper-fremde (Germanin, Salvarsan) gerinnung-shemmende Substanzen in ihrer Beziehung zur Vorstufe des Gerinnungsfermentes (Prothrombin). Z. Ges. Exp. Med. **79**: 18, 1931.

98. Wising, P. J.: The identity of prothrombin and the midpiece of complement. Acta Med. Scand. **94**: 506, 1938.

99. Storti, E., and Vaccari, F.: Studies on the relationship between anticoagulants and hemolysis. Part I. Effect of anticoagulants on hemolysis and on the agglutination of red blood cells by anti-erythrocyte serum. Acta Haemat. (Basel) **15**: 12, 1956.

100. Rosenfield, R. E., Vitale, B., and Kochwa, S.: Immune mechanisms for destruction of erythrocytes in vivo. II. Heparinization for protection of lysin-sensitized erythrocytes. Transfusion **7**: 261, 1967.

101. Ecker, E. E., and Pillemer, L.: Anti-coagulants and complementary activity. An experimental study. J. Immun. **40**: 73, 1941.
102. Roth, K. L.: Notes on the relationship between the therapeutic and anti-complementary effects of heparin in acquired hemolytic anemia. Ann. Allerg. **23**: 83, 1965.
103. Pirofsky, B., Cordova, M. S., and Rigas, D.: The mechanism of streptomycin inhibition of erythrocyte antibodies. Vox Sang. **9**: 653, 1964.
104. Roth, K. L., and Frumin, A. M.: In vitro differentiation between auto- and iso-immune antibodies by protamine and trypsin. Science **120**: 945, 1954.
105. Lalezari, P., Szilagy, A., and Couig, D.: The use of a new method of antibody detection in the blood bank. Paper presented at the Twentieth Annual Meeting of the American Association of Blood Banks, New York, October 23, 1967.
106. Godal, H. C., and Norseth, T.: Inhibition of red cell aggregation by TAME. Scand. J. Haemat. **3**: 383, 1966.
107. Martin du Pan, R.: L'ictère hémolytique, les "hémagglutinines" et les antiagglutinines. Schweiz. Med. Wschr. **78**: 34, 1948.
108. Denys, P., and van den Broucke, J.: Anémie hémolytique acquise et réaction de Coombs. Arch. Franc. Pediat. **4**: 205, 1947.
109. Rosenthal, M. C., and Schwartz, L. I.: Reversible agglutination of trypsin-treated erythrocytes by normal human sera. Proc. Soc. Exp. Biol. Med. **76**: 635, 1951.
110. Spaet, T. H., and Ostrum, B. W.: Studies on the normal serum panhemagglutinin active against trypsinated human erythrocytes. Part I: The mechanism of agglutination reversal. J. Clin. Path. **5**: 332, 1952.
111. Janković, B. D.: An incomplete warm antibody in normal human serum. Acta Med. Iugosl. **8**: 174, 1954.
112. Delage, J. M.: Natural warm auto-antibody. Canad. Med. Ass. J. **78**: 113, 1958.
113. Weiner, W., Tovery, G. H., Gillespie, E. M., Lewis, H. B. M., and Holliday, T. D. S.: "Albumin" autoagglutinating property in three sera. "A pitfall for the unwary." Vox Sang. **1**: 279, 1956.
114. Weiner, W., and Hallum, J.: A further "albumin" auto-agglutinating serum. Vox Sang. **2**: 38, 1957.
115. Moore, B. P. L., Linins, I., and McIntyre, J.: A serum with an albumin active autoagglutinating property. Blood **14**: 364, 1959.
116. Marsh, W. L., and Jenkins, W. J.: A possible specificity of albumin autoantibodies. Nature (London) **190**: 180, 1961.
117. Crowley, L. V., and Hyland, F. R.: The albumin auto-agglutination phenomenon. Amer. J. Clin. Path. **37**: 244, 1962.
118. Hossaini, A. A., Burkhart, C. R., and Hooper, G. S.: A further example of the non-immune auto-agglutinating property of serum. Transfusion **5**: 461, 1965.
119. Hossaini, A. A.: Effects of albumin concentration on compatibility tests for blood transfusion. Amer. J. Clin. Path. **45**: 348, 1966.
120. Kout, M., and Kubickova, Z.: Influence of streptomycin solutions on the interaction between the agglutinating sera and the corresponding red blood cell receptors. Nature (London) **184**: 639, 1959.
121. Boyd, W. C., McMaster, M. H., and Waszczenko-Zacharczenko, E.: Specific inhibition of anti-Rh serum by "unnatural" sugars. Nature (London) **184**: 989, 1959.
122. Pirofsky, B., and Cordova, M. S.: The in vitro neutralization of erythrocyte auto-antibodies and iso-antibodies. Bibl. Haemat. **19**: 550, 1964.
123. Pirofsky, B., and Cordova, M. S.: The in vitro inhibition of erythrocyte antibodies by hexosamine-containing antibiotics. Brit. J. Haemat. **10**: 320, 1964.
124. Gralnick, H. R., and McGinniss, M.: Nature of the Coombs positive reaction with sodium cephalothin. Paper presented at the Twentieth Annual Meeting of the American Association of Blood Banks, New York, October 24, 1967.

Chapter 18

The Demonstration of Warm Acting Erythrocyte Autoantibodies

Warm acting erythrocyte autoantibodies are generally incomplete and they rarely induce spontaneous agglutination or hemolysis of saline suspended erythrocytes. It is therefore necessary to employ additional test systems to demonstrate the presence of such autoantibodies. Three major categories of test procedures are commonly used. These include colloid anisometric macromolecular solutions, the antiglobulin test and various proteolytic enzymes. One point deserves emphasis. Warm acting erythrocyte autoantibodies manifest marked variations of serologic reactivity. It is unduly optimistic to hope that any single test procedure will have the capacity to demonstrate all warm acting erythrocyte autoantibodies. A combination of two or more test systems is recommended for any investigation involving warm acting erythrocyte autoantibodies.

Colloid Anisometric Macromolecular Systems

Bovine Serum Albumin

When erythrocytes coated with incomplete antibodies are suspended in serum, spontaneous agglutination occasionally occurs. This suggests that serum components may be useful in demonstrating incomplete erythrocyte autoantibodies. Wiener (1) in 1945 added albumin to test suspensions of warm acting erythrocyte autoantibodies, and he reported autohemagglutination. The albumin induced reaction was postulated to result from conglutination. It therefore

represented a nonimmunologic effect as required by Wiener's univalent concept of incomplete erythrocyte antibodies (2).

Brüggemann and Hahn (3) noted that a thermal stable serum component was required for the autohemagglutination effect of warm acting incomplete erythrocyte autoantibodies. The patient's own serum could be employed for this purpose (4). Evans and Weiser (5) used a mixture of 30 per cent bovine albumin and patient serum in a test procedure to demonstrate incomplete warm acting erythrocyte autoantibodies. Agglutination was produced in 18 of 41 cases studied. Thirty-seven of the 41 patients, however, had positive antiglobulin tests. A comparative study by van Loghem and associates (6) noted a similar lack of sensitivity of the albumin technique.

Other Reagents

Other solutions containing colloid anisometric molecules have been employed to induce autohemagglutination of erythrocytes coated with incomplete antibodies. Evans and associates (7) successfully employed 2 per cent gum acacia. Heni and Blessing (8) noted the ability of dextran to potentiate the agglutination of antibody coated erythrocytes.

The most extensive study of colloid macromolecular potentiation of hemagglutination was reported by Jandl and Castle (9). In addition to albumin, they tested various human plasma fractions and several synthetic macromolecular solutions. These included dextran, polyvinylpyrrolidone

(PVP) and carboxymethyl cellulose. Their test system depended on agglutination of $Rh_o(D)$ erythrocytes by incomplete anti-$Rh_o(D)$. On the basis of concentration, fibrinogen was the most effective and albumin the least effective additive studied. The synthetic substance PVP was a highly effective reagent for potentiating autoagglutination established by incomplete erythrocyte isoantibodies. A similar observation of the efficiency of PVP had been made by McNeil and associates (10). They established a PVP typing system involving incomplete anti-$Rh_o(D)$. In the study of Jandl and Castle (9) 5 per cent PVP was more efficient than 25 per cent albumin and occasionally appeared to be more sensitive than was the antiglobulin test.

Present Status

Colloidal test solutions employing high concentrations of anisometric macromolecules are currently valuable in limited serologic testing. The albumin procedure has been modified into a high speed centrifugation method for documentation of the D^u factor of erythrocytes (11). Similar techniques have been found to be efficient in demonstrating vast numbers and types of incomplete erythrocyte isoantibodies (12). Recent reports (13) have stressed the advantage of performing the antiglobulin procedure after incubation of test erythrocytes and serum in albumin, rather than in the usual saline suspension. The benefits of this method have not been confirmed by other workers (14). This latter observation more closely follows the experience in our laboratory.

It is extremely difficult to evaluate the current role of techniques employing colloid macromolecular solutions for the demonstration of incomplete erythrocyte autoantibodies. Albumin procedures as used in the past, with slide techniques or low speed centrifugation (1000 r.p.m.), are insensitive and of little value except for an occasional uncommon serum. High speed centrifugation procedures with albumin deserve more detailed consideration. PVP techniques offer great potential in the search for warm acting erythrocyte autoantibodies. This author has observed the use of PVP solutions combined with incomplete anti-$Rh_o(D)$ for routine blood typing in a 12-year period with almost one million blood samples. It is a highly efficient, rapid and inexpensive technique. It appears to be as sensitive as the antiglobulin procedure in determining the presence of the D^u factor.

Antiglobulin Serum

Historical Review and Terminology

In 1944 Wiener (2) and Race (15) independently demonstrated an incomplete or blocking form of anti-erythrocyte antibody. This explained the frequent inability to document an erythrocyte autoantibody in many cases of autoimmune hemolytic anemia. Erythrocytes from patients with autoimmune hemolytic anemia could be coated with incomplete erythrocyte antibodies undemonstrable by available techniques. Additional sensitive serologic procedures were necessary for the analysis of such disease states.

In 1907 and 1908 Friedberger and Moreschi (16) and Moreschi (17) reported a technique to demonstrate the fixation of serum protein molecules to the erythrocyte surface. An antiserum produced against human serum was reacted with erythrocytes coated with human serum components. Hemagglutination was the end point of the reaction. The concept of incomplete erythrocyte antibodies had not been developed and the authors did not apply this technique to erythrocyte antibodies. The procedure was generally forgotten and did not attain widespread usage. In 1945 Coombs and associates (18) independently rediscovered this approach. They postulated that incomplete erythrocyte antibodies were globulin molecules. If erythrocytes were coated with such substances, an antiserum directed against human globulin might induce agglutination. Rabbits were immunized with human serum and with the globulin components of human serum in order to produce an anti-human globulin antiserum. This reagent was then reacted with erythrocytes coated with incomplete anti-$Rh_o(D)$ antibodies. Agglutination resulted, demonstrating the incomplete antibody fixed to the erythrocyte surface.

The rabbit antiserum employed in this reaction has been variously termed anti-human globulin serum, AHG serum, antiglobulin serum and Coombs serum. The test procedure, when employed to demonstrate incomplete antibody fixed to the erythrocyte, has been called a direct anti-human globulin test, a direct AHG test, a direct antiglobulin test or a direct Coombs test. In order to demonstrate unbound incomplete antibodies in the patient's serum, it is necessary to incubate the serum with erythrocytes containing the appropriate antigen and then to employ the rabbit antiserum. This has been termed an indirect anti-human globulin test, indirect AHG test, indirect antiglobulin test or indirect Coombs test.

The phrase "Coombs test" has received the widest usage. This frequently introduces difficulty. Two separate tests are involved and they are employed for different purposes. The clinician who orders a "Coombs test" is requesting the laboratory technologist to decide upon one of two different available procedures. The laboratory must determine whether the intent is to demonstrate an antibody fixed to the red cell or circulating unbound in the serum.

There has been a tendency to use the eponyms "Coombs test" and "Coombs serum" less and less. This is not meant to detract from the brilliant studies of Coombs and his associates. Rather, an awareness of the major contributions of Coombs to the field of immunohematology forces one to avoid the term "Coombs test." The antiglobulin procedure, the I^{131} labeled antibody technique, the mixed agglutination test, the erythrocyte linked antigen test and the various immunoconglutinin procedures are all "Coombs tests" and reflect the fertile ingenuity of R. R. A. Coombs and his associates.

The term anti-human globulin test is clumsy and is not employed unless it is crucial to document the species producing the erythrocyte antibody. For example, in studying the autoimmune phenomenon seen with NZB mice, an anti-mouse globulin test is employed. The abbreviation "AHG test" for anti-human globulin test is to be condemned. AHG can be interpreted as meaning anti-hemophiliac globulin and investigators in coagulation already have a quantitative AHG test. The abbreviations "D.C.T." and "I.C.T." have recently become popular in the British literature. These symbolize a direct Coombs test and indirect Coombs test, respectively. They appear to have little value other than economy and should be avoided as confusing. Most investigators utilize the terms antiglobulin serum and direct and indirect antiglobulin tests.

Types of Antiglobulin Serum

Antiglobulin serum is produced by immunizing various animals, generally the rabbit or goat, with small amounts of normal human serum globulin components. Essentially similar antiglobulin sera are obtained with globulin from normal serum and from sera of patients with either primary or secondary types of autoimmune hemolytic anemia. Eluates obtained from normal erythrocytes or erythrocytes coated with anti-rhesus antibodies or erythrocyte autoantibodies are also immunogenic and produce similar reagents. Antiglobulin sera made in this fashion are termed broad spectrum antiglobulin sera. Modifications of broad spectrum antiglobulin serum may be employed. An anti-gamma-globulin serum may be produced by immunizing the test animal with pure IgG immunoglobulins. The addition of small amounts of pure IgG globulin to broad spectrum antiglobulin serum produces a non-gamma antiglobulin serum. The types of non-gamma antiglobulin sera may be expanded by developing specific antiserum against purified complement components, etc. Radioactive labels may be incorporated in the globulin fraction of the antiglobulin serum. The use of such labeled antiglobulin serum has been reported by several workers with varying claims of success in kinetic studies (19, 20).

Mechanisms of Action

The antiglobulin test is the most important laboratory procedure available for the diagnosis and investigation of autoimmune hemolytic anemia. Although this test is simple to perform, a complex serologic phenomenon is involved. The immunologic principles must be completely understood if the results obtained are to be intelligently interpreted.

The antiglobulin test was developed on the basis of studies performed by Race (15) and Wiener (2). Wiener (2) postulated a univalent antibody structure for incomplete antibodies in order to explain their nonagglutinating blocking action. Antiglobulin serum was produced to supply bivalent antibodies capable of reacting with human globulins. Such antibodies would have the ability to fix to an antigenic determinant of an erythrocyte antibody attached to one erythrocyte. Fixation of the other antibody combining site to a second erythrocyte autoantibody on a second erythrocyte could then occur. This bridging effect of antiglobulin serum would form a lattice framework, leading to erythrocyte aggrega-

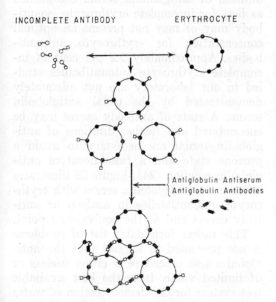

FIGURE 36. The mode of action of antiglobulin serum in inducing agglutination of erythrocytes coated with incomplete erythrocyte antibodies.

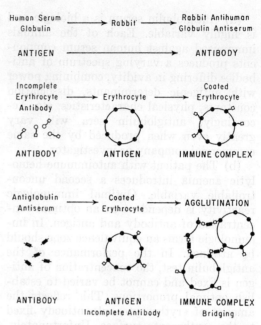

FIGURE 37. The antiglobulin reaction. Incomplete erythrocyte antibody functions as an antibody in combining with erythrocyte antigen. In the antiglobulin reaction, however, the incomplete antibody acts as the globulin antigen.

tion and agglutination. Figure 36 illustrates this relationship.

The antiglobulin test is accordingly dependent on an immunologic interaction between antigen and antibody. It therefore differs from the techniques using colloidal macromolecular solutions and proteolytic enzymes, in which nonimmunologic effects are important. Antiglobulin serum contains antibodies specifically directed against human globulin molecules. The reaction of incomplete erythrocyte antibodies with erythrocytes leads to fixation of the antibody to the cellular surface. In terms of the antiglobulin reaction, the incomplete erythrocyte antibody must be considered as an antigen. Figure 37 illustrates this relationship.

An immunologic interaction between antibody and antigen is the cornerstone of the antiglobulin reaction. This introduces several problems when the procedure is routinely applied in autoimmune hemolytic anemia (21).

(a) Antiglobulin serum is a biologic and is highly variable. Each of the animals immunized against human serum components produces a varying spectrum of antibodies differing in avidity, combining power with antigenic determinants, dissociation constants, physical characteristics, etc. Accordingly, antiglobulin sera will vary greatly even when produced by the same commercial company or investigator.

(b) The patient with autoimmune hemolytic anemia introduces a second uncontrollable variable. Optimal immunologic reactivity is dependent on an optimal concentration of antibody and antigen. In immunologic terms an equivalence zone should be attained. In the performance of the antiglobulin test, the concentration of antigen is fixed and cannot be varied to establish optimal proportions. This reflects the amount of erythrocyte autoantibody fixed to the erythrocyte surface. Unfortunately, each patient with autoimmune hemolytic anemia probably presents a different concentration of antigen (erythrocyte autoantibody) to be reacted with antiglobulin serum.

(c) The marked heterogeneity of erythrocyte autoantibodies (22, 23) creates a further problem in establishing a correct ratio of antiglobulin antibody to erythrocyte antibody (human globulin antigen). Erythrocyte autoantibodies have differences of avidity and of antibody-antigen dissociation constants as well as different rates of erythrocyte antibody dissociation from erythrocytes. All of these factors are involved in arriving at a correct ratio between antibody and antigen. Each patient with hemolytic anemia presents an autoantibody with different kinetics for reaction with the erythrocyte surface and antiglobulin serum.

(d) The problem is further magnified by establishing a fixed concentration of antiglobulin serum. The commercial supply of this reagent creates such a fixed antibody system. When antiserum against human globulin is produced it frequently is in a zone of antibody excess in relation to incomplete warm acting erythrocyte autoantibodies and isoantibodies. It also may appear at equivalence in relationship to cold acting antibodies. Antiglobulin serum is infrequently employed to demonstrate cold acting erythrocyte antibodies. Accordingly, the neat antiserum is diluted out of antibody excess to a level approaching the equivalence point for reaction with warm acting incomplete iso- and autoantibodies. This generally requires a 60- to 100-fold dilution of the neat antiglobulin serum. Most commercial sources establish the dilution ratio of antiglobulin serum as best suited for the demonstration of incomplete anti-Rh_o(D). In recent years an attempt has been made to create a "polyvalent" antiglobulin serum by blending the sera from various immunized animals. Such antiglobulin sera may have a greater capacity to demonstrate other incomplete erythrocyte isoantibodies such as anti-Fy^a, anti-K, anti-Jk^a, etc. It is apparent that a universal dilution to demonstrate optimally every antibody cannot be attained when the erythrocytes of each patient have a different concentration of antibody. This problem is magnified when it is recalled that antibodies of the same specificity also have wide heterogeneity (22, 23). The fixed dilution of antiglobulin serum established as best for incomplete erythrocyte isoantibody may or may not present an optimal concentration for erythrocyte autoantibodies. Approximately 2.2 per cent of incomplete erythrocyte autoantibodies studied in our laboratory are not adequately demonstrated by the usual antiglobulin serum. A state of antibody excess may be encountered and further dilutions of antiglobulin serum are necessary to avoid a prozone state and a false negative antiglobulin reaction (24). Figure 38 illustrates reactions of antiglobulin serum with erythrocyte autoantibodies in antigen or antibody excess and at the equivalence point.

This rather formidable list of problems is not presented to suggest that the antiglobulin test procedure is either useless or of limited value. It is the best available test system for the demonstration of warm acting erythrocyte autoantibodies. Because we are so dependent on this procedure in investigating autoimmune hemolytic anemia, the inadequacies and possible pitfalls have been emphasized. We are fortunate that the antiglobulin procedure works as well as it does in spite of the objections outlined. The clinician and investigator, however, must be aware of the inherent limitations of this test. It is unwarranted to consider a positive antiglobulin test as synonymous with autoimmune hemolytic anemia and a negative test as eliminating the presence of this disease.

Theoretical Concepts

The development of the antiglobulin procedure by Coombs and associates (18) was based on two fundamental assumptions. Experimental data suggested that erythrocytes could be coated with a human globulin acting as a nonagglutinating erythrocyte antibody (2, 15). In addition it was assumed that normal human globulin was not present on the erythrocyte. This latter assumption was necessary to permit the application of an antiglobulin test. Antiglobulin serum contains antibodies directed against normal human globulin, rather than antibodies having the capability to react specifically and exclusively with erythrocyte antibodies. The first assumption has been confirmed. However, the second assumption is in error and suggests that our concept of the mechanism of action of antiglobulin serum deserves reevaluation.

In 1953 Boursnell and associates (25) investigated the kinetics of I^{131} trace labeled erythrocyte isoantibodies. It was noted that erythrocytes were coated with the labeled gamma-globulin preparations independent of antigenic specificity. The elegant studies of Masouredis (26) employing I^{131} trace labeled erythrocyte isoantibodies were similarly complicated by the nonimmunologic binding of globulin molecules onto the erythrocyte surface. Meticulous care had to be exercised to produce erythrocyte antibody eluates which would not coat erythrocytes in a nonimmunologic fashion.

Pirofsky and associates (27) confirmed and expanded these observations. They demonstrated that a substantial number of IgG molecules would fix to the erythrocyte surface in a nonimmunologic fashion. A log-log relationship was shown between

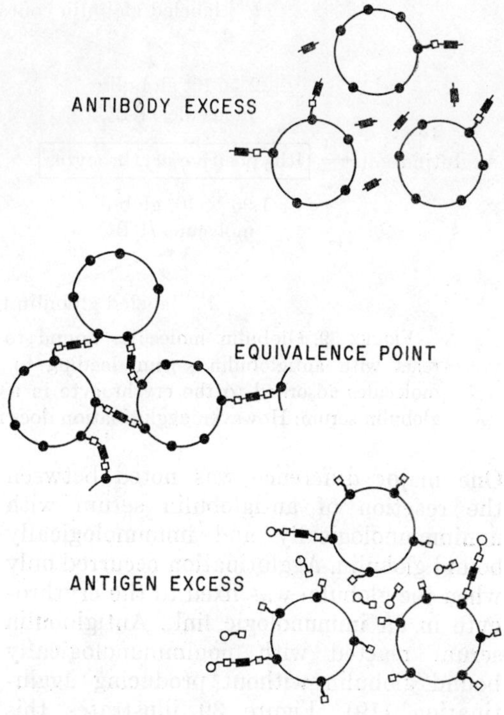

FIGURE 38. The antiglobulin reaction. Schematic representation of the effect of antiglobulin serum and incomplete antibody concentration on hemagglutination. Optimal agglutination occurs at the equivalence zone. Excess antiglobulin serum may inhibit agglutination, creating a prozone phenomenon. Theoretically, a heavy erythrocyte antibody coating may dissociate, inhibiting agglutination through antigen excess.

globulin concentration in the suspending media and globulin fixed to erythrocytes. Approximately 200,000 globulin molecules adsorbed to the erythrocyte at globulin solution concentrations of 1 mg. per ml. The magnitude of this reaction is apparent when it is contrasted with the observation of Masouredis (28) that saturation of $Rh_o(D)$ antigenic sites of homozygous erythrocytes was obtained with approximately 10,000 anti-$Rh_o(D)$ antibody molecules. Antiglobulin serum fixed to nonimmunologically bound globulin at a slightly lesser rate than to antibody bound globulin (19). The difference possibly represented labeled globulin trapped in the agglutinated mass. Elution of nonimmunologically bound globulin from erythrocytes produced globulin solutions able to neutralize antiglobulin serum.

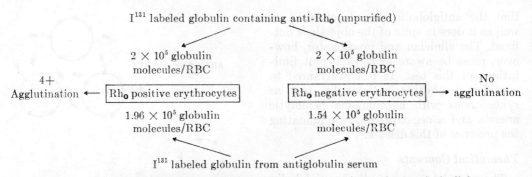

I^{131} labeled globulin containing anti-Rh_0 (unpurified)

2 × 10⁵ globulin
molecules/RBC

2 × 10⁵ globulin
molecules/RBC

4+
Agglutination ← | Rh_0 positive erythrocytes | | Rh_0 negative erythrocytes | → No agglutination

1.96 × 10⁵ globulin
molecules/RBC

1.54 × 10⁵ globulin
molecules/RBC

I^{131} labeled globulin from antiglobulin serum

FIGURE 39. Globulin molecules bound to the erythrocyte in an immunologic linkage react with antiglobulin serum, leading to agglutination. A similar number of globulin molecules adsorbed to the erythrocyte in a nonimmunologic fashion also react with antiglobulin serum. However, agglutination does not occur.

One major difference was noted between the reaction of antiglobulin serum with nonimmunologically and immunologically bound globulin. Agglutination occurred only when the globulin was fixed to the erythrocyte in an immunologic link. Antiglobulin serum reacted with nonimmunologically bound globulin without producing agglutination (19). Figure 39 illustrates this relationship.

No satisfactory explanation for this phenomenon exists at this time. Nonimmunologically bound globulin is firmly fixed to the erythrocyte surface and is not removed after 15 washings. It is possible that the agglutinating specificity of antiglobulin serum relates to the degree or lack of exposure of the Fc fragment of the H chain of the globulin molecule. Different steric relationships may result from immunologic or nonimmunologic binding characteristics. A similar concept has been presented by Gergely and associates (29), who have confirmed the nonimmunologic reaction of globulin to the erythrocyte surface. Nonimmunologic binding appeared to be related to a papain insensitive population of IgG immunoglobulins. It is suggested that a difference of the molecular conformation of the Fc fragment leads to nonimmunologic binding and to papain insensitivity. This hypothesis appears to be tenuous and may have to be discarded. The studies of Eyster and associates (30) clearly show that antiserum directed against L chains may induce agglutination of erythrocytes coated with incomplete antibodies.

The theoretical considerations involved in the action of antiglobulin serum may appear esoteric. However, several aspects are of major importance in the clinical application of the antiglobulin test. Modification of the erythrocyte surface may also modify the manner and effect of normal globulin fixation to the erythrocyte. Positive antiglobulin tests can then occur in the absence of erythrocyte antibodies. Such positive reactions may only reflect the change of erythrocyte surface or globulin molecular characteristics. The nonimmunologic fixation of gamma-globulin may now exist in a physical state permitting an agglutinating antiglobulin serum reaction. Metallic cations, lead, lipoid solvents, phenylhydrazine and reticulocytes all induce false positive antiglobulin reactions. These reactions may reflect this phenomenon. An excellent review of this problem has been presented by Muirhead (31). Alternatively, normal globulin molecules may be directly modified, permitting them to react in an agglutinating pattern with antiglobulin serum, after nonimmunologic fixation to the cellular surface. Cephalothin (32) and trypan blue (33) may be the prototype of this reaction. The basic charge of cephalothin may be the critical factor in creating a globulin-drug complex (34).

Several of the original concepts leading to development of the antiglobulin procedure have now been invalidated. The postulate that incomplete erythrocyte auto-antibodies are univalent must be discarded (35, 36). The assumption that fixation of globulin molecules to erythrocytes occurs only in an immunologic fashion is erroneous (25, 27, 29). Our current theoretical knowledge is insufficient to explain exactly how antiglobulin serum functions. What remains is the clinical observation that the antiglobulin procedure is the most efficient means that we have to demonstrate incomplete erythrocyte autoantibodies fixed to a patient's own erythrocytes. Delineation of the mechanism of antiglobulin serum action may eventually result in the future development of more precise and sensitive tools for the demonstration of incomplete erythrocyte autoantibodies.

The Use of Proteolytic Enzymes

In 1947 Morton and Pickles (37) introduced proteolytic enzymes for the detection of incomplete erythrocyte isoantibodies. The effect of such enzymes was first noted during an analysis of filtrates of *Vibrio cholerae*. It was found that erythrocytes treated with such filtrates were directly agglutinated by incomplete erythrocyte antibodies. These investigators considered the possibility that proteolytic enzymes manufactured by *V. cholerae* modified the erythrocyte surface sufficiently to permit direct agglutination. They investigated the action of various proteolytic enzymes in this test system and selected trypsin as the most reliable agent.

Trypsin System

The trypsin test system to demonstrate incomplete erythrocyte antibodies required pretreatment of the erythrocyte with trypsin. Excess enzyme was then washed out and the trypsinized erythrocytes were exposed to serum containing incomplete antibody. Direct agglutination was searched for. Many investigators compared this test system with the albumin and antiglobulin procedures. It was almost universally conceded that the trypsin pretreatment technique was substantially more sensitive than were plasma-albumin autohemagglutination or the indirect antiglobulin test.

The older literature has been well summarized by Dacie (38). Dausset and Colombani (39) noted that the trypsin procedure was substantially more sensitive than was the antiglobulin technique. The sera of 72 patients with autoimmune hemolytic anemia were tested in duplicate. Two-thirds had positive trypsin tests. Only one-half of these could be documented by the indirect antiglobulin test. Currently, trypsin is rarely if ever used to demonstrate incomplete erythrocyte antibodies. The reagent is expensive and the procedure is time consuming. The presence of a normal serum agglutinin (40, 41) directed against trypsinized erythrocytes also complicates the test. These characteristics have minimized the use of this reagent.

Papain System

Kuhns and Bailey (42) in 1950 introduced the use of papain in a test procedure designed to demonstrate incomplete erythrocyte antibodies. Papain is an inexpensive enzyme preparation obtained from papaya. The papain test system employed an erythrocyte pretreatment phase similar to that used with trypsin. Papainized erythrocytes were incubated with serum containing warm acting incomplete erythrocyte antibodies, and agglutination was determined. The efficiency, lack of expense and ease of handling of papain led to its preferential use over trypsin. The sensitivity of papainized erythrocytes to demonstrate incomplete erythrocyte autoantibodies was repeatedly demonstrated (43). Heller and associates (44) studied the sera obtained from 164 patients with a variety of autoimmune hematologic diseases. Erythrocyte autoantibodies could be demonstrated using papainized cells in 31 per cent of these cases. The antiglobulin technique gave positive results in only 2.4 per cent of cases.

Activated Papain System

Löw in 1955 (45) modified the standard papain technique by adding L-cysteine. This procedure "activated" the enzyme through weak disulfide reduction. With such an activated papain solution it was possible to avoid pretreatment of erythrocytes, substantially shortening the time required to demonstrate incomplete erythrocyte antibodies (46). Löw's activated papain test system consists of the serum to be tested, appropriate erythrocytes, and the addition of activated papain. After incubation the presence of incomplete antibodies is indicated by direct agglutination. The papain and activated papain techniques are extremely sensitive in demonstrating unbound warm acting incomplete erythrocyte autoantibodies. The major problem with this procedure is the extreme lability of the activated reagent. Activated papain must be stored frozen and unused reagents must be discarded after thawing.

Ficin System

Ficin, a proteolytic enzyme extracted from figs, was introduced into immunohematology by Wiener and Katz (47) and Makinodan and Macris (48). The ficin test system is similar to the papain system and utilizes the enzymatic pretreatment of erythrocytes. In addition, a test system similar to the activated papain test may be employed. Incomplete erythrocyte antibodies will induce direct agglutination of erythrocytes under the influence of ficin. This test procedure has been found to be efficient for the demonstration of incomplete warm acting erythrocyte autoantibodies. The ficin dry powder is highly corrosive to mucous membranes. This observation has limited the use of the ficin reagent to selected research laboratories.

Bromelin System

Bromelin is a crude mixture of proteolytic enzymes obtained from the pineapple. Pirofsky and Mangum (49, 50) in 1959 employed this enzyme in a test procedure designed to demonstrate incomplete erythrocyte antibodies. Their studies indicated that bromelin was in an "activated" state and could be used directly without pretreatment of erythrocytes. In addition, the reagent appeared to be stable in solution for weeks at refrigerator temperatures. The bromelin test procedure employed the direct admixture of the serum to be tested, appropriate erythrocytes and the bromelin solution buffered at an acid pH. The

reaction is extremely rapid. Immediate centrifugation may reveal agglutination of erythrocytes by incomplete erythrocyte antibodies. Incubation for 15 minutes at room temperature appears optimal. Both warm and cold acting and incomplete and complete erythrocyte antibodies can be demonstrated. Extensive experience with this procedure indicates that it is a sensitive method to document the presence of erythrocyte autoantibodies (21, 51).

Gray (52) has employed bromelin in a pretreatment technique similar to that used with papain and trypsin. This method appears to be efficient. In addition, Ellis (53) has modified the procedure by adding ethylenediaminetetraacetic acid to the bromelin reagent. The advantage of this additive appears to reside in its acidity which maintains the acid pH obtained by buffers in the system of Pirofsky and Mangum (49, 50). Inattention to the crucial acid pH of this test system creates an unstable reagent and an insensitive test system (43, 54).

Pronase System

Nomoto and associates (55, 56) have extracted and purified a proteolytic enzyme produced by *Streptomyces griseus* which is commonly referred to as pronase. This material contains a number of proteases and has broad specificity (57). Buchanan and Dierich (58) in 1965 employed this material for the detection of incomplete erythrocyte antibodies. The enzyme was found to be rapidly active in a pretreatment system similar to papain and in a direct system comparable to bromelin. Cook and Eylar (59) reported that pronase activity on the erythrocyte surface resulted in the release of *N*-acetylneuraminic acid. This observation has been confirmed by Prager and associates (60) who reviewed the literature and correlated specific activity with the liberation of *N*-acetylneuraminic acid.

Other Systems

For many years the use of proteolytic enzymes remained restricted to the research laboratory. Problems of stability, potency and standardization prevented their general use in the routine laboratory. It has become increasingly apparent that restricting a search for incomplete erythrocyte antibodies to albumin and antiglobulin procedures is unnecessary and dangerous in the routine blood bank and serology laboratory (12, 51, 61, 62). Any combination of procedures devised to document the presence of incomplete erythrocyte iso- or autoantibodies currently must contain an enzyme technique. It is axiomatic that no single procedure is competent to demonstrate all erythrocyte antibodies. The development of practical and standard enzyme preparations and procedures is crucial. This problem has been solved to a great extent by various commercial sources of individual enzymatic reagents and combinations of enzymes designed for use in the routine investigation of erythrocyte antibodies. Such preparations have now made it possible for all laboratories to employ the finest techniques in the search for incomplete erythrocyte antibodies.

The Mechanism of Action of Proteolytic Enzymes

The means by which proteolytic enzymes permit incomplete erythrocyte antibodies to induce direct agglutination of red cells are unknown. Wiener and Katz (47) suggested that digestion removed nonspecific serum proteins which obscured the antigen. Wheeler and associates (63) speculated that proteolytic enzymes modified the erythrocyte surface to rearrange or uncover the antigenic structure. Both of these suggestions would require an increased fixation of incomplete antibody to the erythrocyte. Confirmation of increased antibody binding has been obtained for bromelin (64), papain (65) and ficin (66) treatment of erythrocytes. However, the increased number of antibodies bound to the surface is not responsible for agglutination (64). Pirofsky and associates (64) demonstrated the agglutination of enzyme treated erythrocytes with less than half the number of antibody molecules fixed to unagglutinated erythrocytes which were untreated with enzyme.

In 1951 Ponder (67) observed a decrease in mobility of erythrocytes treated with trypsin. Gottschalk (68) demonstrated that the active principle of the *V. cholerae* filtrates employed by Morton and Pickles (37) was neuraminidase. It was subsequently shown that proteolytic enzymes release mucoids containing N-acylated neuraminic acids from the erythrocyte surface (60, 69–73). The removal of these sialosubstances from the polyanionic charged erythrocyte (74) reduces the electrostatic charge at the erythrocyte surface, decreasing electrophoretic mobility. Seaman and Cook (75) have summarized the mechanisms through which proteolytic enzymes influence the surface charge and mobility of erythrocytes in electrical fields. As discussed in Chapter 17, a similar reduction of the electrophoretic mobility of erythrocytes has been noted following the action of some erythrocyte antibodies. This surface charge lowering effect of erythrocyte antibodies is neither universal nor consistent. Prager and associates (60, 73, 76) have investigated the chemical and serologic events subsequent to proteolytic enzyme treatment. Their studies have resulted in the following conclusions (60): (1) Proteases which induce the serologic effect hydrolyse derivatives of lysine and arginine. (2) Such enzymes are bound to the erythrocyte surface but must be catalytically active to effect the serologic reaction. (3) Neuraminidase duplicates the action of proteolytic enzymes. (4) N-acetylneuraminic acid is released from erythrocytes in a manner correlating with serologic reactivity. (5) The release of N-acetylneuraminic acid is probably responsible for the decrease of erythrocyte surface charge and may be the ultimate factor determining agglutination.

On the basis of such studies several suggestions as to the mode of action of proteolytic enzymes can be made: (1) The enzyme digests the erthyrocyte surface, exposing additional antigenic determinants. This results in the fixation of an increased number of antibody molecules (47, 63). By itself this action is insufficient to explain agglutination (64). (2) The enzyme modifies the erythrocyte surface so that potentially bivalent incomplete antibodies fixed to the cell undergo a change in molecular conformation, exposing a previously unavailable reactive site (77). (3) The enzyme digests the erythrocyte surface and exposes depressed antigenic determinants. In this fashion the smaller, incomplete IgG erythrocyte antibody can project sufficiently from the erythrocyte surface to bridge and link to a neighboring erythrocyte (see Figure 35, Chapter 17). (4) The enzyme releases N-acetylneuraminic acid from the erythrocyte surface (60, 69–73). This decreases the repulsive forces of polyanionic erythrocytes (74, 75). A closer proximity of erythrocytes is thereby possible, enabling smaller IgG incomplete antibodies to bridge between erythrocytes (78).

These explanations are not mutually contradictory, and a combination of several or all of these mechanisms may be involved. At this time a combination of the latter two actions appears to be most likely.

The observation of Prager and associates (76) that proteolytic enzymes fix to and remain attached to the erythrocyte surface suggests an active role of such enzymes in the agglutination process. This observation is compatible with all four of the mechanisms described above. A directly damaging effect of the enzyme on the erythrocyte surface may also occur. Cawley and Goodwin (79) have noted that bromelin produces confluent "holes" in erythrocyte membranes, an effect which appears to be similar to the action of saponin.

Serum components are also necessary for the complete action of proteolytic enzymes in inducing agglutination. Dausset (80) has emphasized the role of serum in the action of trypsin, and Pirofsky (81) found that small quantities of serum were necessary for the function of bromelin. By employing the bromelin test in serum systems the agglutination reaction could be intensified. Isoantibodies generally missed in bromelin tests, such as anti-Fy^a, may be made more reactive.

The Application of Proteolytic Enzyme Test Systems

In autoimmune hemolytic anemia, the majority of studies employing proteolytic enzyme procedures have been directed toward demonstrating unbound erythrocyte autoantibodies. Most laboratories rely exclusively upon the direct antiglobulin procedure to document an erythrocyte autoantibody fixed to the patient's own erythrocytes. The trypsin and standard papain, ficin and pronase procedures are dependent on the pretreatment of erythrocytes with enzymes. Accordingly, they are neither suited nor designed to demonstrate incomplete antibodies already fixed to the erythrocyte surface. In our laboratory we have found that "activated papain" is generally unreliable in a direct procedure. Thirteen eluted autoantibodies were used to coat erythrocytes. Activated papain demonstrated three, had weak reactions with three others and failed to demonstrate seven autoantibodies fixed to the erythrocytes. Unfortunately we have no data concerning the efficacy of either ficin or pronase in this type of test procedure.

Bromelin has been found to be an acceptable reagent for use in a direct test designed to document antibodies fixed to the patient's own erythrocytes (21). In 1960, 42 cases of autoimmune hemolytic anemia were studied with direct antiglobulin and direct bromelin tests (21). In general, parallel results were obtained. The antiglobulin test appeared to be more sensitive in some cases and the bromelin procedure was more sensitive in others. This difference in reactivity was more apparent in weak serologic reactions or after prolonged therapy of the patient. It was not unusual to observe weak direct bromelin reactions and moderately strong antiglobulin tests with the same erythrocytes. The reverse appeared equally true. After therapy one of these two tests may revert to normal while the other remains positive for months or years. This serologic picture does not appear to have clinical significance. Berarida and Giraldi (82) and Vetter (83) have confirmed the efficiency of the direct bromelin test in demonstrating incomplete erythrocyte antibodies bound to the erythrocyte surface. The direct bromelin test must be carefully controlled to rule out false positive reactions. The presence of cold agglutinins in the patient's serum or rouleau formation due to dysgammaglobulinemia may create such false positive reactions (21). Samples obtained from patients with plasma cell myeloma or Waldenström's macroglobulinemia are particularly prone to give erroneous results.

The proteolytic enzyme test procedures have been combined with the antiglobulin test to produce a more sensitive method of detecting incomplete erythrocyte antibodies. Unger (84) utilized the antiglobulin technique with trypsinized erythrocytes to demonstrate anti-rhesus antibodies. Such a combination seemed superior to the individual techniques with occasional antisera. van Loghem and associates (6) evaluated the antiglobulin procedure employing trypsinized and papainized erythrocytes in 38 cases. With papainized erythrocytes 36 sera gave positive reactions. Only 28 positive reactions were found using trypsinized erythrocytes. Buchanan and Dierich (58) utilized the antiglobulin test after treating erythrocytes with pronase. A sensitive procedure was developed. Our laboratory has occasionally used the antiglobulin procedure after bromelin treatment. This approach may have some value with selected incomplete antibodies.

Proteolytic enzymes act on the erythrocyte surface and may digest some antigenic determinants. The loss of M, N and Lu^a specificity of erythrocytes after treatment with influenza virus or receptor destroying enzyme appears similar and apparently results from neuraminidase activity (85). Proteolytic enzymes may therefore induce false negative reactions with certain antibodies. Rosenfield and Vogel (86) suggested that trypsin destroys the MN and Fy^a antigens. Morton (87) reported the destruction of M and N antigens by trypsin, bromelin, ficin and papain. The studies of Seaman and Uhlenbruck (88) suggest an alternative action. They obtained an MN active mucoid from the supernatant fluid of alpha-chymotrypsin treated human erythrocytes. This suggests partial removal or elution of the MN antigen under the influence of enzymatic action. Dodd and associates (89) reported specific inhibition of anti-Rh$_o$(D) by N-acetylneuraminic acid. This suggested that a part of the antigenic determinant of Rh$_o$(D) contains N-acetylneuraminic acid

(90). Such studies have not been confirmed (91–93).

There are no data suggesting that antigenic digestion may invalidate the use of enzyme procedures in the demonstration of erythrocyte autoantibodies. The reverse situation must also be considered. Enzymes may directly digest or denature erythrocyte antibodies. The use of pretreated erythrocytes in the usual trypsin and papain techniques eliminates this problem. With activated papain and bromelin test systems the enzyme is directly mixed with the antibody, and this action must be considered. Dybkjaer (94) has performed comparative studies with papain, bromelin and activated papain procedures employing erythrocyte isoantibodies and the D^u factor. He concluded that papain in a pretreatment technique is the most sensitive procedure and that it avoids the possibility of digestive action on the antibody. Dybkjaer (95) similarly found the antiglobulin test to be unreliable for demonstrating anti-rh"(E) and recommends the two-stage papain procedure. There are no similar studies evaluating this problem with erythrocyte autoantibodies.

Interpretation of Proteolytic Test Data

Many investigators have difficulty interpreting the significance of a positive enzyme test when the antiglobulin test is negative. Do such results indicate that erythrocyte autoantibodies are present or absent? The difficulty appears to be related to an unwarranted assumption of infallibility of the antiglobulin procedure. The antiglobulin test was so superior to other techniques previously available that a positive reaction was automatically assumed to indicate the presence of an antibody. In addition, a negative test was thought sufficient to rule out the presence of an antibody. In recent years most investigators have found that this fine test is susceptible to false positive and negative reactions. Innumerable examples have been accumulated indicating the occasional failure of the antiglobulin procedure to demonstrate incomplete anti-rhesus antibodies (51, 61, 62, 95). The antiglobulin procedure is similarly vulnerable in demonstrating all warm acting incomplete erythrocyte auto-antibodies. The various proteolytic enzymes frequently appear to be more sensitive with both anti-rhesus antibodies and erythrocyte autoantibodies (38, 39). This is not surprising in view of the marked heterogeneity of warm acting erythrocyte auto-antibodies. Such heterogeneity makes it unlikely that any one procedure can demonstrate all such antibodies.

The presence of a negative indirect and a positive direct antiglobulin test in a patient with autoimmune hemolytic anemia illustrates this problem. This does not indicate the absence of unbound erythrocyte autoantibodies. Rather, it suggests that unbound autoantibody exists either in small amounts or in a form not amenable to demonstration by the antiglobulin procedure. The data presented by Evans and associates (96, 97) clearly show that unbound autoantibody always exists in dynamic equilibrium with antibody fixed to the erythrocyte surface. The kinetics may vary greatly with each specific erythrocyte antibody. Positive enzyme tests in indirect procedures with such serum, when adequately controlled, indicate the presence of erythrocyte antibody, irrespective of results obtained with the antiglobulin test.

Status of Tests to Demonstrate Incomplete Erythrocyte Autoantibodies

Enzyme techniques occupy a firm position in any clinical or investigative analysis of incomplete erythrocyte antibodies. Bromelin, papain, activated papain and ficin are the current reagents of choice. An adequate evaluation of pronase is not yet available. When employed to demonstrate unbound warm acting incomplete erythrocyte auto-antibodies, these procedures appear to be equally efficient. They are substantially superior to albumin techniques and are more sensitive than the indirect antiglobulin procedure. In the author's current series, 136 patients had indirect antiglobulin tests and 117 patients had indirect bromelin tests performed on the initial examination (see Chapter 3). Forty-five per cent of the cases had positive indirect antiglobulin tests; 58 per cent had posi-

tive indirect bromelin tests. The difference in sensitivity of these two procedures became more apparent as repeated indirect procedures were performed during therapy, remission and relapse. Sixteen per cent of cases had persistently positive indirect antiglobulin tests. More than twice as many persistently positive indirect bromelin tests were recorded. Table 22 (Chapter 3) summarizes these results. Other investigators have noted the same order of sensitivity with other proteolytic enzyme preparations.

The direct antiglobulin test is the procedure of choice to demonstrate warm acting incomplete erythrocyte autoantibodies fixed to the patient's own erythrocytes. The only proteolytic enzyme test adequately investigated for this purpose is the direct bromelin technique (21, 82, 83). In the present series the direct bromelin test appeared to be inferior in sensitivity to the direct antiglobulin procedure. Parallel trials employing these two tests were carried out in 227 cases on initial examination. Identical reactions were found in both tests in 176 cases or 77.5 per cent of the series. The antiglobulin test failed in nine cases in which direct bromelin tests were positive. The direct bromelin test failed in 42 cases in which positive direct antiglobulin tests were found. In subsequent direct testing during the course of disease, 164 patients were tested with both procedures. Identical results were found in 67 per cent of cases. Positive direct bromelin tests were noted in 19 patients who had negative direct antiglobulin tests. Thirty-five cases had positive direct antiglobulin tests and negative direct bromelin tests. These results are discussed in Chapter 3 and summarized in Tables 19 and 21.

Although these data indicate a greater sensitivity of direct antiglobulin tests, another interpretation deserves emphasis. Neither procedure by itself was capable of consistently demonstrating erythrocyte autoantibodies fixed to the patient's own erythrocytes. Clinicians and investigators are therefore encouraged to use both the antiglobulin procedure and an enzyme technique in any evaluation of incomplete erythrocyte autoantibodies.

BIBLIOGRAPHY

1. Wiener, A. S.: Conglutination test for Rh sensitization. J. Lab. Clin. Med. 30: 662, 1945.
2. Wiener, A. S.: A new test (blocking test) for Rh sensitization. Proc. Soc. Exp. Biol. Med. 56: 173, 1944.
3. Brüggemann, W., and Hahn, F.: Über unvollständige Autoagglutinine (Wärmeagglutinine) beim hämolytischen Ikterus. Aerztl. Wschr. 4: 403, 1949.
4. Wagley, P. F., Shen, S. C., Gardner, F. H., and Castle, W. B.: Studies on the destruction of red blood cells. VI. The spleen as a source of a substance causing agglutination of the red blood cells of certain patients with acquired hemolytic jaundice by an anti-human serum rabbit serum (Coombs' serum). J. Lab. Clin. Med. 33: 1197, 1948.
5. Evans, R. S., and Weiser, R. S.: The serology of autoimmune hemolytic disease. Observations on forty-one patients. Arch. Intern. Med. (Chicago) 100: 371, 1957.
6. van Loghem, J. J., van der Hart, M., and Dorfmeier, H.: Serologic studies in acquired hemolytic anemia. In Proceedings of the Sixth International Congress of the International Society of Hematology. Grune & Stratton, Inc., New York, 1956.
7. Evans, R. S., Duane, R. T., and Behrendt, V.: Demonstration of antibodies in acquired hemolytic anemia with anti-human globulin serum. Proc. Soc. Exp. Biol. Med. 64: 372, 1947.
8. Heni, F., and Blessing, K.: Die Bedeutung der Glutinine für die erworbenen hämolytischen anämien. Deutsch. Arch. Klin. Med. 201: 113, 1954.
9. Jandl, J. H., and Castle, W. B.: Agglutination of sensitized red cells by large anisometric molecules. J. Lab. Clin. Med. 47: 669, 1956.
10. McNeil, C., Trentelman, E. F., Sullivan, W. P., and Agall, C. I.: A new rapid Rh tube test using polyvinylpyrrolidone (PVP). Amer. J. Clin. Path. 22: 1216, 1952.
11. Sturgeon, P.: The Rh₀ variant-Dᵘ. II. Its detection with a direct tube test. Transfusion 2: 244, 1962.
12. Griffitts, J. J., and Schmidt, P.: Effectiveness of techniques in demonstrating the iso-hemagglutinins. Transfusion 2: 385, 1962.
13. Stroup, M., and MacIlroy, M.: Evaluation of the albumin antiglobulin technique in antibody detection. Transfusion 5: 184, 1965.
14. Tobias, K. I., and Hoxworth, P. I.: The practical application of low ionic strength mannitol-saline in the antiglobulin test (a new crossmatch technique). Paper presented at the Nineteenth Annual Meeting of the American Association of Blood Banks, Los Angeles, Oct. 28, 1966.
15. Race, R. R.: An "incomplete" antibody in human serum. Nature (London) 153: 771, 1944.
16. Friedberger, E., and Moreschi, C.: Ueber Häemolyse beschleunigende Immunsubstanzen. Zbl. Bakt. (Orig.) 45: 346, 1907.
17. Moreschi, C.: Neue Tatsachen über die Blutkörperchenagglutination. Zbl. Bakt. (Orig.) 46: 49, 1908.
18. Coombs, R. R. A., Mourant, A. E., and Race, R. R.: A new test for the detection of weak and "incomplete" Rh agglutinins. Brit. J. Exp. Path. 26: 255, 1945.
19. Pirofsky, B., Cordova, M. S., and Imel, T. L.: The mechanism of action of antiglobulin serum. Vox Sang. 7: 348, 1962.
20. Costea, N., Schwartz, R., Constantoulakis, M., and Dameshek, W.: The use of radioactive antiglobulin for the detection of erythrocyte sensitiaztion. Blood 20: 214, 1962.
21. Pirofsky, B.: A new diagnostic test for antiglobulin positive ("auto-immune") haemolytic anaemia. Brit. J. Haemat. 6: 395, 1960.
22. Constantoulakis, M., Costea, N., Schwartz, R. S., and Dameshek, W.: Quantitative studies of the effect of red-blood-cell sensitization on in vivo hemolysis. J. Clin. Invest. 42: 1790, 1963.
23. van der Giessen, M., van der Hart, M., and van der Weerdt, C. M.: Fractionation of sera containing antibodies against red cells or platelets with special reference to anti-D sera. Vox Sang. 9: 25, 1964.
24. van Loghem, J. J., Kresner, M., Coombs, R. R. A., and Fulton Roberts, G.: Observations on a prozone phenomenon encountered using the antiglobulin sensitization test. Lancet 2: 729, 1950.
25. Boursnell, J. C., Coombs, R. R. A., and Risk, V.: Quantitative studies with antisera marked with iodine¹³¹ isotope and their corresponding red-cell antigens. Biochem. J. 55: 745, 1953.
26. Masouredis, S. P.: Reaction of I¹³¹ trace labeled human anti-Rh₀(D) with red cells. J. Clin. Invest. 38: 279, 1959.
27. Pirofsky, B., Cordova, M. S., and Imel, T. L.: The nonimmunologic reaction of globulin molecules with the erythrocyte surface. Vox Sang. 7: 334, 1962.
28. Masouredis, S. P.: Relationship between Rh₀(D) genotype and quantity of I¹³¹ anti-Rh₀(D) bound to red cells. J. Clin. Invest. 39: 1450, 1960.
29. Gergely, J., Horváth, E., Medgyesi, G. A., and Puskás, E.: The papain sensitivity and nonspecific binding capacity of incomplete anti-Rh₀(D) antibodies. Vox Sang. 14: 161, 1968.
30. Eyster, M. E., Nachman, R. L., Christenson, W. N., and Engle, R. L.: Structural characteristics of red cell autoantibodies. J. Immun. 96: 107, 1966.
31. Muirhead, E. E.: The relationship of current transfusion practice to modern immunohematology. Ann. N. Y. Acad. Sci. 127: 926, 1965.

32. Molthan, J., Reidenberg, M. M., and Eichman, M. F.: Positive direct Coombs tests due to cephalothin. New Eng. J. Med. **277**: 123, 1967.

33. Brown, D. V., Boehni, E. M., and Norlind, L. M.: Anemia with positive direct Coombs test induced by trypan blue. Blood **18**: 543, 1961.

34. Gralnick, H. R., and McGinniss, M.: Nature of the Coombs positive reaction with sodium cephalothin. Paper presented at the Twentieth Annual Meeting of the American Association of Blood Banks, New York, October 24, 1967.

35. Pirofsky, B., and Cordova, M. S.: Bivalent nature of incomplete anti-D (Rh₀). Nature (London) **197**: 392, 1963.

36. Stalinsky, P., and Fudenberg, H.: On the univalent fragments of human 7S gamma-globulin. Nature (London) **200**: 856, 1963.

37. Morton, J. A., and Pickles, M. M.: Use of trypsin in the detection of incomplete anti-Rh antibodies. Nature (London) **159**: 779, 1947.

38. Dacie, J. V.: *The Haemolytic Anaemias, Part II,* Ed. 2. Grune & Stratton, Inc., New York, 1962.

39. Dausset, J., and Colombani, J.: The serology and the prognosis of 128 cases of autoimmune hemolytic anemia. Blood **14**: 1280, 1959.

40. Rosenthal, M. C., and Schwartz, L. I.: Reversible agglutination of trypsin-treated erythrocytes by normal human sera. Proc. Soc. Exp. Biol. Med. **76**: 635, 1951.

41. Coffield, K. J., and Spaet, T. H.: Studies on the normal serum panagglutinin active against trypsinated human erythrocytes. V. The nonidentity of the agglutinin with serum trypsin inhibitor and the components of complement. J. Lab. Clin. Med. **54**: 871, 1959.

42. Kuhns, W. J., and Bailey, A.: Use of red cells modified by papain for detection of Rh antibodies. Amer. J. Clin. Path. **20**: 1067, 1950.

43. Lewis, A. J.: Papain, ficin and bromelain in the detection of incomplete rhesus antibodies. Brit. J. Haemat. **3**: 332, 1957.

44. Heller, I., Nelken, D., and Gurevitch, J.: Etudes sérologiques sur les anticorps anti-érythrocytaires, antileukocytaires et anti-plaquettaires dans différentes affections hématologiques. Sang **29**: 17, 1958.

45. Löw, B.: A practical method using papain and incomplete Rh antibodies in routine Rh blood grouping. Vox Sang. **5**: 94, 1955.

46. Stern, K., Busch, S., and Buznitsky, A.: A cross-matching test using activated papain. Amer. J. Clin. Path. **27**: 707, 1957.

47. Wiener, A. S., and Katz, L.: Studies on the use of enzyme-treated red cells in test for Rh sensitization. J. Immun. **66**: 51, 1951.

48. Makinodan, T., and Macris, N. T.: The effect of ficin on the agglutination of human red cells. J. Immun. **75**: 192, 1955.

49. Pirofsky, B., and Mangum, M. E.: Use of bromelin to demonstrate erythrocyte antibodies. Proc. Soc. Exp. Biol. Med. **101**: 49, 1959.

50. Pirofsky, B.: The use of bromelin in establishing a standard cross match. Amer. J. Clin. Path. **32**: 350, 1959.

51. Pirofsky, B., Nelson, H., Imel, T., and Cordova, M.: The present status of the antiglobulin and bromelin tests in demonstrating erythrocyte antibodies. Amer. J. Clin. Path. **36**: 492, 1961.

52. Gray, M. P.: Use of bromelin in blood typing. J. Lab. Clin. Med. **54**: 155, 1959.

53. Ellis, B. C.: A bromelin Rh slide test for rapidly typing patients prior to transfusion. Amer. J. Clin. Path. **39**: 129, 1963.

54. Boorman, K., and Dodd, B. E.: *An Introduction to Blood Group Serology,* Ed. 3. Little, Brown and Company, Boston, 1966.

55. Nomoto, M., and Narahashi, Y.: A proteolytic enzyme of *Streptomyces griseus.* I. Purification of a protease of *Streptomyces griseus.* J. Biochem. **46**: 653, 1959.

56. Nomoto, M., Narahashi, Y., and Murakami, M.: A proteolytic enzyme of *Streptomyces griseus.* VII. Substrate specificity of *Streptomyces griseus* protease. J. Biochem. **48**: 906, 1960.

57. Hiramatsu, A., and Ouchi, T.: On the proteolytic enzymes from the commercial protease preparation of *Streptomyces griseus* (pronase). J. Biochem. **54**: 462, 1963.

58. Buchanan, D. I., and Dierich, K. P.: The use of a proteolytic enzyme of *Streptomyces griseus* (protease G) in blood banking: a preliminary account. Transfusion **5**: 11, 1965.

59. Cook, G. M. W., and Eylar, E. H.: Separation of the M and N blood group antigens of the human erythrocyte. Biochim. Biophys. Acta **101**: 57, 1965.

60. Prager, M. D., Soules, M. L., and Fletcher, M. A.: Further studies on the mechanism of the effect of enzymes on erythrocyte serology with special reference to pronase. Transfusion, **8**: 220, 1968.

61. Grove-Rasmussen, M.: Routine compatibility testing: standards of the AABB as applied to compatibility tests. Transfusion **4**: 200, 1964.

62. Strohm, P. L., and Busch, S.: An evaluation of those proteolytic enzyme preparations commonly used in the detection of blood group antibodies. Paper presented at the Twentieth Annual Meeting of the American Association of Blood Banks, New York, October 24, 1967.

63. Wheeler, W. E., Luhby, A. L., and Scholl, M. L. L.: The action of enzymes in hemagglutinating systems. II. Agglutinating properties of trypsin-modified red cells with anti-Rh sera. J. Immun. **65**: 39, 1950.

64. Pirofsky, B., Cordova, M., and Imel, T. L.: The function of proteolytic enzymes and

tannic acid in inducing erythrocyte agglutination. J. Immun. **89**: 767, 1962.

65. Masouredis, S. P.: Reaction of I[131] anti-Rho(D) with enzyme treated red cells. Transfusion **2**: 363, 1962.

66. Hughes-Jones, N. C., Gardner, B., and Telford, R.: The effect of ficin on the reaction between anti-D and red cells. Vox Sang. **9**: 175, 1964.

67. Ponder, E.: Effects produced by trypsin on certain properties of the human red cell. Blood **6**: 350, 1951.

68. Gottschalk, A.: Neuraminidase: the specific enzyme of influenza virus and *Vibrio cholerae*. Biochim. Biophys. Acta **23**: 645, 1957.

69. Cook, G. M. W., Heard, D. H., and Seaman, G. V. F.: A sialomucopeptide liberated by trypsin from the human erythrocyte. Nature (London) **188**: 1011, 1960.

70. Klenk, E., and Uhlenbruck, G.: On the isolation of mucoids containing neuraminic acid from human erythrocyte stroma, a contribution to the chemistry of agglutinogens. Z. Physiol. Chem. **319**: 151, 1960.

71. Mäkelä, O., Miettinen, T., and Pesola, R.: Release of sialic acid and carbohydrates from human red cells by trypsin treatment. Vox Sang. **5**: 492, 1960.

72. Seaman, G. V. F., and Uhlenbruck, G.: The action of proteolytic enzymes on the red cells of some animal species. Biochim. Biophys. Acta **64**: 570, 1962.

73. Prager, M. D., and Fletcher, M. A.: The effect of enzymatic release of sialic acid from human erythrocytes on Rh agglutinations. J. Immun. **97**: 165, 1966.

74. Seaman, G. V. F., and Heard, D. H.: The surface of the washed human erythrocyte as a polyanion. J. Gen. Physiol. **44**: 251, 1960.

75. Seaman, G. V. F., and Cook, G. M. W.: Modification of the electrophoretic behavior of the erythrocyte by chemical and enzymatic methods. In *Cell Electrophoresis*, edited by E. J. Ambrose. Little, Brown and Company, Boston, 1965.

76. Prager, M. D., Fletcher, M. A., and Efron, K.: Mechanism of the immuno-hematologic effect of papain and related enzymes. J. Immun. **89**: 834, 1962.

77. Pirofsky, B., and Cordova, M. S.: The nature of incomplete erythrocyte antibodies. Vox Sang. **9**: 17, 1964.

78. Pollack, W., Hager, H. J., Reckel, R., Singher, H. O., and Toren, D. A.: A study of the forces involved in the second stage of hemagglutination. Transfusion **5**: 158, 1965.

79. Cawley, L. P., and Goodwin, W. L.: Electron microscopic investigation of the binding of bromelin by erythrocytes. Vox Sang. **13**: 393, 1967.

80. Dausset, J.: The agglutination mechanism of trypsin modified red cells. Blood **7**: 816, 1952.

81. Pirofsky, B.: The influence of a plasma factor on the erythrocyte antibody-antigen-bromelin reaction. Vox Sang. **5**: 442, 1960.

82. Berarida, G., and Giraldi, A.: Il metodo della bromelina nella diagnosi delle anemie emolitiche autoimmuni. Riv. Emoter. Immunoemat. **9**: 310, 1962.

83. Vetter, O.: Vergleichende Untersuchungen über den Coombs- und bromelin-test zum Nachweis erythrozytärer Auto-antikörper. Z. Inn. Med. **10**: 439, 1963.

84. Unger, L. J.: A method for detecting Rho antibodies in extremely low titer. J. Lab. Clin. Med. **37**: 825, 1951.

85. Springer, G. F., and Ansell, N. J.: Inactivation of human erythrocyte agglutinogens M and N by influenza viruses and receptor-destroying enzyme. Proc. Nat. Acad. Sci. USA **44**: 182, 1958.

86. Rosenfield, R. E., and Vogel, P.: The identification of hemagglutinins with red cells altered with trypsin. Trans. N. Y. Acad. Sci. **13**: 213, 1951.

87. Morton, J. A.: Some observations on the action of blood-group antibodies on red cells treated with proteolytic enzymes. Brit. J. Haemat. **8**: 134, 1962.

88. Seaman, G. V. F., and Uhlenbruck, G.: On the effect of chymotrypsin on erythrocytes. Z. Aerztl. Fortbild. (Berlin) **56**: 739, 1962.

89. Dodd, M. C., Bigley, N. J., and Geyer, V. B.: Specific inhibition of Rho(D) antibody by sialic acids. Science **132**: 1398, 1960.

90. Boyd, W. C., and Reeves, E.: Specific inhibition of anti-D antibody by colominic acid. Nature (London) **191**: 511, 1961.

91. Johnson, G. A., and McCluer, R. H.: Relation of sialic acid to Rho(D) antigen. Proc. Soc. Exp. Biol. Med. **107**: 692, 1961.

92. Springer, G. F., Williamson, P., and Brandes, W. C.: Blood group activity of gram negative bacteria. J. Exp. Med. **113**: 1077, 1961.

93. Prager, M. D., and Lowry, M. E.: On the possible relation of sialic acid to the Rh factor. Transfusion **6**: 577, 1966.

94. Dybkjaer, E.: The use of papain and bromelin in one-stage methods in blood-group serology. Sangre (Barc.) **9**: 89, 1964.

95. Dybkjaer, E.: Irregular blood group antibodies. A screening test including a two-stage papain technique. Danish Med. Bull. **13**: 188, 1966.

96. Evans, R. S., Bingham, M., and Boehni, P.: Autoimmune hemolytic disease. Antibody dissociation and activity. Arch. Intern. Med. (Chicago) **108**: 60, 1961.

97. Evans, R. S., Turner, E., and Bingham, M.: Studies of I[131] tagged Rh antibody of D specificity. Vox Sang. **8**: 153, 1963.

Chapter 19

Cold Acting Erythrocyte Autoantibodies

The cold acting erythrocyte autoantibodies are generally complete antibodies capable of agglutinating or lysing saline suspended erythrocytes. They are maximally reactive at low temperatures, although a wide thermal range of activity can frequently be demonstrated. At 37°C. serologic function is minimal if it occurs at all. Cryopathic erythrocyte autoantibodies differ from the warm acting variety in the ease of inducing hemolysis. They frequently lyse normal erythrocytes and will almost always lyse enzyme treated red cells or erythrocytes obtained from patients with paroxysmal nocturnal hemoglobinuria.

Stats and Wasserman (1) have characterized cold hemagglutination as follows: (a) agglutination of homologous or heterologous erythrocytes at low temperatures (25°C. or less in most cases) with complete reversal of the reaction upon warming; chilling of the resuspended cell-serum mixture again results in agglutination; (b) exhaustion of the agglutinin in the serum by adsorption with erythrocytes at low temperatures; and (c) release of the agglutinin from cold agglutinated erythrocytes by raising the temperature toward 37°C.

Cold acting erythrocyte autoantibodies leading to cold hemagglutination as defined above are found in five states. These include: (a) in normal individuals, (b) in individuals suffering from cold hemagglutinin disease, (c) in association with various viral infections such as viral penumonia and infectious mononucleosis, (d) in association with malignancies of the reticuloendothelium and (e) in paroxysmal cold hemoglobinuria. The pertinent clinical syndromes have been discussed in Chapter 11. The serologic characteristics of the erythrocyte autoantibodies found in the first four categories are similar and are discussed together. The Donath-Landsteiner autoantibody found in paroxysmal cold hemoglobinuria has several distinctive characteristics and is reviewed separately. The erythrocyte antigen against which the cryopathic erythrocyte autoantibodies are directed is discussed in Chapter 20.

Cold Acting Gamma M Erythrocyte Autoantibodies

Cold hemagglutination was first described by Landsteiner (2) in 1903. This phenomenon was observed during studies performed on chilled erythrocytes and on sera of normal guinea pigs, chickens, horses, dogs, rabbits and cattle. Landsteiner (2) accurately described cold hemagglutination and was able to prepare almost pure saline solutions of cold acting autoantibodies. A simple procedure was employed. Erythrocytes were agglutinated in the cold and the serum was removed. The agglutinated erythrocytes were suspended in saline and the mixture was warmed in order to release the cold acting autoantibody.

Several fundamental dissimilarities exist between cold acting autoantibodies and the warm acting varieties previously described. The ability to induce autohemagglutination and autohemolysis and the disparity between the thermal ranges of activity of the two types of erythrocyte autoantibodies are obvious differences. Two other remarkable characteristics further distinguish cold from warm acting erythrocyte autoantibodies. These depend on the species specificity of the autoantibody and its relationship to a pathologic state.

Species Specificity

Warm acting erythrocyte autoantibodies are generally considered to be nonspecific because of their capacity to react with all normal human erythrocytes. However, a certain degree of specificity is apparent in their nonreactivity with erythrocytes of most animals species (see Chapter 20). In contrast, cold acting erythrocyte autoantibodies do not demonstrate species specificity, although their reactivity with various animal erythrocytes is variable. Cold acting autoantibodies obtained from human sera were shown by Clough and Richter (3) to react with erythrocytes obtained from the rabbit, guinea pig, hen, sheep and cat. Rosenthal and Corten (4) noted their ability to induce hemagglutination of rabbit and pig erythrocytes. Rabbit, mouse, guinea pig, horse and sheep red cells also are agglutinated by human cold hemagglutinins (5).

Wiener and associates (6) studied the effects of three human sera with high titer cold hemagglutinins. The sera reacted strongly with rhesus monkey, spider monkey, pig and rabbit erythrocytes. Only weak reactions were obtained with chimpanzee, cow, horse and sheep erythrocytes. Schubothe (7) performed similar studies using six sera from patients with cold hemagglutinin disease. Eluates were prepared and tested for the ability to agglutinate various animal erythrocytes. The highest titers were obtained with rabbit, pig, guinea pig and rat erythrocytes. Dog, mouse, horse and sheep erythrocytes presented low titers or an absence of hemagglutination.

Evans and associates (8) studied the cryopathic phenomenon using I^{131} tagged human cold hemagglutinins and various erythrocytes. Adult and cord human erythrocytes were employed, as well as red cells obtained from the rabbit, dog, sheep and rat. Three of seven cold hemagglutinins studied showed an uptake with rabbit erythrocytes which exceeded that of human red cells. The stability of human cold agglutinin fixation to rabbit erythrocytes was variable. One antibody did not appreciably dissociate as the temperature was raised to 50°C. These observations are expanded in Chapter 20 in which the nature of the antigen is discussed.

The Presence of Cryopathic Autoantibodies in Normal Human Beings

The development of a warm acting erythrocyte autoantibody is almost always a pathologic event and is a distinct abnormality. Cold acting erythrocyte autoantibodies have an entirely different connotation. They are a normal constituent of human sera and can probably be demonstrated in all sera. The widespread development of cold acting erythrocyte autoantibodies is not confined to the human being. Wheeler (9) described a similar occurrence in rabbits. Ottenberg and Thalhimer (10) encountered the phenomenon in cats, Walther (11) found it in sheep, monkeys, donkeys and goats and Yu (12) encountered it in various animal species.

The frequent occurrence of cryopathic erythrocyte autoantibodies in the human being is remarkable. Amzel and Hirszfeld (13) found that 47 per cent of 238 sera submitted for Wassermann testing contained cold hemagglutinins. Kettel (14) used a more sensitive procedure and was able to demonstrate cold hemagglutinins in 95 per cent of 600 sera obtained from patients suffering from various chronic diseases. He concluded that cold hemagglutinins could probably be found in all normal human sera. Young (15) studied 130 "normal" medical students and in 63 of them he found cold hemagglutinins at titers over 4. Savonen (16) investigated the sera of 437 normal subjects and found cold hemagglutinin titers of 32 or higher in only 4.5 per cent. Janković (17) investigated 100 normal blood donors and 100 patients not suffering from hematologic disease. In only two of the normal sera were titers as high as 64 obtained. Three of the patients' sera had cold hemagglutinin titers as high as 256. The titers could be elevated substantially by using trypsinized erythrocytes.

Rosenthal and Corten (4) attempted to distinguish the cold hemagglutinins found in normal humans from those found in pathologic states. They suggested that "pathologic cold hemagglutination is not only an increase in the normal but is something different and apart." Proof or disproof of this statement is still not available. The weight of evidence, however, suggests that the same type of antibody is found in both normal and pathologic sera. The early experimental studies in this area are summarized by Stats and Wasserman (1). The major distinguishing feature between normal and pathologic cold hemagglutinins seems to be a difference in degree, rather than the development of entirely different substances. In normal individuals cold hemagglutinin titers are low and generally below 128. According to Kettel (14) their thermal range of reactivity is generally between 0 and 10°C., although 3 per cent of normal sera had cold hemagglutinin activity at 20°C. or higher. The cryopathic erythrocyte autoantibodies found in pathologic states have hemagglutinin titers of 500 or higher and a broad range of thermal activity approaching 37°C. Accordingly, cold acting erythrocyte autoantibodies are a normal constituent of human sera. Their presence in high concentrations and their ability to act at high temperatures apparently convert a harmless autoantibody into one with pathologic potential.

The Distribution of Cryopathic Erythrocyte Autoantibodies

The cold acting erythrocyte autoantibodies are serum proteins and have wide distribution in various body fluids. They have been demonstrated in ascitic fluid (18, 19), in rabbit peritoneal exudates (2), in various transudates and exudates and in blister fluids (20). A blood-brain barrier apparently exists for these substances. Although Montanari (20) found cold hemagglutinins in three of 18 spinal fluids examined, Riebeling (21) was unable to confirm this. Stats and Wasserman (1)

did not find cold hemagglutinin activity in the spinal fluid of a patient with a serum hemagglutinin titer of 32,000.

Cold acting erythrocyte autoantibodies have the capacity to react with various body constituents other than erythrocytes. Such reactions have been described with liver and kidney cells (22), with spermatozoa (23) and with thrombocytes (24). Clough and Richter (3) could not demonstrate cold hemagglutinin activity with epithelial cells of the urinary tract.

Physical and Immunochemical Properties of Cryopathic Erythrocyte Autoantibodies

Landsteiner (2) in his initial 1903 report described rabbit cold autohemagglutinins as serum proteins located in the globulin fraction. Clough and Richter (3) in 1918 precipitated a human serum with 36 volumes per cent saturated ammonium sulfate and removed all cold acting auto antibody activity. Stats and associates (25) and Spaet and Kinsell (26) presented electrophoretic evidence that cold acting autoantibodies were located in the gamma-globulin fraction of human serum.

Gordon (27) performed detailed studies on one human serum containing cold acting erythrocyte autoantibodies. Cold hemagglutinin activity was found in the euglobulin fraction of the serum. Relatively pure solutions of the cryopathic autoantibody were obtained by elution. Electrophoresis demonstrated that 75 per cent of the proteins formed a single peak. Ultracentrifugation analysis revealed that 65 per cent of the eluate proteins had a sedimentation constant coefficient of 18S and contained the cold hemagglutinin. Schubothe (28) in 1954 investigated the serum of a patient with cold hemagglutinin disease and demonstrated a 12 per cent concentration of macroglobulins. Electrophoresis of this serum showed an increase in the beta 2 globulin portion. Rørvik (29) also described a serum obtained from a patient with cold hemagglutinin disease as having a split beta pattern. Both authors suggested that the increased beta 2 globulin concentration reflected the cold hemagglutinin and macro-globulin. Varques and associates (30) in 1955 found an increase in "euglobulin I" in the sera of patients with potent cold hemagglutinins. The increase was as high as 6 times over normal. Cold hemagglutinin titers in the euglobulin fractions were even higher than in the original serum. Weber (31) investigated sera from five patients with cold hemagglutinin disease. Eluates of the cold acting erythrocyte autoantibody were prepared and analyzed in the ultracentrifuge. All preparations were homogeneous and contained macro-globulins with sedimentation coefficients ranging from $(s_{20,w})$ 17.6 to 18.0. The molecular weights were calculated to range between 330,000 and 350,000.

Christenson and Dacie (32) studied 38 patients with hemolytic anemia associated with cryopathic erythrocyte autoantibodies. There were 10 cases of cold hemagglutinin disease included in this group and abnormal serum electrophoretic patterns were noted in nine. All abnormal patterns involved elevations at the gamma 1 globulin area. Beta-globulin was essentially normal and alpha 2 globulin values were variable. Dacie (33) reevaluated these abnormal peaks and localized them to a variable position in the gamma to beta region. Three of these sera contained cryoglobulins migrating as gamma 1 globulins. The remaining 28 patients with paroxysmal cold hemoglobinuria or idiopathic hemolytic anemia and cold hemagglutinins did not have consistent electrophoretic abnormalities. Only one case demonstrated an elevation of the gamma 1 globulin. Christenson and associates (34) expanded this study. The increased gamma 1 globulin in three patients with cold hemagglutin disease was examined by erythrocyte adsorption, elution and isolation with cellulose column electrophoresis. The elevated gamma 1 globulin was identified as the cryopathic erythrocyte autoantibody. Ultracentrifugation studies indicated that the cold hemagglutinin consisted of macromolecules with a sedimentation coefficient of $s_{20,w}$ 16.

The definitive study in this area was carried out by Fudenberg and Kunkel (35) who analyzed eight sera obtained from patients with cryopathic autoimmune hemolytic anemia. In four an abnormal elevation of globulin was documented by serum electrophoresis. The peak of cold hemagglutinin activity corresponded to the abnormal globulin peak and the magnitude roughly correlated with the titer of cold hemagglutinin activity. Electrophoresis localized the various abnormal peaks to the fast gamma through the slow beta range. Density gradient and analytic ultracentrifugation studies identified the cold hemagglutinins as macroglobulins with sedimentation coefficients of 19S. The molecular weights of these macroglobulins were approximately one million.

The above observations suggest that cold acting erythrocyte autoantibodies may be associated with abnormal electrophoretic patterns. Abnormal peaks in the gamma to beta range are particularly significant. These conclusions have been widely confirmed. Mehrotra and Charlwood (36) further confirmed that cold hemagglutinins were macromolecules with sedimentation coefficients $(s_{20,w})$ of 17.1 to 18.8. The pure eluates that these authors analyzed also contained heavier units.

Antiserum has been prepared against purified cold acting erythrocyte autoantibodies in an attempt to characterize them immunochemically (37–39). Reactions of identity between eluted cold hemagglutinins and crude beta-globulin were found using Ouchterlony agar diffusion techniques. Mehrotra (40, 41) in 1960 expanded this type of study and employed anti-human serum antiserum and anti-IgM gamma-globulin antiserum. Cold acting autoantibodies were localized to the beta 2-M region and formed reactions of identity with the gamma 1 electrophoretic peak of the original serum. Cold acting autoantibodies cross reacted with normal human serum components but also had immunologically specific reactivity. Antisera prepared against eluted cold acting autoantibodies formed a single precipitin band with normal sera. Two precipitin bands were formed when they were reacted against autologous and homologous sera containing high titer cold hemagglutinins. Such antisera were adsorbed with normal human serum or the gamma 2 or gamma 1 components of normal serum. The adsorbed antiserum now produced only a single precipitin band when reacted with autologous serum.

Fudenberg and Kunkel (35) noted that warm acting and cold acting erythrocyte antibodies differed in their response to treatment with the disulfide reducing agent 2-mercaptoethanol. Serologic reactivity of warm acting erythrocyte antibodies persisted with little if any change in antibody titers. However, cold acting erythrocyte antibodies lost all or most of their serologic reactivity. Chan and Deutsch (42) in 1960 obtained similar results with various human anti-rhesus antibodies. Mehrotra and Charlwood (36) studied 19 sera obtained from patients with cryopathic varieties of autoimmune hemolytic anemia. 2-Mercaptoethanol treatment of these sera markedly reduced hemagglutinin activity.

Deutsch and Morton (43) in 1957 originally demonstrated that treatment of macroglobulins with 2-mercaptoethanol disrupted disulfide bonds and converted a single 19S macroglobulin into five or six subunits. Each unit had a sedimentation coefficient of approximately 7S. A loss of immunologic activity as a result of such reduction is understandable. Dialyzing the reducing agent out of the reacting system permits recombination of these six units. The 19S macromolecule is accordingly reformed. Restoration of the macromolecular structure does not necessarily restore immunologic reactivity to the level previously present. Some degree of random recombination of the five or six subunits occurs, partially modifying the molecule. Evans and associates (8) found that removal of mercaptanes permitted the restoration of I[131] labeled cold hemagglutinins. The recombined molecule could induce hemagglutination and was adsorbed by erythrocytes. Harboe and Deverill (44) found that 2-mercaptoethanol reduction of a cold hemagglutinin destroyed both the hemagglutinating property and the ability to combine with the antigen at low temperatures. Reassocia-

tion restored the agglutinating activity at a lower titer.

Jacot-Guillarmod and Isliker (45) studied the reduction of cold hemagglutinins induced by thiols and sodium borohydride. Reduction dissociated 19S isohemagglutinins into 6S subunits with a loss of agglutinating activity. Reoxidation did not restore immunologic reactivity when thiols had induced reduction. Removal of sodium borohydride in the presence of oxygen restored hemagglutinating activity which approached 100 per cent in some instances. A mixture of anti-A and anti-B was reduced with sodium borohydride and then reoxidized. Hybrid molecules were found during recombination. "Mixed" antibodies with anti-A and anti-B activity on the same molecule were found.

Anderson (46) has reported a gamma A type cold hemagglutinin. Mild reduction with 2-mercaptoethanol induced a loss of agglutinating activity and antigen binding capacity. Removal of the reducing agent permitted a 25 to 50 per cent return of agglutinating activity. If alkylation was performed immediately after reduction, the loss of immunologic activity was permanent. Accordingly, the IgA type of cold hemagglutinin reacted to reduction and reoxidation procedures in a fashion similar to that of the more common IgM cold hemagglutinin.

L Chain Types of Cold Hemagglutinins

Almost all cold hemagglutinins are gamma M immunoglobulins. Accordingly, mu type H chains appear as a common characteristic. An exception to this general rule is the case reported by Anderson (46) who described an IgA cold hemagglutinin which must contain alpha H chains.

In 1964 Franklin and Fudenberg (47) analyzed the L chains of various antibodies. Anti-rhesus antibodies and rheumatoid factor were found to contain a mixture of kappa and lambda type L chains. By contrast, five cold hemagglutinins were found to consist exclusively of kappa type L chains. This observation of a monotypic kappa type L chain has been repeatedly confirmed (44, 48–51). More than

100 cold hemagglutinins found in cold hemagglutinin disease have been investigated. It accordingly appears to be a general rule that a monotypic kappa type IgM immunoglobulin is characteristic of cold hemagglutinin disease.

Several exceptions to this rule have been noted. Cooper and Worlledge (52) analyzed the sera from six patients with chronic cold hemagglutinin disease. In five a kappa type L chain was present. One cold hemagglutinin was composed of lambda L chains. The specificity of this antibody was anti-"not I." An additional anti-"not I" cold acting antibody had kappa L chains. Harboe and Lind (53) and Costea and associates (54) have reported that cold hemagglutinins of anti-I or anti-i specificity associated with Mycoplasma or viral infections may have either kappa or lambda L chains. Naturally occurring cold hemagglutinins may also have either kappa or lambda chains. Costea and associates (54) have unified these observations and suggest that naturally occurring cold hemagglutinins and the cold hemagglutinins obtained from patients with infectious mononucleosis, *Mycoplasma pneumoniae* infections and systemic lupus erythematosus are bitypic IgM molecules containing kappa and lambda type L chains on the same molecule. Feizi (55) studied three sera from patients with chronic hemolytic anemia and cold hemagglutinins. His results cast some doubt on the postulate of Costea and associates (54). Lambda type L chains were found in all. Two of the cold hemagglutinins were cryoglobulins and were neither I nor i specific. One patient had an *M. pneumoniae* infection and the cold hemagglutinin contained only lambda type L chains.

The demonstration of a monotypic kappa type L chain pattern in cold hemagglutinin disease suggests that the antibody is the product of a single clone of cells. As such, the cold hemagglutinin resembles the paraproteins of monoclonal dysgammaglobulinemia as described by Waldenström. This observation is reinforced by the studies of Schubothe (49, 56) which document the similarities between cold hemagglutinin disease and macroglobulinemia.

Cryoglobulins and Cold Hemagglutinins

Cryoglobulins are cold precipitable proteins of varying immunoglobulin classes. IgG forms are most common. Such substances do not generally manifest immunologic reactivity against erythrocytes. An occasional cryoglobulin has been identified as an IgM type of cold hemagglutinin (34). Firkin and associates (39) observed the simultaneous occurrence of a cryoglobulin and a cold hemagglutinin. Different proteins were involved in these different activities. Harris and Fairley (57) noted that a cold hemagglutinin isolated from a patient with cold hemagglutinin disease had antigenic cross reactivity with a cryoglobulin also present in the serum. Turro and Straface (58) and Gökcen (59) have reported cryoglobulins which function as cold autoantibodies and lead to hemolytic anemia. Feizi (55) reported one such cryoglobulin with a monotypic lambda type L chain structure. Additional studies in this area are necessary.

Serologic Properties of the Cold Hemagglutinins

The usual cold acting erythrocyte autoantibody is a macromolecule with a sedimentation coefficient of 19S. It generally is a gamma M immunoglobulin. It therefore differs from the usual warm acting erythrocyte autoantibody which most often is an IgG immunoglobulin. Gamma M immunoglobulins are formed of monomeric subunits composed of two L and two H chains. Polymerization of five or six monomeric subunits occurs, creating a macromolecule. The resulting large size undoubtedly plays an important role in producing a complete erythrocyte antibody capable of mediating autohemagglutination and autohemolysis (see Chapters 16 and 17).

In general, therefore, warm acting and cold acting erythrocyte antibodies differ in their immunoglobulin class. Different H chains are accordingly present. The H chain, through its Fc fragment, determines the secondary immunologic characteristics of the antibody molecule. It may therefore be anticipated that warm and cold acting erythrocyte antibodies will present different serologic features.

Incomplete Cold Acting Autoantibodies

In 1950 Dacie (60) described an incomplete form of cold acting erythrocyte antibody. He demonstrated that normal erythrocytes exposed to chilled human serum would develop positive antiglobulin reactions. This was more apparent when potent (less diluted) antiglobulin serum was employed. The incomplete cold agglutinin was present in most if not all human sera. The antibodies could only be detected using fresh serum. Heating the serum to 56°C. or using anticoagulants prevented sensitization or fixation to erythrocytes. The incomplete cold agglutinin was firmly bound to the erythrocyte surface, and repeated washings at 37°C. did not elute the antibody. Ferriman and associates (61) demonstrated such incomplete cold agglutinins in patients suffering from cold hemagglutinin disease. On the basis of gamma-globulin neutralization tests, Dacie (62) reported that the incomplete antibodies were of the non-gamma type.

Extensive studies by Dacie and associates (63) clarified the nature of the incomplete cold agglutinin associated with high titer cold hemagglutinins. Incomplete cold agglutinins were simply serologic artifacts. The positive antiglobulin reaction resulted from the interaction of anti-complement antibodies present in antiglobulin serum with components of complement bound to the erythrocyte surface. Such complement components attach to erythrocytes concomitantly with cold acting erythrocyte autoantibodies. Studies by Adinolfi and associates (64) indicated that the normal incomplete cold antibody is not a gamma-globulin. It was not eluted with the gamma-globulin fraction on DEAE cellulose column chromatography. In addition, it was present in 10 of 11 sera obtained from hypogammaglobulinemic patients and was not properdin. Differences were observed from typical IgG antibodies in heat resistance.

Data have accumulated confirming that the positive antiglobulin test is due to complement fixed to the red cell surface. Rosenfield and associates (65) were able to produce positive reactions using specific anticomplement antiserum, even after adsorption with human gamma-globulin. They termed this procedure the complement antiglobulin test. Gandini (66) noted that the reaction would occur in the absence of the $C'2$ component of complement. Pondman and associates (67) confirmed that $C'2$ is not necessary for the reaction. Agglutination could occur with the $C'1,4$ complex alone; $C'4$ apparently acts as the agglutinogen. Leddy and associates (68) investigated the complement reaction and its relationship to IgM antibodies. They rejected the concept that complement was bound to the erythrocyte surface by IgM antibodies in a manner which produced steric hindrance of IgM, thus preventing its detection. It is most likely that complement protein is fixed to the red cell surface by cold hemagglutinins. After complement fixation the antibody is free to dissociate, leaving complement on the erythrocyte surface. Harboe (69) investigated this aspect using I^{131} trace labeled cold hemagglutinins. Strong agglutination reactions were obtained with sensitized erythrocytes using specific antiserum directed against beta 1-E (fourth complement component) and beta 1-C (moiety of third complement component). At the same time anti-IgG and anti-IgM antisera failed to induce agglutination, even though the latter antiserum gave a strong precipitin band with isolated cold hemagglutinins. Boyer (70) found that complete dissociation of the antibody occurs from $EAC'1,4,2$ sites (erythrocyte-antibody-complement complex). $C'1$ and $C'2$ are also removed and $C'4$ remains fixed to the erythrocyte.

Cold acting antibodies fixed to the surface of the erythrocyte are easily removed by heating to 37°C. However, complement which is concomitantly adsorbed remains fixed. Dacie (33) has pointed out that this concept clarifies many confusing aspects of the positive antiglobulin reaction associated with cold acting antibodies. Complement bound to the erythrocyte is responsible for the thermal lability of the reaction, for the inhibiting effect of anticoagulants, for the pattern of reactivity with dilute antiglobulin serum, for the non-gamma antiglobulin reaction and for the inability to elute incomplete cold antibodies.

Such data suggest that incomplete cold antibody does not exist. Harboe (69) has proposed the following sequence of events to account for all of the clinical and experimental observations. At low temperatures cold hemagglutinins interact with red cells, producing agglutination. Complement is fixed to the erythrocyte during this process, if it is present in the reaction mixture. The antibody is eluted from the erythrocyte by warming to 37°C. This leads to a reversal of agglutination. By washing at this temperature the cold acting antibody is removed from the reacting system. Complement remains fixed to the erythrocyte in spite of elution of the cold hemagglutinin. Two of the complement components, C'4 and C'3a, may then react with antiglobulin serum or anticomplement antiserum, resulting in agglutination.

The Role of Complement

The involvement of complement in autoimmune hemolytic anemia is unquestionable. Low serum complement levels are common in cold acting autoimmune hemolytic anemia and are not rare with warm acting varieties. van Loghem and associates (71) reported low serum complement levels in 50 per cent of patients with cryopathic autoimmune hemolytic anemia and in 20 per cent of warm acting autoantibody cases. Dacie (33) noted subnormal to absent serum complement values in all of nine cases of cold acting autoimmune hemolytic anemia and in five of 13 cases of warm acting autoimmune hemolytic anemia. Jonsen and associates (72) found reduced complement values in five patients with cold hemagglutinins. Fife and associates (73) reported reduced complement values as part of experimental runt disease.

Low serum complement levels presumably result from continual in vivo antibody-antigen union. This may not be the only explanation. Dacie (33) described a patient whose serum complement levels remained reduced although hemolysis was decreased by splenectomy. Complement persisted at the abnormally low level in spite of almost complete hematologic remission. Accordingly, a deficiency of complement component synthesis or formation of anticomplementary substances may also play a role. A deficiency of serum complement may be important in retarding hemolysis. Evans and associates (8) have emphasized the dangers of transfusion in patients with depleted complement. Such therapy may supply complement to patients in whom hemolysis has stablized through exhaustion of serum complement. A hemolytic crisis can result. Although circulatory hemolysis may be inhibited by complement depletion, premature death of erythrocytes can still occur through sequestration in the liver and spleen.

The serologic activity of cold acting erythrocyte autoantibodies is greatly modified by complement. Lysis appears as a function of these elements. Cryopathic autoantibodies are thermally stable and can resist heating to 56°C. for 30 minutes. The lytic capability of heated samples, however, is lost and only hemagglutinin activity persists. Complement may also function in firmly fixing the cold acting antibody to the erythrocyte surface (33). Without firm fixation, elution of antibody from erythrocytes could occur prior to lysis as the temperature is raised (33). The supply of complement necessary for hemolysis and firm binding of antibody may be responsible for many variations found in serologic testing. The capacity of complement to resist elution of antibody varies from serum to serum (33). Enzyme treated erythrocytes and erythrocytes from patients with paroxysmal nocturnal hemoglobinuria apparently have the ability to fix sufficient antibody from heated serum to induce hemolysis. Rosse and Dacie (74) studied the role of complement in immune hemolysis employing paroxysmal nocturnal hemoglobinuria erythrocytes. Complement only slightly increased the antibody binding capacity. Lysis was related to a greater efficiency of action of complement complexes acting on the erythrocyte surface. This reflected differences in the later stages of the complement lysis sequence.

Evans and associates (8) employed an I^{131} labeled cold hemagglutinin test system to evaluate the role of complement with cold acting autoantibodies. Complement did not bind the hemagglutinin to the intact cell or influence the association-dissociation equilibrium at temperatures of 5 to 37°C. These authors suggest that the relative resistance of a patient's erythrocytes to hemolysis may be due to two factors in addition to complement concentration. The circulating cells may represent a selected population of resistant erythrocytes. In addition, the coating of erythrocytes by complement may inhibit hemolysis by interfering with the reattachment of cold hemagglutinins.

Harboe (69) also employed a radioactive labeling procedure to demonstrate that complement is directly fixed to the erythrocyte membrane. Interaction of a hemolytic antibody with the red cell and complement forms the complex EAC'1,4,2. Mayer and associates (75) have shown that if insufficient C'3 is available this complex decays, even though a stable union of antibody with erythrocyte is maintained. Evans and associates (8, 76) found that with cold hemagglutinins the complement reaction is transient at body temperatures as a result of dissociation of the complex to A + EC'1,4,2 or EC'1,4,2,3a. This complex is probably rapidly broken down. Erythrocytes coated with such complexes are not hemolyzed by cold hemolysins and ethylene diaminetetraacetic acid treated serum (source of C'3).

The theoretical possibility exists that complement may be attached to the heavy chain of the antibody molecule. Taranta and Franklin (77) showed that the heavy chain of the IgG molecule contains the complement fixing site. Leddy and Vaughan (78) described a macroglobulin distinct from cold hemagglutinins which they termed the "Tr factor." This factor is found in the sera of some patients whose erythrocytes are coated in vivo with complement. Eyster and associates (79) reviewed this problem and they state that the mechanism of complement fixation in the presence of cold hemagglutinins is not clear. Complement may attach to the heavy chain of IgG immunoglobulins, may be fixed directly to the erythrocyte membrane through the action of IgG or IgM antibodies or may adhere nonspecifically to the cell membrane in the absence of antibody.

The Influence of pH

In 1950 Dacie (80) reported the effect of pH changes on the lytic ability of sera containing high titer cold hemagglutinins. Hemolysis of normal erythrocytes occurred if the sera were suitably acidified. A progressive rise in antibody titer was noted as the pH was decreased from 8.2 to 5.8. The optimal pH range was determined to be from 6.5 to 7.0. Lysis was dependent on complement in the reacting system. This observation has been confirmed by many investigators. A great deal of variation has been encountered. Ferriman and associates (61) noted one case in which lysis occurred without acidification but was intensified by acid treatment. Dacie (33) and Bonnin (81) have observed the reverse, with slightly more hemolysis found with unacidified sera than with acid solutions. Schubothe (7) in 1958 documented a progressive increase in binding of antibody to erythrocytes as the pH was lowered from 9.0 to 6.0.

Dacie (33) demonstrated lysis of normal erythrocytes by cold acting autoantibodies in every instance in which acidification procedures were used. The temperature of the reacting system is important. Adsorption of a typical acid hemolysin increased steadily as the pH fell over a range of 8.0 to 5.8. Little or no hemolysis occurred below pH 6.0. The abrupt cessation of hemolysis reflects inhibition of complement at pH levels below 6.0. Cold acting erythrocyte autoantibodies whose lytic action is potentiated by acidification show a reverse effect on agglutination. Agglutination may appear more intense in unacidified sera. Dacie (33) suggests that pH changes do not influence the degree of binding of antibody to erythrocytes. The pH effect is to increase the binding of complement to the cells.

Evans and associates (8) quantitated the influence of pH on the degree of adsorption of cold hemagglutinins by erythrocytes. Their studies were carried out at 25°C. More than twice the amount of cold hemagglutinin was adsorbed and retained at pH 6.6 than at pH 7.6. The intensification of complement hemolysis obtained by acidification may be a pH effect on the equilibrium relationship between cell and cold hemagglutinin. The data of these authors suggest that an increase in hydrogen ion concentration induces a shift in the antigen-antibody equilibrium toward combination.

Temperature Ranges

The temperature range for the action of cryopathic erythrocyte autoantibodies is important from two aspects. It serves to distinguish the cold acting hemagglutinin found in normal sera from that seen in patients with hemolytic anemia. Pathologic cold acting autoantibodies have a greater range of thermal action. The upper limits may even approach 37°C. Most normal sera contain cold hemagglutinins with a narrow thermal range whose upper limit is 15°C. or lower. The correlation between upper thermal ranges of activity and initiation of hemolytic disease has great clinical significance. A high titer cold hemagglutinin with an upper thermal range at 15°C. is not as dangerous as a low titer cold hemagglutinin able to react with erythrocytes at 32°C. The capacity of such antibodies to react with erythrocytes in vivo is the critical factor. The extremities of the human being have skin and subcutaneous temperatures approaching 28°C. with moderate cooling (82).

Evans and associates (8) have performed meticulous quantitative studies on the influence of temperature to erythrocyte binding of cold hemagglutinins. A linear relationship existed between the amount of cold hemagglutinin bound and a temperature range of 5 to 32°C. Their studies suggest that cold hemagglutinins and red cells exhibit a temperature dependent association-dissociation equilibrium. In an ice bath, washed erythrocytes coated with cold hemagglutinins manifested less than 5 per cent dissociation of antibody. With warming of the suspension a progressive increase in antibody dissociation occurred. At 31°C. agglutination disappeared and there was less than 1 per cent of antibody found at 5°C. Although cold acting erythrocyte autoantibodies dissociate from the erythrocyte at temperatures below that found in vivo, the antibody effect may persist. Evans and associates (8) demonstrated complement hemolysis of erythrocytes exposed to pure preparations of cold agglutinins at 37°C. This indicates that cold acting antibodies may react with erythrocytes for a sufficient time to permit complement action.

The in vivo presence of high thermal acting cold hemagglutinins can lead to erythrocyte fixation of such antibodies. This in turn can initiate autohemagglutination and autohemolysis. Stats (83) suggested that lysis of such erythrocytes results from mechanical trauma. Ham and associates (84) demonstrated that mechanical trauma induced the lysis of erythrocytes sensitized by incomplete antibody. Lewis and associates (85) studied the survival of erythrocytes sensitized by a cold acting hemagglutinin at the appropriate temperature. Agglutination was not permanently harmful. When agglutination was reversed, erythrocytes survived normally. The critical factor was the degree of complement binding. Sublytic concentrations of complement bound to the erythrocyte in the cold persisted and led to erythrocyte hepatic sequestration even after agglutination had been reversed. Higher concentrations of complement bound to the cell surface resulted in their early destruction by phagocytosis.

Titer Ranges

Hemagglutination titers of cryopathic erythrocyte autoantibodies are variable and are pH and temperature dependent. They are not necessarily important in the development of clinical hemolytic anemia. Extreme cold hemagglutinin titers have been recorded. Stats (83) mentioned one serum with a cold hemagglutinin titer of 30,000 at 4°C. Heilmeyer and associates (86) noted a 131,072 titer for a cold acting autoantibody whose upper thermal range was 33°C. Johnsson (87) presented a case with a titer of 32,000 at 2°C. which dropped to 2,000 at 37°C. Ferriman and associates (61) described three sera with titers of 32,000 to 128,000 at 2 to 5°C. with an upper thermal range of 29 to 31°C. Rørvik (29) recorded a serum with a cold hemagglutinin titer of 168,000,000. According to Dacie (33) the maximal titers of cold acting erythrocyte autoantibodies generally fall within the range of 8,000 to 64,000. It should be emphasized that the highest titer is only a laboratory curiosity. Of greater clinical significance is the titer obtained at the highest temperature approaching the in vivo state.

Placental Passage

Cold acting erythrocyte autoantibodies differ from warm varieties and generally are not involved in an active placental transport mechanism. The ability to traverse the placental barrier is a secondary immunologic characteristic determined by the Fc fragment of the H chain. Accordingly, placental transport has no specific relationship to optimal antibody temperature reactivity. A cold acting erythrocyte antibody may be a gamma G immunoglobulin and may have the potential to traverse the placental barrier. The Donath-Landsteiner antibody illustrates this state (88, 89). The reverse appears to be equally possible. A warm acting IgM erythrocyte autoantibody would be unable to traverse the placenta. The high degree of variation and the heterogeneity of erythrocyte antibodies makes such a blending of serologic characteristics a not infrequent occurrence.

Kinetic Data

Evans and associates (8) have performed careful quantitative kinetic studies of the cold hemagglutinin reaction. They employed I^{131} labeled purified cold hemagglutinins to determine the speed of interaction with normal chilled erythrocytes. The uptake of antibody in 2 hours was taken as 100 per cent. In 30 minutes 95 per cent of the antibody was fixed to the erythrocyte; 98 per cent was cellularly

bound in 1 hour. The influence of antibody concentration on the rate of erythrocyte adsorption was similarly determined. Maximal uptake representing 505,500 cold hemagglutinin molecules per erythrocyte was obtained with maximal concentration of antibody. Complete saturation of all antigenic sites was not obtained even at this high level of fixation to the cell. A 6-fold dilution of the cold hemagglutinin (original titer 8,000) resulted in a 50 per cent reduction of erythrocyte antibody binding. The volume of eluate containing potent tagged cold hemagglutinins (titer 16,000) was varied from 5 to 100 times the volume of erythrocytes used in the reacting system. These studies indicated that erythrocytes were capable of adsorbing increasing amounts of cold hemagglutinins from solutions up to and including 100 times the volume of cells. From the data of Evans and associates (8) it seems that erythrocyte antigen saturation still had not been reached, although 574,000 cold hemagglutinin molecules were bound per erythrocyte. Boyd and associates (90) similarly did not saturate A antigenic erythrocyte sites with as many as 10^6 anti-A lectin molecules.

Enzyme Treatment

The treatment of erythrocytes with proteolytic enzymes increases their sensitivity to cold acting autoantibodies as manifested by hemagglutination and hemolysis. Pisciotta (91), Janković (17), Schubothe (7) and Dacie (33) reported that trypsinization of erythrocytes accentuated the action of cold hemagglutinins. Evans and associates (8) studied the effect of trypsin and ficin with an I^{131} tagged purified cold hemagglutinin test system. An increased uptake of cold hemagglutinins by treated cells was noted with both enzymes. In addition, the equilibrium between enzyme treated cells and antibody was modified. Complete dissociation of the cold hemagglutinin did not occur until the temperature was elevated to 37°C. or higher. Stroma prepared from enzyme treated erythrocytes was capable of binding an increased amount of cold hemagglutinin. Identical effects were obtained with stroma

TABLE 94. *Contrasting characteristics of warm and cold acting erythrocyte autoantibodies (excluding the Donath-Landsteiner antibody)*

	Cold Acting Autoantibody	Warm Acting Autoantibody
General characteristics		
Species specificity	No	Yes
Naturally occurring	Yes	No
Physical-chemical characteristics		
Serum globulin	Yes	Yes
Immunoglobulin class	IgM	IgG
Sedimentation constant	19S	7S
Molecular weight	890,000	140,000
L chain composition	Monotypic, K type	Mixture of K and L types
Effect of reducing agents	Loss of activity	No loss of activity
Electrophoresis	Abnormal gamma-beta peak	Broad gamma peak
Serologic characteristics		
Type of antibody	Complete	Incomplete
Autohemagglutination	Yes	Rare
Autohemolysis	Common	Rare
Temperature for maximal action	4°C.	37°C.
Agglutination titers	High (>1,000)	Low (<1,000)
Potentiation by acid	Yes	Rare
Complement fixation	Yes	Uncommon
Placental passage	No	Yes
Type of in vivo hemolysis	Circulatory and hepatic sequestration	Splenic sequestration
Antigenic specificity	Yes: anti-I, anti-i	Uncommon: anti-Rh types
Antiglobulin test	Positive	Positive

produced from adult and cord blood human erythrocytes.

It is obvious that cold and warm acting erythrocyte autoantibodies differ in innumerable aspects. Table 94 summarizes the major characteristics considered to be typical of each group. It must again be stated that this grouping does not imply rigid boundaries. Antibodies containing various blends of the listed characteristics will be encountered. The heterogeneity of erythrocyte autoantibodies must always be remembered. Accordingly, the qualities summarized above are simply guidelines to the most frequently observed patterns.

The Cold Acting Erythrocyte Autoantibody of Paroxysmal Cold Hemoglobinuria (Donath-Landsteiner Antibody)

The Donath-Landsteiner antibody characteristic of paroxysmal cold hemoglobinuria is a cold acting erythrocyte autoantibody. It differs markedly, however, from the cold hemagglutinins described above. Antigenic differences are reviewed in Chapter 20. The distinctive physical, chemical and serologic characteristics are described below.

In 1904 Donath and Landsteiner (92) demonstrated that the lysin causing paroxysmal cold hemoglobinuria was located in the patient's serum. Heat inactivation of the serum prevented hemolysis. The addition of fresh serum restored hemolytic activity. The hemolytic reaction in vitro was shown to consist of two phases. A cold dependent reaction led to fixation of a serum constituent (antibody, hemolysin) to the erythrocyte surface. Hemolysis developed in a second phase when the sensitized cells were warmed in the presence of serum complement. These studies were expanded by Donath and Landsteiner (93, 94) and confirmed by Eason in 1906 (95).

Physical and Immunochemical Properties

Jordan and associates (96, 97) carried out extensive studies on the complement and antibody phases of the paroxysmal cold hemoglobinuria reaction. They noted positive antiglobulin reactions, and they separated cold acting autoantibody activity from the C'1, C'3 and C'4 components of complement. Antibody activity was absent in euglobulin fractions insoluble at pH 5.0 to 7.0. Fractionation of serum in an alcohol-water system located antibody activity in the water soluble pseudoglobulin fraction. Gouttas and associates (98) applied electrophoretic techniques to the study of the Donath-Landsteiner antibody. Cold acting autoantibody activity was located in the gamma-globulin fraction. Leonardi and Andolfatto-Zaglia (99) also demonstrated that an eluted Donath-Landsteiner antibody migrated as a gamma 1 globulin on paper electrophoresis. Christenson and Dacie (32) did not note abnormal electrophoretic patterns in the sera of patients with paroxysmal cold hemoglobinuria.

Hinz and associates (100) in 1961 suggested that the Donath-Landsteiner antibody was associated with low molecular weight globulins. In 1963 Hinz (88) studied six sera obtained from patients with paroxysmal cold hemoglobinuria. The antibody was located in the gamma-globulin peak by zone electrophoresis. Paper electrophoresis and immunoelectrophoresis indicated that the antibody migrated as a gamma 2 globulin. Column chromatography employing DEAE cellulose eluted the antibody in the initial fraction typical of IgG immunoglobulins. Sucrose gradient ultracentrifugation studies confirmed the 7S nature of the Donath-Landsteiner antibody. No relationship was found to the Wassermann antibody. Some heterogeneity was noted among the six antibodies studied. In particular, one antibody migrated faster during electrophoresis than did the other five. The 7S nature of the Donath-Landsteiner antibody has been confirmed by the studies of Kissmeyer-Nielson and Schleiner (101), van der Hart and associates (102) and Weiner and associates (103).

Hemagglutination

Hemoglobinuria is the most striking clinical manifestation of this disease. The obvious intravascular hemolysis has oriented many studies toward elucidating the lytic mechanism. It is frequently forgotten that hemagglutination may also be induced by the Donath-Landsteiner antibody. Agglutination is frequently not noted when testing for this antibody in the usual fashion. It can usually be demonstrated, however, if the erythrocytes are suspended in heat inactivated serum. Titers observed are generally low. Stats and Wasserman (1) and Becker (104) noted agglutination titers similar to those found with normal sera. A few reports of titers as high as 320 are available. Hinz (88) noted agglutination reactions with the sera of all six of his patients. Values ranged from 4 to 32 and in each case was lower than the hemolysis titer.

The Role of Complement

Many of the striking serologic characteristics of the Donath-Landsteiner antibody are related to complement. It is therefore not surprising that the role of complement has been intensively investigated. Its influence in both the initial cold sensitizing stage and in the final warm lytic phase has been well documented.

There is no doubt that complement plays a critical role in lysis initiated by warming. Early studies suggested that sufficient complement was adsorbed during the initial cold reaction to induce the lysis observed during warming. This was denied by the data presented by Siebens and associates in 1948 (105). Jordan and associates (96) noted a reciprocal relationship between the amounts of complement needed for the two phases. Employing sensitive test systems they demonstrated that sufficient complement could be adsorbed in the initial cold reaction to produce hemolysis in the warm phase.

Opinion has sharply differed as to the role complement plays during the cold phase. Hoover and Stone in 1908 (106) suggested that complement was necessary for cold fixation of the Donath-Landsteiner antibody to erythrocytes. MacKenzie (107) was not able to confirm this assumption. He noted that the degree of hemolysis obtained upon warming was increased if antibody fixation during the cold phase occurred in the presence of complement. Siebens and associates (105) suggested that Donath-Landsteiner antibody fixation to erythrocytes in the cold required at least one component of complement. The C'4 component was implicated by Jordan and associates (96) as the critical factor.

van Loghem and associates (108) and Schubothe (7) clarified this problem. They used heat inactivated serum during cold interaction and noted a small amount of lysis upon warming. Maximal hemolysis did not occur unless complement was present during chilling of erythrocytes with antibody. Baxter and Jordan (109) found that Mg^{++} ions were not necessary for this reaction. Dacie (33) reported that complement was not crucial for antibody fixation to erythrocytes. However, the presence of complement substantially increases the amount of antibody cellularly bound. Hinz and associates (100, 110) extended these observations, employing normal erythrocytes and erythrocytes obtained from patients with paroxysmal nocturnal hemoglobinuria. Human and guinea pig sera were used as a source of complement. Complement requirement in the cold phase was variable. It depended on the potency of the Donath-Landsteiner antibody and on the sensitivity of erythrocytes (100). The C'1 complement component and Ca^{++} ions were essential for the cold reaction (110). The C'4 component was active in both the cold and warm phases, but was not crucial for cold fixation of the antibody. C'2, C'3 and Mg^{++} ions were necessary for warm lysis to occur (110).

Complement plays a critical role in paroxysmal cold hemoglobinuria. A reduction of serum complement is usual in patients with this syndrome. MacKenzie (107) reported an anticomplementary serum in 1929. Jordan (111) encountered low levels of serum complement in three of four patients he analyzed. van Loghem and associates (71) noted abnormally low levels of serum complement in all 17 patients they investigated. A syphilitic or nonsyphilitic etiology did not appear to be related to the reduction of complement. These observations suggest that complement should be added to the test system when a search is made for the Donath-Landsteiner antibody (33, 100).

Optimal Temperatures

The extremes of temperature required to induce lysis with the Donath-Landsteiner antibody have impressed most workers in this field. Chilling the test system is critical for the initial phase of antibody fixation; warming the test system is equally critical for the development of hemolysis. van Loghem and associates (71, 108), Dausset and associates (112) and Schubothe (7) emphasized this temperature variation by terming the antibody biphasic or bithermic. The Donath-Landsteiner antibody differs in its temperature requirements from the more frequently encountered cold acting hemagglutinins. These substances attach to the erythrocyte and induce lysis at one temperature. They have accordingly been termed monophasic or monothermic cold acting antibodies. Dacie (33) suggests that this distinction is unwarranted. Both antibodies are cold acting and both exhibit increased binding to the erythrocyte as the temperature is progressively lowered to 0°C. He postulates that the temperature differences may simply be quantitative, with the higher titer cold hemagglutinins having greater heterogeneity and a wider thermal reaction range. The force of this hypothesis is blunted by the demonstration of a different immunoglobulin class for the two types of antibodies (88). The H chains differ and different secondary immunologic characteristics are anticipated as a reflection of the different Fc fragments.

Optimal in vitro reactivity of the Donath-Landsteiner antibody is obtained by immersing the test mixtures in crushed ice baths. The maximal temperature permitting sensitization of erythrocytes by the Donath-Landsteiner antibody is variable, although not to the degree seen with cold acting hemagglutinins. MacKenzie (107) noted maximal temperatures of 10 to 12°C. in his three cases. Schubothe (7) considered 20°C. to be the highest sensitization temperature. Dacie (33) noted one unusual case with a maximal temperature of 25°C.

The temperature required to initiate hemolysis by warming sensitized erythrocytes has a similarly narrow variation. Schubothe (7) indicated that more lysis results at 40 than at 30°C. Hinz and associates (100) found 32°C. to be the optimal thermal level and they reported that lysis might occur at temperatures as low as 10°C.

MacKenzie (107) and Siebens and associates (105) felt that heating serum to 56°C. either damaged or destroyed the Donath-Landsteiner antibody. A moderate degree of variation to heat sensitivity was noted by these workers. Jordan and associates (96) suggested that these prior observations did not indicate sensitivity of the antibody to heat, but that rather they were related to the destruction of complement. By employing an excess of complement these authors demonstrated hemolytic activity after heating the antibody to 62°C. for 30 minutes. They also observed that human erythrocytes heated to 56°C. for 15 minutes were capable of adsorbing the Donath-Landsteiner antibody. Schubothe (7) expanded these studies. The Donath-Landsteiner antibody was stable in spite of heating to 60°C. for 10 minutes. Almost all lytic action of the antibody was destroyed by increasing the temperature to 70°C. for 10 minutes. Hinz and associates (100) confirmed the thermal stability of the Donath-Landsteiner antibody. They concluded that prior observations of the inhibition of lysis were due to the anticomplementary action of heat rather than to any direct effect on the antibody.

The Effect of pH

In 1909 Hijmans van den Bergh (113) added carbon dioxide to erythrocytes suspended in the serum of a patient with paroxysmal cold hemoglobinuria. Hemolysis was noted at 16°C. This observation was confirmed by other workers (105). Carbon dioxide apparently exerted its effect on the lytic phenomenon by lowering the pH of the system. Dacie (33, 114)

investigated this effect using dilute hydrochloric acid. The optimal pH for development of lysis with the Donath-Landsteiner antibody was 7.0 to 7.5. Lysis was almost maximal in unacidified sera which Dacie describes as having a pH of 8.0. Hemolysis was inhibited at pH levels over 8.7 and below 6.2. Schubothe (7) has reported essentially the same observations. Hinz and associates (100) found inhibition of lysis at pH values above 9.7 and below 5.2; their optimal range was 7.5 to 8.5. The effect of pH on hemolysis was investigated employing erythrocytes from patients with paroxysmal nocturnal hemoglobinuria. Such cells increased the sensitivity of the reaction and broadened the effective pH range. The optimal pH for the cold phase of the reaction was 6.0 to 8.0; in the warm phase a pH range of 6.5 to 8.5 was effective.

Antiglobulin Reactions

Positive antiglobulin tests have been frequently encountered during study of the Donath-Landsteiner antibody. Siebens and associates (105) used the antiglobulin reaction to demonstrate fixation of the Donath-Landsteiner antibody and complement to the erythrocyte surface. Lysis was inhibited by the action of sulfanilamide and cyanide. Jordan and associates (97) recorded positive antiglobulin reactions in their two cases. In one patient positive direct antiglobulin tests were obtained without evidence of in vivo hemolysis. Lysis did not occur even when such erythrocytes were warmed to 37°C. with added complement. On this basis these authors raised the following questions. What is the nature of the abnormal factor adsorbed in vivo? Is the "cell antibody" detected in the direct antiglobulin test the same as the serum antibody detected in the indirect antiglobulin test? Is the serum antibody detected in the indirect antiglobulin test the same as the hemolysin?

Jordan and associates (97) were unable to elute the erythrocyte coating material responsible for the direct antiglobulin test. The Donath-Landsteiner antibody in serum could be adsorbed onto erythrocytes, creating positive indirect antiglobulin tests. Elution was then successful at 56°C. The studies of these authors and those of van Loghem and associates (108) eliminated a prozone phenomenon in "strong" antiglobulin serum as occurring with the Donath-Landsteiner antibody. These observations were similar to those encountered with other cold acting hemagglutinins. Dacie (33) reported positive direct antiglobulin reactions at the onset of hemolysis in a case of paroxysmal cold hemoglobinuria. With clinical improvement the antiglobulin test became negative, although the Donath-Landsteiner antibody persisted. By contrast, the indirect antiglobulin test paralleled the activity of the Donath-Landsteiner hemolysin.

The studies of Dacie and associates (33, 63) with "incomplete" cold hemagglutinins have clarified this confusing picture. Positive antiglobulin reactions seen in paroxysmal cold hemoglobinuria are due to erythrocyte binding of both complement and Donath-Landsteiner antibody. Irreversibly bound complement creates the direct antiglobulin reaction with the inability to elute an antibody. Indirect antiglobulin reactions, which are best demonstrated with "strong" (potent, undiluted) antiglobulin serum, reflect the adsorption of both complement and Donath-Landsteiner antibody. Strong anti-nongamma antiglobulin reactions are found because of cellularly bound complement. In addition, weak anti-IgG antiglobulin reactions may also be obtained. This demonstrates Donath-Landsteiner antibody irreversibly bound to erythrocytes.

Trypsinized and PNH Erythrocytes

Dacie (33) noted that the use of trypsinized normal erythrocytes in the Donath-Landsteiner test increased lysis approximately 2-fold over that obtained with untreated cells. An even greater sensitivity was obtained using erythrocytes from patients with paroxysmal nocturnal hemoglobinuria (PNH). A similar observation was made by Hinz and associates (100). Hemolysis was increased 4- to 8-fold by employing PNH erythrocytes rather than normal cells. These authors also noted that increasing the ionic strength of the reacting system tended to decrease lytic activity. This effect was more apparent with normal erythrocytes than with PNH erythrocytes. A mechanism for the increased sensitivity of PNH erythrocytes to hemolysis is discussed in Chapter 21.

Kinetic Data

Maximal binding of the Donath-Landsteiner antibody to the erythrocyte surface is a function of temperature. Rapid fixation of the antibody occurs at optimal cold temperatures. Schubothe (7) reported that approximately 50 per cent of maximal binding occurred at 1 minute at 0°C. A gradual increase in binding was noted with longer exposure times extending from 30 to 60 minutes. Dacie (33) found maximal binding of the Donath-Landsteiner antibody to the erythrocyte surface in approximately 20 minutes. Hinz and associates (100) noted almost maximal binding in 10 to 15 minutes, with a gradual increase up to 30 minutes.

Jordan and associates (97) reported elution of the Donath-Landsteiner antibody by heating coated erythrocytes to 56°C. Dacie (33) noted substantial elution at 37°C. Schubothe (7) reported a lesser degree of elution of the Donath-Landsteiner antibody at 40°C.

Placental Passage

The Donath-Landsteiner antibody is a gamma G immunoglobulin (88). The presence of a gamma type H chain suggests that an active placental transport mechanism exists for this antibody. Hoppe and Witte (89) in 1960 reported a clinical case illustrating this state. A mother suffering from paroxysmal cold hemoglobinuria delivered an infant who developed hemolytic anemia and jaundice. The Donath-Landsteiner antibody was shown to be the agent responsible for this unusual form of erythroblastosis. This observation is supported by the demonstration that the sera of frequent aborters may have an antibody with erythrocyte specificity identical to the Donath-Landsteiner antibody (115).

TABLE 95. *Contrasting characteristics of the cold acting hemagglutinins and the Donath-Landsteiner antibody*

	Cold Acting Hemagglutinin	Donath-Landsteiner Antibody
General characteristics		
Species specificity	No	No
Naturally occurring	Yes	Rare
Physical-chemical characteristics		
Serum globulin	Yes	Yes
Immunoglobulin class	IgM	IgG
Sedimentation constant	19S	7S
Molecular weight	890,000	140,000
Electrophoresis	Abnormal gamma-beta peak	Normal
Serologic characteristics		
Type of antibody	Complete	Complete
Agglutination titer	High	Low
Hemolysis titer	Low	High
Effect of temperature	Monothermic	Bithermic
Effect of acidification	Induces hemolysis	Hemolysis without acid
Complement fixation	Yes	Yes
Use of PNH red blood cells	Increases hemolysis	Similar to normal red blood cells; hemolysis increased
Antigenic specificity	Yes: anti-I, anti-i	Yes: anti-P
Placental transfer	No	Yes
Positive anti-gamma antiglobulin test	No	Yes
Positive anti-non-gamma antiglobulin test	Yes	Yes

The cold acting erythrocyte autoantibody (Donath-Landsteiner antibody) characteristic of paroxysmal cold hemoglobinuria has many qualities which serve to distinguish it from other cold acting erythrocyte autoantibodies. Its bithermic nature is unique and it is a member of a different immunoglobulin class. Antigenic specificity is different for these two types of cold acting erythrocyte autoantibodies (see Chapter 20). The contrasting features of the Donath-Landsteiner antibody and other cold acting erythrocyte autoantibodies are summarized in Table 95.

BIBLIOGRAPHY

1. Stats, D., and Wasserman, L. R.: Cold hemagglutination—an interpretive review. Medicine (Balt.) **22**: 363, 1943.
2. Landsteiner, K.: Ueber Beziehungen zwischen dem Blutserum und den Körperzellen. Munchen. Med. Wschr. **50**: 1812, 1903.
3. Clough, M. C., and Richter, I. M.: A study of an autoagglutinin in human serum. Bull. Hopkins Hosp. **29**: 86, 1918.
4. Rosenthal, F., and Corten, M.: Über das phänomen der Autohämagglutination und über die Eigenschaften der kältehämagglutinine. Folia Haemat. (Frankfurt) **58**: 64, 1937.
5. Turner, J. C., and Jackson, E. B.: Serological specificity of an autoantibody in atypical pneumonia. Brit. J. Exp. Path. **24**: 121, 1943.
6. Wiener, A. S., Gordon, E. B., and Gallop, C.: Studies on autoantibodies in human sera. J. Immun. **71**: 58, 1953.
7. Schubothe, H.: *Serologie und Klinische Bedeutung der autohämantikörper.* S. Karger, Basel, 1958.
8. Evans, R. S., Turner, E., and Bingham, M.: Studies with radioiodinated cold agglutinins of ten patients. Amer. J. Med. **38**: 378, 1965.
9. Wheeler, K. M.: Group specific agglutinins in rabbit serum for human cells; cold agglutinins. J. Immun. **34**: 409, 1938.
10. Ottenberg, R., and Thalhimer, W.: Studies in experimental transfusion. J. Med. Res. **28**(N.S.): 213, 1915.
11. Walther, G.: Autohämagglutination, Geldrollenbildung und Senkungsgeschwindigkeit. Folia Haemat. (Frankfurt) **38**: 281, 1929.
12. Yu, I.: Ueber die Frigid-hämagglutinine. Zbl. Bakt. (Orig.) **106**: 388, 1928.
13. Amzel, R., and Hirszfeld, L.: Ueber die

Kälteagglutination der roten Blutkörperchen. Immunitaetsforsch. **43**: 526, 1925.

14. Kettel, K.: *Undersøgelser over Kuldehaemagglutininer. I. Meuneskeserum.* Levin & Munksgaard, Copenhagen, 1930.

15. Young, L. E.: The clinical significance of cold hemagglutinins. Amer. J. Med. Sci. **211**: 23, 1946.

16. Savonen, K.: Cold haemagglutination test and its clinical significance. Ann. Med. Exp. Fenn. **26**: Suppl. 3, 1948.

17. Janković, B. D.: Reaction between incomplete cold autoantibody and trypsin treated red cells. Acta Med. Iugosl. **9**: 28, 1955.

18. Milders, H. D. E.: Bloed transfusie en Autoagglutinatie. Nederl. T. Geneesk. **72**: 4108, 1928.

19. Li, C-P.: Investigation on "cold" or autohemagglutination. J. Immun. **11**: 297, 1926.

20. Montanari, A.: Studi sull'autoemagglutinazione. Riv. Clin. Med. **30**: 659, 1929.

21. Riebeling, C.: Ueber einen Fall von Sog. Panagglutination. Med. Klin. **29**: 1440, 1933.

22. Niu, M.: Ueber die Antigene der Autohaemoagglutinine. J. Chosen M. A., 415, 1928.

23. Debenedetti, E.: La grande autoagglutination des hématies. Presse Med. **37**: 1688, 1929.

24. Benhamou, E., and Nouchy, A.: Grande autoagglutination des hématies. Presse Med. **41**: 27, 1933.

25. Stats, D., Perlman, E., Bullowa, J. G. M., and Goodkind, R.: Electrophoresis and antibody nitrogen determinations of a cold hemagglutinin. Proc. Soc. Exp. Biol. Med. **53**: 188, 1943.

26. Spaet, T. H., and Kinsell, B. G.: Studies on the normal serum panagglutinin active against trypsinated human erythrocytes. II. Relationship to cold agglutination. J. Lab. Clin. Med. **42**: 205, 1953.

27. Gordon, R. S.: The preparation and properties of cold hemagglutinin. J. Immun. **71**: 220, 1953.

28. Schubothe, H.: Kombinationen von Paraproteinämie und Autoantikörperbildung. Schweiz. Med. Wschr. **84**: 1109, 1954.

29. Rørvik, K.: The syndrome of high-titre cold haemagglutination. Acta Med. Scand. **148**: 299, 1954.

30. Varques, R., Zermati, M., and Labrosse, S.: Une agglutinine froide cliniquement définie l'euglobuline I. de Sandor. Sang **26**: 294, 1955.

31. Weber, R.: Molecular weight of cold hemagglutinins. Vox Sang. **1**: 37, 1956.

32. Christenson, W. N., and Dacie, J. V.: Serum proteins in acquired haemolytic anaemia (auto-antibody type). Brit. J. Haemat. **3**: 153, 1957.

33. Dacie, J. V.: *The Haemolytic Anaemias, Part II,* Ed. 2. Grune & Stratton, Inc., New York, 1962.

34. Christenson, W. N., Dacie, J. V., Croucher,

B. E. E., and Charlwood, P. A.: Electrophoretic studies on sera containing high-titre cold haemagglutinins: identification of the antibody as the cause of an abnormal γ_1 peak. Brit. J. Haemat. **3**: 262, 1957.

35. Fudenberg, H. H., and Kunkel, H. G.: Physical properties of red cell agglutinins in acquired hemolytic anemia. J. Exp. Med. **106**: 689, 1957.

36. Mehrotra, T. N., and Charlwood, P. A.: Physico-chemical characterization of the cold auto-antibodies of acquired haemolytic anaemia. Immunology. **3**: 254, 1960.

37. Firkin, B. G., and Blackburn, C. R. B.: Identification of a cold agglutinin as a β-globulin. Aust. J. Exp. Biol. Med. Sci. **34**: 407, 1956.

38. Firkin, B. G.: The nature of the adsorbed antibody in acquired haemolytic anaemia. Aust. J. Exp. Biol. Med. Sci. **36**: 359, 1958.

39. Firkin, B. G., Blackwell, J. B., and Johnston, G. A. W.: Essential cryoglobulinaemia and acquired haemolytic anaemia due to cold antibodies. Aust. Ann. Med. **8**: 151, 1959.

40. Mehrotra, T. N.: Immunological identification of the pathological cold auto-antibodies of acquired haemolytic anaemia as β_2M globulin. Immunology **3**: 265, 1960.

41. Mehrotra, T. N.: Individual specific nature of the cold auto-antibodies of acquired haemolytic anaemia. Nature (London) **185**: 323, 1960.

42. Chan, P. C. Y., and Deutsch, H. F.: Immunochemical studies of human serum Rh agglutinins. J. Immun. **85**: 37, 1960.

43. Deutsch, H. F., and Morton, J. I.: Dissociation of human serum macroglobulins. Science **125**: 600, 1957.

44. Harboe, M., and Deverill, J.: Immunochemical properties of cold haemagglutinins. Scand. J. Haemat. **1**: 223, 1964.

45. Jacot-Guillarmod, H., and Isliker, H.: Scission et réassociation des iso-agglutinines traitées par des agents réducteurs des ponts disulfures. Préparation d'anticorps mixtes. Vox Sang. **7**: 675, 1962.

46. Anderson, B. R.: Gamma A cold agglutinin: importance of disulfide bonds in activity and structure. Science **154**: 281, 1966.

47. Franklin, E. C., and Fudenberg, H. H.: Antigenic heterogeneity of human Rh antibodies, rheumatoid factors, and cold agglutinins. Arch. Biochem. **104**: 433, 1964.

48. Harboe, M., van Furth, R., Schubothe, H., Lind, G., and Evans, R. S.: Exclusive occurrence of kappa chains in isolated cold haemagglutinins. Scand. J. Haemat. **2**: 259, 1965.

49. Schubothe, H.: The cold hemagglutinin disease. Seminars Hemat. **3**: 27, 1966.

50. Costea, N., Yakulis, V., and Heller, P.: Light chain heterogeneity of cold agglutinins. Science **152**: 1520, 1966.

51. van Furth, R., and Diesselhoff-den Dulk, M.:

The formation in vitro of cold auto-hemagglutinins without anti-I specificity. J. Immun. **96**: 920, 1966.
52. Cooper, A. G., and Worlledge, S. M.: Light
chains in chronic cold haemagglutinin disease. Nature (London) **214**: 799, 1967.
53. Harboe, M., and Lind, K.: Light chain types
of transiently occurring cold haemagglutinins. Scand. J. Haemat. **3**: 269, 1966.
54. Costea, N., Yakulis, V., and Heller, P.: The
dependence of cold agglutinin activity on K
chains. J. Immun. **99**: 558, 1967.
55. Feizi, T.: Lambda chains in cold agglutinins.
Science **156**: 1111, 1967.
56. Schubothe, H.: Current problems of chronic
cold hemagglutinin disease. Ann. N. Y.
Acad. Sci. **124**: 484, 1965.
57. Harris, G., and Fairley, C. H.: Immunological identification of a cryomacroglobulin
in a patient with acquired hemolytic anemia associated with a cold antibody. Nature
(London) **194**: 1090, 1962.
58. Turro, O. R., and Straface, R. T.: Anemia
hemolitica aguda par crioaglutininas. Arch.
Argent. Pediat. **63**: 57, 1965.
59. Gökcen, M.: Cryoglobulins behaving as
"cold autoantibodies." Postgrad. Med. **39**:
68, 1966.
60. Dacie, J. V.: Occurrences in normal human
sera of "incomplete" forms of "cold" autoantibodies. Nature (London) **166**: 36,
1950.
61. Ferriman, D. G., Dacie, J. V., Keele, K. D.,
and Fullerton, J. M.: The association of
Raynaud's phenomena, chronic haemolytic
anaemia, and the formation of cold antibodies. Quart. J. Med. **20**: 275, 1951.
62. Dacie, J. V.: Differences in the behaviour of
sensitized red cells to agglutination by antiglobulin sera. Lancet **2**: 954, 1951.
63. Dacie, J. V., Crookston, J. H., and Christenson, W. N.: "Incomplete" cold antibodies:
role of complement in sensitization to antiglobulin serum by potentially haemolytic
antibodies. Brit. J. Haemat. **3**: 77, 1957.
64. Adinolfi, M., Daniels, C., and Mollison, P.
L.: Evidence that "normal incomplete cold
antibody" is not a gamma-globulin. Nature
(London) **199**: 389, 1963.
65. Rosenfield, R. E., Haber, G. V., and Gilbert,
H. S.: Complement and the antiglobulin
test. Vox Sang. **5**: 182, 1960.
66. Gandini, E.: Comportamento dei sieri antiglobuline nell'emoagglutinazione del tipo
cosiddetto non gamma-globulinico. In Proceedings of the Seventh Congress of the
International Society of Blood Transfusion. S. Karger, Basel, 1959.
67. Pondman, K. W., Rosenfield, R. E., Tallal,
L., and Wasserman, L. R.: The specificity
of the complement antiglobulin test. Vox
Sang. **5**: 297, 1960.
68. Leddy, J. P., Hill, R. W., Swisher, S. N., and

Vaughan, J. H.: Observations on the immunochemical nature of red cell autosensitization. In Immunopathology, Third In-
national Symposium, edited by P. Grabar
and P. Miescher. Schwabe and Company,
Basel, 1963.
69. Harboe, M.: Reaction of I¹³¹ trace labeled
cold agglutinin. Ann. N. Y. Acad. Sci. **124**:
491, 1965.
70. Boyer, J. T.: Stability of the antigen-antibody complex. Bibl. Haemat. **23**: 19, 1965.
71. van Loghem, J. J., van der Hart, M., and
Dorfmeier, H.: Serologic studies in acquired
hemolytic anemia. In Proceedings of the
Sixth International Congress of the International Society of Hematology. Grune &
Stratton, Inc., New York, 1958.
72. Jonsen, J., Koss, E., and Harboe, M.: Complement and complement components in
acquired hemolytic anemia with high titer
cold antibodies. Acta Med. Scand. **170**:
725, 1961.
73. Fife, E. H. J., Hook, W. A., and Muschel, L.
H.: Tissue antibody and complement levels
in runt disease. Proc. Soc. Exp. Biol. Med.
110: 524, 1962.
74. Rosse, W. F., and Dacie, J. V.: The role of
complement in the sensitivity of the paroxysmal nocturnal haemoglobinuria red cell
to immune lysis. Bibl. Haemat. **23**: 11,
1965.
75. Mayer, M. M., Levine, L., Rapp, H. J., and
Marucci, A. A.: Kinetic studies of immune
hemolysis. VII. Decay of EAC 142, fixation
of C'3 and other factors influencing the
hemolytic action of complement. J. Immun.
73: 443, 1954.
76. Evans, R. S., Bingham, M., and Turner, E.:
Autoimmune hemolytic disease: observations of serological reactions and disease
activity. Ann. N. Y. Acad. Sci. **124**: 422,
1965.
77. Taranta, A., and Franklin, E. C.: Complement fixation by antibody fragments.
Science **134**: 1981, 1961.
78. Leddy, J. P., and Vaughan, J. H.: Auto-
sensitization of trypsin treated human red
cells by complement. Proc. Soc. Exp. Biol.
Med. **117**: 734, 1964.
79. Eyster, M. E., Nachman, R. L., Christenson,
W. N., and Engle, R. L.: Structural characteristics of red cell autoantibodies. J. Immun. **96**: 107, 1966.
80. Dacie, J. V.: The presence of cold haemolysins in sera containing cold haemagglutinins. J. Path. Bact. **62**: 241, 1950.
81. Bonnin, J. A.: Chronic acquired hemolytic
anemia associated with hemaglobinuria and
Raynaud's phenomena. Blood **9**: 959, 1954.
82. Barcroft, H., and Edholm, O. G.: Temperature and blood flow in the human forearm.
J. Physiol. **104**: 366, 1946.
83. Stats, D.: Cold hemagglutination and cold

hemolysis. The hemolysis produced by shaking cold agglutinated erythrocytes. J. Clin. Invest. **24**: 33, 1945.

84. Ham, T. H., Gardner, F. H., Wagley, P. F., and Shen, S. C.: Studies on the mechanism of hemolytic anemia and hemoglobinuria occurring in patients with high concentrations of serum cold agglutinin. J. Clin. Invest. **27**: 538, 1948.

85. Lewis, S. M., Dacie, J. V., and Szur, L.: Mechanism of haemolysis in the cold-haemagglutinin syndrome. Brit. J. Haemat. **6**: 154, 1960.

86. Heilmeyer, L., Hahn, F., and Schubothe, H.: Hämolytische anämien auf der Basis abnormer serologischer Reaktionen. Klin. Wschr. **24/25**: 193, 1947.

87. Johnsson, S.: On autoagglutinins active at body temperature. Acta Med. Scand. **134**: 180, 1949.

88. Hinz, C. F.: Serologic and physicochemical characterization of Donath-Landsteiner antibodies from six patients. Blood **22**: 600, 1963.

89. Hoppe, H. H., and Witte, A.: Hämolytische Erkrankung eines Neugeborenen bei paroxysmaler Kältehämoglobinurie der Mutter. Vox Sang. **5**: 425, 1960.

90. Boyd, W. C., Bhatia, H. M., Diamond, M. A., and Matsubara, S.: Quantitative study of the combination of lima bean lectin with human erythrocytes. J. Immun. **89**: 463, 1962.

91. Pisciotta, A. V.: Cold hemagglutination in acute and chronic hemolytic syndromes. Blood **10**: 295, 1955.

92. Donath, J., and Landsteiner, K.: Ueber paroxysmale hämoglobinurie. Munchen. Med. Wschr. **51**: 1590, 1904.

93. Donath, J., and Landsteiner, K.: Ueber paroxysmale Hämoglobinurie. Z. Klin. Med. **58**: 173, 1906.

94. Donath, J., and Landsteiner, K.: Weitere Beobactungen über paroxysmale Hämoglobinurie. Zbl. Bakt. (Orig.) **45**: 204, 1908.

95. Eason, J.: The pathology of paroxysmal haemoglobinuria. J. Path. Bact. **11**: 167, 1906.

96. Jordon, W. S., Pillemer, L., and Dingle, J. H.: The mechanism of hemolysis in paroxysmal cold hemoglobinuria. I. The role of complement and its components in the Donath-Landsteiner reaction. J. Clin. Invest. **30**: 11, 1951.

97. Jordan, W. S., Pillemer, L., and Dingle, J. H.: The mechanism of hemolysis in paroxysmal cold hemoglobinuria. II. Observations on the behavior and nature of the antibody. J. Clin. Invest. **30**: 22, 1951.

98. Gouttas, A., Tzevreuis, H., Pouggouras, P., Reniéri, N., and Papathanassion, S.: Hémoglobinurie paroxystique à frigoré avec coëxistence d'un anticorps froid incomplet à

grande marge thermique. Sang **29**: 53, 1958.

99. Leonardi, P., and Andolfatto-Zaglia, G.: Emoglobinuria parossistica a frigore non luetica da anticorpo bifasico tipo Donath e Landsteiner. Minerva. Med. **51**: 453, 1960.

100. Hinz, C. F., Jr., Picken, M. E., and Lepow, I. H.: Studies on immune human hemolysis. I. The kinetics of the Donath-Landsteiner reaction and the requirement for complement in the reaction. J. Exp. Med. **113**: 177, 1961.

101. Kissmeyer-Nielson, F., and Schleiner, P.: Paroxysmal cold haemoglobinuria. Report of a case with haemolytic anaemia and a normal cold agglutinin titer. Danish Med. Bull. **10**: 52, 1963.

102. van der Hart, M., van der Giessen, M., van der Veer, M., Peetom, F., and van Loghem, J. J.: Immunochemical and serological properties of biphasic haemolysins. Vox Sang. **9**: 36, 1964.

103. Weiner, W., Gordon, E. G., and Rowe, D.: A Donath-Landsteiner antibody (nonsyphilitic type). Vox Sang. **9**: 684, 1964.

104. Becker, R. M.: Paroxysmal cold hemoglobinurias. Arch. Intern. Med. (Chicago) **81**: 630, 1948.

105. Siebens, A. A., Zinkham, W. H., and Wagley, P. F.: Observations on the mechanism of hemolysis in paroxysmal (cold) hemoglobinuria. Blood **3**: 1367, 1948.

106. Hoover, C. F., and Stone, G. W.: Paroxysmal hemoglobinuria. Account of two cases. Arch. Intern. Med. (Chicago) **2**: 392, 1908.

107. MacKenzie, G. M.: Paroxysmal hemoglobinuria. A review. Medicine (Balt.) **8**: 159, 1929.

108. van Loghem, J. J., Mendes de Leon, D. E., Frenkel-Tietz, H., and van der Hart, M.: Two different serologic mechanisms of paroxysmal cold hemoglobinuria, illustrated by three cases. Blood **7**: 1196, 1952.

109. Baxter, J. A., and Jordan, W. S.: Role of magnesium ions in Donath-Landsteiner hemolytic reaction of paroxysmal cold hemoglobinuria. Proc. Soc. Exp. Biol. Med. **85**: 648, 1954.

110. Hinz, C. F., Picken, M. E., and Lepow, I. H.: Studies on immune human hemolysis. II. The Donath-Landsteiner reaction as a model system for studying the mechanism of action of complement and the role of C'1 and C'1 esterase. J. Exp. Med. **113**: 193, 1961.

111. Jordan, F. L. J.: The role of complement in immunohemolytic disease. In *Proceedings of the Sixth International Congress of the International Society of Hematology*. Grune & Stratton, Inc., New York, 1958.

112. Dausset, J., Colombani, J., and Evelin, J.:

Technique de recherche des autohémolysines immunologiques. Rev. Franc Etud. Clin. Biol. 11: 735, 1957.

113. Hijmans van den Bergh, A. A.: Ueber die Hämolyse bei der paroxysmalen Hämoglobinurie. Berlin. Klin. Wschr. 46: 1609, 1909.

114. Dacie, J. V.: Hemolysins in acquired hemolytic anemia. Effect of pH on the activity in vitro of a serum hemolysin. Blood 4: 928, 1949.

115. Vos, G. H., Celano, M. J., Falkowski, F., and Levine, P.: Relationship of a hemolysin resembling anti-Tj[a] to threatened abortion in Western Australia. Transfusion 4: 87, 1964.

Chapter 20

The Antigen in the Autoimmune Hemolytic Anemias

The concept of autoantibody formation has been formulated for many years. Only in the last decade, however, have a substantial number of investigators accepted this hypothesis. The inability to define the antigen involved in autoimmune hemolytic anemia was a major factor preventing general acceptance of the autoimmune postulate. No doubt existed that a substance could be produced by a host with the capacity to react with the host's own erythrocytes. In addition, production of this substance was usually related to erythrocyte damage and hemolytic anemia. In spite of these observations there was a reluctance to accept an autoantibody nature of the reacting material. This reluctance was expressed by employing terms such as "erythrocyte coating material" and "antiglobulin positive state" or by placing quotation marks around "autoantibody" (1).

The Antigen in Warm Acting Autoimmune Hemolytic Anemia

Physical, chemical, immunologic and serologic studies demonstrated a marked similarity between incomplete warm acting erythrocyte iso- and autoantibodies. Table 96 summarizes the characteristic features of these two types of erythrocyte antibodies. Both are gamma G immunoglobulins that function serologically in an incomplete fashion, react with antiglobulin serum, can induce autohemagglutination in albumin or other colloid materials, directly agglutinate enzyme treated erythrocytes, pass the placental barrier, do not lose immunologic activity after reduction with 2-mercaptoethanol and have optimal reactivity at 37°C. Two outstanding differences exist between these two antibody varieties. Erythrocyte isoantibodies have easily documented antigenic specificity and their formation can generally be related to immunization of the host producing the antibody. Warm acting erythrocyte autoantibodies generally appear nonspecific and react with all human erythrocytes. Specific examples of immunization leading to autoantibody formation usually cannot be documented.

Two different experimental approaches have been used to determine the antigen in warm acting autoimmune hemolytic anemia. One set of studies relates similarities or dissimilarities of incomplete erythrocyte isoantibodies to autoantibodies. The second experimental approach involves direct documentation of antigenic specificity and identification of the antigen in warm acting autoimmune hemolytic anemia.

Comparative Studies of Erythrocyte Autoantibodies and Isoantibodies

Most comparative studies of warm acting erythrocyte auto- and isoantibodies reveal gross similarities. Differences between the two types of antibodies, however, have been reported.

Roth (2) noted that heparin inhibited the agglutination of autoantibody coated erythrocytes by antiglobulin serum. The

TABLE 96. *The characteristics of warm acting erythrocyte autoantibodies contrasted with those of warm acting erythrocyte isoantibodies*

Serologic Characteristics	Warm Acting Autoantibody (AHA)	Warm Acting Isoantibody (Anti-Rh$_o$(D))
Type of antibody	Incomplete	Incomplete
Agglutination demonstrated with:		
Saline	No	No
Antiglobulin serum	Yes	Yes
Colloidal solutions	Yes	Yes
Proteolytic enzymes	Yes	Yes
Pass placental barrier	Yes	Yes
Complement dependent	No	No
Adsorbed by erythrocytes	Yes	Yes
May be eluted	Yes	Yes
Shortens red blood cell survival time	Yes	Yes
Type of in vivo hemolysis	Splenic sequestration	Splenic sequestration
Physical-chemical characteristics		
Serum globulin	Yes	Yes
Immunoglobulin class	IgG	IgG
Sedimentation constant	7S	7S
Molecular weight	140,000	140,000
Inhibition by streptomycin	Yes	Yes
Effect of disulfide reduction		
Loss of immunologic activity	No	No
Conversion to saline agglutination	Yes	Yes
Saline titer, % of antiglobulin titer	5–10	5–10
General characteristics		
Evidence for sensitization	No	Yes
Antigenic specificity	Uncommon	Yes

inhibitory effect of heparin was not obtained with anti-rhesus antibodies. Roth and Frumin (3) also reported that protamine had different effects on the agglutination of antibody coated erythrocytes, depending on whether iso- or autoantibodies were employed. The heparin effect may result from an anticomplementary action or by increasing the negative charge of the erythrocyte surface. Accordingly, differences between iso- and autoantibodies may not have structural or antigenic implications. This phenomenon deserves detailed reexamination. The significance of the data obtained with protamine is questionable. Basically charged molecules such as protamine agglutinate erythrocytes independently of immunologic mechanisms (4).

Pirofsky (5) studied the quantitative reaction of erythrocyte auto- and isoantibody eluates with antiglobulin serum. Anti-Rh$_o$(D) and anti-rh'(C) were neutralized by and in turn inactivated antiglobulin se-

rum in a soluble test system. Four warm acting erythrocyte autoantibody eluates were similarly studied. They inactivated antiglobulin serum and were neutralized only when erythrocytes were added to the test solution. The differences seen between the two types of antibodies have dubious significance. Iso- and autoantibody eluates were prepared by different methods, and different degrees of denaturation of antibody may have influenced their reactivity. Variations in the concentration of antibody and antiglobulin serum may also have been responsible for the differences observed.

Brodie and Finch (6) studied sera containing erythrocyte autoantibodies in an immune adherence test system. Reactions obtained did not suggest the presence of antibodies. It was postulated that erythrocyte autoantibodies were proteins with an affinity for the erythrocyte surface and that they reflected a dysproteinemic state. Brodie (7) subsequently expanded this study, employing immune adherence. He tested erythrocyte autoantibody eluates for reactivity with autologous leukemic leukocytes and erythrocytes. Immune adherence reactions were noted with autologous leukemic lymphocytes but not with autologous erythrocytes. Brodie (7) concluded that autologous leukemic lymphocytes may be one of the factors that stimulate the development of the autoantibody. This concept had been previously investigated by Pirofsky (8), employing less elegant immunologic procedures, with negative results.

In spite of these dissenting views most studies documented a similarity between warm acting erythrocyte autoantibodies and isoantibodies. Table 96 summarizes this relationship employing incomplete anti-Rh_o(D). Three experimental approaches have been carried out in the author's laboratory to clarify this relationship further.

1. I^{131} Trace Labeling. Kinetic studies were performed using I^{131} trace labeled globulin fractions of normal sera and of sera containing anti-Rh_o(D) (9). These studies confirmed the observation of Boursnell and associates (10) that substantial numbers of gamma-globulin molecules fix to the erythrocyte surface in a nonimmunologic fashion. Elution of nonimmunologically bound globulin makes available reagents able to neutralize antiglobulin sera (11). Globulin bound to the erythrocyte surface in a nonimmune linkage also can combine with antiglobulin serum. However, agglutination does not result from this interaction. This contrasts with the case of immunologically bound globulins such as anti-rhesus antibodies (11). Representative data are presented in Figure 39 (see Chapter 18). Erythrocyte autoantibodies react in a manner similar to that of anti-rhesus antibodies. The interaction with antiglobulin serum does not resemble the pattern seen with globulin molecules fixed to the erythrocyte in a nonimmune fashion. Such studies suggest that the erythrocyte coating material in autoimmune hemolytic anemia functions as an antibody in its reaction with an erythrocyte. The globulin-

erythrocyte linkage does not suggest the presence of a nonspecific dysgammaglobulinemia state (9, 11).

2. Disulfide Reduction Reactions. 2-Mercaptoethanol was employed to disrupt disulfide bonds of incomplete anti-Rh_o(D) in an attempt to change the tertiary molecular structure (12, 13). This reducing procedure converted incomplete anti-Rh_o(D) into saline agglutinating forms. The saline agglutinating titers, however, were only 5 to 10 per cent of titers obtained with antiglobulin serum. This suggests that disulfide reduction only exposes a limited number of potential bivalent reactive sites previously unavailable because of steric obstruction. Similar results have been obtained using Cleland's reagent at a concentration of 0.01 to 0.008 M. Warm acting erythrocyte autoantibodies showed reactions identical to those obtained with anti-Rh_o(D) (14). These data indicate that incomplete anti-Rh_o(D) and incomplete erythrocyte autoantibodies are potentially bivalent. In addition, treatment with reducing agents exposes a similar number of previously inaccessible antibody combining sites. Mandy and associates (15) have obtained similar results, but they feel that a nonimmunologic phenomenon is involved.

3. Inhibition by Hexose Antibiotics. Streptomycin inhibition of erythrocyte antibodies exhibits a certain degree of specificity (16, 17). The agglutinating capacities of anti-A, anti-B, anti-N and anti-M were unaffected by streptomycin. In contrast, streptomycin inhibited the agglutination inducing ability of anti-Rho_o(D), anti-rh' (C), anti-rh" (E), anti-hr'(c) and anti-hr"(e). Inhibition of agglutination occurred with both 2-mercaptoethanol resistant and 2-mercaptoethanol sensitive forms of the antibody. Warm acting erythrocyte autoantibodies were susceptible to streptomycin in a manner similar to that of anti-rhesus antibodies (14).

Boyd and associates (18) suggested that the inhibition capacity of streptomycin is related to the N-methyl-L-glucosamine portion of the molecule. This is assumed to function as an analog of the Rh_o(D) antigen. The high concentration of streptomycin necessary to induce inhibition makes this explanation unlikely. Pirofsky and Cordova (16, 17, 19) demonstrated that the streptidine portion of streptomycin functioned as an inhibiting agent in the absence of N-methyl-L-glucosamine. Streptomycin inhibited agglutination by preventing the anti-Rh_o(D) antibody from fixing to the antigenic site (19). Preliminary studies related inhibition of agglutination to the polar basic charge of the streptomycin molecule. It was suggested that binding of streptomycin to negative groups of the antibody resulted in a streptomycin-globulin complex. This complex possibly induced steric obstruction, preventing combination with the Rh_o(D) antigen.

If the explanation offered by Boyd and associates (18) of streptomycin inhibition were accurate, it would suggest a rhesus antigenic relationship to warm acting erythrocyte autoantibodies. If the hypothesis of Pirofsky and Cordova (19) is true, the molecular structure of anti-rhesus antibodies and that of warm acting erythrocyte antoantibodies are similar. Both types of antibodies must have a general resemblance in molecular charge distribution. In addition, a similar change in molecular charge introduces similar steric obstruction at the antibody combining site.

The three sets of studies outlined above indicate that warm acting erythrocyte autoantibodies are similar to anti-Rh_o(D) in several critical respects (14). These include: (a) type of linkage to the erythrocyte surface, (b) type of reaction with antiglobulin serum, (c) a bivalent status which is not apparent in saline testing, (d) exposure of a similar number of previously inaccessible antibody combining sites by disruption of the tertiary molecular structure, (e) a similar charge distribution of the molecule, (f) a similar steric obstruction of antibody combining sites induced by changing the charge and (g) possibly a similar antibody combining site in relation to the Rh_o(D) antigen. These observations strongly suggest that warm acting erythrocyte autoantibodies are directed against the rhesus antigen. More specific evidence of a relationship to the rhesus antigen is presented below.

Evidence of Specificity of Warm Acting Autoantibodies

Direct evidence of a relationship between warm acting erythrocyte autoantibodies and the rhesus antigen has rapidly accumulated. A documentation of antigenic specificity for erythrocyte autoantibodies is required.

Denys and van den Broucke (20) were the first to encounter an erythrocyte autoantibody with specificity. They tested the serum of a patient with acquired hemolytic anemia against the erythrocytes of 32 normal donors in an indirect antiglobulin procedure. Two samples appeared compatible with negative antiglobulin results. Blood typing data to document autoantibody specificity were not obtained. Kuhns and Wagley (21) encountered a similar case. Studies were performed with a serum containing both cold acting and warm acting hemagglutinins. The warm acting hemagglutinin reacted with the patient's own erythrocytes and with 63 per cent of 156 blood samples compatible in O, A_1, A_2, M, N and rhesus subtypes. Specificity of the autohemagglutinin was not documented to a specific blood group type. The patient received 2,000 ml. of blood without difficulty and had negative compatibility tests 1 month before the hemagglutinin developed.

In 1951 Dameshek (22) reacted erythrocyte autoantibodies with a variety of different erythrocytes. The most intense agglutination reactions were obtained with the patient's own erythrocytes. Dameshek felt that the difference in reactivity was due to previous coating of the patient's erythrocytes with the warm acting erythrocyte autoantibodies. Davidsohn and Oyamada (23) noted the same phenomenon in 1953. They tested each of 26 erythrocyte autoantibody containing sera against the patient's own cells, against cells of a similar Rh type and against group O cells. Agglutination was determined in 20 per cent bovine albumin and occasionally with papain treated erythrocytes. Three different types of serologic reactivity were noted. With 11 sera a similar titer was obtained, irrespective of test erythrocytes. With four sera the patient's own erythrocytes gave the highest agglutination titer. The remaining 11 sera showed an even greater discrepancy between the patient's own erythrocytes and other test cells. Varying agglutination titers were obtained with the patient's own erythrocytes, whereas agglutination was absent with other test cells. The authors concluded that there were both specific and nonspecific erythrocyte autoantibodies. They discarded the explanation that prior coating of erythrocytes by autoantibody increased the fixation of antibody to the cells. Erythrocytes coated with antibody were unable to adsorb additional antibody from potent antisera.

Wiener and associates (24, 25) presented a brilliant set of speculations to explain the apparent lack of specificity of erythrocyte autoantibodies. They accepted the premise that the involved substances were antibodies reacting with host erythrocytes. It was postulated that antigenic material present on all human erythrocytes created the appearance of nonspecificity. Three different antigenic types were suggested to explain the variations of autoantibody action. The ability of cold acting erythrocyte autoantibodies to react with human and animal erythrocytes indicated specificity against antigenic determinants of the ABO blood group. Other erythrocyte autoantibodies demonstrated specificity for antigenic determinants related to the MNS blood group. Two sets of studies were performed with warm acting erythrocyte autoantibodies. Maximal sensitization of human erythrocytes with anti-Rh_o(D) and warm acting autoantibodies gave identical antiglobulin titers. This suggested that anti-Rh_o(D) and the autoantibody were reacting with a similar number of antigenic sites. Three primate erythrocyte types were also reacted with anti-Rh_o(D) and warm acting erythrocyte autoantibodies. Chimpanzee erythrocytes were sensitized with both antibodies and had similar agglutination titers with antiglobulin serum. Erythrocytes obtained from the rhesus monkey and spider monkey were not sensitized by either anti-Rh_o(D) or warm acting erythrocyte autoantibodies. It was therefore postulated that warm acting

erythrocyte autoantibodies were directed against the nucleus of the Rh-hr substance.

Identification of the Antigen

The hypothesis developed in 1953 by Wiener and associates (24, 25) of a relationship between warm acting erythrocyte autoantibodies and the rhesus blood group substance received almost immediate experimental support. Weiner and associates (26) reported a case of autoimmune hemolytic anemia occurring in a patient of rhesus genotype R_1R_1 (CDe/CDe). Eluates made from the antiglobulin positive erythrocytes had a specificity of anti-hr″(e). This therefore appeared as a true erythrocyte autoantibody with specificity directed against a rhesus agglutinogen of the host's erythrocytes. A similar observation was made by Holländer (27) in the same year. A patient of rhesus genotype R_1r (CDe/cde) with autoimmune hemolytic anemia was studied. The serum contained an antibody with specificity for hr′(c). Eluates from the antiglobulin positive erythrocytes contained two antibodies, a nonspecific reacting panhemagglutinin and anti-hr′(c).

Subsequent reports indicated that warm acting erythrocyte autoantibodies with anti-rhesus specificity were not uncommon. Dacie and Cutbush (28) studied 10 cases of warm acting autoimmune hemolytic anemia. One patient of rhesus genotype R_1r (CDe/cde) produced anti-rh′(C) and anti-hr″(e). The remaining nine cases were characterized by a nonspecific panhemagglutinin. In addition to the panhemagglutinin, however, three patients also produced anti-hr″(e) and an additional patient produced anti-Rh_o(D) and anti-hr″(e). All four had a rhesus genotype of R_1r (CDe/cde). Elution revealed the anti-hr″(e) autoantibody in two cases. Dacie and Cutbush (28) employed adsorption procedures in three cases to study the nature of the nonspecific autoantibody. Normal erythrocytes of all groups and types and erythrocytes deleted at the C/c and E/e loci (—D—/—D—) were employed. The nonspecific autoantibodies contained two components. One component was adsorbed with both normal and —D—/—D— deleted erythrocytes. A second component could not be adsorbed with the deleted erythrocytes. This suggested that the rh'(C), hr'(c), rh''(E) and hr''(e) agglutinogens had an antigenic relationship to the autoantibodies. van Loghem and van der Hart (29) studied 10 patients with autoimmune hemolytic anemia. Six autoantibodies were found with isoantigen specificity. They were identified as anti-Rh_o(D), anti-rh'(C), anti-hr'(c), anti-hr''(e) and anti-Jk^a.

The Demonstration of Specificity

Many laboratories (30–35) have confirmed the existence of warm acting erythrocyte autoantibodies with specificity for known erythrocyte isoantigens. Several examples of specific erythrocyte autoantibodies occurring in infants have been recorded (36–38). In general, these reports have supported the original postulate of Wiener and associates (24, 25) that the involved antigen belongs to the rhesus group.

Possible pitfalls in ascribing specificity to warm acting erythrocyte autoantibodies must be mentioned. Demonstration of an isoantigenic specific antibody in the serum of a patient suffering from autoimmune hemolytic anemia is not sufficient to document specificity. Patients with autoimmune hemolytic anemia may produce erythrocyte isoantibodies in addition to autoantibodies. This tendency is probably greater than that seen in other transfused populations. van Loghem and associates (33) found a 10 per cent incidence of isoantibody formation in autoimmune hemolytic anemia. Our laboratory has recently studied a 15-year-old male with ulcerative colitis and autoimmune hemolytic anemia. He had previously received two transfusions. In addition to a nonspecific erythrocyte autoantibody eluted from his erythrocytes, the serum contained anti-Rh_o(D), anti-rh'(C), anti-rh''(E) and anti-Jk^a. Before an unbound serum isoantibody can be accepted as an autoantibody it must be coupled with typing data indicating the presence of the antigen on host erythrocytes. This may not be a simple task.

Accurate typing of erythrocytes coated with incomplete erythrocyte antibody is difficult and frequently impossible. Such erythrocytes may be classified as AB, CDe/cDE (see Chapter 3). The seven antisera used in the typing procedure all induced agglutination of the test erythrocytes. If controls consisting of serum albumin and normal AB serum are employed, agglutination may also be found. Accordingly, the typing data cannot be accepted and may only reflect autohemagglutination of coated erythrocytes suspended in a colloid macromolecular medium. It is obvious that typing procedures relying on antiglobulin serum, proteolytic enzymes or bovine serum albumin are of dubious value with coated erythrocytes. It should be recalled that many commercial typing antisera contain substantial amounts of bovine albumin as an additive.

Elution of the antibody from antiglobulin positive erythrocytes is required to determine specificity of erythrocyte autoantibodies. Even this procedure is not infallible. An Ogata phenomenon may be present (39, 40). Nonimmunologic binding of an isoantibody to host erythrocytes may occur during interaction of the same erythrocytes with panhemagglutinating warm acting autoantibody or cold acting anti-I autoantibody (41).

Recently administered transfusions may produce positive direct antiglobulin reactions with eluates exhibiting isoantibody specificity. Transfused incompatible erythrocytes are coated with an erythrocyte isoantibody produced by the recipient. Elution will obtain and identify the isoantibody with an erroneous interpretation of an autoantibody. This author has seen examples of this phenomenon with two cases of anti-K, one case of anti-Jk^a and one case of anti-Rh_o(D). The latter case is remarkable. A patient with reticulum cell sarcoma was considered to have autoimmune hemolytic anemia. During a 6-month period she was transfused with 18 units of blood. On each occasion the patient was typed as Rh_o(D) positive and received Rh_o(D) positive blood. No transfusion reactions were noted. Direct and indirect antiglobulin reactions were positive and were interpreted as indicating autoimmune hemolytic anemia. The unbound antibody and eluates demonstrated a potent anti-Rh_o(D). Transfusion therapy was withheld for several weeks and the patient was retyped. It was then shown that the patient was actually Rh_o(D) negative. The assumed autoantibody was an anti-Rh_o(D) produced by a patient of genotype cde/cde. The positive Rh_o(D) typing reflected either errors in typing or the presence of transfused Rh_o(D) positive erythrocytes. The positive direct antiglobulin test and eluates of anti-Rh_o(D) specificity represented the presence of an isoantibody coating transfused foreign cells, with long survivals in the circulation.

Other misinterpretations are possible. Whittingham and associates (42) reported the presence of multiple isoantibodies which simulated a panhemagglutinating autoantibody. Croucher and associates (43) documented the formation (restimulation) of multiple isoantibodies days after the transfusion of apparently compatible blood. The coating of the transfused erythrocytes by multiple isoantibodies resulted in positive direct antiglobulin tests and led to the erroneous assumption of autoimmune hemolytic anemia. It is well recognized that a delay in producing isoantibodies may simulate autoimmune hemolytic anemia (44). Our laboratory has inadvertently documented this sequence. Erythrocyte survival studies were performed in a patient who received normal erythrocytes labeled with Cr^{51}. A normal survival time was recorded for the first 10 days when an abrupt shortening of survival was seen. This coincided with the production of anti-M in the NN recipient. The donor erythrocytes were MN.

A too limited testing procedure may also permit an erroneous assumption of autoantibody specificity. This generally reflects an investigator's belief in the infallibility of the antiglobulin test. The antiglobulin test may fail to demonstrate erythrocyte antibodies directed against rhesus agglutinogens. Iso- and autoantibodies are both vulnerable to this problem (see Chapters 3 and 18). Many investigators limit their investigation of incomplete erythrocyte autoantibodies to the antiglobulin procedure. Specificity of eluates may then be assumed because of failure to agglutinate one or several cells in the test panel. Most often a pattern of anti-hr"(e) is obtained. An expansion of the test system to include high speed albumin and proteolytic enzyme procedures will subsequently demonstrate panhemagglutinating ability. Such reactions are frequently interpreted as anti-hr"(e) with false positive proteolytic enzyme or albumin reactions. The reverse is more likely. A panhemagglutinating erythrocyte autoantibody is probably present with failure of the antiglobulin test. A mixture of antibodies may also be encountered with different reactivity in antiglobulin and enzyme procedures.

The antigenic specificity of warm acting erythrocyte autoantibodies is remarkably localized to the rhesus group. Autoantibodies with anti-f specificity have been described (45). van Loghem and associates (33) described single examples of autoantibodies with anti-Jk^a and anti-Fy^a specificities. Autoantibodies with anti-K specificity have been reported by Flückiger and associates (46) and Dausset and Colombani (34). In the latter case an additional warm acting erythrocyte autoantibody with anti-Rh_o(D) specificity was noted. Yokoyama and associates (47, 48) have described an autoantibody with anti-Xg^a specificity in a female presenting with severe anemia.

The Frequency of Specific Forms of Warm Acting Autoantibody

The relative frequency of specific warm acting erythrocyte autoantibodies is difficult to determine and varies greatly among reporting groups. Crowley and Bouroncle (30) noted three examples in 12 tested cases, a 25 per cent incidence. van Loghem and van der Hart (29) found eight specific warm acting autoantibodies in a group of 16, a 50 per cent incidence. A continuation of this study demonstrated 21 of 42 warm acting antibodies with isoantigenic specificity (33). Dausset and Colombani (34) reported seven specific autoantibodies in 18 patient eluates, a specificity frequency of 39 per cent. Dacie (49) noted 10 examples of warm acting autoantibody specificity in 33 cases, an incidence of 30 per cent. Nine

of the 10 also had a nonspecific erythrocyte autoantibody. Only one example of
autoantibody specificity was seen without
an additional nonspecific autoantibody. An
expansion of this study by Worlledge (50)
demonstrated specificity of 13 warm acting
erythrocyte autoantibodies in 41 tested
eluates. None of the above reports indicates
the temporal relationship of transfusion to
analysis of specificity. In several instances
sera rather than eluates were employed to
document specificity.

Dacie (49) summarized the reports of
152 patients with warm acting autoantibodies. Specificity was found in 52, an incidence of 34 per cent. Weiner (51) also
emphasizes the necessity of employing eluates for specificity determinations. He
states that there is a 15 per cent incidence
of specific erythrocyte autoantibodies and
all are directed against the rhesus group.

Erythrocyte autoantibodies with isoantigenic specificity are remarkably frequent
when induced by alpha-methldopa ingestion. In the series of Carstairs and associates (52) specificity of the autoantibody
was seen in 16 of 28 cases, an incidence of
57 per cent. In the series of Worlledge and
associates (53) specificity was documented
in 12 of 18 cases, an incidence of 66 per
cent. In all instances specificity was directed
against rhesus agglutinogens.

Other investigators have not observed
the high frequency of isoantigenic specific
warm acting erythrocyte autoantibodies reported above. Wiener and associates (54)
commented on the rarity of such examples.
Witebsky (55) was unable to confirm specificity of erythrocyte autoantibodies until
1965 when he studied two cases. In this
report he emphasized the difficulty of determining specificity of erythrocyte autoantibodies. A critical requirement in addition to specificity is a demonstration of
reactivity of autoantibody with host
erythrocytes.

In the author's present series, isoantigenic
specificity of warm acting erythrocyte autoantibodies was relatively uncommon. Unbound erythrocyte autoantibodies with isoantigenic specificity were frequently found
in the sera of patients with autoimmune

hemolytic anemia. The proximity of transfusions and the lack of eluate analysis
detracted from the value of this observation. Adequate studies were performed in
89 patients. Isoantigenic specificity of the
erythrocyte autoantibody was noted in
eight cases, an incidence of 9.0 per cent.
The autoantibody was anti-hr″(e) in all
cases. Typing studies documented the hr″(e)
agglutinogen on the patient's own erythrocytes in all instances. The probable genotypes were as follows: R_1R_2 (five), rr (one),
rr′ (one), rr″ (one).

Significance of Specificity of Warm Acting Autoantibodies

It is pertinent to question the degree of
specificity manifested by warm acting
erythrocyte autoantibodies. Reports by
Weiner and associates (56) and Speiser
(57) suggest that specificity can be absolute. In the case studied by Weiner and
associates (56) the autoantibody had a
specificity of anti-rh″(E). The patient's
erythrocytes coated with this antibody
typed as rh″(E) negative. It was assumed
that an in vivo blocking test had occurred
with saturation of rh″(E) sites by incomplete erythrocyte autoantibody. A similar
finding was noted by Speiser (57) with anti-
Rh_o(D) specific erythrocyte autoantibodies.
By contrast, unpublished observations in
our laboratory indicate that panhemagglutinating erythrocyte autoantibodies are unable to saturate the various rhesus antigen
combining sites.

Additional reports suggest that specificity
of warm acting erythrocyte autoantibodies
may be illusory. Many investigators have
documented binding of isoantigenically
specific autoantibodies to erythrocytes not
containing the isoantigens (31, 58–62).
Autoantibodies with an apparent specificity
of anti-Rh_o(D), anti-rh′(C) and anti-
rh″(E) were implicated in this type of reaction. Such autoantibodies were found in
eluates from antiglobulin positive erythrocytes lacking the antigen. Wiener's analogy
(63) offers a possible explanation for this
unusual phenomenon. Many men can put on
a suit; however, the best fit will occur with
the man for whom the suit was tailored.

This interpretation supports the postulate of Wiener and associates (25) of an antigenic relationship of warm acting erythrocyte autoantibodies to a basic structure present on all human erythrocytes. The apparent specificity for a rhesus agglutinogen represents a cross reaction or poor fit for only a portion or related part of the antigenic determinant. The specificity observed may be directed toward an undefined part of the rhesus substance. Similar suggestions have been made by Fudenberg and associates (59). Although serologic testing apparently indicates specificity, a nonspecific or cross reacting system may be activated. Similar occurrences have been reported for individuals not involved in autoimmune hemolytic anemia. Such patients have produced antibodies of apparent specificity for antigenic determinants on their own erythrocytes. This is illustrated in the report of Shapiro (64) describing the production of anti-Rh_o(D) by Rh_o(D) positive individuals. Others have described similar cases with the antibody interacting with host erythrocytes producing positive direct antiglobulin tests (65–67). True autoantibody formation was generally not involved. The most frequent explanation has implicated the Rh_o(D) antigen as either a D^u, Rh^a or Rh^b part of the rhesus mosaic. In the case reported by MacPherson and associates (67) the rhesus variant was D^w. Cross reactions with an imperfect fit as described above are probably responsible for fixation of anti-Rh_o(D) antibodies to such cells. The data of MacPherson and colleagues (67) indicate that such antibody binding does not shorten the red cell survival time or initiate hemolytic anemia.

An alternative explanation for these observations has been offered by Svardal and associates (41). They postulate an Ogata phenomenon (39, 40) for the adsorption of erythrocyte isoantibodies onto erythrocytes not containing the antigen. In such cases nonspecific adhesion of serum isoantibodies occurs on erythrocytes undergoing an additional antigen-antibody reaction. Elution will then release the isoantibody which is erroneously considered an autoantibody. Svardal and associates (41) have demon-

strated this sequence initiated by anti-I cold hemagglutinins present in a subject's serum. This process must always be considered when erythrocyte autoantibodies with isoantigenic specificity are found in eluates.

Human erythrocytes deficient in various rhesus agglutinogens have been employed to study the relationship of warm acting erythrocyte autoantibodies to the rhesus blood group. Dacie and Cutbush (28) utilized erythrocytes deficient at the C/c and E/e loci (—D—/—D— erythrocytes). Weiner and Vos (68) expanded this approach in 1963. Sixty eluates containing "panagglutinating, unspecific" warm acting autoantibodies were reacted with a panel of erythrocytes including the common rhesus genotypes, the rare genotypes Cde/Cde, cdE/cdE, CdE/cde, CDE/CDE, cde/cde KK and the deleted erythrocytes —D—/ —D—, cD—/cD— and ———/——— (Rh null). Some eluates had been prepared in the past and stored frozen and others were produced from frozen erythrocytes. Bovine albumin, the antiglobulin test, papain and bromelin techniques were all utilized. The enzyme procedures were found to be the most sensitive. The results were analyzed after absorption, reelution and titration. An antigenic relationship of these autoantibodies to the common antigens Vel, Ge and U was not found. The autoantibodies did not have anti-LW specificity. Of 60 eluates tested, 32 failed to react with ———/——— (Rh null) cells. In addition, 11 eluates showed less activity against such cells than against erythrocytes with normal rhesus characteristics. The authors concluded that they demonstrated "distinct blood group specificity within the rhesus system in at least 70 per cent." The patterns of reactivity suggested three different erythrocyte autoantibody types. These were termed anti-nl, anti-pdl and anti-dl. The postulated antigenic substance of the rhesus group are nl, pdl and dl. The terminology is based on the use of normal erythrocytes (not deleted, i.e., nl), partially deleted erythrocytes (pdl) and fully deleted erythrocytes (dl). The suggested antigenic makeup of the test erythrocytes reacting with the specific autoantibody is

TABLE 97. *Postulated specificity of warm acting erythrocyte autoantibodies and the hypothesized antigens**

Autoantibody Specificity[†]	Agglutination of Erythrocytes	Postulated Antigens[†]
Anti-nl	Normal erythrocytes	nl
Anti-pdl		pdl
Anti-dl		dl
Anti-pdl	D— —/D— —	pdl
Anti-dl	Dc—/Dc—	dl
Anti-dl	— — —/— — — (Rh null)	dl

* Modified from Weiner and Vos (68).

† nl, Normal cells; pdl, partially deleted cells; dl, fully deleted cells.

given in Table 97, as modified from Weiner and Vos (68).

Reaction of Warm Acting Autoantibodies with Animal Erythrocytes

Cold acting erythrocyte autoantibodies may react with erythrocytes obtained from many animal species. In contrast, human warm acting erythrocyte autoantibodies are generally species specific and unreactive with animal erythrocytes. Negative reactions have been demonstrated with erythrocytes obtained from the mouse, guinea pig, rabbit, rat, fowl, sheep, horse, dog, pigmy goat and gray whale. Primate erythrocytes have not been extensively tested. Sturgeon (69) noted a lack of reaction with rhesus monkey cells, and Komninos and Rosenthal (70) could not demonstrate reactivity of autoantibody eluates with "monkey" cells. Kidd (71) and Evans and Weiser (72) found that rhesus erythrocytes interacted with warm acting erythrocyte autoantibodies. Wiener and associates (25) noted that autoantibodies reacted strongly with chimpanzee erythrocytes and had questionable reactions with rhesus and squirrel monkey red cells.

Even fewer studies have been performed to document rhesus or rhesus related agglutinogens on primate erythrocytes. Wiener and associates (73) demonstrated that anti-Rh_0(D) reacted strongly with chimpanzee erythrocytes. Further studies using

saline and ficin techniques did not reveal agglutination of other New and Old World monkey erythrocytes by various antisera directed against human rhesus agglutinogens (74, 75).

Pirofsky and Pratt (76) investigated the apparent nonspecificity of warm acting erythrocyte autoantibodies utilizing primate and non-primate erythrocytes. Nonprimates tested included the dog, rabbit, guinea pig, mouse, pigmy goat and gray whale. The primates examined were the tree shrew (*Tupala glis*), fulvus lemur (*Lemur fulvus*), ringtail lemur (*Lemur catta*), woolly monkey (*Lagothrix lagotricha*), squirrel monkey (*Saimiri sciurea*), celebes ape (*Cynopithecus niger*), rhesus monkey (*Macaca mulatta*), baboon (*Papio doguera*) and chimpanzee (*Pan satyrus*). Eluates containing erythrocyte autoantibodies were obtained from four cases of autoimmune hemolytic anemia. Elution techniques were also employed to produce human anti-Rh_0(D), anti-rh'(C), anti-rh"(E), anti-hr'(c) and anti-hr"(e) antisera appropriate for testing with animal erythrocytes. Pirofsky and Pratt (76) noted that neither autoantibody eluates nor anti-rhesus isoantibody eluates reacted with nonprimate erythrocytes in either saline, antiglobulin or bromelin techniques. A similar lack of reactivity was found with primate erythrocytes obtained from the tree shrew, fulvus lemur and woolly monkey. However, erythrocytes from the remaining six primate species reacted with both human erythrocyte autoantibodies and anti-rhesus antibodies. Table 98 summarizes these data. The antigenic relationship of primate erythrocytes to various human anti-rhesus antisera is summarized in Table 99. Strong reactions were noted with anti-Rh_0(D) and chimpanzee erythrocytes. In addition, strong reactions with anti-hr'(c) were found with squirrel monkey, celebes ape, rhesus monkey and chimpanzee erythrocytes. The authors concluded that nonspecificity of warm acting erythrocyte autoantibodies is illusory. Specificity is dependent on the presence or absence of rhesus agglutinogens irrespective of the animal species. This strongly suggests that warm acting erythrocyte autoantibodies have specificity for a rhesus antigen (76).

Summary of Specificity

Weiner and Vos (68) have objected strongly to the term "nonspecific" when referring to the action of warm acting erythrocyte autoantibodies. They postulated three specific antigenic determinants on human erythrocytes (nl, pdl, dl) with which autoantibodies may react. Dacie (49) presents an alternative viewpoint. "... The question as to whether an antigen of hypothetical extreme frequency should be called 'nonspecific' or not is a matter of sematics. There seems ... no inherent reason why an antigen common to the vast majority of mankind should not be common to *all* mankind. 'Nonspecific' is certainly a useful term. . . ." This author would have to take an intermediate position. The term nonspecific, when used descriptively to indicate reactivity with all human erythrocytes, is satisfactory. However, warm acting erythrocyte autoantibodies are not globulin molecules which fortuitously have the ability to fix to the erythrocyte surface. Current data strongly suggest that specificity exists, particularly in relation to the rhesus group. In immunologic terms we are not dealing with a nonspecific reaction. There are nonspecific globulin reactions with the erythrocyte surface These differ from autoantibody reactions. This does not imply that one or even three specific rhesus agglutinogens are antigenically involved, as suggested by Weiner and Vos (68). The primate erythrocyte data suggest that a vast array of structurally similar but not identical antigenic rhesus substances can combine with warm acting erythrocyte autoantibodies. The original hypothesis in 1953 of Wiener and associates (25) that autoantibodies react with the "nucleus of the Rh-hr structure" currently offers the most logical explanation. The degree of "fit" of such antibodies with various rhesus antigenic determinants best explains the reactions encountered with primate erythrocytes and the more confusing data seen with human erythrocytes. These include "specific" and "nonspecific" reactions with normal

TABLE 98. *Agglutination of erythrocytes obtained from primates and nonprimates by erythrocyte autoantibodies and antibodies directed against various rhesus agglutinogens*

Source of Erythrocytes	Agglutination Induced by	
	Human anti-rhesus antisera	Human erythrocyte autoantibodies
Nonprimates		
Dog	0	0
Rabbit	0	0
Guinea pig	0	0
Mouse	0	0
Pigmy goat	0	0
Gray whale	0	0
Primates		
Tree shrew	0	0
Fulvus lemur	0	0
Ringtail lemur	+	+
Woolly monkey	0	0
Squirrel monkey	+	+
Celebes ape	+	+
Rhesus monkey	+	+
Baboon	+	+
Chimpanzee	+	+
Human (control)	+	+

erythrocytes, the reaction or nonreaction found with erythrocytes missing portions of the rhesus molecule and the ability of "specific" autoantibodies to bind with host erythrocytes not containing the required antigen.

We may now conclude that the major obstacles preventing the acceptance of warm acting erythrocyte autoantibodies as true antibodies, i.e., nonspecificity and no demonstrable antigen, no longer exists. Specificity is present and is related to the rhesus blood group. This does not preclude the possibility that other blood groups will eventually be shown to have a similar antigenic relationship to warm acting erythrocyte autoantibodies (76).

The Antigen in Cold Acting Autoimmune Hemolytic Anemia

It appeared doubtful that specificity would ever be shown for cold acting erythrocyte autoantibodies. The widespread

TABLE 99. *Presence of rhesus or rhesus-like factors on the erythrocytes of various primates**

Primate Species	Definite	Presumptive	Test System
Tree shrew	0	0	
Fulvus lemur	0	0	
Ringtail lemur	0	$Rh_0(D)$	Bromelin
Woolly monkey	0	0	
Squirrel monkey	hr'(c)	0	
Celebes ape	hr'(c)	$Rh_0(D)$, rh'(C), rh''(E)	Antiglobulin
Rhesus monkey	hr'(c)	0	
Baboon	0	$Rh_0(D)$, rh'(C), rh''(E), hr'(c), hr''(e)	Bromelin
Chimpanzee	$Rh_0(D)$, hr'(c)	rh'(C), rh''(E)	Antiglobulin

* A "definite" relationship is listed if reactions occurred in more than one test system. A "presumptive" category is accepted if equivocal results were found or if a reaction occurred in only one test system; that system is listed in the far right-hand column.

distribution of cold hemagglutinins in most normal human sera, as well as a large number of animal sera, made it unlikely that a specific erythrocyte agglutinogen was antigenically involved. The ability of human cold hemagglutinins to react with all human erythrocytes and with many animal erythrocytes also suggested a lack of specificity. This widespread reactivity led Mino (77) to coin the phrase "panhemagglutinin" to describe nonspecific agglutinating substances.

The Reaction of Cold Agglutinins with Animal Erythrocytes

Animal studies were particularly discouraging in reference to specificity. Cold acting erythrocyte autoantibodies were demonstrated in the sera of the human being and of normal guinea pigs, chickens, horses, dogs, rabbits, cattle, cats, sheep, monkeys, donkeys and goats. In addition, human cold acting erythrocyte autoantibodies agglutinated various animal erythrocytes. The cross adsorption studies with such substances are particularly interesting. Clough and Richter (78) in 1918 described extensive cross reactivity of a high titer human cold hemagglutinin. This substance induced agglutination of rabbit, guinea pig, hen, sheep, cat, and pig erythrocytes. The cold hemagglutinin could be adsorbed by reaction with either human or rabbit erythrocytes. Turner and Jackson (79) studied high titer cold hemagglutinins obtained from seven patients with virus

pneumonia. Such sera cross reacted with erythrocytes obtained from various animal species. Eluates were produced from human erythrocytes sensitized by human cold acting autoantibodies. The eluates induced similar agglutination titers with rabbit and human erythrocytes. Lower agglutination titers were found with guinea pig and pig erythrocytes. Adsorption removed activity against human erythrocytes without significantly affecting the agglutination titer obtained with many animal cells. Finland and associates (80) noted a lack of correlation between agglutination titers induced by human cold hemagglutinins reacting with human and animal cells. Rabbit erythrocytes were most sensitive to agglutination by normal human serum. Cold hemagglutinins found in virus pneumonia produced the highest titer with monkey red cells. Adsorption with rabbit erythrocytes significantly decreased agglutination titers obtained with human and guinea pig erythrocytes. Adsorption with human and guinea pig erythrocytes did not remove hemagglutinins directed against various animal erythrocytes.

Millet and Fincler (81) were unable to adsorb cold hemagglutinins of human sera directed against human erythrocytes using intact rabbit, guinea pig or ox erythrocytes. The antibody was adsorbed using the stroma of these cells. Delage and associates (82) produced severe hemolysis and hemoglobinuria in rabbits by transfusing them with human serum obtained from a patient with cold hemagglutinin disease. Schubothe (83) studied eluates obtained from six patients with cold hemagglutinin disease. A marked variation was observed in the agglutinating ability of human cold hemagglutinins with animal erythrocytes.

Such studies suggest that the term panhemagglutinin is an appropriate description of cold acting erythrocyte autoantibodies. There are no other antibodies with so broad a range of reactivity. It is questionable if any other antibodies possess the ability to cross the species barriers with such ease. An attempt to document antigenic specificity for such a widespread action would appear to be doomed to failure.

The Cold Acting Autoantibodies and the ABO System

Variations in the reactivity of cold acting erythrocyte autoantibodies with human erythrocytes gradually became apparent. Amzel and Hirszfeld (84) emphasized such differences as early as 1925. However, they were unable to demonstrate any dissimilarities of erythrocyte surface receptors through adsorption. Kettel (85) in 1929 reported that cold hemagglutinin titers were lowest in group O sera. Boxwell and Bigger (86) and Wheeler and associates (87) suggested that group O erythrocytes were most sensitive to the agglutinating action of cold hemagglutinins. Stratton (88) and Finland and associates (80) observed that some but not all cold hemagglutinins had an anti-O preferential agglutinating ability. Bird (89) similarly related the action of cold hemagglutinins to the ABO group. His data suggested multiple antibody combining sites with specificity as anti-O, anti-A, anti-B and anti-patient cell. The cold hemagglutinin reaction appeared to be independent of H content.

Turner and Jackson (79), Young (90) and Dacie (91) were all unable to confirm a relationship of cold hemagglutinins to the ABO grouping of erythrocytes. Crookston and associates (92) studied 14 sera with a panel of cells derived from 64 normal individuals. The observed agglutination pattern was variable but was not related to the ABO, Rh, MNS, P, Lutheran, Kell, Lewis, Duffy or Kidd blood groups. The variation of agglutination titers obtained with human erythrocytes was found to have a normal distribution.

More precisely defined examples of specificity have been reported. Hennemann and Rasch (93) demonstrated the presence of cold acting anti-P antibody in the serum of a P positive woman with hemolytic anemia. van Loghem and associates (33) reported three cold acting erythrocyte autoantibodies with specificities of anti-O, anti-B and anti-M, respectively. Crowley (94) studied an incomplete cold acting autoantibody with anti-H specificity.

In 1951 Wiener (63) suggested that cold acting erythrocyte autoantibodies had a heteroimmune origin. He postulated that infections (virus pneumonia, infectious mononucleosis, trypanosomiasis and tropical eosinophilia) and certain foods stimulated antibody formation which cross reacted with an agglutinogen on human erythrocytes. Wiener (63) visualized such cross reacting antibodies as poor fitting with a low avidity for human red cells. He suggested that at body temperatures thermal agitation caused dissociation of weak antigen-antibody combinations. This resulted in cold acting erythrocyte autoantibodies. In 1953 it was postulated that the involved agglutinogen was a member of either the ABO or MNS blood group systems (24, 25).

Cold Acting Autoantibodies and the Ii System

In 1956 Wiener and associates (95) studied an unusual case of acquired hemolytic anemia. A cold hemagglutinin was documented with a titer at refrigerator temperatures of 50,000 employing normal erythrocytes and 200,000 with ficin treated cells. Transfusions with the patient and the blood both warmed led to severe reactions and hemoglobinuria. Donor erythrocytes were strongly agglutinated, whereas the patient's own erythrocytes were unagglutinated at room temperature. This observation was employed in establishing compatibility tests screening a large number of potential blood donors. Over 22,000 donors

TABLE 100. *Reaction of an anti-I cold hemag-glutinin with various erythrocytes (red cells have been selected to illustrate the variation of agglutination seen with enzyme treatment and change in temperature)**

Suggested Classific-ation	Agglutination Titers					
	4°C.		24°C.		37°C.	
	Un-treated	Ficin	Un-treated	Ficin	Un-treated	Ficin
I₁	130,000	500,000	1,600	3,200	0	140
	320,000	500,000	5,000	20,000	0	2,400
I₂	100,000	320,000	320	2,500	0	25
	80,000	250,000	240	1,600	0	5
	80,000	190,000	160	1,900	0	10
I₃	50,000	190,000	20	2,200	0	5
	40,000	190,000	25	960	0	0
i	4,000	64,000	0	120	0	0
Patient†	0	80,000	0	240	0	0

* Modified from Wiener and associates (95).

† Erythrocytes of host producing the tested anti-I cold hemagglutinin.

were examined and five were found to be compatible at room temperature. Blood from these donors was successfully transfused.

The cold acting autoantibody was not related to the ABO, MN, Kell or Rh-hr systems. Its frequency distribution tended to exclude any relationship to the Lewis, Lutheran, Duffy, Kidd or P blood group systems. No resemblance of the antibody to anti-Vel, anti-Tjᵃ, anti-U and an India serum with a specificity of anti-H could be documented. The authors concluded that the cold hemagglutinin was reacting with a blood group factor previously undescribed. The symbol I for the factor and anti-I for the corresponding antibody was selected to emphasize the high degree of individuality of blood specimens failing to react with anti-I serum at room temperature. The rare individual with erythrocytes compatible with anti-I serum at room temperature were designated type i (I negative). Several variants of the I factor were apparent and designated as I₁, I₂, I₃, etc., depending on the intensity and titer of agglutination re-

actions. It should be emphasized that i (I negative) erythrocytes were agglutinated at room temperature if treated with ficin and at 4°C. when untreated. Table 100, modified from Wiener and associates (95), illustrates the titers involved and the effect of ficin treatment and temperature on I and i erythrocytes. Adsorption studies documented a single antibody and eliminated a nonspecific autoantibody reacting with all human cells.

This observation has been amply confirmed by other investigators. Jenkins and associates (96) and Tippett and associates (97) found most pathologic high titer cold hemagglutinins to have anti-I specificity. These investigators also reported additional Caucasian and Negro i (I negative) subjects. Worlledge (50) studied 36 sera containing high titer cold hemagglutinins. Specificity for anti-I was demonstrated in 20 of 21 sera obtained from patients with idiopathic cold hemagglutinin disease. Nine sera obtained from patients with virus pneumonia all revealed anti-I specificity of the cold hemagglutinins. Anti-I specificity was present in three of six cases of cold acting hemolytic anemia associated with malignancies of the reticuloendothelium. The study of Jenkins and associates (96) documented iso-anti-I formation in I negative patients without hemolytic anemia. Wiener and associates (95) had previously unsuccessfully searched for this isoantibody in their five I negative patients. Table 101, modified from Dacie (49) illustrates the characteristics of iso-anti-I and auto-anti-I.

Characteristics of the Ii Blood Group System

Knowledge of the Ii blood group system has rapidly increased. Tippett and associates (97) suggested a relationship of the I substance to the ABO system. Marcus and associates (98) expanded this observation. They postulated that steric interaction of adjacent I and ABO structures existed. Gold (99) reported similarities between anti-O, anti-A₁ and anti-I. Anti-O sera was found to have a spectrum of activity when the I grouping was considered. Gold (99) divided anti-O sera into two major groups. One

TABLE 101. *Characteristics of iso-anti-I and auto-anti-I*

Serologic Characteristics	Auto-anti-I	Iso-anti-I
Autohemagglutination	+	0
Reaction with I(+) cells	Strong +	+
Reaction with I(−) cells	+	0
Acts as agglutinin	+	+
Acts as hemolysin	Potential	Potential
Thermal range	Up to 37°C. with I(+) cells (but not with patient's cells)	Up to 37°C. with I(+) cells
Titer levels	Very high	Moderate
Purification	Single antibody	Single antibody

* Modified from Dacie (49).

group reacted with a theorized antigen OI producing reactivity patterns of anti-O → anti-OI → anti-IO → anti-I. A second group reacted with the theorized antigen Oi producing anti-O → anti-Oi → anti-iO → anti-i reactions. Rosenfield and associates (100) described a serum that they termed anti-H (−i) which is inhibited by saliva but requires the I antigen on cells with which it reacts.

Schmidt and McGinniss (101) expanded this relationship employing anti-H. The reactions of anti-H were very different from anti-O when the I system was considered. Anti-O and anti-H sera had different reactivity with Oi and A₂i cells. Schmidt and McGinniss (101) suggested that this system be termed OI rather than HI. The excellent studies of Yokoyama (102) and Yokoyama and Plocinik (103) support this concept. Using gangliosides isolated from brain tissue, they were able to inhibit anti-A, anti-O and anti-I; anti-H was not inhibited by gangliosides. These studies suggest a close relationship between I and "A" substances. Anti-I was inhibited by purified "A" substance, by "A" secretor saliva and weakly inhibited by intermediate types of "A" secretor saliva. "A" nonsecretor, O secretor, and nonsecretor salivas did not inhibit anti-I. The A and I substances can be differentiated by hemagglutination inhibition studies. Marcus and associates (98) reported that anti-A but not anti-I was inhibited by N-acetylgalactosamine. This was confirmed by Yokoyama (102). A relationship also exists between the I and "B" substances. Tegoli and associates (104)

have described an autoantibody, anti-IB, which detects an antigen produced by the interaction of the I and B genes. Salmon and associates (105) reported eluates of autoantibodies which contained specificities of anti-HI, anti-AI and anti-BI.

In 1952 Unger and associates (106) noted that cord blood erythrocytes were poorly agglutinated by high titer cold hemagglutinins. Mortara and Martinetti (107) confirmed this observation. Jenkins and associates (96) noted that iso-anti-I antiserum reacted very weakly with cord blood erythrocytes. Marsh (108) reported that all newborn infants have an i phenotype (I negative). Normally this changes to the adult I phenotype at approximately 3 weeks of age. Within 18 months the change appears complete. The progressive increase of I substance is accompanied by a progressive decrease in i antigen. This relationship between age and Ii composition is summarized in Figure 40, modified from Marsh (108). Marsh speculates that I negative adults lack a genetically determined factor. The H factor is also deficient in cord blood erythrocytes. This suggests that the postulated genetic factor for the development of I may also involve the development of H substance. Marsh (108) classifies human cells in reference to Ii grouping as follows: I (normal adult cells); I(int) (weakly reacting adult cells that possibly represents heterozygosity for the I development factor); i(cord); i₂; i₁; and i. The i₁ group is rare and is found in Caucasians. The i group is reserved for a theoretically postulated cell which does not contain any I substance.

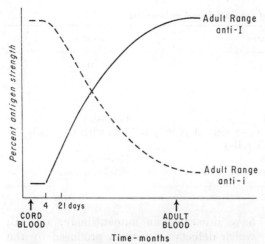

FIGURE 40. The influence of age on the erythrocyte concentration of I and i. Erythrocytes obtained from subjects of various ages are reacted with anti-I and anti-i. (Modified from Marsh (108).)

It is assumed that all human erythrocytes contain a variable amount of both I and i substances. Giblett and Crookston (109) demonstrated that erythrocytes obtained from adult patients with thalassemia and other hematologic abnormalities have an increased reactivity with anti-i antiserum. Erythrocytes, produced more rapidly and released into the circulation of adults under anemic stress, presumably contain an increased amount of i substance.

The late neonatal development of I substance offers a possible explanation for the universal production of cold acting anti-I autoantibodies in normal human beings. Its absence or low concentration during prenatal life may prevent the establishment of normal immune tolerance. I substance is subsequently produced in large amounts during a period when immune competence is developing. The immune apparatus may recognize its presence as foreign, or a state of partial immune tolerance may be created. A limited amount of anti-I erythrocyte autoantibodies will accordingly be produced. This concept may be extrapolated further. Immune competence in the neonatal human is expressed initially through gamma M production. I substance becomes available prior to active synthesis of gamma G immunoglobulins. It may therefore be

anticipated that "natural" anti-I cold hemagglutinins will be IgM antibodies. It can also be predicted that such antibodies will be polyclonal in origin and show a mixture of kappa and lambda type molecules. This will contrast with the monoclonal pathogenesis and pattern of IgM production seen in cold hemagglutinin disease and in Waldenström's macroglobulinemia.

Marsh (108) noted that heating intact erythrocytes to 56°C. reduced agglutination titers with anti-I cold hemagglutinins. Evans and associates (110) confirmed this observation. They demonstrated that the loss of agglutination titer was not due to heat inactivation of the antigen. The red cell receptor, whether I or i, was found in erythrocyte stroma and was resistant to heat at 160°C. Heated intact erythrocytes, although agglutinated to a much lower titer, bound similar amounts of I^{131} labeled cold hemagglutinins as did untreated cells.

Marcus and associates (98) suggested that I and i substances are polysaccharides. The treatment of erythrocytes with beta-galactosidase and beta-glucosaminidase from Clostridium tertium culture filtrates substantially reduced agglutination of I positive erythrocytes by anti-I cold hemagglutinins. The adsorptive capacity of treated I positive erythrocyte stroma for anti-I was also reduced. After enzymatic treatment, galactose and N-acetylglucosamine were found free in the supernatant. Marcus and associates (98) suggested that these two sugars may be structural units of the I antigenic determinant. However, Marcus and associates (98) and Yokoyama and Plocinik (103) were unable to inhibit anti-I with various sugars including galactose and N-acetylglucosamine. Evans and associates (110) noted that vigorous heat treatment of erythrocyte stroma did not destroy the I antigen. This observation supports the hypothesis of a polysaccharide structure for I substance. I^{131} labeled cold hemagglutinin fixation was actually increased with such heated stromas. These authors speculate that increased reactivity may reflect denaturation and removal of surrounding proteins and the subsequent exposure of more polysaccharide antigen receptor sites.

Effect of Disease on the I Blood Group

The incidence of I negative individuals in the normal blood donor population has been estimated to be less than 0.1 per cent. McGinniss and associates (111) surprisingly noted a high incidence of the I negative state in patients with various forms of leukemia. Five of 40 leukemic patients examined were found to have a partial and 10 a total modification of the I antigen. Extensive studies by Schmidt and associates (112) revealed that 38 of 124 patients with leukemia were I negative, an incidence of 30 per cent. Similar observations were made by Ayers and associates (113), who noted nine antigenic abnormalities, mostly involving the I and H locus, in 51 leukemic patients tested. The I antigen was specifically involved in five of 25 leukemic patients. Schmidt and associates (114) were unable to correlate the I negative state with age, peripheral leukocyte counts or ABO grouping. There was no association with levels of fetal hemoglobin, Philadelphia chromosomes or type of leukemia. I antigen reactivity fluctuated during exacerbations and remissions of the leukemic state. This suggests that the I antigen may be blocked or destroyed during the disease process.

Schmidt and associates (112) searched for a possible relationship between various microorganisms and the I negative state seen in leukemia. An in vitro test system was devised employing the products of 45 microbial agents, including Mycoplasma (PPLO or pleuropneumonia-like organisms), viruses and bacteria. The microbial products were incubated with I positive erythrocytes and the washed erythrocytes were subsequently examined for I reactivity. Anti-I agglutination was inhibited by 18 of 25 Mycoplasma strains tested. Only one of 11 viruses tested had trace inhibitory activity. The direct mixing of Mycoplasma material with anti-I antisera was not inhibitory. Inhibition did not appear to result from a serologic cross reactivity between Mycoplasma and anti-I. The data

suggested that Mycoplasma induced an alteration of the I receptor sites of the erythrocyte. Anti-A_1, anti-Le^a and anti-Le^b were not inhibited by Mycoplasma.

Several investigators have demonstrated that Mycoplasma are present in leukemic tissue. There is no evidence that an etiologic relationship exists between Mycoplasma and leukemia. Mycoplasma may act as a secondary invader. Its presence, however, may relate to the production of high titer anti-I cold hemagglutinins seen in reticuloendothelial neoplasia. The ability of such organisms to modify the surface of erythrocytes may play a role in altering cell susceptibility to virus penetration.

Thomas (115) has called attention to the relationship of Mycoplasma infections to autoimmune disease. Autoantibodies directed against lung tissue have been detected in virus pneumonia, particularly when cold hemagglutinins are present. The development of anti-I cold hemagglutinins in leukemic patients who show an altered reactivity of the I antigen site suggests that a termination of tolerance or a modification of the autologous antigen mechanism may be involved.

Smith and associates (116) have reported that the Mycoplasma effect occurs in vivo. Twenty-seven volunteers were experimentally infected with Mycoplasma. Reactivity of the I antigen was transiently reduced in five subjects. Seven volunteers had a rise in titer of cold hemagglutinins. Twelve subjects had an elevation of the thermal amplitude of anti-I cold hemagglutinins.

Costea and associates (117) have presented an in vivo animal system which offers great potential for investigations in this area. The infection of rabbits with a strain of Listeria monocytogenes results in the production of cold hemagglutinins of anti-I specificity.

Anti-i

Cold acting erythrocyte autoantibodies have been described which exhibit a reverse specificity of anti-I. These have been termed anti-i, and they show a higher titer, avidity and thermal amplitude with cord blood erythrocytes than with normal human adult erythrocytes. Marsh and Jenkins (118) reported two examples of anti-i production. The patients were diagnosed as having anemia with reticulosis and reticulum cell sarcoma, respectively. The erythrocyte autoantibodies were cold acting and had an agglutinating capacity transposed from anti-I. They strongly agglutinated cord blood erythrocytes and I negative adult cells. Their reactivity with normal adult erythrocytes (I positive) was weak. van Loghem and associates (119) reported two additional cases of hemolytic anemia associated with anti-i specific cold hemagglutinins.

Evans and associates (110) studied 10 cold hemagglutinins with an I^{131} procedure. Two sera exhibited greater agglutination activity with cord blood and i erythrocytes than with I cells. Anti-i specificity was confirmed by differences in uptake of the labeled purified cold hemagglutinin. The sensitive labeling studies indicated that the 10 cold acting autoantibodies reacted more avidly with either I or i cells. None was neutral with regard to these two factors. van Loghem and associates (120), however, have reported such a neutral state. Evans and associates (110) speculated that this state could occur during transition of i to I. Ii neutral autoantibodies might be directed against the I-i antigen nucleus in a manner similar to that postulated by Wiener and colleagues (25) for warm acting autoantibodies and the rhesus nucleus.

Evans and associates (121) reported in detail a case of hemolytic anemia associated with a cold hemagglutinin of anti-i specificity. A 16-year-old girl had a transient but unusually severe hemolytic anemia following a febrile illness of unknown etiology. No evidence of a reticuloendothelial malignancy was found. A nongamma type of direct antiglobulin reaction was noted. Positive indirect antiglobulin reactions developed after incubating normal erythrocytes with the patient's purified cold hemagglutinin and normal serum. The antiglobulin reaction was dependent on complement factors C′1, C′4 and C′2. A low serum complement level was docu-mented. The hemolytic process rapidly disappeared. Four months later normal serum complement levels were present, antiglobulin tests were negative and anti-i had disappeared.

Anti-i cold hemagglutinins must no longer be considered as rare occurrences. Bell and associates (122) encountered eight examples over a 2-year period in a routine blood transfusion service. The antibodies were discovered during screening procedures employing enzyme treated erythrocytes. Anti-i was found in two normal individuals and in association with pregnancy, ulcerative colitis, metastatic carcinoma, leukemia and myelofibrosis. Rosenfield and associates (123) have demonstrated an unusually high incidence of anti-i cold hemagglutinins in patients with infectious mononucleosis. Thirty-eight sera from patients with infectious mononucleosis were studied. All sera contained heterophile agglutinins resistant to adsorption with either guinea pig or horse kidney antigen but readily adsorbable with boiled ox cells. Twenty-six of these sera, or 68 per cent, contained cold hemagglutinins which reacted with higher titers and greater avidity with cord blood erythrocytes than with normal adult erythrocytes. Erythrocytes obtained from I negative adults were agglutinated by the cold hemagglutinins. The titer of anti-i was only poorly predictable from titers of heterophile agglutinins. Cross adsorption studies clearly separated heterophile and anti-i agglutinins.

Summary

There is adequate evidence that cold acting erythrocyte autoantibodies have antigenic specificity. Most often specificity is directed against the I antigen of erythrocytes. There is suggestive evidence that the I substance is related to the ABO blood group system. Cold hemagglutinins of anti-i specificity also exist and do not appear to be rare. Cold hemagglutinins that are not anti-I or anti-i may also be found. Jenkins and Marsh (124) have termed such cold acting antibodies anti-"not-I." Additional studies delineating the characteristics of the Ii blood group, its distribution in man and animals and its cross reactivity with various antibodies are necessary. The relationship of anti-I and anti-i formation to various infectious agents deserves particular emphasis.

The Antigen in Paroxysmal Cold Hemoglobinuria

The Donath-Landsteiner antibody is a cold acting erythrocyte autoantibody characteristic of paroxysmal cold hemoglobinuria. For many years it was considered to be nonspecific in its ability to lyse all normal human erythrocytes and the patient's own red cells. Schubothe (83) investigated the action of the Donath-Landsteiner antibody with various animal erythrocytes. The antibody had the capacity to cross the species barrier. Lysis was demonstrated with pig erythrocytes at a level comparable to that seen with human cells. Ox, horse and sheep erythrocytes were only weakly lysed by the Donath-Landsteiner antibody. Erythrocytes from the guinea pig, rat, mouse, dog and one of two tested rabbits were resistant to the lytic action of the Donath-Landsteiner antibody. Schubothe (83) noted that human erythrocytes vary in their sensitivity to lysis induced by the Donath-Landsteiner antibody. Quantitative techniques employing a panel of erythrocytes obtained from 10 normal patients revealed a lytic sensitivity ranging from 14 to 62 per cent.

The clinical association of syphilis and paroxysmal cold hemoglobinuria stimulated several attempts to relate reaginic material responsible for the Wassermann test and the Donath-Landsteiner antibody. An etiologic relationship or cross reactivity was not found. Hinz (125) fractionated various human sera containing the Donath-Landsteiner antibody. He was able to document the independent existence of the two serologic substances. Hinz demonstrated that the Donath-Landsteiner antibody is an IgG immunoglobulin, whereas the Wassermann reagin may be either an IgG or IgM molecule.

Specificity Studies

Dacie (49) studied the relationship of the Donath-Landsteiner antibody to the Ii blood group system. He noted no differences in the ability of four separate Donath-Landsteiner antibodies to induce lysis of normal adult I positive erythrocytes, adult I negative (i positive) erythrocytes and cord blood erythrocytes.

Levine and associates (126, 127) reported specificity of the Donath-Landsteiner antibody. This hemolysin lysed all P_1 or P_2 erythrocytes, including the patient's own cells. Four rare blood samples obtained from pp or Tj^a negative patients were unaffected by the Donath-Landsteiner antibody. It was observed that P_1 erythrocytes were somewhat more sensitive to the lytic action than were P_2 cells. A serum containing anti-I cold hemagglutinin and the Donath-Landsteiner antibody was adsorbed. Adsorption with P_1 erythrocytes removed both hemolytic and agglutinating activity. Adsorption with pp erythrocytes left both agglutinating and hemolytic activity directed against P_1 and P_2 cells. However, it removed the anti-I specific cold hemagglutinin. Levine and associates (126, 127) concluded that the Donath-Landsteiner antibody had anti-Tj^a specificity. Preliminary studies indicated neutralization of the Donath-Landsteiner antibody by sheep hydatid cyst fluid containing P_1 substance. The antibody was not neutralized by the P_1 substance partially purified by Morgan and Watkins. One sample of p^k erythrocytes was tested and did not react with three sera containing Donath-Landsteiner antibodies.

Table 102 summarizes the current status of the P blood group system. The P_1 and P_2 phenotypes are common and may be considered almost universal. The remaining two phenotypes are extremely rare. Apparently, p erythrocytes lack all antigens for the P blood group system. The genotype of the p^k erythrocyte is unknown but is usually associated with P_1. P_1 individuals do not produce antibodies against P group antigens. Antibodies produced by P_2 individuals generally have anti-P_1 specificity. The rare pp individuals produce an antibody of anti-$P + P_1 + p^k$ specificity which has previously been termed anti-Tj^a. This antibody reacts with all erythrocytes except pp. Anti-P may occur in the sera of

TABLE 102. *Terminology of the P blood group system and reactivity of anti-P₁ , anti-P+P₁+pᵏ, anti-P and Donath-Landsteiner antibodies with various typed erythrocytes**

P Blood Group System

Pheno-type	Frequency	Geno-type	Red blood cell antigen	Antibody produced by patient with phenotype
P_1	Common	P_1P_1 P_1P_2 P_1p	P_1 , P	None
P_2	Common	P_2P_2 P_2p	p	Anti-P_1 (usually)
p	Rare	pp	None	Anti-P + P_1 + p^k (anti-Tjᵃ)
p^k	Rare	?	p^k, P_1 (usually)	Anti-P

Reactivity of P Blood Group Antibodies

Antibody	Erythrocyte typing			
	P_1	P_2	pp	p^k
Anti-P_1	+	0	0	+ (usually)
Anti-P + P_1 + p^k (anti-Tjᵃ)	+	+	0	+
Anti-P	+	+	0	0
Donath-Landsteiner antibody	+	+	0	0

* Modified from Worlledge and Rousso (128).

p^k individuals and reacts with P_1 and P_2 cells.

Worlledge (50) and Worlledge and Rousso (128) tested 11 sera containing the Donath-Landsteiner antibody against a panel of P_1 , P_2 , p and p^k erythrocytes. The Donath-Landsteiner antibody lysed P_1 and P_2 red cells and did not react with p and p^k erythrocytes. Its action differed from that of anti-P + P_1 + p^k (anti-Tjᵃ) which reacted with p^k but not p erythrocytes. Anti-P found in the sera of p^k positive individuals did not react with p or p^k erythrocytes. Its antibody specificity was accordingly identical to that of the Donath-Landsteiner antibody. These results are summarized in Table 102. Six of the patients with paroxysmal cold hemoglobinuria were typed for various P blood group anti-

gens. The erythrocytes were found to contain P_1 or P_2 in all instances. Worlledge and Rousso (50, 128) concluded that the Donath-Landsteiner antibody has a specificity of anti-P. Paroxysmal cold hemoglobinuria develops when this antibody functions as an autoantibody by being produced in a P_1 or P_2 patient.

Summary

The Donath-Landsteiner autoantibody can no longer be considered to be nonspecific. Reactivity is directed to the P blood group and a specificity of anti-P is present.

All three varieties of erythrocyte autoantibodies have now overcome the immunologic stigma of nonspecificity. Different antigens are involved. Warm acting autoantibodies have an antigenic relationship to the rhesus blood group. Cold acting hemagglutinins have specificity against Ii antigens which are part of or closely related to the ABO blood group. Antigenic specificity of the Donath-Landsteiner antibody is oriented toward the P blood group.

In all instances a panhemagglutinin was previously assumed because of an almost universal reactivity of these antibodies with human erythrocytes. It is now apparent that this broad reactivity reflects the broad distribution of involved antigens, rather than "nonspecificity" of the autoantibody. Hemolytic anemia develops when such antibodies are produced in a host whose erythrocytes contain the pertinent antigen. Such a sequence results in true autoantibody formation. It is apparent that two critical components are necessary to classify erythrocyte antibodies as autoantibodies. The erythrocyte antibody must have isoantigenic specificity. The erythrocytes of the host producing the antibody must contain the specific antigenic determinant. Both of these criteria are usually fulfilled in autoimmune hemolytic anemia.

BIBLIOGRAPHY

1. Dameshek, W.: Theories of autoimmunity. In *Conceptual Advances in Immunology and Oncology.* Hoeber Medical Division, Harper & Row, Publishers, New York, 1963.

2. Roth, K. L.: Interaction of heparin with auto-agglutinins in idiopathic acquired hemolytic anemia. Proc. Soc. Exp. Biol. Med. **86:** 352, 1954.

3. Roth, K. L., and Frumin, A. M.: In vitro differentiation between auto- and iso-immune antibodies by protamine and trypsin. Science **120:** 945, 1954.

4. August, A., and Pirofsky, B.: Interaction of basic polyelectrolytes and human blood: The effect of antiheparin agents. Transfusion **6:** 74, 1966.

5. Pirofsky, B.: Immunologic differences between iso-antibodies and auto-antibodies. Amer. J. Clin. Path. **29:** 120, 1958.

6. Brody, J. I., and Finch, S. C.: Serum factors of acquired hemolytic anemia in leukemia and lymphoma. J. Clin. Invest. **40:** 181, 1961.

7. Brody, J. I.: Reactivity of red cell eluates and serums in patients with acquired hemolytic anemia and chronic lymphocytic leukemia. J. Clin. Invest. **41:** 471, 1962.

8. Pirofsky, B.: Studies on leukemic leukocyte extracts. I. Lack of antigenic relationship in acquired hemolytic anemia. II. The demonstration of a hemolysin and agglutinin. J. Lab. Clin. Med. **48:** 745, 1956.

9. Pirofsky, B., Cordova, M. S., and Imel, T. L.: The nonimmunologic reaction of globulin molecules with the erythrocyte surface. Vox Sang. **7:** 334, 1962.

10. Boursnell, J. C., Coombs, R. R. A., and Rizk, V.: Quantitative studies with antiserum marked with iodine[131] isotope and their corresponding red-cell antigens. Biochem. J. **55:** 745, 1953.

11. Pirofsky, B., Cordova, M. S., and Imel, T. L.: The mechanism of action of antiglobulin serum. Vox Sang. **7:** 348, 1962.

12. Pirofsky, B., and Cordova, M. S.: Bivalent nature of incomplete anti-D (Rh$_o$). Nature (London) **197:** 392, 1963.

13. Pirofsky, B., and Cordova, M. S.: The nature of incomplete erythrocyte antibodies. Vox Sang. **9:** 17, 1964.

14. Pirofsky, B.: The structure and specificity of erythrocyte autoantibodies. Ann. N. Y. Acad. Sci. **124:** 448, 1965.

15. Mandy, W. J., Fudenberg, H. H., and Lewis, F. B.: On "incomplete" anti-Rh antibodies: mechanism of direct agglutination induced by mercaptoethanol. J. Clin. Invest. **44:** 1352, 1965.

16. Pirofsky, B., and Cordova, M. S.: The in vitro inhibition of erythrocyte antibodies by hexosamine-containing antibiotics. Brit. J. Haemat. **10:** 320, 1964.

17. Pirofsky, B., and Cordova, M. S.: The in vitro neutralization of erythrocyte auto-antibodies and iso-antibodies. Bibl. Haemat. **19:** 550, 1964.

18. Boyd, W. C., McMaster, M. H., and Waszczenko-Zacharczenko, E.: Specific inhibition

of anti-Rh serum by "unnatural" sugars. Nature (London) **184:** 989, 1959.

19. Pirofsky, B., Cordova, M. S., and Rigas, D.: The mechanism of streptomycin inhibition of erythrocyte antibodies. Vox Sang. **9:** 653, 1964.

20. Denys, P., and van den Broucke, J.: Anémie hémolytique acquise et réaction de Coombs. Arch. Franc. Pediat. **4:** 205, 1947.

21. Kuhns, W. J., and Wagley, P. F.: Hemolytic anemia associated with atypical hemagglutinins. Ann. Intern. Med. **30:** 408, 1949.

22. Dameshek, W.: Acquired hemolytic anemia. Physiopathology with particular reference to autoimmunization and therapy. In *Proceedings of the Third International Congress of the International Society of Hematology*. William Heinemann, Ltd., London, 1951.

23. Davidsohn, I., and Oyamada, A.: Specificity of auto-antibodies in hemolytic anemia. Amer. J. Clin. Path. **23:** 101, 1953.

24. Wiener, A. S., and Gordon, E. B.: Quantitative test for antibody-globulin coating human blood cells and its practical applications. Amer. J. Clin. Path. **23:** 429, 1953.

25. Wiener, A. S., Gordon, E. B., and Gallop, C.: Studies on autoantibodies in human sera. J. Immun. **71:** 58, 1953.

26. Weiner, W., Battey, D. A., Cleghorn, T. E., Marson, F. G. W., and Meynell, M. J.: Serological findings in a case of haemolytic anaemia, with some general observations on the pathogenesis of this syndrome. Brit. Med. J. **2:** 125, 1953.

27. Holländer, L.: Specificity of antibodies in acquired haemolytic anaemia. Experientia **9:** 468, 1953.

28. Dacie, J. V., and Cutbush, M.: Specificity of auto-antibodies in acquired haemolytic anaemia. J. Clin. Path. **7:** 18, 1954.

29. van Loghem, J. J., and van der Hart, M.: Varieties of specific auto-antibodies in acquired haemolytic anaemia. Vox Sang. **4:** 2, 129, 1954.

30. Crowley, L. V., and Bouroncle, B. A.: Studies on the specificity of autoantibodies in acquired hemolytic anemia. Blood **11:** 700, 1956.

31. Meuli, H. C.: Über blutgruppenspezifische antierythrocytäre Autoantikörper. Blut. **3:** 270, 1957.

32. Kissmeyer-Nielsen, F.: Specific auto-antibodies in immunohaemolytic anaemia. With a note on the pathogenesis of autoimmunization. In P. H. Andressen: *Papers in Dedication of His Sixtieth Birthday*. Levin & Munksgaard, Copenhagen, 1957.

33. van Loghem, J. J., van der Hart, M., and Dorfmeier, H.: Serologic studies in acquired hemolytic anemia. In *Proceedings of the Sixth International Congress of the International Society of Hematology*. Grune & Stratton, Inc., New York, 1958.

34. Dausset, J., and Colombani, J.: The serology

and the prognosis of 128 cases of autoimmune hemolytic anemia. Blood **14**: 1280, 1959.

35. Weiner, W.: Probleme der autoimmunhämolytischen Anämien. Klin. Wschr. **38**: 885, 1960.

36. Laski, B., Wake, E. J., Gunson, H., and Bain, H. W.: Idiopathic acquired anemia in two young infants. Amer. J. Dis. Child. **100**: 524, 1960.

37. Gross, S., and Newman, D. J.: Autoimmune anti-D specificity in infancy. Amer. J. Dis. Child. **108**: 181, 1964.

38. DiPiero, G., Mencarini, L., and Stegagno, G.: Anemia emolitica autoimmune con autoanticorpi anti-c in lattante. (Guarigione clinical dopo 23 mesi). Rev. Clin. Pediat. **77**: 305, 1966.

39. Ogata, T., and Matuhasi, T.: Problems of specific and cross reactivity of blood group antibodies. In *Proceedings of the Eighth Congress of the International Society of Blood Transfusion*. S. Karger, Basel, 1962.

40. Ogata, T., and Matuhasi, T.: Further observations on the problems of specific and cross reactivity of blood group antibodies. In *Proceedings of the Ninth Congress of the International Society of Blood Transfusion*. S. Karger, Basel, 1964.

41. Svardal, J. M., Yarbro, J., and Yunis, E. J.: Ogata phenomenon explaining the unusual specificity in eluates from Coombs positive cells sensitized by autogenous anti-I. Vox Sang. **13**: 472, 1967.

42. Whittingham, S., Jakobowicz, R., and Simmons, R. T.: Multiple antibodies imitating the presence of a panagglutinin in the serum of a patient suffering from haemolytic anaemia. Med. J. Aust. **48**: 205, 1961.

43. Croucher, B. E. E., Crookston, M. C., and Crookston, J. H.: Delayed haemolytic transfusion reactions simulating auto-immune haemolytic anaemia. Vox Sang. **12**: 32, 1967.

44. Joseph, J. I., Awer, E., Laulight, M., and Scudder, J.: Delayed hemolytic transfusion reaction due to appearance of multiple antibodies following transfusion of apparently compatible blood. Transfusion **4**: 367, 1964.

45. Meara, J. F., Hoffman, G. C., and Hewlett, J. S.: Autoimmune hemolytic anemia associated with anti-f: report of a case. Transfusion **7**: 48, 1967.

46. Flückiger, P., Ricci, C., and Usteri, C.: Zur Frage der Blutgruppenspezifität von Autoantikörpern. Acta Haemat. (Basel) **13**: 53, 1955.

47. Yokoyama, M., Eith, D. T., and Bowman, M.: The first auto-Xg^a antibody in a female. Hawaii Med. J. **25**: 328, 1966.

48. Yokoyama, M., and McCoy, J. E.: Further studies on auto-anti-Xg^a antibody. Vox Sang. **13**: 15, 1967.

49. Dacie, J. V.: *The Haemolytic Anaemias, Part II*, Ed. 2. Grune & Stratton, Inc., New York, 1962.

50. Worlledge, S. M.: Serologic aspects of the auto-immune haemolytic anaemia. In *Autoimmunity*, edited by R. W. Baldwin and J. H. Humphrey. Blackwell Scientific Publications Ltd., Oxford, 1965.

51. Weiner, W.: The specificity of the antibodies in acquired hemolytic anemias. Bibl. Haemat. **23**: 24, 1965.

52. Carstairs, K. C., Breckenridge, A., Dollery, C. T., and Worlledge, S.: Incidence of a positive direct Coombs test in patients on α-methyldopa. Lancet **2**: 133, 1966.

53. Worlledge, S., Carstairs, K. C., and Dacie, J. V.: Autoimmune haemolytic anaemia associated with α-methyldopa therapy. Lancet **2**: 135, 1966.

54. Wiener, A. S., Gordon, E. B., and Russow, E.: Observations on the nature of the autoantibodies in a case of acquired hemolytic anemia. Ann. Intern. Med. **47**: 1, 1957.

55. Witebsky, E.: Acquired hemolytic anemia. Ann. N. Y. Acad. Sci. **124**: 462, 1965.

56. Weiner, W., Whitehead, J. P., and Walkden, W. J.: Acquired haemolytic anaemia: Clinical and serological observations of two cases. Brit. Med. J. **1**: 73, 1956.

57. Speiser, P.: Ueber eine beobachtete temporäre Ausnahme von der Ehrlichschen Regel des Horror autotoxicus bei idiopathischer hämolytischer Anämie. Wien. Klin. Wschr. **69**: 149, 1957.

58. Spielmann, W.: Spezifische Autoantikörper bei hämolytischen Anämien. Klin. Wschr. **34**: 248, 1956.

59. Fudenberg, H. H., Rosenfield, R. E., and Wasserman, L. R.: Unusual specificity of auto-antibody in auto-immune hemolytic disease. J. Mount Sinai Hosp. **25**: 324, 1958.

60. Stratton, F., and Renton, P. H.: *Practical Blood Grouping*. Blackwell Scientific Publications Ltd., Oxford, 1958.

61. Hubinont, P. O., Massart-Guiot, T., Bricoult, A., and Ghysdael, P.: Immunological specificity of eluates from "Coombs positive" erythrocytes. Vox Sang. **4**: 419, 1959.

62. Muirhead, E. E.: The relationship of current transfusion practice to modern immunohematology. Ann. N. Y. Acad. Sci. **127**: 926, 1965.

63. Wiener, A. S.: Origin of naturally occurring hemagglutinins and hemolysins: a review. J. Immun. **66**: 287, 1951.

64. Shapiro, M.: ABO, MN, P and Rh blood group systems in the South African Bantu. Genetic study. S. Afr. Med. J. **25**: 187, 1951.

65. Anderson, L. D., Race, G. J., and Owen, M.: Presence of anti-D antibody in Rh(D) positive person. Amer. J. Clin. Path. **30**: 228, 1958.

66. Chown, B., Kaita, H., Lewis, M., Roy, R. B., and Wyatt, L.: A "D-positive" man who produced anti-D. Vox Sang. **8**: 420, 1963.

67. MacPherson, C. R., Stevenson, T. D., and Gayton, J.: Anti-D in a D-positive man, with positive direct Coombs test and normal red cell survival. Amer. J. Clin. Path. **45:** 748, 1966.

68. Weiner, W., and Vos, G. H.: Serology of acquired hemolytic anemias. Blood **22:** 606, 1963.

69. Sturgeon, P.: A new antibody in serum of patients with acquired hemolytic anemia. Science **106:** 293, 1947.

70. Komninos, F. D., and Rosenthal, M. C.: Studies on antibodies eluted from the red cells in autoimmune hemolytic anemia. J. Lab. Clin. Med. **41:** 887, 1953.

71. Kidd, P.: Elution of an incomplete type of antibody from the erythrocytes in acquired haemolytic anaemia. J. Clin. Path. **2:** 103, 1949.

72. Evans, R. S., and Weiser, R. S.: The serology of autoimmune hemolytic disease. Observations on forty-one patients. Arch. Intern. Med. (Chicago) **100:** 371, 1957.

73. Wiener, A. S., Moor-Jankowski, J., and Gordon, E. B.: Blood groups of apes and monkeys. IV. The Rh-hr blood types of anthropoid apes. Amer. J. Hum. Genet. **16:** 246, 1964.

74. Wiener, A. S., Gavan, J. A., and Gordon, E. B.: Blood group factors in anthropoid apes and monkeys. II. Further studies on the Rh-hr factors. Amer. J. Phys. Anthrop. **11:** 39, 1953.

75. Wiener, A. S.: Blood groups in man and lower primates: a review. Transfusion **3:** 173, 1963.

76. Pirofsky, B., and Pratt, K.: The antigen in autoimmune hemolytic anemia. I. Reactivity of human autoantibodies with primate and non-primate erythrocytes. Amer. J. Clin. Path. **45:** 75, 1966.

77. Mino, P.: La panemoagglutinina del sangue umane. Policlinico (Prat.) **31:** 1355, 1924.

78. Clough, M. C., and Richter, I. M.: A study of an autoagglutinin occurring in a human serum. Johns Hopkins Hosp. Bull. **29:** 86, 1918.

79. Turner, J. C., and Jackson, E. B.: Serological specificity of an auto-antibody in atypical pneumonia. Brit. J. Exp. Path. **24:** 121, 1943.

80. Finland, M., Peterson, O. L., and Barnes, M. W.: Cold agglutinins. III. Observations on certain serological and physical features of cold agglutinins in cases of primary atypical pneumonia and of hemolytic anemia. J. Clin. Invest. **24:** 474, 1945.

81. Millet, M., and Fincler, L.: Remarques sur les affinités de l'auto-agglutinine (cold agglutinin) du sérum humain. C. R. Soc. Biol. (Paris) **140:** 1226, 1946.

82. Delage, J. M., Gauvreau, L., and Simard, J.: Les anémies hémolytiques par auto-anti-corps. Etude clinique et expérimentale. Un. Med. Canada **85:** 132, 1956.

83. Schubothe, H.: *Serologie und Klinische Bedeutung der Autohämantikörper.* S. Karger, Basel, 1958.

84. Amzel, R., and Hirszfeld, L.: Ueber die Kälteagglutination der roten Blutkörperchen. Z. Immunitaetsforsch. **43:** 526, 1925.

85. Kettel, K.: Recherches sur les agglutinines au froid dans les sérums humains. C. R. Soc. Biol. (Paris) **100:** 371, 1929.

86. Boxwell, W., and Bigger, J. W.: Autohemagglutination. J. Path. Bact. **34:** 407, 1931.

87. Wheeler, K. M., Gallacher, H. J., and Stuart, C. A.: An unusual case of autoagglutination. J. Lab. Clin. Med. **24:** 1135, 1939.

88. Stratton, F.: Some observations on autohaemagglutination. Lancet **1:** 613, 1943.

89. Bird, G. W. G.: Observations on haemagglutinin "linkage" in relation to iso-agglutinins and auto-agglutinins. Brit. J. Exp. Path. **34:** 131, 1953.

90. Young, L. E.: The clinical significance of cold hemagglutinins. Amer. J. Med. Sci. **211:** 23, 1946.

91. Dacie, J. V.: The serology of acquired haemolytic anaemia. Sang **25:** 675, 1954.

92. Crookston, J. H., Dacie, J. V., and Rossi, V.: Differences in the agglutinability of human red cells by the high-titre cold antibodies of acquired haemolytic anaemia. Brit. J. Haemat. **2:** 321, 1956.

93. Hennemann, H., and Rasch, L. H.: Kälteagglutination durch ein spezifisches Blutfaktorensystem mit besonderem klinischem Erscheinungsbild. Z. Ges. Inn. Med. **4:** 535, 1949.

94. Crowley, L. V.: Blood group specific autoantibodies in acquired hemolytic anemia. Amer. J. Clin. Path. **29:** 426, 1958.

95. Wiener, A. S., Unger, L. J., Cohen, L., and Feldman, J.: Type-specific cold auto-antibodies as a cause of acquired hemolytic anemia and hemolytic transfusion reactions: biologic test with bovine red cells. Ann. Intern. Med. **44:** 221, 1956.

96. Jenkins, W. J., Marsh, W. L., Noades, J., Tippett, P., Sanger, R., and Race, R. R.: The I antigen and antibody. Vox Sang. **5:** 97, 1960.

97. Tippett, P., Noades, J., Sanger, R., Race, R. R., Sausais, L., Holman, C. A., and Buttimer, R. J.: Further studies of the I antigen and antibody. Vox Sang. **5:** 107, 1960.

98. Marcus, D. M., Kabat, E. A., and Rosenfield, R. E.: The action of enzymes from *Clostridium tertium* on the I antigenic determinants of human erythrocytes. J. Exp. Med. **118:** 175, 1963.

99. Gold, E. R.: Observations on the specificity of anti-O and anti-A_1 sera. Vox Sang. **9:** 153, 1964.

100. Rosenfield, R. E., Schroeder, R., Ballard, R., van der Hart, M., Moes, M., and van

Loghem, J. J.: Erythrocytic antigenic determinants characteristic of H, I in the presence of H (IH), or H in the absence of i [H(−i)]. Vox Sang. **9**: 415, 1964.

101. Schmidt, P. J., and McGinniss, M. H.: Differences between anti-H and anti-OI red cell antibodies. Vox Sang. **10**: 109, 1965.

102. Yokoyama, M.: Close relationship between A and I blood groups. Nature (London) **206**: 411, 1965.

103. Yokoyama, M., and Plocinik, B. A.: Ganglioside inhibition of blood group antibodies with special reference to blood group I. Z. Immun. Allergieforsch. **129**: 137, 1965.

104. Tegoli, J., Harris, J. P., Issitt, P. D., and Sanders, C. W.: Anti-IB, an expected "new" antibody detecting a joint product of the I and B genes (abstract). Nineteenth Annual Meeting of the American Association of Blood Banks, Los Angeles, October 26, 1966.

105. Salmon, C., Homberg, J. C., Liberge, G., and Delarue, F.: Autoanticorps A spécificités multiples, anti-HI, anti-AI, anti-BI dans certains éluats d'anémie hémolytique. Rev. Franc. Etud. Clin. Biol. **10**: 522, 1965.

106. Unger, L. J., Wiener, A. S., and Dolan, D.: Anémie autohémolytique chez un nouveau-né. Rev. Hemat. (Paris) **7**: 495, 1952.

107. Mortara, M., and Martinetti, L.: Su di un caso di anemia emolitica cronica con sindrome di Raynaud e crioagglutinazione. G. Clin. Med. **36**: 1791, 1955.

108. Marsh, W. L.: Anti-i: A cold antibody defining the Ii relationship in human red cells. Brit. J. Haemat. **7**: 200, 1961.

109. Giblett, E. R., and Crookston, M. C.: Agglutinability of red cells by anti-i in patients with thalassemia major and other haematological disorders. Nature (London) **201**: 1138, 1964.

110. Evans, R. S., Turner, E., and Bingham, M.: Studies with radioiodinated cold agglutinins of ten patients. Amer. J. Med. **38**: 378, 1965.

111. McGinniss, M. H., Schmidt, P. J., and Carbone, P. P.: Close association of I blood group and disease. Nature (London) **202**: 606, 1964.

112. Schmidt, P. J., Barile, M. F., and McGinniss, M. H.: Mycoplasma (pleuro-pneumonialike organisms) and blood group I; association with neoplastic disease. Nature (London) **205**: 371, 1965.

113. Ayers, M., Salzano, F. M., and Ludwig, O. K.: Blood group changes in leukemia. J. Med. Genet. **3**: 180, 1966.

114. Schmidt, P. J., Yokoyama, M., McGinniss, M. H., and Carbone, P. P.: Effect of disease on an expression of blood group I. In *Proceedings of the Tenth Congress of the International Society of Blood Transfusion.* S. Karger, Basel, 1965.

115. Thomas, L.: Circulating autoantibodies and human disease. With a note on primary atypical pneumonia. New Eng. J. Med. **270**: 1157, 1964.

116. Smith, C. B., McGinniss, M. H., and Schmidt, P. J.: Changes in erythrocyte I agglutinogen and anti-I agglutinins during *Mycoplasma pneumoniae* infection in man. J. Immun. **99**: 333, 1967.

117. Costea, N., Yakulis, V., and Heller, P.: Experimental production of cold agglutinins in rabbits. Blood **26**: 323, 1965.

118. Marsh, W. L., and Jenkins, W. J.: Anti-i: a new cold antibody. Nature (London) **188**: 753, 1960.

119. van Loghem, J. J., Peetoom, F., van der Hart, M., van der Veer, M., van der Giessen, M., Prins, H. K., Zurcher, C., and Engelfriet, C. P.: Serological and immunochemical studies in haemolytic anemia with high titre cold agglutinins. Vox Sang. **8**: 33, 1963.

120. van Loghem, J. J., van der Hart, M., Veenhoven-van Riesz, E., van der Veer, M., Engelfriet, C. P., and Peetoom, F.: Cold auto-agglutinins and haemolysins of anti-I and anti-i specificity. Vox Sang. **7**: 214, 1962.

121. Evans, R. S., Bingham, M., and Turner, E.: Autoimmune hemolytic disease: observations of serological reactions and disease activity. Ann. N. Y. Acad. Sci. **124**: 422, 1965.

122. Bell, C. A., Zwicker, H., and Sacks, H. J.: Anti-i: identification of the "non-specific" cold agglutinin (abstract). Nineteenth Annual Meeting of the American Association of Blood Banks, Los Angeles, October 25–28, 1966.

123. Rosenfield, R. E., Schmidt, P. J., Calvo, R. C., and McGinniss, M. H.: Anti-i, a frequent cold agglutinin in infectious mononucleosis. Vox Sang. **10**: 631, 1965.

124. Jenkins, W. J., and Marsh, W. L.: Glandular fever and cold agglutinins. Lancet **1**: 1158, 1966.

125. Hinz, C. F.: Serologic and physicochemical characterization of Donath-Landsteiner antibodies from 6 patients. Blood **22**: 600, 1963.

126. Levine, P., Celano, M. J., and Falkowski, F.: The specificity of the antibody in paroxysmal cold hemoglobinuria (P.C.H.). Transfusion **3**: 278, 1963.

127. Levine, P., Celano, M. J., and Falkowski, F.: The specificity of the antibody in paroxysmal cold hemoglobinuria (P.C.H.). Ann. N. Y. Acad. Sci. **124**: 456, 1965.

128. Worlledge, S. M., and Rousso, C.: Studies on the serology of paroxysmal cold haemoglobinuria (P.C.H.), with special reference to its relationship with the P blood group system. Vox Sang. **10**: 293, 1965.

Chapter 21

The Effect of Immune Reactions on the Erythrocyte

The erythrocyte coating materials found in autoimmune hemolytic anemia have been shown to be antibodies. They exhibit isoantigenic specificity, and the erythrocytes of a host producing the antibody contain the pertinent antigen. Immunologic interactions therefore occur. Do such reactions damage the red cell? If so, what mechanisms are involved? Such questions are fundamental to the central problem of how autoantibody production is related to the clinical picture of hemolytic anemia. This chapter is designed to examine this aspect of erythrocyte immune interactions.

Autoimmune hemolytic anemia has been presented as an end stage syndrome resulting from many different etiologic and pathophysiologic mechanisms. It is probable that a single pathologic sequence is not universally present in autoimmune hemolytic anemia. At least four different erythrocyte-globulin relationships exist which may lead to erythrocyte damage. These include the following: (a) nonimmune fixation of globulin molecules to the erythrocyte surface, (b) modification of autologous erythrocyte antigens and binding of an autologous antibody to the red cell, (c) the innocent bystander role of the erythrocyte in an unrelated immunologic event, and (d) interaction of an autoantibody with its erythrocyte isoantigen.

The bulk of knowledge concerning the nature and effect of immune interactions on the erythrocytes has been derived from heteroimmune and isoimmune studies. By analogy this information has been transposed into autoimmune systems. Although this approach is probably generally accurate, several fundamental differences exist between antiglobulin positive and autoimmune hemolytic anemia and isoimmune and heteroimmune hemolytic anemia. The first two states present a clinical picture of gradual hemolysis which is in contrast to the rapid and massive hemolysis seen with heteroimmune and isoimmune hemolytic anemia. In addition, a chronic hemolytic element is the rule in the autoimmune syndromes, rather than the transient acute episodes which characterize isoimmune hemolytic states. These clinical characteristics must be superimposed on the more accurately gathered data obtained in isoimmune and heteroimmune systems.

The Normal Maintenance of Erythrocyte Survival

Jandl (1) has emphasized that erythrocyte survival depends on the ability of the erythrocyte to preserve its size, shape, plasticity and stickiness within relatively narrow limits. Ponder (2) stated that the metabolic activity of the erythrocyte is designed to perpetuate its morphologic continuity. The energy for preserving morphology and withstanding wear in the mature erythrocyte is derived entirely from the metabolism of glucose. Two mechanisms are involved. Oxidation-reduction homeostasis is maintained through formation of reduced pyridine nucleotides and generation of the high energy compound adenosine triphosphate (ATP). Both oxidative and anerobic metabolic pathways are activated. ATP formation is crucial to the maintenance of cell volume, size, shape and plasticity and is generated purely by anerobic pathways. The erythrocyte has no appreciable reserve of glycogen (3) or high energy compounds such as phosphocreatine (4). In addition, during aging there is a decline in several critical glycolytic enzymes (5, 6). Accordingly, the overt evidence of erythrocyte damage may be strongly influenced by age dependent factors.

The Active Transport Pumping System

Relatively complex controls are necessary to maintain erythrocyte volume. Water crosses the red cell membrane rapidly without evidence of an osmotic gradient (7, 8). The small "physiologic" anions such as Cl^- and HCO_3^- also cross the erythrocyte membrane rapidly and distribute according to the Donnan equilibrium. Cations such as Na^+ and K^+ only slowly penetrate the erythrocyte membrane. The half-exchange time for K^+ is over 30 hours (9); this should be compared to half-exchange times of 0.2 seconds for Cl^- and 0.004 seconds for water (10). A high concentration of impermeable molecules within the erythrocyte creates an unbalanced osmotic force. Hemoglobin is the principal constituent and acts as a polyanion contributing about 5 mEq. of anion per liter of cells (11). The erythrocyte maintains volume control in spite of the osmotic asymmetry by an active "pumping" of cations, principally Na^+. This cation is removed from the cell at a rate sufficient to balance the limited rate of entry of Na^+. During the process the erythrocyte maintains a remarkable consistency of gradients for individual cations. Intracellular-extracellular ratios of K^+ (25:1) and Na^+ (1:12) are preserved (12, 13). The active transport pumping system clearly distinguishes these two cations, although biologically the difference is not apparent.

The erythrocyte is a partially collapsed sphere in its normal state. Substantial swelling can occur before the complete spherical shape is assumed. This point, which is known as the hemolytic volume and is characterized by rupture of the cell, occurs when the volume is increased 60 to 70 per cent (1). Cell injury may reduce the surface area as well as affect the ionic exchange. Such damage may reduce the hemolytic volume to as little as 20 per cent (2, 14). A loss of surface lipids can assume importance in lowering the hemolytic volume (15, 16).

The active transport of ions and molecules against electrochemical gradients is critical to the erythrocyte's ability to resist hemolysis. The "pumping in" of K^+ and the "pumping out" of Na^+ are related processes with the rate controlled by concentration of intracellular Na^+ or extracellular K^+. Energy for the process is supplied by an adenosine triphosphate enzymatic (ATPase) mechanism located in the erythrocyte cell membrane. This mechanism is particularly sensitive to the action of small amounts of cardiac glycosides such as ouabain (17).

Colloid Osmotic Hemolysis

Hemolysis can result from a breakdown in osmotic regulation and volume control through either of two fundamental changes: (a) a diminished active cationic transport or (b) increased membrane permeability. The concept of colloid osmotic hemolysis was developed by Wilbrandt (18) to describe the effect of a hemolytic agent on cell permeability. The primary mechanism concerned is an increased rate of cation entry into the erythrocyte. This disturbance of the ionic gradient permits an inward flow of water and the gradual swelling of the cell into a sphere. As swelling continues, permeability of the erythrocyte membrane increases, eventually leading to leaking of hemoglobin. The loss of K^+ from the erythrocyte and the inflow of Na^+ are characteristic of this process.

The normal pores of the erythrocyte membrane are estimated to have a radius of 3 to 4 Å. This is sufficiently small to retard the entry of K^+ and Na^+ and to prevent the transport of Ca^{++}, Mg^{++}

and sucrose. Increasing the suspending medium concentration of large colloid molecules such as albumin, dextran and polyvinylpyrrolidone counteracts the osmotic gradient introducing water into the erythrocyte. Erythrocytes suspended in such media will exhibit retarded hemolysis. Figure 41 illustrates the lysis of erythrocytes through colloid osmotic hemolysis.

The above survey has closely followed the analytical review of Jandl (1). This excellent presentation should be consulted for further information and reference material.

Immune Damage to the Erythrocyte

The mechanisms through which erythrocyte surface immune reactions create cellular damage are complex. The complexity is magnified by the fact that in vivo hemolysis can differ fundamentally from in vitro hemolysis. Swisher (19) emphasized that in vivo hemolysis resulting from the action of erythrocyte antibodies may involve a two-phase system. The initial erythrocyte damage reflecting the immediate antibody action may not be sufficient to induce rapid lysis. However, damaged erythrocytes can be removed from the circulation and hemolysis will follow after a variable delay. A period of time and several additional mechanisms may be involved between the stages of initial antibody action and final erythrocyte destruction. Swisher (19) states that "it seems important to recognize that the events which initiate in vivo loss of erythrocytic viability are of primary significance in such a hemolytic process; actual disruption of red cell structure may be a matter of lesser interest, and indeed, may proceed by several mechanisms."

Four well defined pathologic sequences have been documented to explain the effect of antibody-antigen union involving the erythrocyte. These include the action of complement, the production of subtle abnormalities in the glycolytic and cation gradient pumping systems, the sequestration of antibody coated erythrocytes and erythrophagocytosis. Excellent reviews of this subject have been presented by Jandl (1, 20), Swisher (19, 21), Rifkind (22),

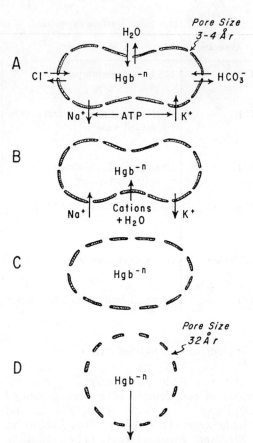

FIGURE 41. Diagramatic representation of colloid osmotic hemolysis. The inflow of water creates a spherocyte and enlarges the pore size sufficiently to permit the release of hemoglobin (Hgb).

Dourmashkin and Rosse (23) and Weed and Reed (16).

The Effect of Complement

Complement was discovered and established as an immunologic entity at the turn of the century. Early investigations demonstrated it to be a heat labile factor destroyed by heating at 56°C. for 30 minutes. Complement is present in normal serum and appears to be essential for the lytic action of antibodies. Serum levels of complement are not influenced by immunization and are relatively constant in the adult of a given species. Complement is unable to react with either antibody or antigen alone; rather, the reaction of complement is dependent on the presence of

TABLE 103. *Various components of complement (C') and their characteristics**

Component	Identification	Characteristic
C'0	11S human serum protein	Binds at 0°C. in the presence of EDTA. Relation to or part of C'1 complex
C'1	Euglobulin (insoluble fraction in distilled water)	Heat labile. Exists as proesterase and is activated by contact with immune complex. Three components. C'0 may be one part
C'2	Pseudoglobulin (soluble fraction in distilled water)	Heat labile. May function as the substrate for C'1 esterase activity
C'3a	Euglobulin, beta 1-C globulin	Decay, spontaneous or after interaction with immune complex. Breakdown produces a smaller beta 1-A globulin
C'3 other	Not well characterized	Not well characterized. At least three additional components present
C'4	Pseudoglobulin, beta 1-E globulin	Heat stable. Inactivated by ether, ammonia or hydralazine. C'1 esterase will destroy it in solution

* Modified from Swisher (21).

immune complexes. Excellent recent reviews of complement have been presented by Borsos and Mayer (24), Plescia and Heidelberger (25), Osler (26), Lachmann (27) and Swisher (21). The following summary closely follows the presentation of Swisher (21).

Complement Components

Four basic components of complement (C') have been recognized for many years. This number has been expanded to at least six well standardized components. Additional C'3 components are postulated, and possibly 12 or more components actually exist. Table 103 summarizes the well established six components which are briefly described here. C'0 was described by Müller-Eberhard (28) in 1961 and has been prepared in pure form. It is an 11S serum component that may be removed from serum by immune complexes using ethylenediaminetetraacetic acid (EDTA) at 0°C. C'1 is a heat labile euglobulin destroyed by heating at 56°C. for 30 minutes. It occurs as a proesterase and is activated by immune complexes (29). C'2 is a heat labile pseudoglobulin fraction of serum

(30). C'3 is a heat stable group of components primarily found in the euglobulin fraction of serum. It spontaneously decays at room temperature and is inactivated by zymosan under conditions which will not affect other complement components. Four components of C'3 have been described (31). The C'3a portion has been purified by Müller-Eberhard and found to be a beta 1-A globulin (32). The C'4 component is a heat stable pseudoglobulin fraction that may be inactivated by ammonia, hydralazine or ether. It is destroyed by C'1 esterase in solution (33). Figure 42 presents the postulated sequence of action of complement components reacting with an erythrocyte (E) in the presence of an antibody (A). This sequence, as originally developed by Mayer (34), has been modified by Osler (26) and Lachmann (27).

The amount and availability of the C'2 and C'3 complement components are critical for the eventual development of hemolysis. The C'3 reaction appears to be the slowest, at least when guinea pig C' is used. This influences the end stage of immune hemolysis. A formation-decay equilibrium is established between the EAC'0,1,4 and

EAC'0,1,4,2 complexes. As the latter complex is formed, two alternative sequences can occur. If C'3 is available in adequate amounts the reaction can go to completion, resulting in hemolysis. If C'3 is unavailable or present in inadequate amounts the EAC'0,1,4,2 complex will decay, inactivating C'2. A continuation of this process will eventually exhaust C'2. The reaction between EAC'0,1,4,2 and C'3 may be artificially inhibited. Mills and Levine (35) demonstrated that salicylaldoxime is a moderately potent inhibitor. Rodriguez and Osler (36) found that both phlorizin and phloretin were active inhibiting agents. Lepow and Ross (37) have emphasized that the C'1 esterase component is critical in initiating immune cytotoxicity. Employing human amnion cells and rabbit antiserum it was found that cytotoxicity required Mg^{++}, Ca^{++} and C'1 esterase (38).

The binding site of complement components in relationship to the erythrocyte-antibody complex is still unknown. The Fc fragment of the H chain appears to be responsible for complement fixation. Accordingly, it may be theorized that complement can be bound to either the erythrocyte membrane or to the heavy chain of the antibody molecule. Harboe (39), on the basis of in vitro studies, suggests that complement is fixed to the erythrocyte membrane. Müller-Eberhard and Lepow (40) obtained data which indicate direct activation of complement components on the red cell membrane. Taranta and Franklin (41) demonstrated a complement fixing site located on the H chain of IgG antibodies. Leddy and associates (42) have shown that eluted IgG autoantibodies may cause in vitro complement fixation to erythrocytes. This suggests that complement components are fixed to the sensitizing eluted antibody.

The fixation of complement components to the erythrocyte surface differs from antibody fixation in one crucial respect. Although antibodies may be eluted from erythrocytes by various procedures, complement appears to be irreversibly bound. The end stage of hemolysis seems to be related to the fixation of complement.

1. E (erythrocyte) + A (antibody) ⟶ EA

2. EA + C'0 $\xrightarrow{\text{Divalent cations not required}}$ EAC'0

3. EAC'0 + C'1 $\xrightarrow{\quad CA^{++} \quad}$ EAC'0,1

4. EAC'0,1 + C'4 $\xrightarrow{\qquad\qquad}$ EAC'0,1,4

5. EAC'0,1,4 + C'2 $\xrightarrow{\quad Mg^{++} \quad}$ EAC'0,1,4,2

6. EAC'0,1,4,2 + C'3c $\xrightarrow{\qquad}$ EAC'0,1,4,2,3c

7. EAC'0,1,4,2,3c + other C'3 (b,a,d) $\xrightarrow{\qquad}$ E* (damaged erythrocyte)

8. E* $\xrightarrow{\qquad\qquad}$ Ghost cells + hemoglobin

FIGURE 42. The sequential reactions of complement (C') components after an erythrocyte (E) has combined with an antibody (A).

Antibody or antibody-antigen complexes appear to be unnecessary for eventual cellular destruction. The in vivo delay between cellular damage and eventual immune hemolysis, however, minimizes the significance of this observation. The interaction of complement with antibody may produce the defects necessary to permit lysis to result in the absence of antibody. The development of globulin aggregates may be important for this reaction.

The Alteration of the Erythrocyte by Complement

Complement induced in vivo immune hemolysis may occur through three different mechanisms. The role of complement components in erythrophagocytosis and sequestration of antibody coated erythrocytes is discussed separately below. The major lytic action of complement is related to the establishment of certain biophysical changes of the erythrocyte membrane. The postulated sequence of events is as follows.

Antibodies which fix complement can induce cellular lysis through the mechanism of colloid osmotic hemolysis. Ellem (43) noted that antibody and complement binding to the cell surface induced an immediate swelling of target cells. A change in membrane permeability occurs, with leaking out of inorganic K^+ and loss of organically bound K^+. Green and associates (44), Goldberg (45) and Green (46) investigated the effect of antibody and complement on lysis of Krebs ascites tumor cells and erythrocytes. Antibody alone produced local structural changes in the cell membrane which reflected the in situ formation of antibody-antigen complexes. The addition of complement led to marked swelling of the endoplasmic reticulum and mitochondria. Within a few minutes there was a marked loss of cellular potassium, free amino acids, cellular proteins and ribonucleotides. This suggests that the action of antibody and complement on cellular surfaces initiates two effects. Metabolic death of the cell must occur. In addition, disruption of the cationic gradient across the membrane prevents the cell from preserving its normal osmotic relationship. The membrane damage permits a rapid loss of small intracellular molecules, while the defect is insufficient in size for the passage of large molecules such as hemoglobin. The unopposed osmotic pressure results in a rapid flow of water into the cell with subsequent swelling. Swelling further increases the membrane pore size defects until a hemolytic volume is reached, with leaking of hemoglobin and hemolysis. Such studies suggest that antibody and complement acting on an erythrocyte create functional "holes" or pore defects in the cell membrane. This type of cellular damage may be related to the fine cracks on the erythrocyte surface described by Latta (47).

Sears and associates (48) attempted to quantitate this defect. A heteroimmune erythrocyte antibody was prepared in rabbits by immunizing with group O human erythrocytes. This antiserum was reacted with human erythrocytes. Hemolysis was inhibited by employing a size graded series of dextran polymers and albumin in the suspending medium. This procedure permitted determination of the size of the membrane defect induced by antibody-complement action. The membrane defect appeared to have an effective radius of somewhat less than 32 Å. In addition, diffusion of hemoglobin is dependent on a pore defect radius of approximately 32 Å. Accordingly, hemolysis in this system resulted from swelling and initiation of a colloid osmotic hemolysis sequence. It was observed that complement dependent human anti-A and rabbit anti-human A antisera induced hemolysis of A erythrocytes without a prior stage of swelling. Membrane defects with an effective radius greater than 32 Å were initially produced, permitting the diffusion of hemoglobin. Such large defects can occur through one of two mechanisms. Single defects of this size may be directly induced by an antibody-complement complex. Alternatively, large defects may represent a coalition of multiple small defects which develop in close proximity.

Scott and associates (49) have employed the same antisera with various sources of animal complement. A membrane defect of similar size was produced, although hemolytic activity of the different complements varied. This suggests that the size of the membrane defect primarily reflects characteristics of the cellular antigen. Swisher (21) speculates that the defect produced by complement fixation may be uniform, irrespective of the antibody involved. The morphologic lesion may therefore represent the loss of a membrane structural unit. Alternatively, complement fixation may induce cleavage of major structural membrane bands which form pore defects without a loss of membrane substance.

Rosse and associates (50) and Dourmashkin and Rosse (23) have performed similar quantitative studies of the membrane defects leading to lysis. Their data suggest that the species of the complement rather than the antibody type determines the size of the membrane pore defect. Human complement produced pore defects with a diameter of 103 Å, irrespective of the antibody used. The defects induced by guinea pig complement had an average diameter of 88 Å. The appearance of the membrane defects was not influenced by either the source or the immunoglobulin type of antibody. They noted that the number of "holes" produced varied with the different antibody-antigen systems employed. Some of the numerous holes produced could coalesce and prevent the protective effect of large molecules in the surrounding media. Electron microscopy studies by Humphrey and Dourmashkin (51) suggest that the holes have a diameter of 80 to 100 Å. The defects appear to be circular and fairly uniform in size. Coalescent defects appear in clusters. These workers suggest that the membrane defect occurs in the lipid layer.

The geographic distribution of antigenic material on the erythrocyte surface may play an important part in hemolysis induced by complement fixation and antibody-antigen union. Techniques mapping antigenic site density in relationship to pore size and functional membrane units are highly desirable. Rebuck (52) estimated the antigen site in acquired hemolytic anemia as 30 μ in diameter with the A antigen site 24 times this size.

In vitro immune hemolysis may require the action of only a single antigen site-antibody-complement complex. Mayer (34) has presented evidence of this "one hit" theory of immune lysis. A single membrane pore defect may be sufficient to cause increase cellular permeability and lysis through a colloid osmotic sequence. Humphrey and Dourmashkin (51) suggest that a single IgM molecule may produce the required pore defect. In contrast, several thousand IgG molecules may be required for the same effect.

Weinrach and associates (53) postulated that antibody molecules must occupy two relatively close antigenic sites before complement is fixed. Ishizaka and associates (54) have quantitated the fixation of the C'1a component of complement by various immunoglobulin antibody types. One molecule of an IgM type of anti-A fixed one molecule of C'1a to human A erythrocytes. Two molecules of an IgG type of anti-A were required to fix a single C'1a molecule to human A red cells. Low molecular weight antibodies such as the sheep red cell hemolysins studied by Stelos and Talmage (55) may require a larger number of related antigen sites. These authors suggest that a tetramolecular antibody-four-antigen site complex may be necessary for stability and complement fixation. Swisher (19) hypothesizes that under these circumstances complement fixation and hemolysis assume a statistical character. Since antibody molecules redistribute from cell to cell, and presumably from antigen site to antigen site, there is a rising probability with time that the required geographic distribution of antibody molecules and antigenic sites will be attained. When a large number of antigen sites are occupied by antibody, it becomes certain that the required complex will be formed, resulting in complement fixation and immune hemolysis.

Complement and antibody fixation to erythrocytes can induce hemolysis through two related mechanisms. The initial membrane damage may create a pore size with an effective diameter insufficient to permit direct extravasation of hemoglobin. Water diffuses into such an erythrocyte and swelling occurs through colloid osmotic hemolysis. Hemolysis will develop when a sufficient pore size is reached through swelling. Alternatively, the initial membrane damage may produce large pore openings of sufficient diameter to permit direct seepage of hemoglobin without swelling and spherocytosis. This latter sequence is particularly apparent when erythrocytes from patients with paroxysmal nocturnal hemoglobinuria (PNH) are exposed to acid hemolysins. Yachnin and Ruthenberg (56, 57) demonstrated that hemolysis at an acid pH can be induced by C'3 alone. This extreme sensitivity may result from a nonimmunologic structural abnormality. The increased affinity of the erythrocyte membrane for C'3 possibly creates more numerous pores than is seen with normal erythrocytes. Such an effect would result in an all-or-none action of complement, with hemolysis occurring without spherocytosis. Dourmashkin and Rosse (23) state that the type of membrane pore defects produced by complement acting on PNH erythrocytes is similar to that seen with normal erythrocytes. Rosse and Dacie (58) found that the binding of antibody to PNH erythrocytes was only slightly increased over the binding with normal erythrocytes. The increased lytic sensitivity of PNH cells reflected a greater efficiency of binding of complement complexes to the red cell membrane and their increased tendency to induce hemolysis.

The ability of proteolytic enzymes to potentiate the action of erythrocyte iso- and autoantibodies may also be related to the creation of membrane defects. The enzyme treatment of erythrocytes renders them directly agglutinable by incomplete warm acting erythrocyte antibodies. In addition, enzyme treated erythrocytes will usually lyse when exposed to cold acting autoantibodies in the presence of complement. Cawley and Goodwin (59) demonstrated by electron microscopy that bromelin produces relatively large confluent holes in the erythrocyte membrane. Ferritin tagged bromelin was visualized around and between the holes.

Metabolic Abnormalities

The integrity of the erythrocyte membrane is dependent on maintenance of the cationic gradient pump mechanism and the anerobic glycolytic cycle producing ATP. Various chemicals can interfere with these mechanisms. Jacob and Jandl (14) demonstrated that sulfhydryl inhibitors may induce hemolysis in this fashion. Blockage of membrane sulfhydryl groups increases by several fold the leak rate of cations. An accelerated glycolysis develops on a compensatory basis, presumably to increase the active transport mechanism. When the cation diffusion rate exceeds the transport mechanism, the sequence of colloidal osmotic hemolysis occurs. Damage produced by sulfhydryl inhibitors apparently creates pore sizes with radii of less than 4.4 Å. The radii of the pore defects are increased with swelling until a hole is formed large enough to permit extravasation of hemoglobin molecules (i.e., presumably over 32 Å).

Several varieties of nonimmune hemolytic anemia and positive antiglobulin tests may develop hemolysis through similar mechanisms. These include the effect of metallic cations, lead intoxication, trypan blue, phenylhydrazine and lipid solvents. Different initiating surface phenomena are probably involved, such as a loss of membrane substance with lipid solvents. However, their effect on cationic gradients and glycolysis with production of large pore defects through colloid osmotic hemolysis may be a common denominator. Modified globulin molecules produced in monoclonal or polyclonal dysgammaglobulinemia may exert a similar abnormal erythro-

cyte effect, thereby simulating antibody action.

Hemolytic anemia resulting from various hereditary defects of the erythrocyte involves similar abnormalities. The shortened survival of erythrocytes in hereditary spherocytosis and nonspherocytic forms of hemolytic anemia reflects membrane instability resulting from deficiencies of the gradient pump mechanism and glycolysis.

Antibody Induced Metabolic Defects

Similar mechanisms may be postulated as responsible for the detrimental action of antibodies on erythrocytes. Such a sequence would be particularly useful to explain the activity of noncomplement dependent antibodies. Erythrocyte antibodies are large molecules unable to penetrate the cell membrane. If complement does not induce cellular damage, the antibody itself may influence the erythrocyte through comparatively subtle metabolic injuries of the cell membrane. Only incomplete and contradictory evidence to support this hypothesis is available.

Storti and associates (60) and Abrahamov and Diamond (61) reported a decreased utilization of glucose by erythrocytes coated with anti-Rh_o (D). Storti and associates (60) found that a 25 to 30 per cent reduction of in vivo glycolysis may occur independently of agglutination. Young (62), Altman and associates (63) and Nicolau and Teitel (64) all suggested that disturbances of carbohydrate metabolism result from antibody action on erythrocytes. Pipitone and associates (65) employed heteroimmune anti-erythrocyte antiserum in experimental animals and documented a reduction of ATPase activity and glycolysis in rabbit erythrocytes. Kaplan and associates (66) found a reduction of erythrocyte acetylcholinesterase activity in ABO hemolytic disease of newborns. The defect was not present in erythroblastosis caused by rhesus antibodies and it could not be produced in vitro with anti-A and anti-B. Brabec and associates (67) studied the metabolic changes occurring in erythrocytes during hemolysis and reticulocytosis. An increase of glucose 6-phosphate dehydrogenase, acid phosphatase and respiration in the presence of methylene blue was documented. Erythrocytes with positive antiglobulin tests exhibited a reduction of acetylcholinesterase, irrespective of the degree of hemolysis.

Greenwalt and associates (68, 69) studied the phosphate metabolism of erythrocytes obtained from normal adults and newborns and from newborn infants with erythroblastosis due to anti-Rh$_o$ (D). Their data are difficult to reconcile with the suggestion that antibodies induce impaired glycolysis in erythrocytes. They noted that erythrocytes from erythroblastotic infants had an increased amount of 2,3-diphosphoglycerate (nonhydrolyzable phosphate) when compared with erythrocytes from normal newborns; the levels approximated values seen in the normal adult. The uptake and turnover rates of phosphorous by erythrocytes of erythroblastotic and normal newborns were similar. When this relationship was studied on a time basis, erythroblastotic erythrocyte phosphate turnover was approximately 2-fold that of normal erythrocytes in the first 20 minutes of incubation. The direction of flow was primarily from cell to plasma. Langley (70) analyzed erythrocytes obtained from two cases of autoimmune hemolytic anemia. He noted that glycolytic intermediates and ATP levels were normal. However, total lipids, cholesterol and phospholipids were elevated. In vitro incubation at 37°C. indicated a marked loss of cell lipids. During this period there was reduction of 2,3-diphosphoglycerate followed by a reduction of ATP. Langley (70) suggests that the labile lipids of erythrocytes are susceptible to alteration by noncomplement dependent antibodies.

Tishkoff (71) investigated erythrocyte mucoids in autoimmune hemolytic anemia. Erythrocytes obtained from seven cases of autoimmune hemolytic anemia and from 13 cases of nonantibody induced anemia with similar reticulocyte levels were studied. Stromata from these erythrocytes were analyzed. The stroma protein content was elevated in all cases and paralleled the reticulocyte elevation. Levels of fucose and sialic acid were normal. The antiglobulin positive stroma had a statistically signifi-

cant decrease in the ratios of sialic acid to protein and fucose to protein. Tishkoff (71) suggests that noncomplement dependent autoantibodies induce alterations of the carbohydrate moiety of the erythrocyte membrane. He postulates that antibody-antigen union may activate proteases in the cell membrane.

Vulpis (72) analyzed the water soluble protein fractions obtained from ghost forms of normal human erythrocytes and from erythrocytes obtained from patients with hereditary spherocytosis and autoimmune hemolytic anemia. Antisera were produced against the various proteins (S proteins) obtained. No immunochemical differences were found between normal erythrocytes and those obtained in hereditary spherocytosis. However, specific precipitins were found for the S protein fractions obtained from erythrocytes involved in autoimmune hemolytic anemia.

Modification of the cationic active transport mechanism by noncomplement dependent antibodies has also been suggested. Goldstein and Desforges (73) reported a K$^+$ leak occurring from erythrocytes coated with incomplete antibodies. Langley and Felderhof (74) investigated this system with incomplete anti-Rh$_o$ (D) and human erythrocyte ghost membranes free of hemoglobin. They were unable to show any effect of the antibody on the sodium-potassium dependent ATPase activity. A K$^+$ leak could not be demonstrated with intact erythrocytes.

Jandl (20) investigated possible subtle changes in glycolysis or cationic pumping resulting from the action of noncomplement binding antibodies. He employed six anti-A sera, seven anti-Rh$_o$ (D) sera and two sera containing erythrocyte autoantibodies. There was no demonstrable effect on total glucose consumption, lactic acid formation or glucose-1-C^{14} to C^{14}O$_2$ by hexose monophosphate shunt activity. All sera tested contained high titer antibodies and were analyzed after equilibration of pH and content of glucose ions. In addition, no changes were noted in cell size, osmotic fragility, glutathione content, cation levels or cation flux. Letarte and associates (75) studied adenosine triphosphatase activity in 70 normal individuals and in 22 patients with hemolytic disease. Five had acquired hemolytic anemia and five had hemolysis induced by anti-Rh_o (D) and anti-A. No quantitative or qualitative differences in adenosine triphosphatase activity were found in any of these patient groups.

The Sequestration of Erythrocytes

Erythrocyte antibodies may induce hemolysis by complement fixation or by creating subtle metabolic abnormalities of the erythrocyte membrane. However, many clinically important erythrocyte antibodies apparently do not exert their detrimental action through such mechanisms. In particular, warm acting incomplete erythrocyte autoantibodies and non-complement dependent drug - antibody erythrocyte surface reactions generally cannot be explained by such pathologic pathways. The major hemolytic mechanism activated by such antibodies is the sequestration of antibody coated erythrocytes. The trapping or removal from the circulation of such erythrocytes involves the pooling of cells into areas where they cannot be freely and constantly perfused. The involved sites are portions of the reticuloendothelial system with the liver and spleen appearing prominent. These areas are characterized by sinusoidal patterns of circulation.

On the basis of anatomic location, two major sites of in vivo hemolysis may be documented. The sequences leading to these different areas of erythrocyte destruction have been termed intravascular and extravascular hemolysis. This terminology is unfortunate as both mechanisms involve destruction of erythrocytes within the vascular bed. More accurate and descriptive terms can be suggested with "circulatory hemolysis" substituted for intravascular and "sequestration hemolysis" employed in place of extravascular. Different laboratory and clinical findings characterize the two states and differentiation is frequently important. The destruction of erythrocytes through such mechanisms has been extensively reviewed by Mollison (76). This

excellent survey should be consulted by all students of hemolysis.

Circulatory Hemolysis

The lytic effect of complement dependent erythrocyte antibodies is frequently manifested through a circulatory form of hemolysis. This event is characterized by the rapid destruction of circulating erythrocytes with direct extravasation of hemoglobin into the plasma. The pyrogenic reactions which frequently accompany this type of erythrocyte destruction do not appear to be exclusively dependent on antibody-antigen union. Fever is present only when cell destruction occurs and may be related to the release of nonparticulate antibody-antigen complexes (77). Globulin aggregation and deformed antibody molecules may be important. The violent transfusion reactions seen with ABO incompatibilities are typical of this category. Severe hemolytic episodes with hemoglobinuria may result from this type of in vivo hemolysis. This is commonly seen as a result of the action of potent cold acting autoantibodies.

Sequestration Hemolysis

The removal of erythrocytes from the circulation and their sequestration in the reticuloendothelium leads to a form of hemolysis which differs from that described above. This has been termed sequestration hemolysis and it is characterized by a rate of lysis considerably slower than that seen in the circulatory variety. The explosive character of hemolysis, which frequently dominates clinical manifestations of the circulatory type, is absent. Hemoglobinuria is not classically found. Chills, abdominal and flank pain and shocklike episodes with immediate anaphylactoid reactions generally do not occur. Jandl and Tomlinson (77) suggest that leukopenia and pyrogenic reactions may result from sequestration hemolysis taking place in the spleen. Free hemoglobin in the plasma is neither marked nor characteristic of this type of reaction. Either direct catabolism of hemoglobin occurs prior to its release into the plasma, or else the rate of hemoglobin release is sufficiently low to ensure its catabolism or effective renal clearance (19). The binding of hemoglobin to haptoglobin can usually be demonstrated in such cases.

Although differentiation between circulatory and sequestration hemolysis can frequently be made, distinguishing characteristics may not be readily apparent (19, 76). A valid differentiation is sometimes not possible or even indicated. The destruction of sequestered erythrocytes can occasionally occur rapidly with the production of free plasma hemoglobin. Hemolysis resulting from a sequestration mechanism is generally slower than that seen in the circulation variety. However, it should not be assumed that fewer erythrocytes are destroyed in the process. Although the time period may be prolonged, the total number of erythrocytes destroyed through the sequestration route may be greater than through circulatory hemolysis. Many complement dependent erythrocyte antibodies induce hemolysis through circulatory hemolysis. In contrast, sequestration hemolysis generally results from the action of noncomplement dependent erythrocyte antibodies. There is no reason to assume that the type of antibody or complement itself directly initiates the specific variety of erythrocytic destruction. The type of hemolysis appears to be dependent on the degree of erythrocyte damage sustained through antibody action, with or without complement (19–21, 76). Noncomplement dependent erythrocyte antibodies which cause extreme erythrocyte damage can initiate rapid circulatory hemolysis with hemoglobinuria.

The sequestration of erythrocytes sensitized by antibodies occurs through two pathophysiologic mechanisms. These include the filtration of agglutinated erythrocytes and the direct participation of reticuloendothelial sinusoidal cells.

Erythrocyte Filtration, Hepatic Type

Red cell filtration is visualized as a purely physical phenomenon. It involves the removal of agglutinated masses of erythrocytes from the general circulation by sequestration in the reticuloendothelial sinusoidal circulation (76, 78). Two different pathophysiologic pathways may be distinguished on the basis of anatomic and clinical characteristics. Complete antibodies and high titer complement dependent incomplete erythrocyte antibodies initiate rapid clearance of involved red cells (19, 20, 76, 78). The liver functions as the major area for sequestration of such sensitized cells. The rapid clearance of these erythrocytes from the circulation correlates with the liver receiving 20 to 25 per cent of the cardiac output (76). The clearance rate of such sensitized cells, even when complement fixation occurs, may be so rapid that hepatic sequestration can occur before circulatory hemolysis results (20). During this process circulating granulocytes are decreased. Fever is minimal if the hemolytic episode is transient. According to Jandl (20) fever and chills may be marked with a prolonged hemolytic process.

Jandl and associates (78) employed a Millipore test system and demonstrated that erythrocytes agglutinated by anti-A were completely retained in a filter having uniform, nonbranching capillary pores 5 μ in diameter at diffusing pressures of 4 mm. of mercury. Lewis and associates (79) demonstrated that agglutination itself did not permanently damage erythrocytes. After dispersion of such cells hepatic sequestration did not occur unless complement had been fixed irreversibly to the erythrocyte surface. As a general rule the rate of sequestration parallels the degree of antibody titer and avidity. With heavy erythrocyte damage, hepatic sequestration is marked. Lesser degrees of sensitization lead to splenic sequestration and to more prolonged survival times (80–83). It is apparent that a single erythrocyte antibody may destroy incompatible erythrocytes through many mechanisms. The quantitative relationships between antibody and antigen assume importance (19). It is possible to infuse relatively large amounts of agglutinating antibody and incomplete noncomplement dependent antibody without inducing erythrocyte destruction (80, 83–86). Mollison and Hughes-Jones (87) quantitated the in vivo onset and rate of destruction of Rh_o (D) erythrocytes exposed to anti-Rh_o (D). The rate of destruction was proportional to the square root of the amount of antibody fixed to the erythrocyte.

Erythrocyte Filtration, Splenic Type

Erythrocytes sensitized by the usual type of noncomplement dependent, warm acting, incomplete antibody are generally sequestered in the spleen. In addition, erythrocytes sensitized with low titer complete agglutinins and weak complement dependent incomplete erythrocyte antibodies may also manifest splenic sequestration (19, 20, 76, 78). The rate of clearance of such sensitized erythrocytes is partially dependent on the magnitude of the splenic circulation. This is substantially less than the hepatic circulation. Mollison and Cutbush (82) calculated that the half-time splenic clearance rate of sensitized erythrocytes would approximate 25 minutes if 3 per cent of the cardiac output passed through the spleen. Jandl and Kaplan (80) found that the unsaturated spleen could remove erythrocytes coated with incomplete antibodies at a rate of 3 ± 1 per cent per minute. This observation correlates with the slower hemolytic process generally observed in splenic sequestration. The number of erythrocytes destroyed in this process may equal that seen with complete acting antibodies, although a longer time is required.

Experimental studies strongly supported these concepts. Mollison (83) and Cutbush and Mollison (88) found that the half-time removal of sensitized erythrocytes by hepatic sequestration approximated 2 to 6 minutes. Potent complete or complement dependent incomplete erythrocyte antibodies were the sensitizing agents. Weakly agglutinating noncomplement dependent erythrocyte antibodies were also employed to sensitize red cells. Splenic sequestration resulted, with the sensitized erythrocytes having half-time clearances of 20 minutes or more. Incomplete erythrocyte antibodies also led to splenic sequestration of the sensitized erythrocytes. Half-time clearance rates of 15 to 22 minutes were obtained.

The liver and spleen do not function independently of each other in sequestration. Hepatic sequestration may occur with incomplete noncomplement dependent erythrocyte antibodies. Massive antibody sensitization and saturation of the splenic system are generally present. This fact is probably responsible for clinical observations made in warm acting autoimmune hemolytic anemia. Splenectomy in such cases may be followed by rapid enlargement of the liver and by hepatic sequestration. The reverse situation also occurs. Minimal sensitization of erythrocytes by complete or complement fixing incomplete antibodies may primarily result in splenic sequestration. An identical pattern is seen with nonimmune erythrocyte damage. Mild injury to erythrocytes usually leads to splenic sequestration; heavier damage activates an hepatic sequestration mechanism (20). Protamine sulfate and Polybrene may fix to erythrocytes in a nonagglutinating reaction and lead to erythrocyte destruction through hepatic sequestration (89).

The sequestration of agglutinated antibody sensitized erythrocytes is simple to visualize on the basis of physical filtration (78). It is more difficult to explain the sequestration of erythrocytes coated with incomplete noncomplement dependent antibodies. Jandl and Castle (90) suggested that the ability of erythrocytes coated with incomplete erythrocyte antibodies to survive correlates best with the degree of agglutination which may be induced by plasma or various colloidal anisometric molecules. In the dog, splenic protein concentrations may be increased $1\frac{1}{2}$ times over those seen in normal plasma (91). Hemoconcentration may magnify this tendency. The fibrinogen concentration in the reticuloendothelium may play a crucial role in these processes. Wagley and associates (92) and Wright and associates (93) suggested that splenic antibody production may increase the coating of splenic sequestered erythrocytes. It is therefore possible that nonagglutinating incomplete erythrocyte antibodies may induce in vivo agglutination. This in turn may lead to mechanical filtration and to sequestration. Jandl and associates (81) noted that splenic blood samples may contain agglutinated erythrocytes when obtained from patients with positive direct antiglobulin tests. In addition, agglutinated cells may occasionally be found in the circulation of subjects transfused with unagglutinated antibody coated erythrocytes (20).

The Action of Reticuloendothelial Cells

It is still not proved that unagglutinated erythrocytes coated with incomplete erythrocyte antibodies undergo in vivo agglutination. Accordingly, true mechanical filtration may not be involved with such sensitized erythrocytes. An alternative mechanism to explain sequestration is therefore required. The function of reticuloendothelial cells may assume importance in this regard. It may be postulated that antibody induced erythrocyte surface changes predispose such erythrocytes to stick to the reticuloendothelium (94, 95). This mechanism implies the active participation of reticuloendothelial sinusoidal cells in the sequestration process. The hypothesis is supported by the observation that erythrocytes altered by nonimmunologic means such as sulfhydryl inhibition (14), heat (96) and protamine or Polybrene (89) are readily sequestered by the reticuloendothelium in the absence of agglutination.

The action of protamine and Polybrene on erythrocytes offers a potential explanation for this phenomenon (89). Such substances are highly basically charged molecules which bind to the polyanionic erythrocyte. The net result of this interaction is a reduction of the zeta potential of the erythrocyte surface. If a sufficient number of molecules is adsorbed by the erythrocyte, agglutination occurs. A lesser number of molecules reduces the surface charge of the erythrocyte without producing agglutination. Such erythrocytes have a shortened survival and exhibit sequestration in the reticuloendothelium. Hepatic

sequestration is prominent. This reaction may be considered to be a prototype of erythrocyte antibody function. The adsorption of some incomplete erythrocyte antibodies onto the erythrocyte surface may result in a reduction of the zeta potential of the cell (97). This may correlate with the release of N-acetyl neuraminic acid from the erythrocyte membrane, reflecting antibody binding to the erythrocyte (98). The change in erythrocyte surface charge may ultimately lead to sequestration.

The Destruction of Erythrocytes by Sequestration

It is still not known how sequestration of antibody sensitized erythrocytes leads to their destruction. Early hypotheses considered the activation of tissue lysins as the major hemolytic mechanism. Ponder (99), however, pointed out that many tissue lysins are artificially produced and in a sense are only laboratory creations. It has been suggested that tissue enzymes may increase the sensitivity of erythrocytes to the action of autoantibodies. Leroy and Spurrier (100) emphasized the role of beta-glucuronidase in this regard. Magalini and associates (101) suggested the role of long chain fatty acids. Torp (102) stated that acetylcholine can induce a fall in pH and that this may result in hemolysis.

More current concepts suggest that an abnormal perfusion of sequestered erythrocytes limits the availability of critical metabolic substrates. This results in a metabolic deficiency which subsequently leads to membrane damage. This sequence would eventually inactivate the cationic gradient control mechanism and induce metabolic death. Ham and Castle (103) emphasized the role of erythrostasis in inducing metabolic abnormalities. The loss of membrane substance during sequestration has been postulated in hereditary spherocytosis (104). This defect could permit the hemolytic volume to be reached even at plasma levels of osmotic pressure.

Nicolau and associates (105) demonstrated that the fixation of incomplete antibodies to the erythrocyte surface impaired the ability of erythrocytes to pass through filter paper. The loss of filterability of erythrocytes was considered to result from an alteration of erythrocyte plasticity. Seventeen patients with acquired hemolytic anemia were studied. In 16 an altered plasticity of the erythrocyte was found. This modification of the biophysical property of red cells was suggested as playing a role in sequestration and destruction of sensitized erythrocytes. The exact mechanism by which antibodies induce changes in membrane plasticity is unknown. However, such changes may indicate a significant modification of the erythrocyte membrane which affects their sensitivity to sequestrational hemolysis.

Studies by Jandl (20) indicate that three levels of cellular sensitivity are involved in reticuloendothelial sequestration. The spleen appears as the most sensitive filter mechanism. When the erythrocyte damage is marked, or when the splenic system approaches saturation, hepatic sequestration occurs. The bone marrow may offer a third system for sequestration. Keene and Jandl (106) and Jandl and Kaplan (80) demonstrated that bone marrow sequestration does not normally occur in the rat. When such animals are made hypoplastic, or when the reticuloendothelial system is blocked by carbon or cortisone, the ability of the bone marrow to sequestrate erythrocytes markedly increases. In the rat the number of phagocytic cells in the liver, spleen and bone marrow are of the same magnitude. Accordingly, the marked differences in sequestration ability of these three organ systems depend on blood flow, placement and cellular avidity rather than on the number of functioning cells.

One additional element of the sequestration phenomenon deserves emphasis. Splenic hyperplasia and hepatic hyperplasia may occur in the presence of chronic hemolytic anemia. The hyperplasia appears to be partially related to the immunologic reaction and it reflects splenic hematopoiesis. Increased hematopoiesis is not seen with nonimmune but otherwise damaged erythrocytes involved in sequestration (20). The trapping of injured erythrocytes stimulates proliferation in the outer part of the lymphatic follicle. This occurs even in the absence of immunologically mediated erythrocyte damage. The new cells migrate into the red pulp and may present as clusters of round cells in the sinusoids. A similar but much more restrictive cytoproliferative response can involve the Kupffer cells of the liver (20). The net result of such proliferation is an increased capacity of the reticuloendothelium to sequestrate damaged cells. Accordingly, hemolysis increases the efficiency for further hemolysis. The sequestration ability is concomitantly expanded to trap leukocytes and thrombocytes. This may result in peripheral blood pancytopenia. The hyperplasia also involves an increased production of lymphocytes and plasma cells. Hypergammaglobulinemia may eventually develop. This suggests that hemolysis can potentiate the ability of the spleen to engage in antibody production. Jandl (20) speculates that the enhanced immunologic reactivity of the hyperplastic spleen may take two pathways. It could initiate immunologic responses directed against related or coincidental antigens of the erythrocyte. In addition, it may convert reactions which are initially nonimmune into immune forms. This latter mechanism could possibly permit metabolically modified antigenic determinants to be recognized as "foreign." In this way it would supply the background for the autoimmune state described as an enhanced sensitivity of antibody forming tissues. Splenic hyperplasia creating these two antibody producing states could result in an immune relationship which is autocatalytic and which would appear as autoimmune hemolytic anemia.

Erythrophagocytosis

Erythrophagocytosis supplies an additional mechanism to remove damaged erythrocytes. The exact role and importance of erythrophagocytosis in immune interactions are still to be determined. Wright and Douglas (107) in 1903 demonstrated that phagocytosis was dependent upon a serum component they termed "opsonin." Dean (108) in 1907 showed that opsonins included heat labile and heat stable factors and suggested that phagocytosis involved antibody-complement systems. Blood leukocytes and fixed macrophages of the reticuloendothelium initiate erythrophagocytosis in vivo. In vitro, neutrophiles, eosinophiles and monocytes all phagocytose erythrocytes under the influence of opsonizing antibodies (19).

Levaditi (109) in 1902 pointed out that fixed tissue macrophage erythrophagocytosis is a prominent part of experimentally induced hemolytic anemia. Mohn and associates (110) noted striking in vivo erythrophagocytosis by blood leukocytes in experimental human isoimmune hemolytic anemia. This phenomenon is also observed in human autoimmune hemolytic anemia. Erythrophagocytosis may be produced simply by incubating erythrocytes with fresh human serum incompatible in the ABO system. It is seen with regularity during Ehrlich tests performed on patients with paroxysmal cold hemoglobinuria. Normal reticuloendothelial tissues will generally demonstrate erythrophagocytosis. Accordingly, this process undoubtedly supplies a normal mechanism for the removal of damaged or dying erythrocytes. Erythrophagocytosis is increased in the reticuloendothelial tissues of patients with autoimmune hemolytic anemia. Erythrophagocytosis may therefore play an important role in the hemolysis noted with antibody induced erythrocyte disease.

Erythrophagocytosis occurs in normal individuals and in patients with a variety of hematologic diseases. Weed and Reed (16) divide this phenomenon into four categories: (a) attraction between damaged erythrocytes and phagocytic cells, (b) adhesion between cells, (c) ingestion and (d) digestion. Fixed macrophages as found in the splenic cords of Billroth are in intimate contact with erythrocytes and do not require attraction. Circulating phagocytic cells, however, require the migration of such cells to the damaged erythrocyte. The attraction mechanism is still obscure. Bessis (111) documented the release of material from damaged cells, which stimulates the migration of leukocytes. This process was termed "necrotaxis" and it was interpreted as evidence that an active damaging process must be occurring. Previously lysed ghost cells did not stimulate migration. Adhesive forces probably do not operate at distances in excess of 5 Å (112). Changes in erythrocyte surface charge and membrane plasticity resulting from erythrocyte antibody activity may modify adhesiveness (113, 114). Jensen and Moreno (115) have questioned the role of a reduction of erythrocyte surface charge in phagocytosis. Bangham (114) suggests that the opposition of small pseudopods may permit Ca^{++} anion bridging or the operation of van der Waals forces.

Jandl and associates (116) noted that morphologic evidence of erythrophagocytosis may be delayed for several hours after splenic sequestration. The erythrocyte can be phagocytosed intact or in fragments. Cohn and Weiner (117, 118) demonstrated the synthesis and intracellular redistribution of acid phosphatase, cathepsin, ribonuclease, lysozyme and lipase following bacterial phagocytosis. Extraction of hemoglobin from the erythrocyte is the first evidence of digestion and is followed by dissolution of the membrane. Acid phosphatase is important in this action (119) and this enzyme is present in splenic cells in the Billroth cords but not in the sinusoids (120). Within 6 hours of the onset of hemolysis, iron is released from the digested hemoglobin, bound to transferrin, transported and made available to the bone marrow for the synthesis of new hemoglobin (81).

The relationship of complement to erythrophagocytosis is still unclear. Although specific components have not been identified, complement has been implicated in the phagocytosis of various particulate antigens. Ludány and associates (121) noted that phlorizin, an inhibitor of C'3, suppressed phagocytosis. Gelzer and Suter (122) on the other hand question the necessity for complement in phagocytosis. The relationship of complement to erythrophagocytosis in the immunohemolytic anemias is similarly obscure. Marked in vivo erythrophagocytosis was noted by Mohn and associates (110) using noncomplement dependent anti-rh'(C) and anti-Rh_o (D).

Dacie (123) also noted erythrophagocytosis resulting from the action of nonlytic warm acting anti-rhesus antibodies that were potent agglutinins; they presumably did not fix complement. Marked erythrophagocytosis may be found in the lymphomas, particularly in Hodgkin's disease. The degree correlates somewhat with hemolytic anemia, even though erythrocyte autoantibodies cannot be demonstrated. Swisher (21) suggests that erythrophagocytosis assumes importance in immunohemolytic anemia when the antibody alone cannot destroy erythrocytes. As such, this mechanism would be important in the majority of cases of warm acting autoimmune hemolytic anemia and in anti-rhesus types of isoimmune hemolytic anemia. Dacie (123) visualizes erythrophagocytosis as functioning in the removal of erythrocytes coated with complement but not lysed. It may have little effect on erythrocytes binding only incomplete erythrocyte autoantibodies.

Clarification of the role of opsonization and erythrophagocytosis in immunohemolytic anemia depends on the development of accurate quantitative techniques. Such procedures are not as yet available. In vitro test systems are markedly influenced by a variety of physical and chemical factors. Corticosteroids have been found to influence quantitation. Their administration to leukocyte donors or the direct addition of such materials to in vitro systems inhibits erythrophagocytosis (124). Bonnin and Schwartz (125) studied erythrocyte autoantibodies and anti-A antibodies in an in vitro test. Erythrophagocytosis in their system generally correlated with erythrophagocytosis observed in buffy coat peripheral blood preparations. The development of erythrophagocytosis was primarily dependent on the action of complete or complement fixing antibodies. Greendyke and associates (126) documented several parameters of in vitro erythrophagocytosis of antibody coated erythrocytes. Antibody opsonization of erythrocytes in the presence of complement and Mg^{++} appeared to be necessary for phagocytosis.

BIBLIOGRAPHY

1. Jandl, J. H.: Leaky red cells. Blood 26: 367, 1965.
2. Ponder, E.: *Hemolysis and Related Phenomena*. Grune & Stratton, Inc., New York, 1948.
3. Prankerd, T. A. J.: *The Red Cell*. Blackwell Publications, Ltd., Oxford, 1961.
4. Eggleton, G. P., and Eggleton, P.: A method of estimating phosphagen and some other phosphorus compounds in muscle tissue. Brit. J. Physiol. 68: 193, 1929.
5. Bernstein, R. E.: Alterations in metabolic energetics and cation transport during aging of red cells. J. Clin. Invest. 38: 1572, 1959.
6. Brewer, G. J., and Powell, R. D.: Hexokinase activity as a function of age of the human erythrocyte. Nature (London) 199: 704, 1963.
7. Paganelli, C. V., and Solomon, A. K.: The rate of exchange of tritiated water across the red cell membrane. J. Gen. Physiol. 41: 259, 1957.
8. Williams, T. F., Fordham, C. C., Hollander, W., and Welt, L. G.: A study of the osmotic behavior of the human erythrocyte. J. Clin. Invest. 38: 1587, 1959.
9. Sheppard, C. W., and Martin, W. R.: Cation exchange between cells and plasma of mammalian blood. I. Methods and application to potassium exchange in human blood. J. Gen. Physiol. 33: 703, 1950.
10. Whittam, R.: *Transport and Diffusion in Red Blood Cells*. Edward Arnold Publishers, Ltd., London, 1964.
11. Dick, D. A. T.: The effect of the anomalous osmotic coefficient of haemoglobin on the osmotic behavior of erythrocytes. Exp. Cell Res. 14: 608, 1958.
12. Czaczkes, J. W., Ullmann, T. D., Ullman, L., and Bar-Kochba, Z.: Determination of the red blood cell content of water, sodium, and potassium in normal subjects. J. Lab. Clin. Med. 61: 873, 1963.
13. Valberg, L. S., Holt, J. M., Paulson, E., and Szivek, J.: Spectrochemical analysis of sodium, potassium, calcium, magnesium, copper, and zinc in normal human erythrocytes. J. Clin. Invest. 44: 379, 1965.
14. Jacob, H. S., and Jandl, J. H.: Effects of sulfhydryl inhibition on red blood cells. I. Mechanism of hemolysis. J. Clin. Invest. 41: 779, 1962.
15. Prins, H. K., Oort, M., Loos, J. A., Zürcher, C., and Beckors, T.: Congenital nonspherocytic hemolytic anemia, associated with glutathione deficiency of the erythrocytes. Hematologic, biochemical and genetic studies. Blood 27: 145, 1966.
16. Weed, R. I., and Reed, C. F.: Membrane alterations leading to red cell destruction. Amer. J. Med. 41: 681, 1966.
17. Charnock, J. S., and Post, R. L.: Evidence of

the mechanism of ouabain inhibition of cation activated adenosine triphosphate. Nature (London) **199**: 910, 1963.

18. Wilbrandt, W.: Osmotische Natur sogenannter nicht-osmotischer Hämolysen. (Kolloidosmotische Hämolyse). Pflueger. Arch. Ges. Physiol. **245**: 22, 1941.

19. Swisher, S. N.: Immune hemolysis. Ann. Rev. Med. **15**: 1, 1964.

20. Jandl, J. H.: Mechanisms of antibody-induced red cell destruction. Series Haemat. **9**: 35, 1965.

21. Swisher, S. N.: Cell survival in the presence of antibody. Ann. N. Y. Acad. Sci. **127**: 901, 1965.

22. Rifkind, R. A.: Destruction of injured red cells in vivo. Amer. J. Med. **41**: 711, 1966.

23. Dourmashkin, R. R., and Rosse, W. F.: Morphological changes in the membranes of red blood cells undergoing haemolysis. Amer. J. Med. **41**: 699, 1966.

24. Borsos, T., and Mayer, M. M.: Mechanism of action of guinea pig complement. In *Mechanism of Cell and Tissue Damage Produced by Immune Reactions* (Second International Symposium on Immunopathology), edited by P. Grabar and P. Miescher. Schwabe and Company, Basel, 1962.

25. Plescia, O. J., and Heidelberger, M.: Complement. In *Functions of the Blood*, edited by R. G. MacFarlane and A. H. T. Robb-Smith. Academic Press, New York, 1961.

26. Osler, A. G.: Functions of the complement system. Advances Immun. **1**: 132, 1961.

27. Lachmann, P. J.: Complement. In *Clinical Aspects of Immunology*, edited by P. G. H. Gell and R. R. A. Coombs. F. A. Davis Company, Philadelphia, 1962.

28. Müller-Eberhard, H. J.: Chemical aspects of human complement components. In *Mechanism of Cell and Tissue Damage Produced by Immune Reactions* (Second International Symposium on Immunopathology), edited by P. Grabar and P. Miescher. Schwabe and Company, Basel, 1962.

29. Wirtz, G. H., and Becker, E. L.: Studies of the reaction between the sensitized erythrocyte and the first component of complement. Immunology **4**: 473, 1961.

30. Stroud, R., and Austen, K.: Report of workshop on complement and hemolysis. Science **141**: 738, 1963.

31. Nelson, R. A.: Complement and body defense. Transfusion **3**: 250, 1963.

32. Müller-Eberhard, H. J., and Nilsson, U.: Relation of a B1-glycoprotein of human serum to the complement system. J. Exp. Med. **111**: 217, 1960.

33. Müller-Eberhard, H. J., and Biro, C. E.: Isolation and description of the fourth component of human complement. J. Exp. Med. **118**: 447, 1963.

34. Mayer, M. M.: Studies on the mechanism of hemolysis by antibody and complement. Progr. Allerg. **5**: 215, 1958.

35. Mills, S. E., and Levine, L.: The inhibition of immune haemolysis by salicylaldoxime. Immunology **2**: 368, 1959.

36. Rodriguez, E., and Osler, A. G.: Studies on the inhibition of immune hemolysis by phlorizin. J. Immun. **85**: 347, 1960.

37. Lepow, I. H., and Ross, A.: Studies of immune cellular injury. II. Functional role of C'1 esterase in immune cytotoxicity. J. Exp. Med. **112**: 1107, 1960.

38. Ross, A., and Lepow, I. H.: Studies on immune cellular injury. I. Cytotoxic effects of antibody and complement. J. Exp. Med. **112**: 1085, 1960.

39. Harboe, M.: Interactions between 131-I trace-labeled cold agglutinin, complement and red cells. Brit. J. Haemat. **10**: 339, 1964.

40. Müller-Eberhard, H. J., and Lepow, I. H.: C'1 esterase effect on activity and physicochemical properties of the fourth component of complement. J. Exp. Med. **121**: 819, 1965.

41. Taranta, A., and Franklin, E. C.: Complement fixation by antibody fragments. Science **134**: 1981, 1961.

42. Leddy, J. P., Bakemeier, R. F., and Vaughan, J. H.: Fixation of complement components to autoantibody eluted from human R.B.C. J. Clin. Invest. **44**: 1066, 1965.

43. Ellem, K. A. O.: Some aspects of the ascites tumor cell response to a heterologous antiserum. Cancer Res. **18**: 1179, 1958.

44. Green, H., Barrow, P., and Goldberg, B.: Effect of antibody and complement on permeability control in ascites tumor cells and erythrocytes. J. Exp. Med. **110**: 699, 1959.

45. Goldberg, B.: Mechanisms of immune injury in mammalian cell systems. In *Immunopathology, Third International Symposium*, edited by P. Grabar and P. Miescher. Schwabe and Company, Basel, 1963.

46. Green, H.: Molecular events in the immune lysis of mammalian cells. In *Injury, Inflammation and Immunity*. The Williams & Wilkins Company, Baltimore, 1964.

47. Latta, H.: Surface of mammalian erythrocyte; electron microscope study of effect of lipid solvents, fixatives, hypotonicity, and hemolysin (amboceptor) and complement. Blood **7**: 508, 1952.

48. Sears, D. A., Weed, R. I., and Swisher, S. N.: Differences in the mechanism of in vitro immune hemolysis related to antibody specificity. J. Clin. Invest. **43**: 97, 1964.

49. Scott, J. G., Weed, R. I., and Swisher, S. N.: Further studies on the mechanism of in vitro hemolysis: specificity of complement. J. Immun. **96**: 119, 1966.

50. Rosse, W. F., Dourmashkin, R., and Humphrey, J. H.: Immune lysis of normal human and paroxysmal nocturnal hemoglobinuria

(PNH) red blood cells. J. Exp. Med. **123**: 969, 1966.

51. Humphrey, J. H., and Dourmashkin, R. R.: Electron microscope studies of immune cell lysis. In *Complement*, edited by G. E. W. Wolstenholme and J. Knight. Little, Brown and Company, Boston, 1965.

52. Rebuck, J. W.: Structural changes in sensitized human erythrocytes observed with the electron microscope. Anat. Rec. **115**: 591, 1953.

53. Weinrach, R. S., Lai, M., and Talmage, D. W.: The relation between hemolysin concentration and hemolytic rate as measured with chromium[51] labeled cells. J. Infect. Dis. **102**: 60, 1958.

54. Ishizaka, T., Ishizaka, K., Borsos, T., and Rapp, H. C'1 fixation by human isoagglutinins: fixation of C'1 by γ-G and γ-M but not by γ-A antibody. J. Immun. **97**: 716, 1966.

55. Stelos, P., and Talmage, D. W.: The separation by starch electrophoresis of two antibodies to sheep red cells differing in hemolytic efficiency. J. Infect. Dis. **100**: 126, 1957.

56. Yachnin, S.: The hemolysis of red cells from patients with paroxysmal nocturnal hemoglobinuria by isolated subcomponents of the third complement component. J. Clin. Invest. **44**: 114, 1965.

57. Yachnin, S., and Ruthenberg, J. M.: pH optima in immune hemolysis: a comparison between guinea pig and human complement. J. Clin. Invest. **44**: 149, 1965.

58. Rosse, W. F., and Dacie, J. V.: The role of complement in the sensitivity of the paroxysmal nocturnal haemoglobinuria red cell to immune lysis. Bibl. Haemat. **23**: 11, 1965.

59. Cawley, L. P., and Goodwin, W. L.: Electron microscopic investigation of the binding of bromelin by erythrocytes. Vox Sang. **13**: 393, 1967.

60. Storti, E., Vaccari, F., and Baldini, E.: Changes in red cell metabolism in presence of incomplete antibodies. Experientia **12**: 108, 1958.

61. Abrahamov, A., and Diamond, L. K.: Erythrocyte glycolysis in erythroblastic newborns. Amer. J. Dis. Child **99**: 202, 1960.

62. Young, L. E.: Hemolytic disorders: some highlights of 20 years of progress. Ann. Intern. Med. **49**: 1073, 1958.

63. Altman, K. I., Tabechian, H., and Young, L. E.: Some aspects of the metabolism of red blood cells from patients with hemolytic anemias. Ann. N. Y. Acad. Med. **57**: 142, 1959.

64. Nicolau, C. T., and Teitel, P.: Über eine Verbesserung der osmotischen Resistenz von antikörperbeladenen Erythrozyten durch Stoffwechseleffekte des Insulins. Z. Ges. Inn. Med. **14**: 40, 1959.

65. Pipitone, V., Russo, R., Crispo, A., and Dailly,

L.: Anemia emolitica sperimentale da eteroantisieri. (ii) Comportomento della glicolisi eritrocitaria. Boll. Soc. Ital. Biol. Sper. **35**: 1268, 1959.

66. Kaplan, E., Herz, F., and Hsu, K. S.: Erythrocyte acetylcholinesterase activity in ABO hemolytic disease of the newborn. Pediatrics **33**: 205, 1964.

67. Brabec, V. V., Bicanová, J., Friedmann, B., Kout, M., Mirčevová, L., Palek, J., Vopatova, M., and Volek, V.: Stoffwechselveränderungen in Erythrozyten bei der autoimmunen hämolytischen Krankheit. Acta

68. Greenwalt, T. J., and Ayers, V. F.: Phosphate partition in the erythrocytes of normal newborn infants and infants with erythroblastosis. IV. Ion exchange chromatography. Blood **22**: 589, 1963.

69. Greenwalt, T. J., Ayers, V. F., and Morell, S. A.: Phosphate partition in the erythrocytes of normal newborn infants and infants with erythroblastosis fetalis. III. P[32] uptake and incorporation. Blood **19**: 468, 1962.

70. Langley, G. R.: Effects of autoantibody on erythrocyte metabolism. Canad. Med. Ass. J. (abstract) **90**: 478, 1964.

71. Tishkoff, G. H.: Erythrocyte mucoids in acquired autoimmune hemolytic anemia. Blood **28**: 229, 1966.

72. Vulpis, N.: Studies on the antigens of red cell ghost. Differences in antigenic specificity of human normal adult hereditary spherocytosis and autoimmune hemolytic anemia S protein. Acta Haemat. (Basel) **30**: 280, 1963.

73. Goldstein, M. A., and Desforges, J. F.: Hemolytic anemia and erythrocyte K+ leak. Clin. Res. **13**: 273, 1965.

74. Langley, G. R., and Felderhof, C. H.: Anti-Rh$_0$(D) and human erythrocyte membrane. Canad. Med. Ass. J. (abstract) **92**: 357, 1965.

75. Letarte, J., Shahidi, N. T., and Hitzig, W. H.: L'activité de l'adénosine-triphosphatase chez les individus normaux et les malades atteints d'anémie hémolytique. Schweiz. Med. Wschr. **95**: 1440, 1965.

76. Mollison, P. L.: *Blood Transfusion in Clinical Medicine*, Ed. 4. Blackwell Scientific Publications, Ltd., Oxford, 1967.

77. Jandl, J. H., and Tomlinson, A. S.: The destruction of red cells by antibodies in man. II. Pyrogenic, leukocytic and dermal responses to immune hemolysis. J. Clin. Invest. **37**: 1202, 1958.

78. Jandl, J. H., Simmons, R. L., and Castle, W. B.: Red cell filtration and the pathogenesis of certain hemolytic anemias. Blood **18**: 133, 1961.

79. Lewis, S. M., Dacie, J. V., and Szur, L.: Mechanism of haemolysis in the cold haemagglutinin syndrome. Brit. J. Haemat. **6**: 154, 1960.

80. Jandl, J. H., and Kaplan, M. E.: The destruc-

tion of red cells by antibodies in man. III. Quantitative factors influencing the pattern of hemolysis in vivo. J. Clin. Invest. **39:** 1145, 1960.

81. Jandl, J. H., Richardson Jones, A., and Castle, W. B.: The destruction of red cells by antibodies in man. I. Observations on the sequestration and lysis of red cells altered by immune mechanisms. J. Clin. Invest. **36:** 1428, 1957.

82. Mollison, P. L., and Cutbush, M.: Use of isotope-labeled red cells to demonstrate incompatibility in vivo. Lancet **1:** 1290, 1955.

83. Mollison, P. L.: Blood group antibodies and red-cell destruction. Brit. Med. J. **2:** 1035, 1123, 1959.

84. Mollison, P. L., and Paterson, J. C. S.: Survival after tranfusion of Rh-positive erythrocytes previously incubated with Rh antibody. J. Clin. Path. **2:** 109, 1949.

85. Young, L. E., Christian, R. M., Ervin, D. M., Swisher, S. N., O'Brien, W. A., Stewart, W. B., and Yuile, C. L.: Erythrocyte-isoantibody reactions in dogs. In *Proceedings of the Third International Congress of the International Society of Hematology.* William Heinemann, Ltd., London, 1951.

86. Jennings, E. R., and Hindmarsh, C.: The significance of the minor cross-match. Amer. J. Clin. Path. **30:** 302, 1958.

87. Mollison, P. L., and Hughes-Jones, N. C.: Clearance of Rh-positive red cells by low concentrations of Rh antibody. Immunology **12:** 63, 1967.

88. Cutbush, M., and Mollison, P. L.: Relation between characteristics of blood-group antibodies in vitro and associated patterns of red-cell destruction in vivo. Brit. J. Haemat. **4:** 115, 1958.

89. August, A., and Pirofsky, B.: Interaction of basic polyelectrolytes and human blood: the effect of anti-heparin agents. Transfusion **6:** 74, 1966.

90. Jandl, J. H., and Castle, W. B.: Agglutination of sensitized red cells by large anisometric molecules. J. Lab. Clin. Med. **47:** 669, 1956.

91. Jandl, J. H.: Sequestration by the spleen of red cells sensitized with incomplete antibody and with metallo-protein complexes. J. Clin. Invest. **34:** 912, 1955.

92. Wagley, P. F., Shen, S. C., Gardner, F. H., and Castle, W. B.: Studies on the destruction of red blood cells. VI. The spleen as a source of a substance causing agglutination of the red blood cells of certain patients with acquired hemolytic jaundice by an anti-human serum rabbit serum (Coombs serum). J. Lab. Clin. Med. **33:** 1197, 1948.

93. Wright, C.-S., Dodd, M. C., Bouroncle, B. A., Doan, C. A., and Zollinger, R. M.: Studies of hemagglutinins in hereditary spherocytosis and in acquired hemolytic anemia: their relationship to the hypersplenic mechanism. J. Lab. Clin. Med. **37:** 165, 1951.

94. Crosby, W. H.: Normal functions of the spleen relative to red blood cells. A review. Blood **14:** 399, 1959.

95. Teitel, P.: Disk-sphere transformation and plasticity alterations of red blood cells. Nature (London) **206:** 409, 1965.

96. Wagner, H. N., Razzak, M. A., Baertner, R. A., Caine, W. P., and Feagin, O. T.: Removal of erythrocytes from the circulation. Arch. Intern. Med. (Chicago) **110:** 90, 1962.

97. Seaman, G. V. F., and Uhlenbruck, G.: Die elektrophoretische Beweglichkeit von Erythrocyten nach Behandlung mit verschiedenen Enzymen und Antiserum. Klin. Wschr. **40:** 699, 1962.

98. Seaman, G. V. F., and Cook, G. M. W.: Modification of the electrophoretic behavior of the erythrocyte by chemical and enzymatic methods. In *Cell Electrophoresis,* edited by E. J. Ambrose. Little, Brown and Company, Boston, 1965.

99. Ponder, E.: Certain hemolytic mechanisms in hemolytic anemia. Blood **6:** 559, 1951.

100. Leroy, E. P., and Spurrier, W.: Hemolytic property of some carbohydrases; their possible role in red cell destruction. Blood **10:** 912, 1955.

101. Magalini, S. I., Blumenthal, W., and Stefanini, M.: A splenic hemolytic system of lipidic nature in man. Clin. Res. Proc. **4:** 81, 1956.

102. Torp, H. E.: Has the enzyme system acetylcholine-cholinesterase any significance for physiological hemolysis in the spleen? Scand. J. Clin. Lab. Invest. **8:** 84, 1956.

103. Ham, T. H., and Castle, W. B.: Mechanism of hemolysis in certain anemias: significance of increased hypotonic fragility and of erythrostasis. J. Clin. Invest. **19:** 788, 1940.

104. Reed, C. F., and Swisher, S. N.: Abnormalities of in vitro behavior of structural lipids of red blood cells from patients with hereditary spherocytosis. J. Clin. Invest. **39:** 1019, 1960.

105. Nicolau, C. T., Teitel, P., Fotino, M., Butoianu, E., and Taigar, S.: Alterations of erythrocyte plasticity in blood diseases. (A three years' clinical experience with the erythrocyte filtrability test (E.F.T.).) Sangre (Barc.) **9:** 282, 1964.

106. Keene, W. R., and Jandl, J. H.: Studies of the reticuloendothelial mass and sequestering function of rat bone marrow. Blood **26:** 157, 1965.

107. Wright, A. E., and Douglas, S. R.: An experimental investigation of the role of the blood fluids in connection with phagocytosis. Proc. Roy. Soc. (Biol.) **72:** 357, 1903.

108. Dean, G.: Phagocytosis and bactericidal action. Brit. Med. J. **2:** 1409, 1907.

109. Levaditi, C.: Contribution à l'étude de l'anémie expérimentale. Etat de la cytase hémolytique dans le plasma des animaux nor-

maux. Ann. Inst. Pasteur (Paris) **16**: 233, 1902.

110. Mohn, J. F., Lambert, R. M., Bowman, H. S., and Wells Brason, F.: Experimental production in man of autoantibodies with Rh specificity. Ann. N. Y. Acad. Sci. **124**: 477, 1965.

111. Bessis, M.: Cellular mechanisms for the destruction of erythrocytes. Hematologica **2**: 59, 1965.

112. Weiss, L.: The structure of fine splenic arterial vessels in relation to hemoconcentration and red cell destruction. Amer. J. Anat. **111**: 131, 1962.

113. Pethica, B. A.: The physical chemistry of cell adhesion. Exp. Cell Res. **8**: 123, 1961.

114. Bangham, A. D.: The adhesiveness of leukocytes with special reference to zeta potential. Ann. N. Y. Acad. Sci. **116**: 945, 1964.

115. Jensen, W. N., and Moreno, G.: Etude de l'érythrophagocytose après traitement des cellules par la neuraminidase. Nouv. Rev. Franc. Hemat. **4**: 483, 1964.

116. Jandl, J. H., Files, N. M., Barnett, S. B., and MacDonald, R. A.: Proliferative response of the spleen and liver to hemolysis. J. Exp. Med. **122**: 299, 1965.

117. Cohn, Z. A., and Weiner, E.: The particulate hydrolases of macrophages. I. Comparative enzymology, isolation and properties. J. Exp. Med. **118**: 991, 1963.

118. Cohn, Z. A., and Weiner, E.: The particulate

119. Essner, E.: An electron microscopic study of erythrophagocytosis. J. Biophys. Biochem. Cytol. **7**: 329, 1960.

120. Dorfman, R. F.: Nature of the sinus lining cells of the spleen. Nature (London) **190**: 1021, 1961.

121. Ludány, G., Döklen, A., and Tóth, E.: Die Beeinflussung der Leukozytenphagozytose mit Phlorrhizin. Experientia **13**: 409, 1957.

122. Gelzer, J., and Suter, E.: The effect of antibody on intracellular parasitism of *Salmonella typhimurium* in mononuclear phagocytes in vitro. J. Exp. Med. **110**: 715, 1959.

123. Dacie, J. V.: *The Haemolytic Anaemias, Part II*, Ed. 2. Grune & Stratton, Inc., New York, 1962.

124. Packer, J. T., Greendyke, R. M., and Swisher, S. N.: The inhibition of erythrophagocytosis in vitro by corticosteroids. Trans. Ass. Amer. Physicians **73**: 93, 1960.

125. Bonnin, J. A., and Schwartz, L.: The combined study of agglutination, hemolysis and erythrophagocytosis. With special reference to acquired hemolytic anemia. Blood **9**: 773, 1954.

126. Greendyke, R. M., Brierty, R. E., and Swisher, S. N.: In vitro studies on erythrophagocytosis. Blood **22**: 295, 1963.

hydrolases of macrophages. II. Biochemical and morphological response to particle ingestion. J. Exp. Med. **118**: 1009, 1963.

Chapter 22

The Relationship of Erythrocyte Autoantibodies to Autoimmune Hemolytic Anemia

The autoimmune hemolytic anemias are characterized by premature destruction of erythrocytes and by an antibody bound to the erythrocyte surface. It would appear axiomatic to connect these characteristics to each other in a cause and effect relationship. This simple association, however, is not always apparent. It is therefore necessary to examine closely the role of erythrocyte autoantibodies in autoimmune hemolytic anemia. In this chapter the problem is analyzed from three aspects. Experimentally induced autoimmune hemolytic anemia, spontaneous autoimmune hemolytic anemia in animals and the interrelationships observed in human autoimmune hemolytic anemia are all important and are summarized below.

Experimental Autoimmune Hemolytic Anemia

Five major techniques have been employed for the production of experimental autoimmune hemolytic anemia. These include modification of erythrocytes, production of cross reacting antibodies, creation of anti-antibodies, induction of graft-host disease and interference with the role of the thymus gland in establishing a normal immune system.

Modification of Erythrocytes

In 1918 Lüdke (1) noted the development of iso- and autolysins in nine of 11 dogs injected with their own lysed erythrocytes. In 1949 Wagley and Castle (2) investigated this phenomenon in four dogs. Defibrinated blood was frozen, thawed and incubated with streptococcal toxins. Two dogs were immunized intraperitoneally with the modified blood. Lysed blood was incubated with *Staphylococcus aureus*, filtered and employed to immunize the remaining two dogs. No antibody production was noted. Further injections of autologous blood mixed in Freund's adjuvant were employed. In one of the four dogs a positive direct antiglobulin reaction was noted 25 days after the last injection. The positive antiglobulin test persisted until the 35th postinjection date. Neither anemia, reticulocytosis, icterus nor a fall of serum complement accompanied the positive antiglobulin test.

In 1952 Liu and Evans (3) studied a patient with a ruptured ectopic pregnancy and a positive antiglobulin test. They postulated that the intraperitoneal distribution of blood might induce erythrocyte changes leading to antibody production. This hypothesis was tested experimentally. Twenty milliliters of blood were obtained by cardiac puncture from each of 12 rabbits. Autologous blood was intraperitoneally administered without anticoagulant to the donor rabbit. Immunization was repeated weekly. Three of 12 rabbits developed positive antiglobulin tests which persisted for 2 weeks. Neither anemia, reticulocytosis nor an increase in mechanical or osmotic fragility developed. Positive antiglobulin tests did not follow mixing erythrocyte stromata with beta hemolytic streptococcal filtrates, kidney emulsions or liver emulsions.

Motulsky and Crosby (4) performed similar studies in guinea pigs. Autologous erythrocytes were incubated with influenza virus or mixed with Freund's adjuvant and then injected subcutaneously. After six weekly injections positive antiglobulin reactions were noted in seven of 14 animals receiving virus treated cells. Ten of 18 animals that received autologous cells mixed with Freund's adjuvant also developed positive antiglobulin tests. The antiglobulin test reverted to negative a few weeks after injections were discontinued. Booster injections of the same material led to a return of the antiglobulin positive state. Anemia did not occur in the experimental animals developing positive antiglobulin tests. Similar studies have been reported by Cajano and associates (5) and Stadsbaeder (6). Anemia generally did not follow such immunization procedures. Two of the guinea pigs studied by Stadsbaeder (6) developed anemia and positive antiglobulin tests. However, both animals also had pneumococcal infections.

Hamamoto and Yoshikawa (7) immunized rabbits with autologous erythrocytes treated with formalin. Hemolytic anemia developed with positive antiglobulin tests. In some cases antibodies developed only against the formalinized erythrocytes. In other instances an autoantibody was formed which reacted with normal erythrocytes. The authors suggest that erythrocyte autoantibody formation may be initiated as a response to modification of host erythrocyte antigens.

The Production of Cross Reacting Antibodies

Wiener (8) postulated that human anti-A and anti-B antibodies and cold acting autoantibodies resulted from heteroimmune antigenic stimulation. Antigenic stimuli supplied by virus pneumonia, infectious mononucleosis, trypanosomiasis, tropical eosinophilia and various foods led to anti-

body formation. Such antibodies cross reacted with antigenic constituents of the erythrocyte membrane. Smallpox vaccination may create similar cross reacting antibodies. High titer anti-A produced by individuals infected with *Toxocara canis* is probably an example of the same phenomenon.

A similar pathogenesis has been postulated to explain the development of autoimmune hemolytic anemia associated with malignant tumors. Stefanini and associates (9) and Kissmeyer-Nielsen and associates (10) suggested the presence of serologically related antigens on erythrocytes and malignant cells. Aubert and Brendemoen (11) and Wiener and associates (12) have extracted cold agglutinins from tumor cells. Serum carry-over and contamination cannot be excluded in these studies.

Two important experimental studies have utilized these concepts. Suzuki (13) studied rabbits after prolonged immunization with egg albumin. Banti's syndrome developed and was characterized by portal hypertension and splenomegaly. Many animals had an associated anemia, increase in osmotic fragility and positive antiglobulin tests. In addition to anti-egg albumin antibodies, autoantibodies directed against phospholipid components of the liver, spleen and erythrocytes were produced.

In 1957 Korn and associates (14) noted that rabbits formed cold hemagglutinins when immunized with heat killed *Listeria monocytogenes*. Costea and associates (15) expanded this observation and presented detailed studies of the resulting cold hemagglutinin. They immunized rabbits with various types of heat killed *L. monocytogenes*. The highest cold hemagglutinin titers were produced in response to serum type 4b. Three other types did not produce cold hemagglutinins and only weak cold hemagglutinins were found with type 4a. All serum types induced high titers of specific anti-*L. monocytogenes* agglutinins. Physical-chemical studies of the cold hemagglutinin identified the antibody as an IgM immunoglobulin. Cold hemagglutinin titers ranged from 256 to 4096. One serum was tested extensively. It reacted with erythrocytes from 40 normal rabbits at a titer of 1024. It also reacted with 29 of 30 samples of human erythrocytes at titers ranging from 256 to 1024. The rabbit cold hemagglutinins had anti-I specificity. Partial inactivation of the cold hemagglutinin was accomplished by in vivo administration of penicillamine. A mild normochromic normocytic anemia was noted in the immunized animals. Erythrocyte survival time studies suggested two populations of cells with different sensitivities. Hemolysis appeared to be complement dependent. A remarkable similarity was apparent between experimentally produced rabbit cold hemagglutinins and cold hemagglutinins seen in human diseases. This cross reacting system offers great potential in the study of autoimmune hemolytic phenomena. A similar cross reacting system relating human cold autoantibody production to Mycoplasma infections has been mentioned in Chapter 20 (16).

Zmijewski (17) presented a cross reacting system utilizing primates. Chimpanzees were immunized with human blood products. As expected, a circulating antibody was produced against human erythrocytes. In addition, autoantibodies were produced by chimpanzees and were directed against chimpanzee erythrocytes. The erythrocyte autoantibodies fixed complement but did not lead to increased cell destruction.

The Production of Anti-antibodies

Samaille and associates (18) reported the production of positive antiglobulin tests in dogs injected with rabbit antiserum directed against canine erythrocytes. The dog erythrocytes were coated with both dog and rabbit globulin. The authors concluded that the autologous protein coating erythrocytes probably represented anti-antibody formation, although complement fixation could not be ruled out. Identical results were obtained in guinea pigs, using rabbit antiserum. Muratore and associates (19) also employed a guinea pig system in similar studies. Hemolytic anemia with erythrocyte binding of autologous globulin and rabbit globulin was noted. They implicated both the heteroimmune antibody and an auto-

antibody as responsible for the hemolytic state. Lille-Szyszlkowicz and Chojnacka (20) in 1955 observed the same sequence of events and concluded that hemolytic anemia resulted from the action of anti-antibodies functioning as autoantibodies.

A comparable human experimental system has been reported by Bowman and associates (21) and Mohn and associates (22). In these studies the authors transfused human isoantibody containing sera into human volunteers whose erythrocytes contained the related antigen. An expected isoimmune hemolytic anemia developed. In one recipient the prolonged exposure to isoantibodies eventually led to production of an autoantibody of anti-rh″(E) specificity. Anti-antibody formation is probably not related to this phenomenon. A termination of tolerance or cross reacting antibody formation initiated by damaged erythrocytes appears to be more likely.

The Production of a Graft-host (Runt Disease) Syndrome

Although the three approaches discussed above have produced positive antiglobulin tests, experimentally they bear little resemblance to the clinical picture of autoimmune hemolytic anemia. In many instances anemia was absent. In other cases, anemia probably resulted from either heteroimmune or isoimmune antibodies. An isolated abnormality characterized by positive antiglobulin tests was generally observed. The multisystem disease pattern characteristic of the autoimmune state was not produced. In recent years experimental autoimmune hemolytic anemia has been induced as part of a systemic disease.

In 1957 Billingham and Brent (23) demonstrated that immunologically immature mice developed a fatal wasting disease after receiving transplants of immunologically competent homologous spleen cells. Experiments carried out with irradiated adult animals gave similar results and suggested that the wasting disease resulted from graft tissue acting on the host. This phenomenon has been variously termed graft-host disease, runt disease, secondary disease, wasting disease and homologous disease. Simonsen (24) in 1953 noted the development of positive antiglobulin tests in a dog which received a transplanted spleen. He suggested that antibody formation initiated against host antigenic constituents by transplanted immunocompetent splenic cells resulted in the erythrocyte antibody. Muirhead and Groves (25) also noted positive antiglobulin tests in one of several dogs receiving kidney grafts. The antiglobulin test became positive 5 to 10 days after establishment of the graft and it correlated with rejection of the graft.

In 1957 Simonsen (26) clarified many aspects of this graft-host syndrome and firmly established it as an immunologic event. He demonstrated that transplantation of adult chicken spleen cells into chicken embryos resulted in hemolytic anemia and death of the recipient in the 1st or 2nd week of life. The grafted immunocompetent cells recognized the host as foreign and initiated antibody production against various host constituents. These studies were expanded by Cock and Simonsen (27) and Simonsen and Jensen (28) who again demonstrated positive antiglobulin tests as part of the graft-host disease syndrome.

Porter (29, 30) investigated this phenomenon with two different techniques. Fetal rabbits and adult rabbits made immunologically incompetent by radiation therapy were inoculated with homologous spleen cells. Positive antiglobulin tests developed. Chromium^{51} studies indicated a shortening of the life span of host erythrocytes but not of donor erythrocytes. The erythrocyte antibodies were incomplete and elution demonstrated them to be specific for host blood groups. Piomelli and Brooke (31) also employed radiation to prevent rejection of transfused bone marrow in rabbits. Positive antiglobulin tests developed and death eventually occurred in many animals. Several rabbits survived and in such animals the antiglobulin test reverted to negative. Meier and Brown (32) similarly noted immune hemolytic anemia as a complication of a graft-host syndrome.

Trentin (33) in 1958 introduced another model system for the development of a graft-host reaction. He demonstrated that introduction of spleen cells from one parent into an F_1 hybrid inbred mouse strain would lead to a runting syndrome. This has been termed allogenic disease. The inability of the host to destroy the transplanted immunocompetent cell established a cell population which recognized host constituents as foreign and permitted antibody production. Oliner and associates (34) utilized this model test system to study experimental autoimmune hemolytic anemia. They documented the hematologic abnormalities of the graft-host reaction and emphasized its widespread systemic nature and resemblance to human disease patterns. Similarities to human autoimmune hemolytic anemia were striking. In several surviving animals anemia disappeared although the antiglobulin test remained positive. Three animals relapsed after 6 months, suggesting that the prior remission had followed the establishment of a new level of immune homeostasis. The homeostatic state could be disturbed, leading to recurrence of the immune disease. This sequence is reminiscent of the activation of hemolytic anemia following chemotherapy for leukemia and lymphoma (35). Harriss and associates (36) used a similar although not identical F_1 hybrid test system. Allogenic disease and anemia occurred. Cr^{51} studies indicated that both hybrid and parenteral cells were destroyed.

Stastny and associates (37) utilized graft-host reactions as a model for human autoimmunization. They employed inbred strains of Sprague-Dawley and Fisher rats and noted significant abnormalities in the hemopoietic system, joints, heart and skin. Significant degrees of anemia, leukopenia and thrombocytopenia were observed. The antiglobulin test employing host erythrocytes was positive in six of 10 animals studied. One-half of the animals developed polyarthritis. Inflammation of a varying degree was noted in the hearts of almost all animals examined. The mitral and aortic valves were most frequently involved. Myocardial, epicardial and perivascular lesions were also present. A variety of skin lesions were observed and appeared to result from immunologic reactions directed at the host's skin. Histologic relationships to lupus erythematosus and scleroderma were noted. Circulating antibodies directed against host lymphoid cells were demonstrated, using a complement binding system and fluorescent rabbit anticomplement antiserum.

The significance of the graft-host syndrome has been expanded by the detailed studies of Schwartz and associates (38, 39). The ultimate effect of transplanting immunocompetent cells into a foreign host extends beyond the creation of a widespread immunologic disease. A number of such animals eventually develop malignancies of the reticuloendothelium, particularly reticulum cell sarcoma. The exact relationship between an autoimmune state and the eventual appearance of reticuloendothelial malignancy is still to be determined.

Although the experimental graft-host syndrome is similar to human autoimmune hemolytic anemia in many aspects, it differs in one major area. Antibody producing cells are obtained from another animal in the experimental systems. Billingham (40) in 1959 suggested that maternal lymphoid cells may traverse the placenta and survive in the fetus. The eventual proliferation of such cells could then result in a graft-host disease syndrome. Green and associates (41) have also postulated a maternal transfer of immunocompetent cells as leading to chimerism and neoplasia. Schapiro (42) recently described a fascinating family with many siblings involved in immunologic diseases. At least one sibling had autoimmune hemolytic anemia. A striking similarity to graft-host disease was noted in the affected siblings. The author suggests that the process originated in transplacental transfers of immunologically competent cells from the mother to the fetuses, with bacterial or viral infections as precipitating causes of the illness or as terminal complications. Pirofsky and associates (43) theorized that the transfusion of large amounts of viable lymphocytes during open heart surgery may be responsible for transient hemolytic anemia and positive antiglobulin reactions.

The Role of the Thymus in Autoimmunity

The thymus gland plays a significant role in the establishment of a normal immune apparatus. In 1956 Metcalf (44)

documented the presence of a lymphocyte stimulating factor in the thymus gland. This important observation reawakened interest in the function of this organ. It stimulated detailed investigations as to the possible role of the thymus gland in immunologic processes.

Extirpation of the Thymus. The immunologic function of the thymus gland was suggested by studies involving surgical removal of this organ. Thymectomy in the adult animal was found to have little if any effect on the ability to establish humoral or delayed hypersensitivity immunologic responses (45). Metcalf (46) reported that thymectomy in adult life was followed by a blood and tissue deficiency of lymphocytes. Although the ability to produce antibodies was not particularly influenced by adult thymectomy, the capacity of the immune apparatus to recover from damage was impaired (47). Adult mice thymectomized and irradiated had persistently low lymphocyte populations and they failed to regain their capacity for producing immune reactions.

When thymectomy was performed at birth a marked impairment of the immune apparatus was noted. Archer and Pierce (48) reported that humoral antibody formation was inhibited in neonatal thymectomized rabbits. Rats thymectomized shortly after birth had a diminished capacity to develop Arthus sensitivity or to form circulating antibody (49). Neonatal thymectomy also influenced delayed hypersensitivity. Miller (50), Martinez and associates (51) and Arnason and associates (52) reported a marked delay in skin homograft rejection in animals thymectomized in the immediate neonatal period. Complete extirpation of the thymus in mice up to 30 days old resulted in the prolongation of skin grafts (51). Complete extirpation of the neonatal mouse thymus permitted the survival of homotransplanted skin across the strongest histocompatibility barriers. Rats thymectomized within 1 week of birth had a compromised capacity to develop tuberculin sensitivity and delayed reactivity against bovine serum albumin (49, 53). Such thymectomized rats were incapable of developing experimental allergic encephalomyelitis, a laboratory produced autoimmune disease (52, 53).

The morphologic counterpart of the immune deficiency following neonatal thymectomy in the rat has been documented by Waksman and associates (53, 54). There is a depletion of small lymphocytes from the blood, spleen and lymph nodes. In contrast, germinal centers, plasma cells and reticuloendothelial elements are preserved. Plasma protein values, including IgG, are normal by paper electrophoresis.

The Influence of the Thymus Gland on the Immune Apparatus. Extensive studies were designed to document the relationship of the thymus gland to the immune apparatus. Good and associates (55) summarized many of these as follows. (a) Thymectomized mice are unable to reject homografts from donors differing even at the H_2 locus. (b) They have defective capacities to produce circulating antibody. (c) They are deficient in the capacity to produce delayed hypersensitivity. (d) Spleen cells from thymectomized mice are immunologically inadequate and fail to induce a graft-host reaction. (e) Such spleen cells are also a poor source of cells for protecting syngeneic recipients from radiation death. (f) Thymectomized animals develop a wasting disease with retarded growth and a high mortality. (g) This wasting disease and the defective immune function can be prevented by transplanting syngeneic thymus in the neonatal period. (h) Syngeneic thymic transplants performed on neonatally thymectomized mice more than 4 to 6 weeks old do not restore the animals. (i) Allogenic thymus grafts placed in the neonatal period reconstitute neonatally thymectomized mice. (j) Immunologic activity restored by allogenic thymus grafts have characteristics of both host and donor cells; the host cells appear to predominate. (k) The cells of the thymus graft enter into the peripheral lymphoid tissue. The major influence of the graft, however, is to restore the host's lymphoid competence and the production of his own lymphoid cells. (l) The thymus can act by means of a humoral substance which permits the development of the host's lymphoid cells and his immune capacity. (m) Fully dispersed thymic and splenic cells can completely restore the immune competence of neonatal thymectomized mice. Immunologic characteristics are then dependent on the cell type of the donor. (n) The thymus can therefore operate in two ways, i.e., a humoral effect and a means of providing cells with immunologic potential. (o) The wasting disease characterizing neonatal thymectomy can be reversed by fully dispersed spleen or thymic cells. (p) In certain inbred mouse strains thymectomy appears to prevent the development of immunologic potentials far beyond the neonatal period.

Central Lymphoid Structures. The influence of the thymus gland on immunologic capacity appears to be partially species dependent. Glick (56) carried out a series of studies on a lymphoid organ located at the posterior end of the intestines in chickens. This organ, the bursa of Fabricius, had been called the cloacal thymus by Jolly (57) in 1915. Glick (56) noted that removal of the bursa in the newly hatched chicken interfered with its capacity to form antibody. Extensive studies performed on chickens revealed the following (55): (a) A hormonal bursectomy could be produced by administration of 19-nortestosterone. (b) A chicken either surgically or hormonally bursectomized had a diminished capacity to form circulating antibody and IgG immunoglobulins. (c) Thymectomy in the chicken had little effect on either immunogenesis or leukomogenesis. (d) Removal of the bursa of Fabricius had little effect on the ability to develop or to express delayed allergic reactions or rejection of skin grafts. (e) Thymectomy and bursectomy depressed the capacity to develop delayed allergic reactions. Conflicting data as to the effect of skin homotransplants are available.

Such data suggest that the influence of the thymus gland on immune capacity is modified by the presence of a central lymphoid apparatus and by the time of peripheralization of lymphocytes. In the dog, cat and man peripheralization of lymphocytes occurs prior to parturition. Neonatal thymectomy may only have a minimal effect upon the development of lymphoid tissue and immunologic capacity. In the mouse the thymus gland is the only lymphoid structure at birth. Neonatal thymectomy therefore has a profound effect on the immune apparatus. Good and associates (55) suggest that the rabbit appendix may also function as a central lymphoid apparatus independent of the thymus gland.

The Thymus, Self-recognition and Autoimmunity. Three possible modes of action are involved in the role of the thymus gland in establishing the lymphoid and immune apparatus. The thymus may function by providing the cells producing the immune response. It may act by elaborating a humoral factor necessary for maturation of potentially immunologically competent cells. In addition, it may prevent an autoimmune rejection of lymphoid tissue.

The influence of the thymus gland on self-recognition and autoimmune disease is of great importance. Burnet (58) and Burnet and Holmes (59) approached this problem by incorporating the activity of the thymus gland within the theory of clonal selection. Self-recognition was postulated as dependent on the exposure of self-antigens to immunocompetent cells in the thymus, prior to peripheralization of lymphocytes. Germinal follicles were described in the thymus gland of patients with various autoimmune syndromes (60) and in the NZB mice (59). Thymectomy was occasionally found beneficial in infant forms of autoimmune hemolytic anemia (see Chapter 12).

Neonatal thymectomized mice exhibit a poor growth curve, a hunched position and weight loss. Death occurs 1 to 4 months after birth (55, 61). This wasting disease may be prevented or even reversed by the administration of a sufficiently large dose of syngenetic thymus cells (62). Miller and associates (63) noted that neonatally thymectomized mice suffering from the wasting syndrome could develop positive antiglobulin reactions. Kellum and associates (64) found that rabbits thymectomized and appendectomized at birth spontaneously developed a wasting disease with positive antiglobulin tests, anemia, diarrhea, generalized plasmacytosis and severe amyloidosis involving the splenic follicles, kidneys, lymph nodes and liver.

Such observations suggest that the thymus gland functions in the establishment of a state of immune self-recognition. There is a striking resemblance between the wasting disease seen in neonatal thymectomized mice and that in graft-host disease (55, 63). This suggests that some of the lesions found in thymectomized animals may result from antihost activity and that they therefore may be autoimmune. It may therefore be postulated that the thymus gland is necessary for the establishment of self-recognition and that thymectomy prevents the development of tolerance to host antigenic tissues. Thymectomy may be considered as creating a state of autoimmunization. In the course of the antiself-immune reaction, lymphoid atrophy, reticuloendothelial hyperplasia and incompetence of the immune apparatus develop. Figure 43 diagrammatically illustrates the proposed sequence of events. The clinical association of thymoma and hemolytic anemia in the human supports this association (see Chapter 6). Cases 6, 20 and 30 present the protocols of three such patients.

Miller and associates (63) have challenged the postulate that the primary function of the thymus gland is to establish self-recognition. They would further deny that the immunologic deficiency following neonatal thymectomy results from lymphoid atrophy reflecting an autoimmune process. The immune deficiency following neonatal

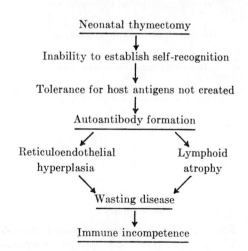

FIGURE 43. The sequence of events through which neonatal thymectomy may create autoimmune disease. The thymus is assumed to function in establishing self-recognition.

thymectomy is apparent by 6 days of age in mice, well before wasting disease and lymphoid aplasia develop. The restoration of immune competence by supplying adult thymic cells also is incompatible with a loss of tolerance. If lymphoid cell autoantibodies were present, donor lymphoid cells of an identical strain should also be destroyed. Miller and associates (63) suggest that autoimmunity in the thymectomized animal may occur as an epiphenomenon. In the absence of a normal humoral thymus mechanism, normal maturation of immunocompetent cells may not occur, establishing a defective immune reactivity. Clones of cells with abnormal functions or different genetic characteristics may arise either as the result of somatic mutations or through virus infections. Normally an animal could effectively resist such virus infections or destroy aberrant clones of cells through immune homeostasis. In thymectomized animals the immune deficiency may inter-

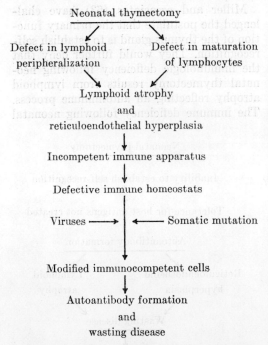

FIGURE 44. The sequence of events through which neonatal thymectomy may create autoimmune disease. The thymus does not function in self-recognition. Autoimmune patterns reflect an immunodeficient state.

fere with normal immune homeostasis, permitting the establishment of such clones. In support of this hypothesis these authors (63) state that thymectomized animals have a particular susceptibility to virus infections. Miller and associates (65) have reported one instance in which a virus caused the appearance and proliferation of cells with a distinct antigenic structure in a thymectomized animal. Such modified cells would have been destroyed by a normal immune mechanism. These observations suggest that the wasting disease and autoimmune phenomena seen in neonatal thymectomized animals may occur through the action of viruses. They also suggest that vertical transmission of a virus may occur in inbred strains of mice which regularly develop autoimmune disease, thereby simulating a genetic transmission. Figure 44 depicts the relationship of thymectomy to autoimmunization employing these concepts. The reports of Jacox and associates (66) and Mongan and associates (67) describing disseminated cytomegalic viruses in the presence of a thymoma and varying immunologic deficiencies, including hemolytic anemia, support this concept. The experimental studies of Mellors and Huang (68, 69) documenting virus particles in NZB mice and transmission of the autoimmune defects by such viruses illustrates this hypothesis. It is also apparent that the system suggested by Miller and associates (63) offers an ideal mechanism to explain the development of malignancies in thymectomized animals.

Spontaneous Autoimmunity in Animals

Frequent attempts have been made to create an animal counterpart of human autoimmune hemolytic anemia. However, an exact animal model system has not been experimentally produced. The observation that animals may spontaneously develop a disease syndrome characterized by positive antiglobulin tests, hemolytic anemia and other autoimmune phenomena therefore assumes great importance. Such animal models offer an exciting potential for future experimental studies. Two well documented animal systems are currently available.

Autoimmune Hemolytic Anemia in the Dog

In 1957 Miller and associates (70) reported the spontaneous occurrence of autoimmune hemolytic anemia in a dog. This observation was confirmed and expanded by Lewis and associates (71, 72) in 19 such animals. They established the clinical features of canine autoimmune hemolytic anemia and emphasized four major groups of abnormalities: (a) those related to anemia which included pallor, weakness, loss of stamina, shortness of breath and collapse, (b) those resulting from increased erythrocyte destruction such as icterus and dark urine, (c) abnormalities secondary to thrombocytopenia, which included epistaxis, hemorrhages into the skin and melena and (d) evidence of an acute systemic disease. Anorexia, fever, malaise, polydypsia, vomiting and diarrhea were prominent. In addition, splenomegaly was noted in 10 of the 19 animals and lymphadenopathy was noted in eight. A severe macrocytic anemia with reticulocytosis, nucleated erythrocytes, bone marrow erythrocytic hyperplasia and autohemagglutination (in 25 per cent of the cases) was found. Positive antiglobulin tests were obtained in all 19 animals. Erythrocyte autoantibodies were successfully eluted from involved red blood cells. Thrombocytopenia was present in 15 animals in spite of adequate numbers of megakaryocytes in the bone marrow. Accordingly, the condition observed in these animals simulated a human Evans' syndrome. Corticosteroid therapy induced remissions in such animals with frequent recurrences noted. Splenectomy led to varying results with three cases developing prolonged remissions. In contrast to human autoimmune hemolytic anemia, the antiglobulin tests reverted to normal as soon as remission was induced. In addition, relapse was frequently heralded by a return to positive antiglobulin tests.

Lewis and associates (73) have recently described an additional form of canine autoimmune disease which closely resembles systemic lupus erythematosus in man. In seven dogs (two poodles, one cocker spaniel, one fox terrier, one German shepherd, one wire haired terrier and one mongrel) a pattern of autoimmune hemolytic anemia, thrombocytopenia and membranous glomerulonephritis was noted. Positive antiglobulin tests were obtained in all seven animals. Positive lupus erythematosus (LE) cell tests were found in six of seven, antithyroid antibodies in four of six, and rheumatoid factor in two of six dogs examined. Hypergammaglobulinemia was not observed. Thrombocytopenia was documented in six of seven animals. Megakaryocytes were found in the bone marrow and a complicating Evans' syndrome or idiopathic thrombocytopenic purpura was diagnosed. Albuminuria was found in six of the seven animals and azotemia was noted in five of six examined. All animals initially responded to prednisone therapy, with four demonstrating recurrent hemolytic episodes. These animals were treated by splenectomy. Positive and negative antiglobulin reactions correlated with the clinical status of the animals. The antiglobulin tests reverted to normal at the start of remission and became positive at the onset of relapse.

Autoimmune Hemolytic Anemia in the Mouse

In 1959 Bielschowsky and associates (74) reported the development of spontaneous autoimmune disease in an NZB/BL (NZB) inbred strain of mice. These animals had been selectively bred for cancer research on the basis of black coat color. Helyer and Howie (75) described two clinical syndromes in the mice. The first occurred more frequently in males and in animals 6 to 9 months of age. It was characterized by hepatosplenomegaly, moderate anemia and jaundice. The second syndrome was more common in females and started after 12 months of age. Progressive anemia and cachexia with mild or absent jaundice and minimal splenomegaly were noted. In the early stages of the disease the mice assumed a hunched posture with ruffling of the fur and narrowing of the palpebral fissure. Alopecia and indolent ulcerations with various orbital infections were seen as the disease progressed.

Erythrocyte autoantibodies were demonstrable in 100 per cent of the animals by 15 months of age. Such autoantibodies were rarely present at 3 months of age. At 6 months of age approximately 20 per cent of the mice showed erythrocyte autoantibody formation. Helyer and Howie (75) noted that female mice develop erythrocyte autoantibodies several weeks earlier than do males. Holmes and Burnet (76) reported that male mice developed positive antiglobulin tests slightly earlier than did females. Positive antiglobulin tests could be produced in young isologous mice by the transfer of living spleen cells from adult antiglobulin positive donors.

Helyer and Howie (75) found unbound erythrocyte autoantibodies in the sera of all animals when tested with ficin treated erythrocytes. Erythrocyte bound autoantibodies were demonstrated by elution. The autoantibody was incomplete and could be demonstrated by albumin techniques. It appeared to be warm acting with optimal reactivity between 18 and 37°C. The autoantibody was noncomplement dependent and was unaffected by heating to 56°C. for 30 minutes or prolonged storage at −10°C. Fifty per cent of the animals developed a weak complete antibody with occasional spontaneous autohemagglutination.

Holmes and Burnet (76) successfully employed papain treated erythrocytes and the antiglobulin test. Elution of the autoantibody was accomplished. Such eluates created positive indirect antiglobulin tests with mouse cells of any strain. Slight reactivity of the mouse autoantibody with rat erythrocytes was noted, but no reaction was found with erythrocytes from five other species. Limited cross adsorption tests did not indicate any particular mouse strain specificity. Holborow and associates (77) reported an additional erythrocyte autoantibody in the sera of NZB mice. This substance reacted with human erythrocytes as well as with mouse red cells. The antigen was not abundant but was stable and could be demonstrated on erythrocyte stromata and dried blood smears. The erythrocyte

autoantibody fixed complement. Adoptive immunization of young NZB mice was carried out with suspensions of viable spleen cells from older NZB mice with spontaneous autoimmune hemolytic anemia (78). The mouse erythrocyte autoantibody and the cross reacting human antibody were produced in recipient animals. Destruction of erythrocytes occurred through excessive hepatic and splenic sequestration.

Adrenocorticotrophic hormone (75), cortisone acetate (79) and betamethazone (80) therapy may induce dramatic hematologic remissions. Positive direct and indirect antiglobulin tests may be reduced in intensity or converted to negative. Splenectomy failed as a therapeutic procedure in the presence of active disease and in mice 6 months of age or older (75). Splenectomy performed in mice younger than 3 months of age modified the eventual clinical picture. Both pathologic and hematologic manifestations of the subsequent disease were less dramatic (75). Denman and associates (81) used antilymphocyte antiserum in NZB mice from age 2 months on. They were able to suppress the development of positive antiglobulin tests and hemolytic anemia. Antilymphocyte antiserum had no effect on adult mice with active disease.

In 1961 Helyer and Howie (75) noted positive LE cell preparations in approximately 4 per cent of the NZB mice. Norins and Holmes (82) demonstrated antinuclear factors in about 40 per cent of adult animals. The death of some animals from renal failure was concomitantly noted. Changes were found in the kidneys which resembled human lupus nephritis. Holmes and Burnet (76) described these changes as membranous glomerulonephritis. Howie and Helyer (83) also demonstrated renal hemosiderosis and hyalinization throughout the tufts of the glomeruli. The hyaline material was not fibrinoid and did not have the staining characteristics or distribution of amyloid. Hybridization procedures were performed by Howie and Helyer (83) using seven different New Zealand inbred strains. In each of the F_1 hybrids some form of autoimmune disorder developed. These authors suggested that the autoimmune characteristic was expressed in the heterozygous state and is inherited as a dominant trait. Hybrids obtained from NZB parentage on either the male or female side did not differ in the development of autoimmune disease. Transmission of the autoimmune abnormalities was not sex linked and a milk factor was ruled out. No linkage was apparent to the black coat color. In four of the hybrids (NZB × NZC, NZB × NZWZ, NZB × NZCW, NZB × NZG) an autoimmune hemolytic pattern developed similar to that found in the original NZB group. In the remaining three hybrids (NZB × NZW, NZB × NZY, NZB × NZF) the clinical disease pattern was altered. These F_1 hybrids had mild or transient autoimmune hemolytic anemia. The predominant clinical finding, however, was progressive azotemia with proteinuria. Positive LE cells were frequent and the kidney presented typical changes of lupus erythematosus. A 35 per cent incidence of positive LE cells was found in the NZB × NZY hybrids. A distinct sex difference was noted. LE cells were found in 55 per cent of females and in 18 per cent of males. An inverse relationship of age and severity of the pathologic state was noted. The NZB × NZW F_1 hybrid had striking pathologic lesions and a short life span. The NZB × NZF F_1 hybrids had more chronic appearing pathologic lesions and the longest life span. Female hybrids generally demonstrated stronger serologic tests which developed earlier than in the male hybrids. In addition, female hybrids had more marked pathologic lesions and more acute clinical courses. Preliminary studies suggested that the autoimmune defects can be transmitted into the F_2 generation. Additional hybridization studies have been reported by Holmes and Burnet (84–86).

The thymus gland showed proliferative changes in over 95 per cent of NZB mice 8 months or older (76). Developing germinal centers were found in expanding medullary areas. Such thymic germinal centers in the adult are distinctly abnormal and resemble normal germinal centers in the spleen and lymph nodes of the same mice. The time of appearance of thymic lesions was variable.

Fifty per cent of males showed recognizable thymic lesions in 240 days. The 50 per cent level of thymic lesions was reached at 175 days in female mice.

Howie and Helyer (83) investigated the role of the thymus gland in the immune process. The original NZB strain with autoimmune hemolytic anemia and NZB × NZW hybrids with a high incidence of lupus nephritis were employed. Neonatal thymectomy did not prevent the autoimmune disease from developing in the two groups. Neonatal thymectomy followed by transplantation of a normal newborn thymus also failed to prevent the development of autoimmune complications. Neonatal exchange grafting of thymus glands from the autoimmune strain into normal nonautoimmune mice created autoimmune diseases in the normal animals. Howie and Helyer speculate that epithelial reticular cells of the thymus carry the abnormal characteristics. These cells may induce their effect by means of a humoral substance acting on the host's lymphoid cells. It was noted that the autoimmune disease induced in grafted normal animals was consistent and unrelated to the strain of NZB mice or the F_1 hybrid employed. The development of a hemolytic or a lupus nephritis form of autoimmune disease was determined by the recipient animal rather than by the donor.

Bielschowsky and Bielschowsky in 1962 (87) noted the spontaneous occurrence of various tumors, i.e., thymoma, lymphocytic leukemia and reticulum cell sarcoma, in the 42nd generation of brother-sister mating of NZB mice. Exposure to the carcinogen 2-aminofluorene increased the incidence of malignancy 5-fold. Some of the tumors were successfully transplanted. Helyer and Howie (75) noted hyperplasia of the reticuloendothelium of NZB mice but could not document malignant transformation. Holmes and Burnet (76) recorded marked hyperplasia and possible malignancies which resembled plasmacytomas, reticulum cell tumors or leukemia. The incidence of lymphoid hyperplasia or tumor in NZB mice older than 400 days was 33 per cent in males and 50 per cent in females. East and associates (88) similarly noted malignant transformations in elderly NZB mice. Mellors (89) sacrificed 20 NZB mice of the 61st generation at 9 to 11 months of age. Reticulum cell sarcoma and pleomorphic malignant lymphomas were demonstrated in four animals. The tumors could be transplanted to other NZB recipients. East and associates demonstrated that the serial passage of lymphoid tissue from aging NZB mice produced reticulum cell neoplasia in BALB/c recipients (90) and in young NZB mice (91). Mellors (89) indicates that the stage of autoimmunization precedes the development of malignancy. Mellors and Huang (68, 69) and East and associates (91) described virus-like particles in the tumors found in NZB mice. Cell free extracts of such tumors were given to Swiss mice, which are free of the autoimmune stigma characteristic of the NZB group (69). The Swiss mice subsequently developed the autoimmune abnormalities as well as malignant transformations. These studies strongly suggest that the genetic implications developed by analysis of NZB mice may be erroneous and may reflect the vertical transmission of a virus. Prosser (92) has similarly documented virus particles in NZB and NZB × NZW F_1 hybrids. It is suggested that the virus is transmitted through the germ cells or placenta. Transmission of neoplasia by such viruses has not been accomplished, although spleen and lymph node cells will transfer reticulum cell neoplasia. It is suggested that neoplasia is cell mediated rather than virus mediated (92).

Other Spontaneous Autoimmune Animal Systems

The development of other spontaneous autoimmune animal systems is highly desirable. Jubb and Kennedy (93) and Lewis and associates (72) have reported histopathologic lesions suggestive of polyarteritis nodosa in cattle, sheep, hogs, horses, dogs, deer, mink and cats. Idiopathic thrombocytopenia purpura has been reported in dogs (94, 95). Lewis and associates (72) quote additional workers as having encountered autoimmune hemolytic anemia in domestic animals. Ristic (96) demon-

strated the presence of autoantibodies directed against bovine erythrocytes in cattle infected with *Anaplasma marginale*. Weber and Marshak (97) have implicated an autoimmune pathology as responsible for the anemia seen with bovine lymphosarcoma. Hemolytic anemia with a positive direct antiglobulin test was reported by Shadduck and Weickert (98) in a dog suffering from disseminated histoplasmosis.

Erythrocyte Autoantibodies and Human Autoimmune Hemolytic Anemia

For many years investigators have been aware of discrepancies between clinical and serologic aspects of human autoimmune hemolytic anemia. The qualitative and quantitative documentation of erythrocyte autoantibodies in the usual serologic testing frequently has little relationship to clinical evidence of hemolysis. Such variations have both theoretical and clinical significance.

Experience in Other Autoimmune Diseases

The demonstration of circulating autoantibodies directed against various host tissue components aroused tremendous interest. Such observations were extensively used in postulating etiologic mechanisms for many human diseases. The original enthusiasm has now been tempered with the realization that the presence or the level of circulating autoantibody may have no relationship to the clinical state of the patient. The lack of correlation between clinical and serologic features is particularly apparent with circulating thyroid autoantibodies and antigastric parietal cell antibodies and in lupus erythematosus.

The studies of Cammarata and associates (99) illustrate this problem. Anti-gamma-globulin factors were found in the sera of 16 per cent of 325 elderly subjects. Antinuclear factors were demonstrated in 36 per cent of 255 of these elderly subjects selected only upon the basis of age. Serafini and associates (100) have also recorded the presence of autoantibodies in normal subjects. As early as 1950 Thomas and associates (101) and Lumsdem and associates (102) demonstrated a lack of relationship between complement fixing anti-brain autoantibodies and experimentally induced encephalomyelitis. Paterson and associates (103) have expanded these observations. They noted that antibrain autoantibodies may actually exert a beneficial or protective effect in nervous tissue sensitization.

Clinical Experience in the Autoimmune Hemolytic Anemias

A direct relationship between erythrocyte autoantibodies and erythrocyte destruction appears logical and generally has been accepted for many years. This simple relationship, however, does not withstand close and critical scrutiny. A crude relationship does exist. The more severe degrees of hemolysis are frequently associated with strong antiglobulin and proteolytic enzyme reactions. In addition, the presence of unbound erythrocyte autoantibodies roughly correlates with marked erythrocyte destruction. This relationship is by no means universal. Discrepancies are sufficiently frequent to place in question the interrelationship between erythrocyte autoantibodies and erythrocyte destruction.

Many investigators have noted that antiglobulin testing, as an index of erythrocyte autoantibody production, may have little correlation with clinical hemolysis. Several clinical and serologic patterns are apparent. Acquired hemolytic anemia indistinguishable from autoimmune varieties can occur without demonstrable circulating erythrocyte autoantibodies. Erythrocyte autoantibodies can be found without hemolytic disease. When both conditions are present, therapy frequently results in correction of the hemolytic stage while autoantibody production continues. Identical hemolytic episodes can occur in the same patient and may be characterized by positive antiglobulin tests during one period and negative tests during another episode.

Weiner (104) has encountered a number of normal blood donors who presented with positive antiglobulin tests in the absence of disease. Twenty-one individuals were found in a donor population of 60,000. Seventeen subjects were males. None of

these has developed hematologic disease, although positive antiglobulin reactions may have persisted for many years. An erythrocyte survival time performed on one of these cases by Mollison (105) did not indicate premature destruction of erythrocytes. Speiser (106) also encountered three blood donors with positive antiglobulin tests in the absence of disease.

Erythrocyte destruction may not even occur with isoantibody sensitization (see Chapter 21). Quantitative antigen-antibody relationships are important (107–109). Wiener and Brancato (110) emphasized that factors other than erythrocyte antibodies and antigen containing erythrocytes are involved in hemolytic disease. They reported a newborn $Rh_o(D)$ infant with a strong positive direct antiglobulin reaction and high titer unbound anti-rhesus antibody who did not develop hemolysis during 2 months of observation. Similar observations have been made with isoantigen specific autoantibodies formed during alpha-methyldopa administration (111) and with the spontaneous development of auto anti-hr'(c) (112). Moller (113) reported that immunization of mice with erythrocytes incompatible at the H_2 locus led to antibody formation without destruction of erythrocytes. Transfusion of incompatible erythrocytes into animals containing antibodies resulted in the destruction of only a portion of the transfused red cells. The observations of Doljanski and associates (114) may be pertinent. They concluded that at least two distinct erythrocyte populations exist on the basis of size.

Evans and Duane (115) attempted to correlate erythrocyte survival with sensitization by erythrocyte autoantibodies. They employed serial dilutions of antiglobulin serum as a quantitative technique. A rough correlation was found between antiglobulin titer and activity of disease. A relationship was not apparent in all patients. In addition, positive antiglobulin tests persisted after 1 year of remission induced by splenectomy. Dameshek (116) noted a rough correlation between unbound erythrocyte autoantibody titers and erythrocyte survival times. Fudenberg and associates (117) studied eluates of erythrocyte autoantibodies and found a rough correlation between eluted N and antibody titers. Young and Miller (118) performed long term studies on patients with autoimmune hemolytic anemia. Nine of 23 did not manifest sufficient hemolysis to require therapy in spite of persistent positive antiglobulin tests. Holländer (119) transfused hr'(c/c) erythrocytes into an rh'(C) positive patient who was producing an anti-rh'(C) autoantibody. Normal erythrocyte survivals were noted. Culp and Chaplin (120) sensitized appropriate erythrocytes with erythrocyte autoantibodies and anti-Rh_o(D). Sequestration hemolysis was found with the isoantibody system. Erythrocytes sensitized with autoantibodies did not demonstrate premature destruction. Wiener and Brancato (110) reported a patient with a potent erythrocyte autoantibody who was studied for 2 years without evidence of hemolysis. Hennemann (121) also encountered patients with positive antiglobulin tests and minimal or no evidence of hemolysis. This pattern is repeatedly described in the clinical section of this volume.

The most extensive analysis of this problem was performed by Constantoulakis and associates (122) in 1963. They employed I^{131} labeled antiglobulin serum to quantitate iso- and autoantibodies bound to the erythrocyte surface. The accuracy of this technique is questionable; it was found unsatisfactory for quantitation by Pirofsky and associates (123) and Rossi and Bianchini (124). It is questionable whether Constantoulakis and associates (122) successfully solved this problem. Their results are striking, however, and clarify many aspects of erythrocyte antibody-erythrocyte reactions. In extreme antibody excess, seven molecules of antiglobulin serum combined with one warm acting antibody molecule. A marked heterogeneity of erythrocyte isoantibodies was noted. Biologic and serologic characteristics appeared to be unrelated. Similar amounts of anti-Rh_o(D) and anti-K fixed to erythrocytes led to entirely different erythrocyte survival times. The T/2 (half-life) of anti-Rh_o(D) coated red cells was 11

days; the T/2 of anti-K coated erythrocytes was 45 minutes. Two different anti-Rh_o(D) antibodies were studied and T/2 survival times of 11 days and of less than 1 day, respectively, were found. Constantoulakis and associates obtained 4+ direct antiglobulin reactions with anti-Rh_o(D) coated erythrocytes demonstrating normal survival times. Antibody sensitization in excess of 0.9 μg. of antibody N per ml. of red blood cells (RBC) induced pronounced effects on erythrocyte survival. Complete antigenic saturation was not necessary. Thirty per cent of antigenic saturation with anti-Rh_o(D) led to rapid erythrocyte destruction.

These investigators (122) studied 17 cases of autoimmune hemolytic anemia. Fifteen had shortened erythrocyte survival times and two were in remission. No correlation was found between red cell survival and the amount of autoantibody fixed to the erythrocyte surface. One case had a T/2 survival of only 3.5 days with only 0.4 μg. of antibody N per ml. of RBC. In contrast, other cases with mild hemolysis had as much as 5 μg. of antibody N per ml. of RBC.

The discrepancy between serologic activity and clinical disease is incontrovertible. Three possible explanations for this lack of correlation may be formulated.

Humoral Erythrocyte Autoantibodies Are Unrelated to the Hemolytic Process

In many autoimmune disease syndromes, circulating autoantibody has little if any causative significance. A similar lack of relationship exists in autoimmune hemolytic anemia. All humans produce cold acting erythrocyte autoantibodies. Hemolytic anemia due to such substances is rare. Warm acting erythrocyte autoantibodies can also be produced in normal healthy individuals without premature erythrocyte destruction (104, 106). When hemolysis does occur in the presence of erythrocyte autoantibodies these two factors may not exhibit any correlation. It can therefore be postulated that humoral erythrocyte autoantibody formation is unrelated to erythrocyte damage.

Acceptance of this hypothesis requires

an additional mechanism to explain erythrocyte destruction. Such mechanisms may be nonautoimmune or may involve autoimmune sequences unrelated to humoral antibody production. Waksman (125) reviewed experimental autoallergic diseases involving the central and peripheral nervous system, the thyroid gland, the adrenal gland, the testi and the lens and uvea of the eye. The pathologic lesions in such experimental conditions appear basically similar and strongly suggest delayed hypersensitivity. Waksman distinguishes these conditions from acquired hemolytic anemia, idiopathic thrombocytopenic purpura, systemic lupus erythematosus and paroxysmal cold hemoglobinuria, which may not involve delayed hypersensitivity.

van Loghem (126) has extended this viewpoint. He suggests that the abnormality in warm acting autoimmune hemolytic anemia is the proliferation of abnormal clones of immunocompetent cells producing both humoral and cell bound antibody. He emphasizes that "there is no relation between the severity of blood destruction and the autoantibody titer...." van Loghem postulates that delayed hypersensitivity or a fixed tissue form of immune interaction may be the primary immune mechanism responsible for red cell damage. A similar suggestion is pertinent to many autoimmune syndromes (127, 128).

Humoral Erythrocyte Autoantibodies Are Only Partially Related to the Hemolytic Process

Positive antiglobulin tests and erythrocyte damage may result from immune but not autoimmune mechanisms. This has been termed antiglobulin positive hemolytic anemia. Antibody formation following the modification of erythrocyte surface antigens is prominent in this category. This sequence would relegate erythrocyte antibodies to the status of a secondary phenomenon. The influence of such antibodies in producing a hemolytic state would be highly variable. The underlying pathologic state modifying the erythrocyte may be completely responsible for erythrocyte destruction. Erythrocyte antibody formation would then be causally unrelated to erythrocyte damage. The reverse may also exist. The initial modification of erythrocytes may not adversely influence cell survival. Erythrocyte antibody formation reflecting red cell antigenic modifications would then be entirely responsible for cell damage and hemolysis. Many variations may exist between these two extremes. Underlying cell damage and anti-erythrocyte antibodies may both contribute to cell destruction. The relative magnitudes of their influences will be reflected in clinical and serologic correlations and will result in the observed variations.

Humoral Erythrocyte Autoantibodies Are Responsible for the Hemolytic Process

The mechanisms discussed above are theoretical possibilities. Until such concepts receive experimental support it must be assumed that humoral erythrocyte autoantibodies induce hemolysis. Accepting this, we still must explain the lack of correlation between serologic testing and hemolysis. Three excellent reasons exist for this lack of correlation.

(a) **Validity of Serologic Tests.** The direct and indirect antiglobulin tests are the most frequently used procedures to demonstrate erythrocyte autoantibodies. Such tests are not designed to supply quantitative information indicating the number of antibody molecules bound to the erythrocyte surface (122–124, 129). Agglutination is the end point of this reaction. However, hemagglutination is only partially dependent on the actual number of antibody molecules. The pH and ionic strength of the medium and the zeta potential of the erythrocyte surface all contribute to the reaction. Agglutination can result from the manipulation of several of these nonimmunologic characteristics in the complete absence of erythrocyte autoantibodies (130). The situation is further confused by the presence of globulin molecules bound to the erythrocyte surface in a nonimmunologic fashion (131). Such globulins have the ability to bind antiglobulin serum without inducing agglutination (123).

Establishing a completely standard test system controlling these variables would not solve the problem of quantitation. Both autoantibodies and antiglobulin serum are variables in this test system. The interaction of these two substances takes place in an immunologic setting. In order to obtain quantitative figures, the reaction should be determined at the equivalence point. This is impossible to attain with current testing. Each antiglobulin serum differs in reactivity, and autoantibodies are heterogeneous in their reaction with antiglobulin serum and the erythrocyte surface (see Chapter 18).

The direct antiglobulin test is particularly ill suited for quantitative interpretation. Positive reactions are graded as 1+ to 4+ agglutination. A patient who has had a 4+ reaction may be retested after therapeutic remission and still reveal a 4+ reaction. Although the number of antibody molecules fixed to the erythrocyte surface may be substantially reduced, there still may be a sufficient number to induce the strong reaction. The reverse problem also exists. Can we interpret a 2+ direct antiglobulin reaction as indicating a smaller number of antibody molecules fixed to the erythrocyte than the number found in a 4+ reaction? If the antiglobulin serum is diluted 4-fold the first case may now have a 4+ reaction while the second example has a 2+ reaction. Which erythrocytes have more antibody fixed to the erythrocyte surface?

The direct antiglobulin test may be performed with varying dilutions of antiglobulin serum. Can results obtained with such dilutions be used to quantitate the reaction? The same problem arises. Such dilutions are valuable only to approximate the equivalence zone of antibody-antigen union. The strongest reaction obtained would approximate the equivalence zone, and quantitative studies may be performed at this level. However, this determination loses its significance as soon as different antiglobulin reagents are employed or different autoantibodies are studied.

This review suggests that the degree of agglutination of antibody coated erythrocytes by antiglobulin serum reflects so many variables that quantitation is impossible. The magnitude of agglutination does not necessarily reflect the number, avidity or biologic activity of the erythrocyte antibody (122). Serologic procedures based on the antiglobulin reaction cannot be employed to estimate the degree of antibody fixation. It is not surprising that antiglobulin testing does not correlate with the degree of hemolysis.

Enzyme procedures are also inadequate for obtaining quantitative data concerning antibody fixation to the erythrocyte surface. The above described limitations of agglutination reactions are again applicable. Evidence has been presented that bromelin (132), papain (133) and ficin (134) substantially increase the fixation of antibody molecules to erythrocytes. However, such enzymes may induce agglutination with fewer incomplete autoantibodies fixed to the erythrocyte surface than were initially present and not agglutinating untreated cells (132).

The enzyme procedures offer the advantage of not being biologic. This permits the establishment of a reproducible standard reagent. Proteolytic enzyme test systems are thought not to show a prozone phenomenon as was described for antiglobulin serum. This observation must be questioned. The author has seen the inhibition or reduction of hemagglutination in both bromelin and papain systems. These can be eliminated by further dilutions of the antibody containing serum. This occurrence is uncommon, however, when compared to the frequency with which it is seen in undiluted antiglobulin serum. Enzyme procedures are not dependent on immunologic reactions. Accordingly, the limitations of quantitation at the equivalence point required for antiglobulin serum do not necessarily apply. The avoidance of prozones, the availability of a standard reagent and the ability to function in a nonimmune setting suggest that proteolytic enzymes may supply adequate quantitative systems. Such systems have been established for erythrocyte isoantibodies using the AutoAnalyzer (135). A direct quantitation of numbers of antibody molecules inducing agglutination has been possible with such approaches. The expansion of these important studies into the routine quantitation of erythrocyte autoantibodies offers great potential benefits.

(b) Heterogeneity of Erythrocyte Autoantibodies. Even if we might accurately and routinely determine the numbers of autoantibodies bound to the erythrocyte surface, it still might not be possible to correlate clinical hemolysis with the serologic test. Such erythrocyte autoantibodies are heterogeneous and will vary in avidity for the erythrocyte and in their biologic property of inducing damage (122). Erythrocyte autoantibodies probably have an additional point of variation. Warm acting erythrocyte autoantibodies may have molecular structures complementary to parts of the rhesus antigenic molecule. Accordingly they differ from isoantibodies reacting with a specific antigenic determinant. If this hypothesis is true, then the degree of "fit" of erythrocyte autoantibody assumes a major role in the kinetics of antibody association and dissociation with erythrocyte surface antigens. It appears logical to assume also that the degree of fit will play a significant role in initiating erythrocyte damage. This would have maximal influence with noncomplement fixing warm acting erythrocyte autoantibodies.

The ratio of autoantibody production to erythrocyte formation must also be considered. The antiglobulin test and proteolytic enzyme procedures are exquisitely sensitive. Although antibody production may easily be demonstrated by such agglutinating tests, the biologic activity of such antibodies must function in the presence of huge amounts of antigenic substances. The avidity and toxicity of such antibodies in the presence of antigen excess will influence cellular destruction independently of the agglutination reaction.

(c) In Vitro Testing and in Vivo Hemolysis. Hemolysis is the end state of several pathophysiologic processes, rather than a simple reflection of antibody action. The age of erythrocytes involved in immunologic damage will influence the degree of hemolysis. Older erythrocytes, with a lack of reserve for glycolytic homeostasis, may be more vulnerable to the action of some antibodies. This sensitivity of older cells may be unimportant in the action of other antibodies. Excessive antibody induced damage may initiate the random destruction of all erythrocytes irrespective of age.

The capacity of the reticuloendothelium to sequestrate and destroy antibody coated erythrocytes is probably the most important in vivo variable. Experimental heteroimmune and isoantibody systems reflect the destructive action of a single massive in vivo introduction of antibody. Human autoimmune hemolytic anemia differs by presenting a chronic hemolytic process. In such states the capability of the spleen to destroy erythrocytes may be saturated to a greater or lesser extent. The activation of hepatic sequestration or even bone marrow sequestration offers a further variable. All of these in vivo factors combine to influence the degree of correlation observed between serologic testing and clinical hemolytic anemia.

The experimental studies of Jandl and Kaplan (108), Mollison (105) and Mollison and Hughes-Jones (109) indicate that the level of isoantibody erythrocyte sensitization correlates with the degree and rate of erythrocyte destruction. Fudenberg and associates (117) studied erythrocyte autoantibody eluates and suggested that a similar relationship exists in autoimmune hemolytic anemia.

When routine serologic tests are employed to indicate the degree of erythrocyte sensitization, the correlation appears less impressive (136). Evans and associates (129, 137) have emphasized the inability of the usual test systems to evaluate accurately a patient with autoimmune hemolytic anemia. They suggest that a more accurate determination of erythrocyte autoantibody activity can be obtained by quantitating the dissociation of autoantibody from the erythrocyte surface. Their data indicate that hemolysis in warm acting autoimmune hemolytic disease reflects the concentration of antibodies fixed to the cell and free in the plasma (129, 137). The free and the adsorbed warm acting erythrocyte autoantibodies are in dynamic equilibrium.

Changes in concentration of one phase are reflected by changes in concentration of the other. This concept is supported by the observation that strong positive direct antiglobulin tests may persist in the presence of therapeutic remissions. In such cases the indirect antiglobulin test generally becomes negative, indicating a reduction of dissociated antibody. Evans and associates (129, 137) suggest that the dissociation rate of autoantibody from the erythrocyte surface correlates best with the clinical state of the disease. In contrast, the degree of positivity of the direct antiglobulin test may not reflect hemolysis. Little or no dissociation of erythrocyte autoantibody from coated erythrocytes indicates a small amount of cell bound antibody. However, even such small amounts of antibody may produce 4+ agglutination reactions with antiglobulin serum. Goodman and Masaitus (138) have attempted to document the factors involved in antibody association to and dissociation from cellular surfaces.

Summary of the Relationship of Erythrocyte Autoantibody to In Vivo Hemolysis

There are insufficient data to establish conclusively a quantitative causative relationship between erythrocyte autoantibodies and erythrocyte destruction. In vitro test tube determinations of autoantibody titers and the degree of positivity of direct antiglobulin or proteolytic enzyme tests are of little value in predicting the severity of the hemolytic disease. It may be true that erythrocyte autoantibodies are simply a secondary phenomenon and not primarily related to red cell destruction. Possibly we have even been studying the wrong immunologic test system. Cell bound antibody functioning in delayed hypersensitivity may be the primary mechanism for cell damage. However, it is premature to discard humoral erythrocyte autoantibody formation as the single most important factor inducing erythrocyte damage in autoimmune hemolytic anemia.

Current serologic tests are inadequate for the accurate quantitation of erythrocyte autoantibody activity. This fact should act as a stimulus to devise more precise test systems relating the immunologic event to the clinical disease. In vivo hemolysis is a complex pathophysiologic state, and the autoantibody exerts its influence within this complex state. An awareness of these limitations in the role of the antibody and, therefore, of tests employed to demonstrate the antibody is important in monitoring patients with autoimmune hemolytic anemia. The clinician should not make the error of ascribing too much significance to a single laboratory test procedure. Autoantibody heterogeneity, variations in the reticuloendothelium, the compensatory capacity of the bone marrow and the presence of associated pathologic states must all be considered concomitantly with the results of serologic tests in order to obtain a meaningful, composite picture of autoimmune hemolytic anemia.

BIBLIOGRAPHY

1. Lüdke, H.: Klinische und experimentelle Untersuchungen über den hämolytischen Ikterus. Munchen. Med. Wschr. 65: 1098, 1918.
2. Wagley, P. F., and Castle, W. B.: Destruction of red blood cells. VII. Apparent autosensitization to dog red blood cells. Proc. Soc. Exp. Biol. Med. 72: 411, 1949.
3. Liu, C. K., and Evans, R. S.: Production of positive antiglobulin serum test in rabbits by intraperitoneal injection of homologous blood. Proc. Soc. Exp. Biol. Med. 79: 194, 1952.
4. Motulsky, A. G., and Crosby, W. H.: Experimental production of red cell autoimmunization (abstract). Amer. J. Med. 17: 102, 1954.
5. Cajano, A., Miller, A., Finch, S. C., and Ross, J. F.: Autoimmunization to blood cells. Sang. 26: 141, 1955.
6. Stadsbaeder, S.: Différences des auto-anticorps au cours des anémies hémolytiques. Acta Clin. Belg. 11: 78, 1956.
7. Hamamoto, Y., and Yoshikawa, S.: Experimental auto-immune hemolytic anemia. Hematological observation. Acta Haemat. Jap. 26: 650, 1963.
8. Wiener, A. S.: Origin of naturally occurring hemagglutinins and hemolysins: a review. J. Immun. 66: 287, 1951.
9. Stefanini, M., Magalini, S. I., and Patterson, J. H.: The relation of neoplastic tissue antigens to "autoimmune" hematologic syndromes (abstract). Clin. Res. Proc. 4: 82, 1956.

10. Kissmeyer-Nielsen, F., Bichel, J., and Bjerre Hanson, P.: Specific autoantibodies in immunohaemolytic anaemia. Acta Haemat. (Basel) 15: 189, 1956.
11. Aubert, A., and Brendemoen, O. J.: Acquired hemolytic anemia and lymphoblastoma. Scand. J. Clin. Lab. Invest. 1: 95, 1949.
12. Wiener, A. S., Gordon, E. B., and Gallop, C.: Studies on autoantibodies in human sera. J. Immun. 71: 58, 1953.
13. Suzuki, T.: Morbus banti and autoimmune hemolytic anemia. In Proceedings of the Seventh International Congress of the International Society of Hematology. Il Pensiero Scientifico, Rome, 1960.
14. Korn, R. J., Yakulis, V. J., Lemke, C. E., and Chomet, B.: Cold agglutinins in Listeria monocytogenes infections. Arch. Intern. Med. (Chicago) 99: 573, 1957.
15. Costea, N., Yakulis, V., and Heller, P.: Experimental production of cold agglutinins in rabbits. Blood 26: 323, 1965.
16. Smith, C. B., McGinniss, M. H., and Schmidt, P. J.: Changes in erythrocyte I agglutinogen and anti-I agglutinins during Mycoplasma pneumoniae infection in man. J. Immun. 99: 333, 1967.
17. Zmijewski, C. M.: The production of erythrocyte autoantibodies in chimpanzees. J. Exp. Med. 121: 657, 1965.
18. Samaille, J., Ropartz, C., and Eyquem, A.: Anémie hémolytique expérimentale par hétéro-immunsérums chez le chien. Mise en évidence à l'aide de la réaction directe de Coombs, de la fixation des protéins de l' animal sur ses propres globules rouges. Ann. Inst. Pasteur (Paris) 85: 48, 1953.
19. Muratore, E., Cervellera, G., and Gardai, G.: Role of incomplete auto-antibodies in production of experimental haemolytic anaemia induced by small doses of haemolytic serum. Acta Haemat. (Basel) 10: 233, 1953.
20. Lille-Szyszlkowicz, I., and Chojnacka, J.: Anémie hémolytique expérimentale. Etude sérologique. Sang 26: 13, 1955.
21. Bowman, H. S., Brason, F. W., Mohn, J. F., and Lambert, R. M.: Experimental transfusion of donor plasma containing blood-group antibodies into incompatible normal human recipients. II. Induction of isoimmune hemolytic anemia by a transfusion of plasma containing exceptional anti-CD antibodies. Brit. J. Haemat. 7: 130, 1961.
22. Mohn, J. F., Lambert, R. M., Bowman, H. S., and Brason, F. W.: Experimental production in man of autoantibodies with Rh specificity. Ann. N. Y. Acad. Sci. 124: 477, 1965.
23. Billingham, R. E., and Brent, L.: A simple method for inducing tolerance of skin homografts in mice. Transplant. Bull. 4: 67, 1957.
24. Simonsen, M.: Biological incompatibility in kidney transplantation in dogs. II. Serologi-cal investigations. Acta Path. Microbiol. Scand. 32: 36, 1953.
25. Muirhead, E. E., and Groves, M.: Homogenous renal transplantation in dogs, associated positive Coombs test and anemia. Arch. Path. (Chicago) 59: 223, 1955.
26. Simonsen, M.: The impact on the developing embryo and newborn animal of adult homologous cells. Acta Path. Microbiol. Scand. 40: 480, 1957.
27. Cock, A. G., and Simonsen, M.: Immunological attack on newborn chickens by injecting adult cells. Immunology 1: 103, 1958.
28. Simonsen, M., and Jensen, E.: The graft vs. host assay in transplantation chimeras. In Biological Problems of Grafting, ed. by F. Albert and P. B. Medawar. Blackwell Scientific Publications, Ltd., Oxford, 1959.
29. Porter, K. A.: Immune haemolysis in rabbit radiation-chimaeras. Brit. J. Exp. Path. 41: 72, 1960.
30. Porter, K. A.: Immune hemolysis: A feature of secondary disease and runt disease in the rabbit. Ann. N. Y. Acad. Sci. 87: 391, 1960.
31. Piomelli, S., and Brooke, M. S.: An immune hemolytic anemia as a component of secondary disease in rabbit radiation chimeras. Transplant. Bull. 7: 428, 1960.
32. Meier, H., and Brown, B.: The "runt disease" syndrome associated with immune hemolytic anemia and splenomegaly. Sang 30: 776, 1959.
33. Trentin, J. J.: An entity resembling homologous disease induced by transplantation of lymphoid tissue in unirradiated mice (abstract). Fed. Proc. 17: 461, 1958.
34. Oliner, H., Schwartz, R., and Dameshek, W.: Studies in experimental autoimmune disorders. I. Clinical and laboratory features of autoimmunization (runt disease) in the mouse. Blood 17: 20, 1961.
35. Lewis, F. B., Schwartz, R. S., and Dameshek, W.: X-radiation and alkylating agents as possible "trigger" mechanisms in the autoimmune complications of malignant lymphoproliferative disease. Clin. Exp. Immun. 1: 1, 1966.
36. Harriss, E., Currie, C., Kriss, J. P., and Kaplan, H. S.: Studies on anemia in F₁ hybrid mice injected with parenteral strain lymphoid cells. J. Exp. Med. 113: 1095, 1961.
37. Stastny, P., Stembridge, V. A., Vischer, T. L., and Ziff, M.: Homologous disease, a model for autoimmune disease. Ann. N. Y. Acad. Sci. 124: 158, 1965.
38. Schwartz, R. S., and Beldotti, L.: Malignant lymphomas following allogenic disease: transition from an immunological to a neoplastic disorder. Science 149: 1511, 1965.
39. Armstrong, M. Y., Andre-Schwartz, J., and Schwartz, R. S.: Immunological homeostasis and leukemia: an experimental model

in the mouse. In *Perspectives in Leukemia.* Grune & Stratton, Inc., New York, 1968.

40. Billingham, R. E.: Immune tolerance and autoimmune disease. Paper presented at the Second Annual Meeting of the American Society of Hematology, St. Louis, November 23, 1959.

41. Green, I., Inkelas, M., and Allen, L. B.: Hodgkin's disease: a maternal-to-foetal lymphocyte chimera? Lancet 1: 30, 1960.

42. Schapiro, M.: Familial autohemolytic anemia and runting syndrome with Rh₀ specific antibody. Transfusion 7: 281, 1967.

43. Pirofsky, B., Sutherland, D. W., Starr, A., and Griswold, H. E.: Hemolytic anemia complicating aortic-valve surgery. New Eng. J. Med. 272: 235, 1965.

44. Metcalf, D.: The thymic origin of the plasma lymphocytosis stimulating factor. Brit. J. Cancer 10: 442, 1956.

45. MacLean, L. D., Zak, S. J., Verco, R. L., and Good, R. A.: The role of the thymus in antibody production: an experimental study of the immune response in thymectomized rabbits. Transplant. Bull. 4: 21, 1957.

46. Metcalf, D.: The effects of thymectomy on the lymphoid tissues of the mouse. Brit. J. Haemat. 6: 324, 1960.

47. Miller, J. F. A. P., Doak, S. M. A., and Cross, A. M.: Role of the thymus in the recovery of the immune mechanism of the irradiated adult mouse. Proc. Soc. Exp. Biol. Med. 112: 785, 1963.

48. Archer, O., and Pierce, J. C.: Role of thymus in development of the immune response. Fed. Proc. 20: 26, 1961.

49. Janković, B. D., Waksman, B. H., and Arnason, B. G.: Role of the thymus in immune reactions in rats. I. The immunologic response to bovine serum albumin (antibody formation, arthus reactivity, and delayed hypersensitivity) in rats thymectomized or splenectomized at various times after birth. J. Exp. Med. 116: 159, 1962.

50. Miller, J. F. A. P.: Immunological function of the thymus. Lancet 2: 748, 1961.

51. Martinez, C., Kersey, J., Papermaster, B. W., and Good, R. A.: Skin homograft survival in thymectomized mice. Proc. Soc. Exp. Biol. Med. 109: 193, 1962.

52. Arnason, B. G., Janković, B. D., and Waksman, B. H.: Effect of thymectomy on "delayed" hypersensitive reactions. Nature (London) 194: 99, 1962.

53. Arnason, B. G., Janković, B. D., Waksman, B. H., and Wennersten, C.: Role of the thymus in immune reactions in rats. II. Suppressive effect of thymectomy at birth on reactions of delayed (cellular) hypersensitivity and the circulating small lymphocyte. J. Exp. Med. 116: 177, 1962.

54. Waksman, B. H., Arnason, B. G., and Janković, B. D.: Role of the thymus in immune reactions in rats. III. Changes in

the lymphoid organs of thymectomized rats. J. Exp. Med. 116: 187, 1962.

55. Good, R. A., Peterson, R. D. A., Martinez, C., Sutherland, D. E. R., Kellum, M. J., and Finstad, J.: The thymus in immunobiology: with special reference to autoimmune disease. Ann. N. Y. Acad. Sci. 124: 73, 1965.

56. Glick, B.: Growth and function of the bursae of Fabricius. Poult. Sci. 34: 1196, 1955.

57. Jolly, J.: La bourse de Fabricius et les organes lympho-épithéliaux. Arch. Anat. Micr. Morph. Exp. 16: 363, 1915.

58. Burnet, F. M.: The immunological significance of the thymus: an extension of the clonal selection theory of immunity. Aust. Ann. Med. 11: 79, 1962.

59. Burnet, F. M., and Holmes, M. C.: Immunological function of thymus and bursa of Fabricius. Thymus lesions in an autoimmune disease of mice. Nature (London) 194: 146, 1962.

60. Burnet, F. M., and MacKay, I. R.: Lympho-epithelial structures and autoimmune disease. Lancet 2: 1030, 1962.

61. Miller, J. F. A. P.: Role of the thymus in transplantation immunity. Ann. N. Y. Acad. Sci. 99: 340, 1962.

62. Yunis, E. J., Hilgard, H. R., Martinez, C., and Good, R. A.: Studies on immunologic reconstitution of thymectomized mice. J. Exp. Med. 121: 607, 1965.

63. Miller, J. F. A. P., Osoba, D., and Dukor, P.: A humoral thymus mechanism responsible for immunologic maturation. Ann. N. Y. Acad. Sci. 124: 95, 1965.

64. Kellum, M. J., Sutherland, D. E., Eckert, E., Peterson, R. D. A., and Good, R. A.: Wasting disease, Coombs-positivity, and amyloidosis in rabbits subjected to central lymphoid tissue extirpation and irradiation. Int. Arch. Allerg. 27: 6, 1965.

65. Miller, J. F. A. P., Ting, R. C., and Law, L. W.: Influence of thymectomy on tumor induction by polyoma virus in C57 Bl mice. Proc. Soc. Exp. Biol. Med. 116: 323, 1964.

66. Jacox, R. F., Mongan, E. S., Hanshaw, J. B., and Leddy, J. P.: Hypogammaglobulinemia with thymoma and probable pulmonary infection with cytomegalovirus. New Eng. J. Med. 271: 1091, 1964.

67. Mongan, E. S., Kern, W. A., and Terry, R.: Hypogammaglobulinemia with thymoma, hemolytic anemia, and disseminated infection with cytomegalovirus. Ann. Intern. Med. 65: 548, 1966.

68. Mellors, R. C., and Huang, C. Y.: Immunopathology of NZB/Bl mice. V. Virus-like (filterable) agent separable from lymphoma cells and identifiable by electron microscopy. J. Exp. Med. 124: 1031, 1966.

69. Mellors, R. C., and Huang, C. Y.: Immunopathology of NZB/Bl mice. VI. Virus sep-

arable from spleen and pathogenic for Swiss mice. J. Exp. Med. **126**: 53, 1967.

70. Miller, G., Firth, F. W., Swisher, S. N., and Young, L. E.: Studies on the destruction of red blood cells by canine autoantibodies in normal dogs and in a dog with naturally occurring autoimmune hemolytic disease. Amer. J. Dis. Child. **93**: 35, 1957.

71. Lewis, R. M., Henry, W. B., Thornton, G. W., and Gilmore, C. E.: A syndrome of autoimmune hemolytic anemia and thrombocytopenia in dogs. Sci. Proc. Amer. J. Vet. Ass. **1**: 140, 1963.

72. Lewis, R. M., Schwartz, R. S., and Gilmore, C. E.: Autoimmune diseases in domestic animals. Ann. N. Y. Acad. Sci. **124**: 178, 1965.

73. Lewis, R. M., Schwartz, R., and Henry, W. B.: Canine systemic lupus erythematosis. Blood **25**: 143, 1965.

74. Bielschowsky, M., Helyer, B. J., and Howie, J. B.: Spontaneous hemolytic anemia in mice of the NZB/Bl strain. Proc. Univ. Otago Med. Sch. **37**: 9, 1959.

75. Helyer, B. J., and Howie, J. B.: Spontaneous autoimmune disease in NZB/Bl mice. Brit. J. Haemat. **9**: 119, 1963.

76. Holmes, M. C., and Burnet, F. M.: The natural history of autoimmune disease in NZB mice. Ann. Intern. Med. **59**: 265, 1963.

77. Holborow, E. J., Barnes, R. D. S., and Tuffrey, M.: A new red-cell autoantibody in NZB mice. Nature (London) **207**: 601, 1965.

78. Barnes, R. D. S., and Tuffrey, M.: Sites of red cell destruction in the haemolytic anaemia of adoptively immunized NZB mice. Brit. J. Haemat. **12**: 717, 1966.

79. Giltinan, P. J., Holmes, M. C., and Burnet, F. M.: Cortisone acetate treatment of haemolytic anaemia in NZB mice. Aust. J. Exp. Biol. Med. Sci. **43**: 523, 1965.

80. Casey, T. P., and Howie, J. B.: Autoimmune hemolytic anemia in NZB/B1 mice treated with the corticosteroid drug betamethasone. Blood **25**: 423, 1965.

81. Denman, A. M., Denman, E. J., and Holborow, E. J.: Suppression of Coombs positive haemolytic anaemia in NZB mice by anti-lymphocytic globulin. Lancet **1**: 1084, 1967.

82. Norins, L. C., and Holmes, M. C.: Antinuclear factor in mice, J. Immun. **93**: 897, 1964.

83. Howie, J. B., and Helyer, B. J.: Autoimmune disease in mice. Ann. N. Y. Acad. Sci. **124**: 167, 1965.

84. Holmes, M. C., and Burnet, F. M.: The inheritance of autoimmune disease in mice: a study of hybrids of the strains NZB and C3H. Heredity (London) **19**: 419, 1964.

85. Burnet, F. M., and Holmes, M. C.: Genetic

86. Burnet, F. M.: The Harben lectures 1966. Implications for autoimmune disease in man of studies on NZB mice and their hybrids. 1. Autoimmune hemolytic anemia. J. Roy. Inst. Public Health **29**: 87, 1966.

87. Bielschowsky, M., and Bielschowsky, F.: Reaction of the reticular tissue of mice with autoimmune haemolytic anaemia to 2-aminofluorene. Nature (London) **194**: 692, 1962.

88. East, J., de Sousa, M. A. B., and Parrott, D. M. V.: Immunopathology of New Zealand black (NZB) mice. Transplantation **3**: 711, 1965.

89. Mellors, R. C.: Autoimmune disease in NZB-B1 mice. II. Autoimmunity and malignant lymphoma. Blood **27**: 435, 1966.

90. East, J., and Prosser, P. R.: Autoimmunity and malignancy in New Zealand Black mice. Proc. Roy. Soc. Med. **60**: 823, 1967.

91. East, J., de Sousa, M. A. B., Prosser, P. R., and Jaquet, H.: Malignant changes in New Zealand black mice. Clin. Exp. Immun. **2**: 427, 1967.

92. Prosser, P. R.: Particles resembling murine leukaemia virus in New Zealand black mice. Clin. Exp. Immun. **3**: 213, 1968.

93. Jubb, K. V. F., and Kennedy, P. C.: *Pathology of Domestic Animals*. Academic Press, New York, 1963.

94. Magrane, H. J., Magrane, W. G., and Ross, J. R.: ITP in a dog: a case report. J. Amer. Vet. Med. Ass. **135**: 520, 1959.

95. Waye, J. W.: ITP in a dog. Canad. Vet. **1**: 569, 1960.

96. Ristic, M.: Studies in anaplasmosis. III. An autoantibody and symptomatic macrocytic anemia. Amer. J. Vet. Res. **22**: 871, 1961.

97. Weber, W. T., and Marshak, R. K.: A correlative study of bone marrow and peripheral blood in bovine lymphosarcoma. Amer. J. Vet. Res. **24**: 515, 1963.

98. Shadduck, J., and Weickert, J.: Acute disseminated histoplasmosis accompanied by anemia. Speculum **16**: 5, 1963.

99. Cammarata, R. J., Rodman, G. P., and Fennell, R. H.: Serum anti-γ-globulin and anti-nuclear factors in the aged. J. A. M. A. **199**: 455, 1967.

100. Serafini, U., Torrigiani, G., and Masala, C.: L'incidenza degli auto-anticorpi nella popolazione normale. Folia Allerg. (Roma) **12**: 79, 1965.

101. Thomas, L., Paterson, P. Y., and Smithwick, B.: Acute disseminated encephalomyelitis following immunization with homologous brain extracts. I. Studies on the role of a circulating antibody in the production of the condition in dogs. J. Exp. Med. **92**: 133, 1950.

102. Lumsden, C. E., Kabat, E. A., Wolf, A., and Bezer, A. E.: Studies on acute dissemi-

nated encephalomyelitis produced experimentally in rhesus monkeys. V. Complement-fixing antibodies. J. Exp. Med. **92:** 253, 1950.

103. Paterson, P. Y., Jacobs, A. F., and Coia, E. M.: Complement-fixing antibrain antibodies and allergic encephalomyelitis. II. Further studies concerning their protective role. Ann. N. Y. Acad. Sci. **124:** 292, 1965.

104. Weiner, W.: "Coombs positive" "normal" people. Bibl. Haemat. **23:** 35, 1965.

105. Mollison, P. L.: *Blood Transfusion in Clinical Medicine,* Ed. 4. Blackwell Scientific Publication, Ltd., Oxford, 1967.

106. Speiser, P.: Some remarks on human erythrocytic autoantibodies. Z. Immunitaetsforsch. **132:** 113, 1967.

107. Mollison, P. L., and Paterson, J. C. S.: Survival after transfusion of Rh positive erythrocytes previously incubated with Rh antibody. J. Clin. Path. **2:** 109, 1949.

108. Jandl, J. H., and Kaplan, M. E.: The destruction of red cells by antibodies in man. III. Quantitative factors influencing the pattern of hemolysis in vivo. J. Clin. Invest. **39:** 1145, 1960.

109. Mollison, P. L., and Hughes-Jones, N. C.: Clearance of Rh-positive red cells by low concentrations of Rh antibody. Immunology. **12:** 63, 1967.

110. Wiener, A. S., and Brancato, G. J.: Rh hemolytic disease and autohemolytic disease. The possible role of agents other than antibodies in their pathogenesis. Exp. Med. Surg. **19:** 344, 1961.

111. Carstairs, K. C., Breckenridge, A., Dollery, C. T., and Worlledge, S. M.: Incidence of a positive direct Coombs test in patients on alpha-methyldopa. Lancet **2:** 133, 1966.

112. Bell, C. A., Zwicker, H., and Sacks, H. J.: Auto anti-hr' in the absence of anemia. Transfusion **7:** 51, 1967.

113. Möller, G.: Resistance of erythrocytes to isoantibody effects in vivo and in vitro. Bibl. Haemat. **23:** 203, 1965.

114. Doljanski, F., Zajicek, G., and Naaman, J.: The size distribution of normal human red blood cells. Life Sci. **5:** 2095, 1966.

115. Evans, R. S., and Duane, R. T.: Acquired hemolytic anemia. I. The relation of erythrocyte antibody production to activity of the disease. II. The significance of thrombocytopenia and leukopenia. Blood **4:** 1196, 1949.

116. Dameshek, W.: Acquired hemolytic anemia. Physiopathology with particular reference to autoimmunization and therapy. In *Proceedings of the Third International Congress of the International Society of Hematology.* William Heinemann, Ltd., London, 1951.

117. Fudenberg, H., Barry, I., and Dameshek, W.: The erythrocyte-coating substance in autoimmune hemolytic disease: its nature and significance. Blood **13:** 201, 1958.

118. Young, L. E., and Miller, G.: The long term picture in auto-immune hemolytic disease. Trans. Ass. Amer. Physicians **66:** 190, 1953.

119. Holländer, L.: Study of the erythrocytes survival time in a case of acquired haemolytic anaemia. Vox Sang. **4:** 164, 1954.

120. Culp, N. W., and Chaplin, H.: The effects of concentrated eluted anti-red blood cell antibodies on the in vivo survival of normal red blood cells. Blood **15:** 525, 1960.

121. Hennemann, H. H.: Positiver Coombs-test als einziger Befund: klinische Aspekte. Bibl. Haemat. **23:** 30, 1965.

122. Constantoulakis, M., Costea, N., Schwartz, R. S., and Dameshek, W.: Quantitative studies of the effect of red-blood-cell sensitization on in vivo hemolysis. J. Clin. Invest. **42:** 1790, 1963.

123. Pirofsky, B., Cordova, M. S., and Imel, T. L.: The mechanism of action of antiglobulin serum. Vox Sang. **7:** 348, 1962.

124. Rossi, V., and Bianchini, E.: Studies on the antiglobulin reaction with ^{131}I-labelled antibodies. Brit. J. Haemat. **8:** 163, 1962.

125. Waksman, B. H.: *Experimental Allergic Encephalomyelitis and the "Auto-allergic" Diseases.* S. Karger, Basel, 1959.

126. van Loghem, J. J.: Some comments on autoantibody induced red cell destruction. Ann. N. Y. Acad. Sci. **124:** 465, 1965.

127. Hall, R.: Immunologic aspects of thyroid function. New Eng. J. Med. **266:** 1204, 1962.

128. Roitt, I. M., and Doniach, D.: Delayed hypersensitivity in auto-immune disease. Brit. Med. Bull. **23:** 66, 1967.

129. Evans, R. S., Bingham, M., and Boehni, P.: Autoimmune hemolytic disease. Antibody dissociation and activity. Arch. Intern. Med. (Chicago) **108:** 60, 1961.

130. August, A., and Pirofsky, B.: Interaction of basic polyelectrolytes and human blood: the effect of antiheparin agents. Transfusion **6:** 74, 1966.

131. Pirofsky, B., Cordova, M., and Imel, T. L.: The nonimmunologic reaction of globulin molecules with the erythrocyte surface. Vox Sang. **7:** 334, 1962.

132. Pirofsky, B., Cordova, M., and Imel, T. L.: The function of proteolytic enzymes and tannic acid in inducing erythrocyte agglutination. J. Immun. **89:** 767, 1962.

133. Masouredis, S. P.: Reaction of I[131] anti-Rh₀(D) with enzyme treated red cells. Transfusion **2:** 363, 1962.

134. Hughes-Jones, N. C., Gardner, B., and Telford, R.: The effect of ficin on the reaction between anti-D and red cells. Vox Sang. **6:** 175, 1964.

135. Rosenfield, R. E., and Kochwa, S.: Immunochemical studies of the Rh system. III. Quantitative hemagglutination that is rel-

atively independent of source of Rh antigens and antibodies. Cold Spring Harbor Symposia on Quantitative Biology **29:** 427, 1964.

136. Pirofsky, B.: Serologic and clinical findings in autoimmune hemolytic anemia. Series Haemat. **9:** 47, 1965.

137. Evans, R. S., Bingham, M., and Turner, E.:

Autoimmune hemolytic disease: observations of serological reactions and disease activity. Ann. N. Y. Acad. Sci. **124:** 422, 1965.

138. Goodman, H. S., and Masaitus, L.: The dissociation of hemolytic antibody from sensitized cells as measured by cell to cell transfer. J. Immuno. **85:** 391, 1960.

Index

Etiology—*continued*
 multisystem immunologic disease, 9, 39, 44, 83, 177, 222, 321, 363, 373, 479
  with associated diseases, 139, 149
Euglobulin, 437, 446
Evans' syndrome, 47, 73, 82, 507
 association
  autoimmune hemolytic anemia, 47
  systemic lupus erythematosus, 82
Experimental syndromes
 animals, *see* Animals, experimental phenomena
 humans, autoimmune diseases, 377

Familial distribution, *see* Genetic predisposition
Fibrinoid degeneration, collagen, 175
Ficin test, 426
Fixation to erythrocyte surface
 agents (*see also under specific agents*)
  autoantibody, 54, 406
  complement, 343, 440, 446, 483
  Donath-Landsteiner antibody, 449
  immunoglobulins, 406, 423
  incomplete antibody, 7
  metallic cations, 339
 demonstration, 418, 425 (*see also specific procedures*)
  nonimmunologic, 338, 406, 423
  mechanism, 421, 441
Folic acid deficiency, 51, 204, 208
Forbidden clone of cells, 29, 332, 363, 367
 theory, 367, 373
Foreign clone of cells, 132, 140, 331, 363
 establishment, 230, 240, 331
 in malignancy, 230
 in tumor formation, 230, 240
 theory, 363, 373
Freund's adjuvant, erythrocyte damage, 354, 376, 500
Fungus infections, 167

Gamma M immunoglobulins, *see* Immunoglobulins, types, gamma M
Gamma-globulin
 abnormalities, 66
 acting as nonagglutinating erythrocyte antibody, 423
 as erythrocyte coating material, 400, 402, 411 (*see also* Immunoglobulins, types)
 formation in hepatitis, 199
 molecular structure, 388
 serum, *see* Antiglobulin serum
Gamma-globulin neutralization test, 400, 408, 440
Gastrointestinal tract, 198 (*see also specific organ and disease*)
 disease, relation
  autoimmune mechanisms, 198
  hypersensitivity and allergic mechanisms, 198
Gaucher's disease, 251
Genetic predisposition, 5, 12, 26, 177, 222
 aberrations, immune apparatus, 24, 30, 140, 215, 222, 332, 371, 507
 abnormalities, inbred mice, 141, 507
 Addisonian pernicious anemia, 216
 autoimmune hemolytic anemia, 30, 140, 215, 222, 332, 371, 507

 idiopathic, 77
 autoimmune syndromes, 26, 77, 177, 369 (*see also specific disease*)
 diabetes, 369
 dysgammaglobulinemia, 339
 pernicious anemia, 216
 systemic lupus erythematosus, 178
 thyroid disease, 230
 ulcerative colitis, 215
 virus transmission, 141, 332, 369, 506, 510
Globulin (*see also* Immunoglobulins)
 antihemophiliac, 84
 antilymphocyte, 306
 molecular structure, 389, 392, 398, 402, 405
 nonimmunologically bound, 424
 relationships with erythrocytes leading to erythrocyte damage, 479
Glucose metabolism, in erythrocyte maintenance, 479, 486
Glycolysis, 486
Gout, 253
Graft-host disease, 132, 363, 367, 371
 experimentally produced, 501
 significance, 503
Granulocytes
 in erythrocytic type of autoimmune hemolytic anemia, 80
 in phagocytic process, 49
Guillain-Barré syndrome, *see* Landry-Guillain-Barré syndrome
GVH disease, *see* Graft-host disease

Hapten formation, 15, 328, 355
 drug induced, 342, 374
Haptoglobin, 36
Hashimoto's disease, 192, 230
Heart surgery, mechanical damage of erythrocytes by prosthetic devices, 10, 242, 354, 377
Heavy chain disease, 393
Heinz body formation, 339
Hemagglutination (*see also* Agglutination erythrocytes)
 bacteriogenic, 346, 351
 cold, 262, 434
 enzymatic sequence, 352
 immune, 6
 viral, 266, 351
Hemagglutinins, cold acting, 262, 408, 434
 anti-I, 439
 anti-i, 439, 471
 anti-"not I," 439
 differentiation, normal and pathologic, 436
 incomplete, 449
 titers in diagnosis, 54
Hematocrit, in diagnosis, 44, 56
Hemoclastic crisis, 274
Hemoglobulinuria, paroxysmal
 cold, 270, 441, 445
  antigen, 473 (*see also* Donath-Landsteiner antibody)
  clinical characteristics, 272
  relation, syphilis, 274, 473
  temperature sensitivity, 273
  therapy, 305